2024 IEEE 4th International Conference on Electronic Communications, Internet of Things and Big Data

2024 IEEE 4th International Conference on Electronic Communications, Internet of Things and Big Data

Volume Editors

Teen-Hang Meen
Shu-Han Liao
Cheng-Fu Yang

MDPI

Basel • Beijing • Wuhan • Barcelona • Belgrade • Novi Sad • Cluj • Manchester

Volume Editors

Teen-Hang Meen
National Formosa University
Yunlin
Taiwan

Shu-Han Liao
Tamkang University
New Taipei City
Taiwan

Cheng-Fu Yang
National University of Kaohsiung
Kaohsiung
Taiwan

Editorial Office
MDPI AG
Grosspeteranlage 5
4052 Basel, Switzerland

This is a reprint of the Proceedings, published open access by the journal *Engineering Proceedings* (ISSN 2673-4591), freely accessible at: https://www.mdpi.com/2673-4591/74/1.

For citation purposes, cite each article independently as indicated on the article page online and as indicated below:

Lastname, A.A.; Lastname, B.B. Article Title. *Journal Name* **Year**, *Volume Number*, Page Range.

ISBN 978-3-7258-3105-0 (Hbk)
ISBN 978-3-7258-3106-7 (PDF)
https://doi.org/10.3390/books978-3-7258-3106-7

Contents

About the Editors

Teen-Hang Meen

Dr. Teen-Hang Meen was born in Tainan, Taiwan, on Aug. 1, 1967. He received his BS degree from the Department of Electrical Engineering, National Cheng Kung University (NCKU), Tainan, Taiwan, in 1989, and obtained his MS and PhD degrees from the Institute of Electrical Engineering, National Sun Yat-Sen University (NSYSU), Kaohsiung, Taiwan, in 1991 and 1994, respectively. He was the chairman of the Department of Electronic Engineering from 2005 to 2011 at National Formosa University, Yunlin, Taiwan. He received the excellent research award of National Formosa University in 2008 and 2014. Currently, he is a lifetime distinguished professor with the Department of Electronic Engineering, National Formosa University, Yunlin, Taiwan. In addition, he is the president of the International Institute of Knowledge Innovation and Invention (IIKII), and the chair of the IEEE Tainan Section Sensors Council. He has published more than 188 SCI and SSCI papers in recent years.

Shu-Han Liao

Dr. Shu-Han Liao was born in Taipei, Taiwan, Republic of China, on September 18, 1982. He received his M.S.C.E. degree from Feng Chia University in 2008 and a Ph.D. degree in electrical engineering from Tamkang University, Taipei, Taiwan, in 2013. From 2014 to 2022, he was a Senior Engineer with the Advanced Communication System Center at the Smart & Network System Institute at the Institute for Information Industry, Taipei. In 2022, he joined the Department of Electrical Engineering, Tamkang University, where he is now an Assistant Professor. Dr. Liao serves as a Chairperson for the Committee of eCloud Mobile, Chinese Professional Management Association of Hsinchu, Hsinchu. He also served as a Deputy Secretary-General for Asia IoT Alliance, Taiwan. Dr. Liao holds 20 patents and has published more than 50 SCI and EI papers in international journals and conference proceedings. His current research interests include the Internet of Things, next-generation (B5G/6G) mobile systems, ESG, smart healthcare, and the Metaverse.

Cheng-Fu Yang

Dr. Cheng-Fu Yang was born in Taiwan on July. 12, 1964. Yang gained his BS, Master's degree, and PhD in 1986, 1988, and 1993 from the Department of Electrical Engineering of Cheng Kung University. Since February 2004, he has served as a Professor of Chemical and Materials Engineering at the National University of Kaohsiung. He received "The Outstanding Contribution Awards of the Chinese Ceramic Society" in 2009. In January 2010, he was the first person to obtain the status of Distinguished Professor at NUK and was the sole recipient of this honor. In August 2014, he was named a fellow of "The Institution of Engineering and Technology" (IET). In May 2015, he became the "The Mingjiang Scholar and Chair Inviting Professor" of Jimei University, Xiamen, Fujian, China, and he has been the "Honorary Chair Professor" of Chaoyang University of Technology since August 2020. He has served as an editorial board member and guest editor for more than 15 international journals, including *Coatings, Materials, Applied Sciences*, etc., and he is the current Chief Editor of *Applied Functional Materials*. So far, he has published more than 390 SCI and SSCI journal papers, more than 140 EI journal papers, and over 300 domestic and international conference papers.

engineering proceedings

MDPI

Editorial

Preface of 2024 IEEE 4th International Conference on Electronic Communications, Internet of Things and Big Data (IEEE ICEIB 2024) †

Teen-Hang Meen [1,*], Shu-Han Liao [2] and Cheng-Fu Yang [3,4,*]

1 Department of Electronic Engineering, National Formosa University, Yunlin 632, Taiwan
2 Department of Electrical Engineering, Tamkang University, New Taipei City 251, Taiwan; shliao@gms.tku.edu.tw
3 Department of Chemical and Materials Engineering, National University of Kaohsiung, Kaohsiung 811, Taiwan
4 Department of Aeronautical Engineering, Chaoyang University of Technology, Taichung 413, Taiwan
* Correspondence: thmeen@gs.nfu.edu.tw (T.-H.M.); cfyang@nuk.edu.tw (C.-F.Y.)
† Presented at the 2024 IEEE 4th International Conference on Electronic Communications, Internet of Things and Big Data, Taipei, Taiwan, 19–21 April 2024.

Citation: Meen, T.-H.; Liao, S.-H.; Yang, C.-F. Preface of 2024 IEEE 4th International Conference on Electronic Communications, Internet of Things and Big Data (IEEE ICEIB 2024). *Eng. Proc.* **2024**, *74*, 82. https://doi.org/10.3390/engproc2024074082

Published: 12 December 2024

This volume presents the proceedings of the 2024 IEEE 4th International Conference on Electronic Communications, Internet of Things, and Big Data (IEEE ICEIB 2024). This conference was organized by Tamkang University, the Institute of Electrical and Electronics Engineers (IEEE), and the International Institute of Knowledge Innovation and Invention (IIKII), and was held at Tamkang University, New Taipei City, Taiwan, on 19–21 April 2024. The conference provided a unified communication platform for researchers in a wide range of topics, such as Big Data and Cloud Computing, Technologies and Applications of Artificial Intelligence, Robotics Science and Engineering, the Internet of Things and Sensor Technology, Intelligent Big Data Analysis and its Applications, and other related fields. In recent years, the rapid development of electronic and microelectronic technologies has brought about a new fundamental and universal revolution in technology. The continuous revolution of electronic technology not only limited to very large-scale integrated (VLSI) circuits and computers but also extends to the development of modern communication technologies. Electronics and communication engineering involve information and communication systems, electronic science and technology, communication and information systems, signal and information processing, circuits and systems, electromagnetic fields and microwave technology, physical electronics and optoelectronics, microelectronics, and solid-state electronics, just to name a few. Related research contents include information transmission, information exchange, information processing, signal detection, integrated circuit design and manufacture, electronic components, microwave and antenna, instrumentation technology, computer engineering, applications, and others. The analysis and application of big data improve the efficiency of existing products and allow new products to be developed. Recent technological breakthroughs have greatly reduced the cost of data storage and computing, making the storage of huge amounts of data considerably less complicated and expensive than in the past. With the increasing volume of data being stored day-by-day and coupled with lower costs and easier access, using big data helps to make more precise business decisions that have been difficult previously.

IEEE ICEIB 2024 was held in a hybrid form, with both on-site and online presentations. Figure 1 shows a group photo of the conference opening. Figure 2 shows the first keynote speech, entitled "Bahasa Rojak: A Research Journey", presented by director and Professor Lim Tong Ming from the Centre of Business Incubation and Entrepreneurial Ventures, Tunku Abdul Rahman University of Management and Technology (TARUMT), Malaysia. He emphasized that Bahasa Rojak is a form of coded mixed language used by internet users to post text on social media platforms. This talk shares the different research methods used and outcomes generated. Challenges faced by the researchers are highlighted. The solutions and remedies produced in the works conducted for the past few years will be presented.

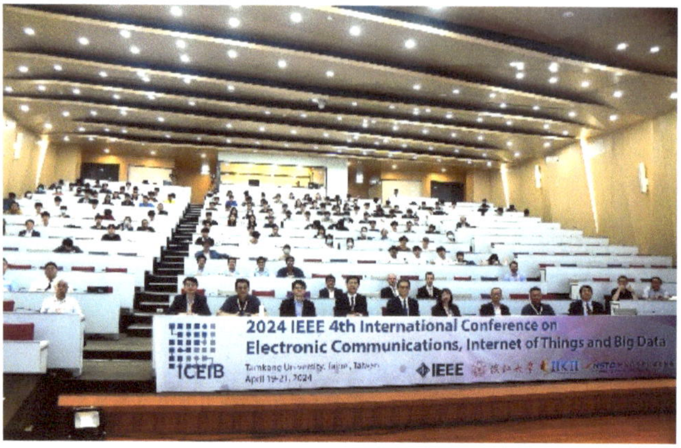

Figure 1. Group photo at the opening ceremony of IEEE ICEIB 2024.

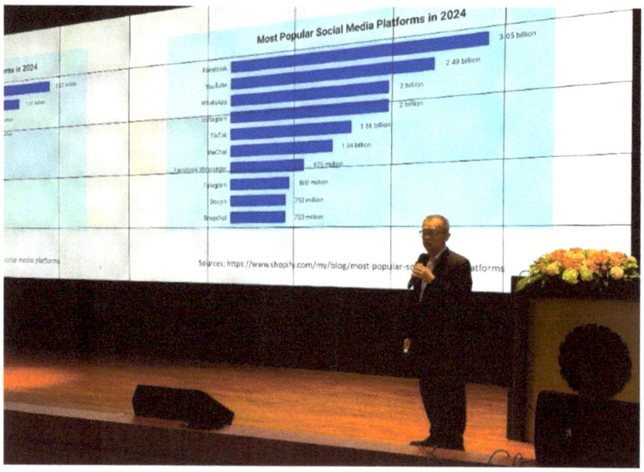

Figure 2. The photo of the first keynote speech at IEEE ICEIB 2024.

Figure 3 shows the second keynote speech entitled "Future Semiconductor IC Technologies for Enabling B5G/6G and AI Revolutions" presented by Chair Professor Donald Y.C. Lie, an IEEE fellow from the Department of Electrical and Computer Engineering, Texas Tech University, United States. He briefly introduced how fifth-generation (5G) mobile network technologies promise to deliver 10 Gbps peak data rates for 5G eMBB (enhanced Mobile Broadband) applications, sub-1ms latency and ultra-reliability for 5G mMTC (ultra-reliable machine type communication), and massive network capacity with increased availability to enable IoE (Internet-of-Everything) with x100 more wireless connected devices compared to 4G for 5G mMTC (massive machine type communication). To accomplish these challenging goals, it is imperative to move up from the sub-6 GHz 5G FR1 band to the higher-frequency bands, which has propelled massive R&D efforts and commercial investments into research on the millimeter-wave (mm-Wave) 5G FR2 band and product developments (i.e., mostly from 24.25 to 52.6 GHz). However, the design requirements of mm-Wave 5G hardware are considerably tougher and consume a bit more power compared to their sub-6 GHz 5G counterparts, especially challenging regarding their power-added efficiency (PAE), linearity, bandwidth, and cost. For the next-generation 6G that utilizes Terahertz (THz) communication (e.g., using D-band), its hardware design specs are expected to be even more challenging, putting a tremendous amount of pressure on IC (integrated circuit) semiconductor device technologists, as well as on the RF/mm Wave hardware IC design and system design communities. The performance and cost of RF hardware will become even more challenging and differentiating as the industry evolves into the AI (artificial intelligence)-centric 6G technologies.

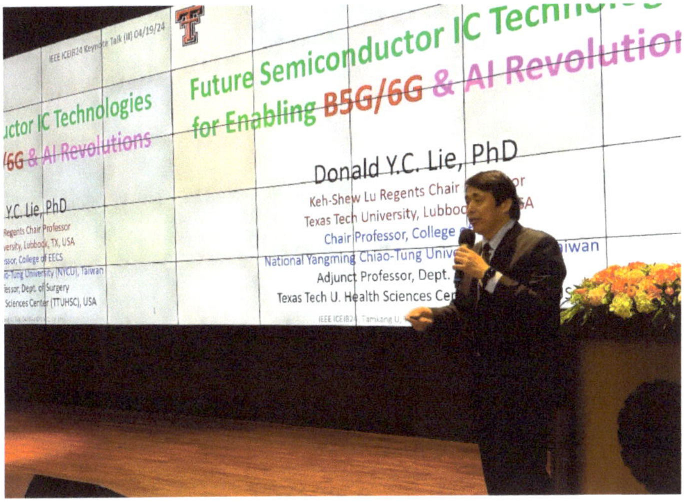

Figure 3. Photo of the second keynote speech at IEEE ICEIB 2024.

IEEE ICEIB 2024 provided eight Regular Sessions including 183 papers, covering Big Data and Cloud Computing, Technologies and Application of Artificial Intelligence, Robotics Science and Engineering, the Internet of Things and Sensor Technology, Intelligent Big Data Analysis and Applications, and other related fields. Figures 4 and 5 show on-site and online oral presentation sessions.

Many substantial results were shared at IEEE ICEIB 2024 by enthusiastic participants and 80 excellent papers about relevant engineering fields to the conference were selected through peer review for publication in *Engineering Proceedings* (ISSN: 2673-4591, indexed by Scopus). The proceedings of IEEE ICEIB 2024 are expected to accelerate the interdisciplinary collaboration of science and engineering technologists in the academic and industrial fields, as well as promote international networking.

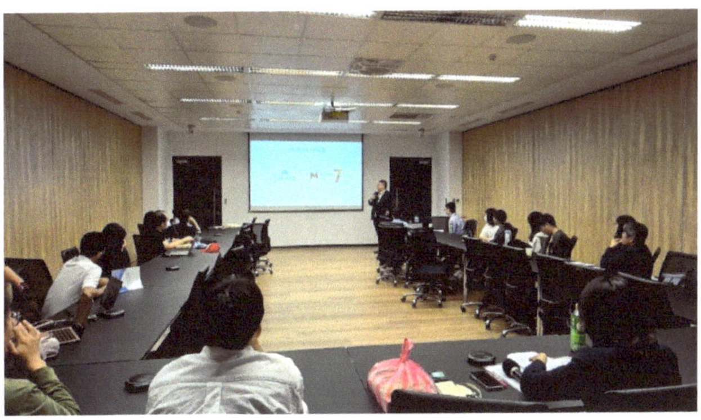

Figure 4. Presentation at an on-site session of IEEE ICEIB 2024.

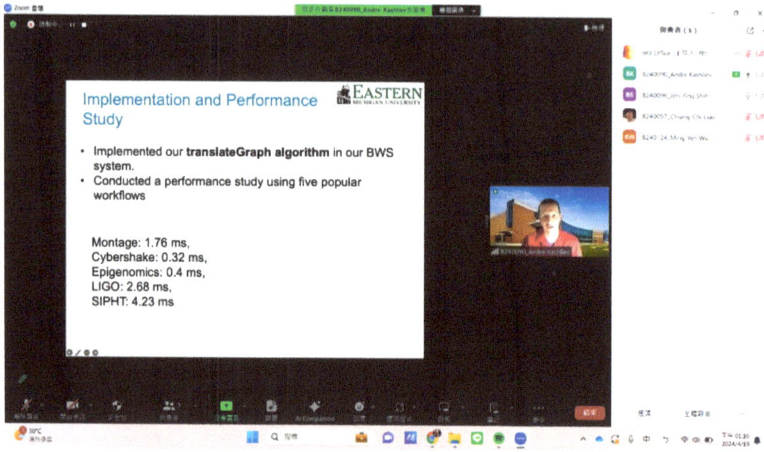

Figure 5. Online presentation at IEEE ICEIB 2024.

Conflicts of Interest: The authors declare no conflicts of interest.

engineering proceedings

MDPI

Editorial

Statement of Peer Review †

Teen-Hang Meen [1,*], Shu-Han Liao [2] and Cheng-Fu Yang [3,4,*]

1 Department of Electronic Engineering, National Formosa University, Yunlin 632, Taiwan
2 Department of Electrical Engineering, Tamkang University, New Taipei City 251, Taiwan; shliao@gms.tku.edu.tw
3 Department of Chemical and Materials Engineering, National University of Kaohsiung, Kaohsiung 811, Taiwan
4 Department of Aeronautical Engineering, Chaoyang University of Technology, Taichung 413, Taiwan
* Correspondence: thmeen@gs.nfu.edu.tw (T.-H.M.); cfyang@nuk.edu.tw (C.-F.Y.)
† Presented at the 2024 IEEE 4th International Conference on Electronic Communications, Internet of Things and Big Data, Taipei, Taiwan, 19–21 April 2024.

In submitting conference proceedings of the 2024 IEEE 4th International Conference on Electronic Communications, Internet of Things and Big Data (IEEE ICEIB 2024) to *Engineering Proceedings*, the volume editors of the proceedings certify to the publisher that all papers published in this volume have been subjected to peer review administered by the volume editors. Reviews were conducted by expert referees to the professional and scientific standards expected of a proceedings journal.

- Type of peer review: single-blind;
- Conference submission management system: http://www.iceib.asia/;
- Number of submissions sent for review: 183;
- Number of submissions accepted: 80;
- Acceptance rate: 0.437;
- Average number of reviews per paper: 2;
- Total number of reviewers involved: 50;
- Any additional information on the review process: please refer to Figure 1.

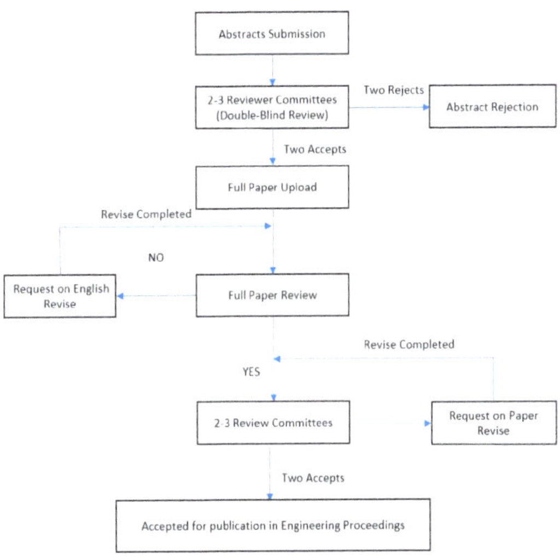

Figure 1. Review process for conference proceedings of the 4th IEEE International Conference on Electronic Communications, Internet of Things and Big Data 2024 (IEEE ICEIB 2024).

Citation: Meen, T.-H.; Liao, S.-H.; Yang, C.-F. Statement of Peer Review. *Eng. Proc.* **2024**, *74*, 81. https://doi.org/10.3390/engproc2024074081

Published: 12 December 2024

Conflicts of Interest: The authors declare no conflicts of interest.

engineering proceedings

Proceeding Paper

Transcendental Equations for Nonlinear Optimization in Hyperbolic Space †

Pranav Kulkarni [1,*] **and Harmanjot Singh** [2]

1 Vice Provost for Undergraduate Education, Stanford University, Palo Alto, CA 94305, USA
2 Independent Researcher, Jammu 180011, Jammu and Kashmir, India; harmanjotsingh.in@gmail.com
* Correspondence: pranavsk@stanford.edu
† Presented at the 2024 IEEE 4th International Conference on Electronic Communications, Internet of Things and Big Data, Taipei, Taiwan, 19–21 April 2024.

Abstract: We present a novel application of transcendental equations for nonlinear distance optimization in hyperbolic space. Through asymptotic approximations using Fourier and Taylor series expansions, we obtain approximations for the transcendental equations with non-zero real values on the boundary λ. The series expansion of the logarithmic form of our equations around two arbitrary points P_1 and P_2 can be used to find values close to definite coordinates on λ. Applying principles from the Poincaré hyperbolic disk—a non-Euclidean space with constant negative curvature—we construct optimization methods following λ of our transcendental equations.

Keywords: nonlinear optimization; hyperbolic space; transcendental equations; Poincaré hyperbolic disk; inverse hyperbolic trigonometry

Citation: Kulkarni, P.; Singh, H. Transcendental Equations for Nonlinear Optimization in Hyperbolic Space. *Eng. Proc.* **2024**, *74*, 1. https://doi.org/10.3390/engproc2024074001

Academic Editors: Shu-Han Liao, Teen-Hang Meen and Cheng-Fu Yang

Published: 26 August 2024

1. Introduction

In *"The Klein, Hilbert and Poincaré metrics of a domain"* by *A.F. Beardon*, Beardon discusses Poincaré distance in the hyperbolic plane, geodesics, and the Hilbert metric in the real coordinate space. Specifically, Beardon noted that for larger distances in the hyperbolic plane, the shape resembles a geodesic. Moreover, in the convex domain on the hyperbolic plane, Beardon determined several key important features with the Hilbert metric, notably, a distance formula using hyperbolic connections between two points in the Euclidean space with a subsequent parameter restriction. On a similar note, the paper *"A Euclidean Model for Euclidean Geometry"* by *Adolf Mader* presents a model of Euclidean geometry. This model is a realization of the Euclidean axioms in a non-Euclidean space and shows that the parallel postulate is not a necessary axiom of Euclidean geometry. The connection between the Mader model and the Poincaré hyperbolic disk model (as detailed in *"Bounded Models of the Euclidean Plane"* by *R. L. Swain, David Gans, and K. O. May*) shows that both models can be used to represent the same set of geometric axioms.

2. Theories

2.1. Hyperbolic Space

Hyperbolic space is a n-dimension non-Euclidean metric space (denoted by $\mathbb{H}^n$, where $n \in \mathbb{N}$ and $n \geq 2$) of constant negative (sectional) curvature denoted by K, where $K < 0$. The n-dimensional unit sphere in Euclidean space can be defined as the set ($x \in \mathbb{R}^{(n+1)} : x \cdot x = 1$). Thus, $\mathbb{H}^n$ is the set $x \in \mathbb{R}^{(n+1)} : x \cdot x = 1$.

2.2. Hyperbolic Trigonometry

The inverse hyperbolic functions, denoted as arccosh, arcsinh, and arctanh [1,2], are the function that maps real numbers to hyperbolic angles. For this research, we are interested in the properties of the inverse hyperbolic cosine function (arccosh) defined as

$$\operatorname{arccosh}(x) = \ln\left(x + \sqrt{x^2 - 1}\right), \cdot \{x \in \mathbb{R} : x \geq 1\} \tag{1}$$

2.3. Hyperbolic Geometry and Distances

In hyperbolic geometry, distances, angles, and geometric properties are based on the hyperbolic metric which defines the distance function between any two points in $\mathbb{H}^n$. The hyperbolic metric satisfies the properties of a metric space, including non-negativity, the identity of indiscernibles, symmetry, and triangle inequality. Nonlinear distance optimization in hyperbolic space is constrained by boundary conditions, such as the unit disk of the Poincaré model, limiting the range of possible distances. The unit disk models of the hyperbolic space (Poincaré and Beltrami–Klein) [3] provide no direct comparison with the Euclidean space limited by the key issue of distance preservation. Additionally, the boundary conditions of the hyperbolic trigonometric functions constrain arccosh(x)'s $x \in \mathbb{R} : x \geq 1$ boundary.

2.4. Transcendental Equation and λ Boundary Conditions in Poincaré and Mader Models

2.4.1. Poincaré Model

The Poincaré disk model [4] represents the hyperbolic plane using a unit disk, $\mathbb{D}$, in the complex plane $\mathbb{C}$. A point, $z \in \mathbb{D}$, is represented by its complex coordinates $z = x + yi$, where x and y are real numbers, satisfying $x^2 + y^2 < 1$. Applying principles from the Poincaré hyperbolic disk, we construct a novel optimization model consisting of the transcendental arcosh equation bound by the λ boundary function, denoted as λ(r) to represent real values in the complex hyperbolic plane. The equation is defined as

$$\operatorname{arcosh}(x + y) = \ln\left[(x + y) + \sqrt{(x + y)^2 - 1}\right] \tag{2}$$

where x and y are coordinates of points belonging to the Poincaré disk $\mathbb{D}$. The domain for the function is $x + y > 1$, and the range is the set of all real numbers. The boundary λ to which this function is constrained is given by the following function:

$$\lambda(r) = \frac{1 - r^2}{1 + r^2} \tag{3}$$

where $r = \sqrt{x^2 + y^2}$ is the Euclidean norm of the point z in the disk. This function λ provides a mapping between the Poincaré disk and Mader models representing the boundary of the unit disk $\mathbb{D}$ where the real values of the function arccosh($x + y$) lie.

2.4.2. Mader Model

The λ boundary function, denoted as λ(r), connects the Poincaré disk model to the Mader model of Euclidean space [5]. The λ boundary function acts as a bijective mapping function $\mathbb{D} \to \mathbb{F}$ where $\mathbb{F}$ is a model in Euclidean space. The Mader model, denoted as $\mathbb{F}$, is defined as the interior of a unit disk ω in the standard Euclidean plane. Points inside the disk are represented by coordinates (x,y). The boundary of the disk (the circle) represents points where $x^2 + y^2 = 1$. The λ boundary function preserves distances between the Euclidean plane $\mathbb{E}$ and the Poincaré disk $\mathbb{D}$ via the bijections $\mathbb{E} \to \mathbb{F}$ and $\mathbb{D} \to \mathbb{F}$.

3. Novel Model for Hyperbolic Transformation

Our novel model acts as a unified space that correlates the geodesic pathways among Mader, Poincaré, and Euclidean geometries by employing transcendental arccosh equations, boundary conditions λ, and series approximations.

Given the Euclidean, Mader, and Poincaré distance metrics d_E, d_M, and d_P, respectively, we establish bijective transformations that allow us to navigate between these geometric spaces [6].

$$\Psi_E : \mathbb{R}^2 \to E\,,\ \Psi_M : \mathbb{R}^2 \to M\,,\ \text{and}\ \Psi_P : \mathbb{R}^2 \to P$$

The model employs Taylor series approximations in the transcendental arccosh function and the λ boundary conditions. Specifically, we use the Taylor series expansion of the natural logarithm form of the transcendental equations to provide approximations for values near the expansion points, P_1 and P_2.

3.1. *Poincaré Model, λ Boundary Transformation, and Transcendental Arccosh*

In the Poincaré disk model, each point within the unit disk $\mathbb{D}$, in the complex plane $\mathbb{C}$, is characterized by complex coordinates $z = x + yi$, where $x, y \in \mathbb{R}$ and $x^2 + y^2 = 1$.

$$\operatorname{arcosh}(x+y) = \ln\left[(x+y) + \sqrt{(x+y)^2 - 1}\right] \tag{4}$$

Proof. Let $y = \cosh(x)$:

$$2y = e^x + e^{-x},$$

$$2y = e^x + e^{-x},$$

Substituting $u = e^x$, we obtain a quadratic equation in u:

$$2yu - u^2 - 1 = 0.$$

Solving the equation using the quadratic formula:

$$\begin{aligned} u &= \tfrac{-2y \pm \sqrt{(2y)^2 - 4(-1)(-1)}}{2(-1)} \\ &= y \pm \sqrt{y^2 - 1}. \end{aligned}$$

Since $u = e^x > 0$, choosing the positive root:

$$e^x = y + \sqrt{y^2 - 1}.$$

Taking the natural logarithm of both sides:

$$x = \ln\left(y + \sqrt{y^2 - 1}\right).$$

Since $y = \cosh(x)$ and $\operatorname{arccosh}(y) = x$:

$$\operatorname{arcosh}(z) = \ln\left(z + \sqrt{z^2 - 1}\right).$$

Substituting $z = x + y$:

$$\operatorname{arcosh}(x+y) = \ln\left((x+y) + \sqrt{(x+y)^2 - 1}\right),$$

for all x and y such that $x + y \geq 1$, which is the domain of the arcosh function.

$$r = \sqrt{x^2 + y^2}$$

$$\lambda(r) = \ln\left[r + \sqrt{r^2 - 1}\right]$$

$$\therefore \text{arcosh}(x+y) = \lambda(r) = \ln\left[(x+y) + \sqrt{(x+y)^2 - 1}\right]$$

The function $\lambda(r)$ sets the boundary conditions, effectively constricting the solution space of the transcendental equation within the constraints of the Poincaré disk model. □

3.2. Mader to Euclidean Transformation, Distance Function d_e

The Mader model is integrated by transformation function Ψ that bridges the distance along the diameter (denoted by r) with the Euclidean distance d_e.

$$r = \Psi(d_e) = \frac{d_e}{d_e + \sqrt{d_e^2 + 1}} \quad (5)$$

Proof. Given the Poincaré metric:

$$ds = \frac{2\,dx}{1 - x^2}$$

To find the hyperbolic distance r from 0 to d_e, we integrate:

$$r = \int_0^{d_e} \frac{2\,dx}{1 - x^2}$$

Using trigonometric substitution:
Let $x = \tan\text{h}(u)$ imply $dx = \sec\text{h}^2(u)\,du$.
When $x = 0$, $u = 0$ and $x = d_e$, $u = \text{artanh}(d_e)$.
Thus,

$$r = \int_0^{\text{artanh}(d_e)} 2\sec\text{h}^2(u)\,du$$

$$r = 2u|_0^{\text{artanh}(d_e)} = 2\text{artanh}(d_e)$$

Using the identity for the inverse hyperbolic tangent,

$$\text{arctanh}(x) = \frac{1}{2}\log\left(\frac{1+x}{1-x}\right)$$

$$r = \log\left(\frac{1+d_e}{1-d_e}\right)$$

$$e^r = \frac{1+d_e}{1-d_e}$$

$$d_e = \frac{1-e^r}{e^r+1}$$

Multiplying both the numerator and denominator by $e^{-\frac{r}{2}}$:

$$d_e = \frac{e^{-\frac{r}{2}} - e^{\frac{r}{2}}}{e^{-\frac{r}{2}} + e^{\frac{r}{2}}}$$

Using the identity $e^r = \cos h(r) + \sin h(r)$:

$$d_e = \frac{\sin h(\frac{r}{2})}{\cos h(\frac{r}{2})}$$

Using the hyperbolic identities:

$$\sin h(x) = \frac{e^x - e^{-x}}{2}$$

$$\cos h(x) = \frac{e^x + e^{-x}}{2}$$

$$d_e = \frac{e^{\frac{r}{2}} - e^{-\frac{r}{2}}}{e^{\frac{r}{2}} + e^{-\frac{r}{2}}}$$

Multiplying the numerator and denominator by $e^{-\frac{r}{2}}$:

$$d_e = \frac{1 - e^{-r}}{1 + e^{-r}}$$

$$r = \ln\left(\frac{d_e + 1}{d_e}\right)$$

Squaring both sides:

$$r^2 = \ln^2\left(\frac{d_e + 1}{d_e}\right)$$

Taking the positive square root (since $r > 0$ for $d_e > 0$):

$$r = \frac{d_e}{\sqrt{d_e^2 + 1}}$$

We assume that

$$d_e \ll \sqrt{d_e^2 + 1}$$

$$\therefore r = \frac{d_e}{d_e + \sqrt{d_e^2 + 1}}$$

$$\Psi(R) = \frac{R}{R + \sqrt{R^2 + 1}}$$

This transformation function Ψ enables a bijection between Mader and Euclidean geometries, connecting these two models using our model. □

3.3. Hyperbolic, Euclidean Distance and Mapping Function

We map the hyperbolic distance, d_h, in the Poincaré disk model through the Euclidean norm of z, $||z||$, using the mapping function Φ.

$$d_h = \Phi(||z||) = \text{arccosh}\left(1 + \frac{2||z||^2}{1 - ||z||^2}\right) \quad (6)$$

Proof. The distance formula in the Poincaré disk model for two points, z_1 and z_2, is

$$d_h(z_1, z_2) = \text{arccosh}\left(1 + \frac{2||z_1 - z_2||^2}{\left(1-||z_1||^2\right)\left(1-||z_2||^2\right)}\right)$$

For the distance between the origin 0 and a point z:

$$d_h(0,z) = \operatorname{arccosh}\left(1 + \frac{2||z||^2}{1-||z||^2}\right)$$

Using the Euclidean norm for $z = x + yi$:

$$||z|| = \sqrt{x^2 + y^2}$$

$$d_h = \operatorname{arccosh}\left(1 + \frac{2(x^2+y^2)}{1-(x^2+y^2)}\right)$$

$$\therefore d_h = \Phi(||z||) = \operatorname{arccosh}\left(1 + \frac{2||z||^2}{1-||z||^2}\right)$$

□

3.4. Mapping Function

Consider an arbitrary point P in the Poincaré disk model $\mathbb{D}$. Let the coordinates of P be (x, y), where $x^2 + y^2 < 1$. We define a mapping $\Psi : \mathbb{D} \to \mathbb{M}$, such that a point P in $\mathbb{D}$ is mapped to a point P' in $\mathbb{M}$, the Mader model.

$$\Psi(x,y) = (h(x), h(y)) \tag{7}$$

$$h(z) = \operatorname{arccosh}(\ln(1+z)) \tag{8}$$

For z in $\mathbb{D}$, the function h effectively translates each coordinate from $\mathbb{D}$ to a corresponding coordinate in $\mathbb{M}$.

3.5. Distance Function

Given two points, P_1' and P_2', in $\mathbb{M}$, which correspond to P_1 and P_2 in $\mathbb{D}$, the distance between P_1' and P_2' in the Mader model, $d_{\mathbb{M}}(P_1\prime, P_2\prime)$, is defined in terms of the distance between P_1 and P_2 in the Poincaré disk model, $d_{\mathbb{D}}(P_1, P_2)$, as follows:

$$d_M(\Psi(x_1,y_1), \Psi(x_2,y_2)) = h(d_D((x_1,y_1),(x_2,y_2))) \tag{9}$$

The transformation Ψ offers a one-to-one mapping between the Poincaré disk $\mathbb{D}$ and Mader model $\mathbb{M}$ using the function h defined in (7). By making use of the function h and the transformation Ψ, this continuous mapping preserves the underlying geometric structures to compare the geometric properties between $\mathbb{D}$ and $\mathbb{M}$.

4. Series Expansions for Approximations

Understanding the behavior of the function $\lambda(r)$ and the hyperbolic distance d_h under different geometrical transformations is critical. To address this, we employ Taylor series expansion to approximate these functions around the point P.

$$f(x+y) = \ln[(x+y) + \sqrt{(x+y)^2 - 1}$$

The Taylor series expansion of a function f about a point P is represented as

$$f(x+y) \approx f(P) + f'^{(P)(x+y-P)} + \frac{f''(P)}{2!}(x+y-P)^2 + \frac{f'''(P)}{3!}(x+y-P)^3 + \cdots$$

$$f(P) = \ln\left[P + \sqrt{P2-1}\right] \tag{10}$$

The hyperbolic distance function d_h can be approximated using a series expansion around the point P in the Poincaré disk model.

$$d_h = \Phi(||z||) = \operatorname{arccosh}\left(1 + \frac{2||z||^2}{1-||z||^2}\right) \tag{11}$$

$$\approx \Phi(P) + (||z|| - P)\Phi'(P) + \frac{(||z|| - P)^2}{2}\Phi''(P) + \cdots \tag{12}$$

The general term for the series expansion about the point P is

$$\frac{\Phi^n[P]}{n!}[||z|| - P]^n \tag{13}$$

where $\Phi^{(n)}[P]$ represents the nth derivative of Φ concerning $||z||$, evaluated at P.

5. Applications

Simple Distance Optimization Application

In the Mader model, P_1 and P_2 are transformed into points within the unit disk. We calculate the Euclidean distances, denoted as d_{e1} and d_{e2}, of these points from the origin. Using the mapping function Ψ from the Mader model to the Poincaré model, these points are translated to the Poincaré disk.

$$\Psi(r) = \frac{2r}{1+r^2} \tag{14}$$

We calculate the hyperbolic distances d_{h1} and d_{h2} for P_1 and P_2, respectively, in the Poincaré disk model.

$$d_{h1} = \operatorname{arccosh}\left(1 + \frac{2d_{e1}}{1 - d_{e1}^2}\right) \tag{15}$$

$$d_{h2} = \operatorname{arccosh}\left(1 + \frac{2d_{e2}}{1 - d_{e2}^2}\right) \tag{16}$$

The hyperbolic geodesic distance between points P_1 and P_2 is computed by the integration of the Poincaré metric over the shortest path represented as a segment of a circle orthogonal to the boundary of the disk in the Poincaré model.

$$\int_{P_1}^{P_2} \frac{2|dz|}{1 - |z|^2} \tag{17}$$

To approximate the complex integral, a Taylor series expansion is employed around the shortest path between P_1 and P_2. The optimal path corresponds to the minima of the hyperbolic distance. The optimal hyperbolic path is then translated back to the Mader model using the inverse mapping function Ψ^{-1} and subsequently to the Euclidean model to provide a real-world trajectory for objects such as airplanes, ships, and the like.

6. Diagrams

For a system modeling shortest-path trajectories in Euclidean space, the metric utilized is the Euclidean distance, given by

$$d_E = \sqrt{(x_2 - x_1)^2 + (y_2 - y_1)^2}.$$

The transformation function, Φ, transforms the system's trajectories from Euclidean space $\mathbb{R}^2$ into the unit disk $\mathbb{D}$, following the condition $\Phi(\mathbb{R}) = z$ in $\mathbb{D}$, with $z = x + yi$.

The geodesic distance in the Poincaré disk, representing the shortest path between two points in hyperbolic space is

$$d_H = \operatorname{arccosh}\left(1 + \frac{2|z_2 - z_1|^2}{\left(1 - |z_1|^2\right)\left(1 - |z_2|^2\right)}\right) \tag{18}$$

- Original trajectory (Euclidean): Figure 1a displays the shortest path between two points using the standard Euclidean metric, represented as a straight line;
- Transformed trajectory (Poincaré disk model): In Figure 1b, the direct line in Euclidean space transforms, resulting in a curved path in the Poincaré disk called a geodesic. This geodesic demonstrates the hyperbolic shortest path, emphasizing that the Poincaré distance is strictly less than the corresponding Euclidean distance for the same two points on the bounded unit circle.

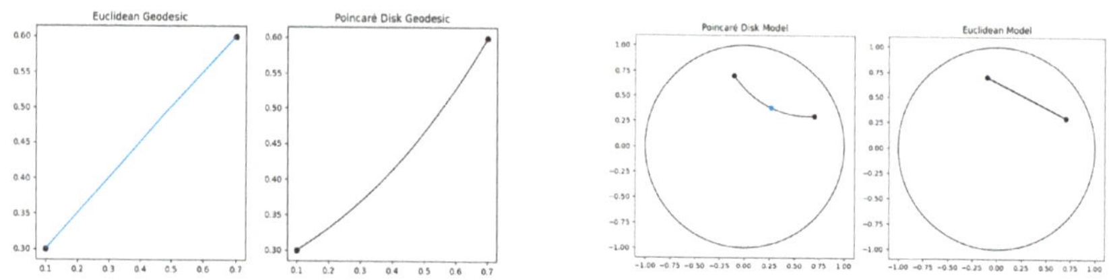

(a) (b)

Figure 1. (**a**) Shortest path trajectory on a Cartesian plane. (**b**) Shortest path trajectory on the Poincaré disk.

Overall, for our diagrams, we employed mathematical transformations to analyze different physical systems from a hyperbolic perspective. We used the numpy, matplotlib, and hypertiling packages in Google Colab to aid with visualizations of our models. Using the Poincaré disk model, we defined a mapping function Ψ to transform Euclidean spaces into hyperbolic spaces. Hyperbolic geodesic distances were calculated using a definite integral over the Poincaré metric. Taylor series expansions were utilized in approximating complex integrals, especially when computing distances. For thermodynamic systems, a 6n-dimensional phase space was transformed using the Ψ function. The pendulum system's dynamics, characterized in a 2D phase space, were explored through a transformation relation capturing angular position and momentum.

7. Conclusions

We established a novel application of transcendental equations for modeling and optimization in hyperbolic space. Utilizing the Poincaré disk model, we defined the boundary function $\lambda(r) = \frac{1-r^2}{1+r^2}$ and transformation functions Φ and Ψ, with specific expressions for hyperbolic distance calculations. A key limitation of the proposed model in this study lies in the Taylor series approximations and assumptions of underlying geometries. However, the error remains negligibly small within the model's defined constraints. Future research is necessary to apply this model to higher-dimensional non-Euclidean surfaces, improving geometric analysis in differential geometry and topological mapping.

Author Contributions: Conceptualization, P.K. and H.S.; formal analysis, P.K.; software, H.S.; writing, P.K. and H.S. All authors have read and agreed to the published version of the manuscript.

Funding: This research received no external funding.

Institutional Review Board Statement: Not applicable.

Informed Consent Statement: Not applicable.

Data Availability Statement: The data that support the findings of this study are available from the corresponding author upon reasonable request.

Conflicts of Interest: The authors declare no conflict of interest.

References

1. Girg, P.; Kotrla, L. Generalized trigonometric functions in complex domain. *Math. Bohem.* **2015**, *140*, 223–239. [CrossRef]
2. Aprahamian, M.; Higham, N.J. Matrix inverse trigonometric and inverse hyperbolic functions: Theory and Algorithms. *SIAM J. Matrix Anal. Appl.* **2016**, *37*, 1453–1477. [CrossRef]
3. Beardon, A.F. The Klein, Hilbert and Poincaré metrics of a domain. *J. Comput. Appl. Math.* **1999**, *105*, 155–162. [CrossRef]
4. Simić, D.; Marić, F.; Boutry, P. Formalization of the Poincaré disc model of hyperbolic geometry. *J. Autom. Reason.* **2020**, *65*, 31–73. [CrossRef]
5. Mader, A. A euclidean model for euclidean geometry. *Am. Math. Mon.* **1989**, *96*, 43. [CrossRef]
6. Swain, R.L. Bounded models of the Euclidean plane. *Am. Math. Mon.* **1954**, *61*, 21. [CrossRef]

engineering proceedings

MDPI

Proceeding Paper

Motivated Learning Strategies and Critical Thinking: Evaluating the Effectiveness of WebQuest-Based EFL Teaching in Taiwanese Higher Education †

Ruei-Teng Hung *, Hsin-Yi Liao, Kate Tzu-Ching Chen and Yun-Sin Chuang

Department of Applied English, Chaoyang University of Technology, Taichung 413310, Taiwan
* Correspondence: hb865777@gmail.com

† Presented at the 2024 IEEE 4th International Conference on Electronic Communications, Internet of Things and Big Data, Taipei, Taiwan, 19–21 April 2024.

Abstract: We delved into the various studying approaches adopted through a survey of 56 undergraduates majoring in English using the WebQuest platform. How eagerly the students participated in learning with Pintrich's Motivated Strategies was investigated. In the survey, a questionnaire was created and used as an assessment tool. In the course structure, the WebQuest methodology was used, supplemented by the Learning Object Review Instrument. The participants employed critical thinking abilities more regularly than effort-based tactics with WebQuest interactions. This demonstrates a direct link between the study approaches employed and the student's motivation. The results have significant implications for educators, signifying that motivated studying in the WebQuest framework boosts the effectiveness of technology-assisted foreign language learning.

Keywords: motivated learning strategies; Motivated Strategies for Learning Questionnaire (MSLQ); WebQuest; EFL; higher education

Citation: Hung, R.-T.; Liao, H.-Y.; Chen, K.T.-C.; Chuang, Y.-S. Motivated Learning Strategies and Critical Thinking: Evaluating the Effectiveness of WebQuest-Based EFL Teaching in Taiwanese Higher Education. *Eng. Proc.* **2024**, *74*, 2. https://doi.org/10.3390/engproc2024074002

Academic Editors: Shu-Han Liao, Teen-Hang Meen and Cheng-Fu Yang

Published: 26 August 2024

1. Introduction

Efficient learning methods are pivotal in student success and impact learners' motivation [1]. However, different learning tactics have differing effects on students. Instructional assistance proves helpful in assisting learners in applying suitable strategies [2]. Pupils who consistently use learning techniques attain more notable outcomes than their peers who do not [3]. This highlights the importance of grasping and implementing suitable tactics in educational paradigms. Furthermore, pupils who actively employ various learning approaches on varying assignments retain knowledge more effectively than those relying on just one or two methods. The most dedicated students systematically focus on the course materials and discussions with peers to gain diverse viewpoints on the studied topics [4].

While previous studies have been extensively focused on the impact of studying strategies, more information is still needed regarding how these strategies are adopted in technology-enhanced settings. In today's era, where education and technology are intertwined to a higher degree, educators need to integrate helpful tools into their teaching. These instruments must be efficient and align with sound pedagogical principles. Thus, assessing their effectiveness is crucial to improve students' inspiration in technology-rich environments [5].

Educators are exploring different routes beyond standard instruction due to the increasing demand for skilled English speakers and are trying to find the most impactful strategies in English as a Foreign Language (EFL) learning. It is necessary to identify diverse and inspired studying strategies for university students to acquire successful language skills. Additionally, learners' viewpoints regarding their experiences in the WebQuest environment need to be understood as digital learning increasingly is used in language study. Such results would provide a valuable basis on which to improve the productivity of language teaching in a consistently evolving educational environment. Thus, this study aims to enhance the present knowledge by offering precise and valuable information for educators, curriculum designers, and policymakers. The results of this study reveal the impacts and future of EFL teaching when connecting theoretical knowledge with practical application. Such a connection is vital in developing practical teaching strategies in EFL education.

2. Literature Review

2.1. Motivated Learning Strategy

Learning strategies facilitate long-lasting information acquisition. While focusing less on negative responses to errors, effective teaching techniques significantly impact student motivation. Current education emphasizes the reinforcement of strategies that prioritize enhancing engagement [6]. Motivated learning approaches are integral to student achievement. The evaluation of such approaches offers a basis for an understanding of the knowledge-gaining process so as to enhance the quality and efficacy of education. Implementing appropriate and inspiring instructional practices increases students' motivation and strengthens their understanding.

Motivated learning style strategies influence an individual's determination and the entire educational environment. Applying such approaches bolsters student motivation and contributes to enhancing learning outcomes. Comprehending and integrating these strategies into pedagogical methods is pivotal for successful teaching. This methodology fosters an atmosphere where pupils are actively involved in their learning, rather than passively receiving information. The shift towards a student-centered approach in education is pivotal. Aligning educational practices with students' diverse learning needs and preferences improves the overall quality and efficiency of education.

Motivated learning strategies signify a transition to a comprehensive educational approach that cultivates an immersive and participatory learning setting. These strategies are beneficial in nurturing a sense of ownership and responsibility among students in education. They emphasize the student's role in the knowledge-gaining process, allowing them to proactively engage in their education and develop a stronger and more personal connection with the material. Consequently, this results in a more meaningful and long-lasting educational experience, underscoring the vital role of motivated learning strategies in shaping the future of academic practices.

2.2. Motivated Strategies for Learning Questionnaire (MSLQ)—Learning Strategy Scale

Pintrich's MSLQ incorporates a learning strategy scale with nine fundamental factors regarding how students regulate their learning processes.

The MSQL comprises a scale assessing the factors related to acquisition approaches. Each component is related to beneficial knowledge about how pupils engage and manage their cognitive processes. The initial method is "Rehearsal", which involves reiterating data to boost memory retention. Furthermore, "Elaboration" enables students to connect fresh information and their preexisting knowledge, promoting more profound comprehension. "Organization" refers to the premeditated and systematic arrangement of information to enhance one's understanding and retention. The scale progresses to "Critical Thinking", which requires students to scrutinize, assess, and amalgamate information. Next is "Meta-Cognitive Self-Regulation", a capacity in which students actively monitor and modify their acquisition to achieve improved outcomes. "Time and Study Environmental Management" emphasizes optimizing the study conditions and efficiently allocating one's time, which is essential in achieving academic success. Moreover, "Effort Regulation" refers to the ability to modify the amount of effort exerted under the requirements of different tasks, ensuring that students maintain their adaptability and resilience throughout their learning. The last two factors encompass "Peer Learning" and "Help Seeking". "Peer Learning" prioritizes the significance of cooperative learning and the interchange of ideas among students, cultivating a communal acquisition atmosphere. "Help Seeking", however, signifies the essential skill of students to actively seek assistance when necessary, recognizing the significance of support in learning.

These factors encompass a wide range of deliberate strategies that students use to improve their learning, comprehension, and academic achievement. Instructors greatly benefit from a comprehensive understanding of these strategies, as it equips them with crucial insights to improve the overall student learning experience.

2.3. MSLQ—Motivated Scale

The creation of the MSLQ by Pintrich represented a significant advancement in educational research. This tool is used to effectively evaluate various aspects of student motivation and learning strategies. The MSLQ's motivation scale comprises six fundamental elements:

1. Intrinsic goal orientation to evaluate students' intrinsic motivation;
2. Extrinsic goal orientation to emphasize external incentives such as academic grades and rewards;
3. Task value to assess the perceived significance of tasks;
4. Control of learning beliefs to manifest students' confidence in influencing their learning;
5. Self-efficacy for learning and performance related to task accomplishment;
6. Test anxiety to quantify the levels of stress experienced during evaluations.

The conception of Pintrich's MSQL signified a formidable step forward in educational evaluation. In this innovative method, various facets of student motivation and study techniques are examined, offering a comprehensive framework for assessment. Renowned for thoroughly scrutinizing the intricate characteristics of student motivation, the MSLQ significantly enhances our comprehension of the ways in which learners participate in educational processes.

In the MSLQ, the motivation scale contains six fundamental elements. In "Intrinsic Goal Orientation", a student's inherent enthusiasm and curiosity are examined to learn about its benefits. "Extrinsic Goal Orientation" is focused on incentives such as marks and rewards. "Task Value" is a pivotal factor that evaluates learners' views of the importance and applicability of academic tasks. "Control of Learning Beliefs" is related to how students perceive their ability to impact their learning results. "Self-Efficacy for Learning and Performance" is used to analyze pupils' faith in their capacity to finish tasks and overcome difficulties. At the same time, "Test Anxiety" is determined as the level of stress and anxiety that learners experience during evaluations.

Pintrich's MSLQ has played a pivotal role in enhancing the understanding of students' motivation and learning mechanisms. Using the MSLQ, instructors and researchers can obtain indispensable knowledge to make educational methodologies more productive. The MSLQ approach is used to evaluate students' motivation and study strategies, which are essential instruments in academic inquiry and influence teaching practices and learner-focused educational environments.

2.4. Digital Learning Strategies in CALL

The digital realm of language pedagogy has been radically transformed during the past half-century, with computers progressively permeating linguistic instruction. Chen [7] argued that an educational technology's value must be judged based on whether positive pedagogical results are actualized. The evolution of educational technology reflects the rising popularity and proven usefulness of digital education in online learning systems, alongside the anticipated requirement for scholarly strategies [8]. While technological integration has accelerated language acquisition, implementation strategies need to benefit all learners. Thus, it is necessary to address such issues and opportunities in this digital age.

Computers have been repositioned in education from an extra tool to an indispensable one. Zhang, Wei, and Cao examined digital language learning apps in data technology and categorized the apps into two categories: those producing instructional materials—for instance, websites, emails, and online assets—and those applying learning management systems [9]. The web's accessibility has prompted a significant shift in academic methods, as pupils at all levels of education, from kindergarten to college, are increasingly taking part in digital language study. Access to this vast expanse of knowledge has transformed methods of learning, enabling independent study via digital means such as structured online courses. Younger learners have embraced diverse apps to complement traditional modes of education, strategically blending digital and in-person learning techniques [10].

While the technologies for instruction have advanced learning, the debate continues around their impact on language acquisition [11]. Students embrace digital tools enthusiastically in their studies and lives, providing opportunities to modernize language education. However, the transformation of curricula requires pedagogical trade-offs with technologies [12]. Universities aim to serve students effectively. Recognizing the changing preferences, many experts have argued about blended approaches. The incorporation of digital aids aligns practices with the ways in which younger generations build skills. However, such changes risk being too "tech-friendly". Thus, guiding technological change with learners' long-term development in mind remains paramount. Each approach is appropriate for different groups of students. However, discussing technology's role openly from different viewpoints strengthens diverse programs. Prioritizing inclusion and understanding influences instead of assumptions can lead to well-rounded reforms based on evidence. With the cooperation of stakeholders with different perspectives, language education can benefit from technology while avoiding potential pitfalls.

3. Method

3.1. Participants

A total of 56 undergraduates from the Department of Applied Foreign Languages at Taiwan's Chaoyang University of Technology were recruited in this study. Participation was voluntary. Students joined a course called "Online Resources for English Educators" to grasp and master internet tools for the learning of English. The participants showed varied progress. Eleven participants were juniors, while 45 were seniors. The mixed group of participants offered diverse perspectives that enabled us to understand how internet resources are implemented and affect the effectiveness of English teaching.

3.2. Instruments

Three separate instruments were used to gather and analyze the data. We implemented the Learning Objective Review Instrument (LORI) for evaluation. The Zimmer Twins website was selected as it complements the methods in the WebQuest platform. The various content on the website offered short lessons and challenging materials. We assessed students' motivation in using the website by using an updated version of MSQL. The Learning Objective Review Instrument played a pivotal role in assessing the suitability of different websites for this research project. After employing the LORI, we assessed whether Zimmer Twins was an appropriate source to ensure that the digital resources used in the study supported its aims. The selection process emphasized matching educational materials with instructional purposes. After validating the suitability of the chosen website, we investigated engaged learning strategies and practices for students in the WebQuest framework. The revised MSQL was used as it enables us to comprehend how pupils interact with and capitalize on the implemented approaches. The updated MSLQ was validated for its internal consistency and reliability, with a Cronbach's alpha coefficient of 0.96. This ensured the significance of the results of this study.

4. Results

4.1. Learning Strategies in WebQuest Environment

Table 1 outlines the participants' mean scores for various learning factors. For rehearsal, they scored 4.84 on average, with a standard deviation (SD) of 1.17, while, for elaboration, they scored 5.24 with an SD of 0.26, suggesting consistent preferences. The average scores for organization and critical thinking were 4.92 and 5.57, with SDs of 1.11 and 0.82. For meta-cognition and self-regulation, the participants scored 5.12 and 4.95, with SDs of 0.85 and 0.69. Critical thinking exhibited the highest average score of 5.57, highlighting students' strong inclination towards analytical and evaluative approaches. Self-efficacy, peer learning, and help seeking showed average scores of 4.13, 4.73, and 5.16 and SDs of 0.93, 1.24, and 1.05, respectively. The participants preferred critical thinking (5.57 with an SD of 0.82) to elaboration, help seeking, meta-cognition, self-regulation, time and study management, organization, rehearsal, and peer learning. This preference profile reflects the participants' learning styles and strategic priorities

Table 1. Frequency and distribution of learning strategies of participants.

Strategy	M	SD
Critical thinking	5.57	0.82
Elaboration	5.21	0.86
Help seeking	5.16	1.05
Meta-cognition and self-regulation	5.12	0.85
Time and study management	4.95	0.69
Organization	4.92	1.11
Rehearsal	4.84	1.17
Peer learning	4.73	1.24

4.2. Students' Perceptions of Learning Experiences in WebQuest Environment

We examined the connection between the diverse learning techniques and the inspiration of the participants who were studying English in an online environment. Pearson itemized connection coefficients were used to determine the significance of the relations. Connections between different learning systems and student inspiration were found, as shown in Table 2. A positive relationship between broadening and motivation (r = 0.73) and between broadening and essential thinking (r = 0.69) was found. The correlation coefficient between meta-cognition and self-efficacy was 0.68. The learning procedures of rehashing and peer learning, and their association, had positive relations with inspiration, with coefficients of r = 0.58, 0.50, and 0.42, respectively.

Table 2. Correlations between learning strategies and motivation.

Strategy	Coefficient	Significance
Critical thinking	0.69	0.000 ***
Elaboration	0.73	0.000 ***
Help seeking	0.29	0.036 *
Meta-cognition and self-regulation	0.68	0.000 ***
Time and study management	0.21	0.128
Organization	0.42	0.002 ***
Rehearsal	0.58	0.000 ***
Peer learning	0.50	0.000 ***

Note. *** $p < 0.001$, * $p < 0.05$.

The results showed that the association between help seeking and motivation was moderate, with a coefficient of 0.29. Help seeking was a part of the learning process and impacted inspiration, but it was not as powerful as other systems. There was a correlation between time and study management and motivation, demonstrated by a coefficient of 0.21. Because of the weak relationship, time and study management was excluded from this study. The results can be used to study the correlations between different learning procedures and the differing levels of impacts on English language learning.

5. Discussion and Conclusions

We studied the diverse learning approaches utilized by university students majoring in English who actively used the WebQuest learning platform. Emphasizing the importance of critical thinking, the results showed that WebQuest improved their reasoning abilities. Elaboration, critical thinking, meta-cognition, and self-regulation influenced the learning process and the achievement of the participants' learning goals in complex ways. These approaches motivated the participants through interconnections between the data and their prior learning, improving their cognitive capacities and encouraging independent study. Meta-cognition and self-regulation were important and reflected extrinsic goal orientation. These approaches necessitate attentive planning and the clear comprehension of the study process and they enhance students' inspiration in striking ways. Critical thinking plays a vital role in developing self-efficacy. This individualized strategy facilitate spontaneous and imaginative thinking and enhances students' inspiration and accomplishments. In contrast, routine rehearsal significantly reduces anxiety. This indicates how regular practice strengthens students' self-assurance and eases pressure. These results emphasize the implementation of nuanced approaches with varying motivations to optimize the results. The intricate links between learning strategies and diverse motivating aspects are important and reflect a delicate and tailored academic approach.

The results of this study encourage administrators to deploy technologies that reflect the multiple facets of student motivation. Educators need to develop engaging and relevant educational methods by personalizing their instruction to support each student's unique motivations and preferences. A sophisticated method with which teachers can customize their teaching to align with individual motivations is needed considering students' preferred learning styles. Such a focused strategy would help to create an environment where students are inspired and proactively participate. Based on the results of this study, well-informed teaching methods can be established to enhance the quality and effectiveness of English as a Foreign Language education on the WebQuest platform.

Author Contributions: Conceptualization, R.-T.H. and H.-Y.L.; methodology, R.-T.H.; software, K.T.-C.C.; validation, R.-T.H., H.-Y.L., and Y.-S.C.; formal analysis, H.-Y.L.; investigation, R.-T.H.; resources, H.-Y.L.; data curation, K.T.-C.C.; writing—original draft preparation, R.-T.H.; writing—review and editing, H.-Y.L.; visualization, K.T.-C.C.; supervision, R.-T.H.; project administration, R.-T.H.; funding acquisition, H.-Y.L. All authors have read and agreed to the published version of the manuscript.

Funding: This research received no external funding.

Institutional Review Board Statement: Not applicable.

Informed Consent Statement: Informed consent was obtained from all subjects involved in the study.

Data Availability Statement: Data sharing is not applicable to this article as no datasets were generated or analyzed during the study.

Conflicts of Interest: The authors declare no conflict of interest.

References

1. Pintrich, P.R.; Smith, D.A.F.; Garcia, T.; McKeachie, W.J. *A Manual for the Use of the Motivated Strategies for Learning Questionnaire (MSLQ)*; University of Michigan, National Center for Research to Improve Postsecondary Teaching and Learning: Ann Arbor, MI, USA, 1991.
2. Nesbit, J.; Belfer, K.; Leacock, T. Learning Object Review Instrument (LORI), Version 1.5. E-Learning Research and Assessment (eLera) and the Portal for Online Objects in Learning (POOL). 2007. Available online: https://www.slideshare.net/slideshow/lori-learning-object-review-instrument/243950974 (accessed on 1 August 2024).
3. Mobo, F.D. Motivated Strategies for Learning and Online Learning Readiness of Students in Maritime Institution in Central Luzon, Philippines. *Mt. J. Sci. Interdiscip. Res. (Former. Benguet State Univ. Res. J.)* **2022**, *82*, 118–131.
4. Bansal, R.; Dutt, S. Using WebQuest Based Instruction to Enhance Students' Critical Thinking. *Issues Ideas Educ.* **2020**, *8*, 1–8. [CrossRef]
5. Bayram, D.; Gökçe, K.; Derin, A. The implementation of webquest-supported critical thinking instruction in pre-service english teacher education: The Turkish context. *Particip. Educ. Res.* **2019**, *6*, 144–157. [CrossRef]
6. Chen, C. Effects of the Application of WebQuest to Technology Education on Business Management Students' Critical Thinking Psychology and Operation Capability. *Contemp. Educ. Technol.* **2021**, *13*, ep290. [CrossRef] [PubMed]
7. Chen, K.T.-C. Identifying barriers faced by university EFL instructors in integrating mobile-assisted language learning. *Contemp. Educ. Technol.* **2023**, *15*, ep467. [CrossRef] [PubMed]

8. Zhang, H.; Wei, W.; Cao, Y. Using computer-assisted language teaching technologies to develop multiple levels of medical vocabulary knowledge for second language medical students. *Comput. Assist. Lang. Learn.* **2022**, *35*, 1–21. [CrossRef]
9. Tejani, S.B.A.; Ejaz, S.; Shamsy, S. Psychometric Features of Motivated Strategies for Learning Questionnaire (MSLQ) among the Students of Higher Education Sector in Karachi–Pakistan. *Rev. Manag. Sci.* **2021**, *3*, 85–100. [CrossRef]
10. Sari, F.M. Study-from-home program: Motivational beliefs of college students in the online learning environment. *ETERNAL (Engl. Teach. Learn. Res. J.)* **2021**, *7*, 350–358.
11. Hew, K.F.; Huang, W. Promoting engagement in online learning beyond COVID-19: Possible strategies and directions for future research. *Future Educ. Res.* **2023**, *1*, 27–49. [CrossRef]
12. Liang, W.; Fung, D. Development and evaluation of a WebQuest-based teaching programme: Students' use of exploratory talk to exercise critical thinking. *Int. J. Educ. Res.* **2020**, *104*, 101652. [CrossRef] [PubMed]

engineering proceedings

MDPI

Proceeding Paper

To Satisfy or Clarify: Enhancing User Information Satisfaction with AI-Powered ChatGPT †

Chung Jen Fu [1], Andri Dayarana K. Silalahi [2,*], I-Tung Shih [1], Do Thi Thanh Phuong [2,3], Ixora Javanisa Eunike [4] and Shinetseteg Jargalsaikhan [1]

1 Department of Business Administration, College of Management, Chaoyang University of Technology, Taichung 411310, Taiwan; drfucj@gmail.com (C.J.F.); itungshih99@gmail.com (I.-T.S.); shinee.jargalsaikhan@gmail.com (S.J.)
2 Department of Marketing and Logistics Management, Chaoyang University of Technology, Taichung 411310, Taiwan; phuong.dothanh904@gmail.com
3 Department of Distribution Management, National Chin-Yi University of Technology, Taiping 411030, Taiwan
4 Master of Management Program, Graduate School, University of Technology, Medan 20235, Indonesia; ixorajavanisa1902@gmail.com
* Correspondence: andridksilalahi@gmail.com
† Presented at the 2024 IEEE 4th International Conference on Electronic Communications, Internet of Things and Big Data, Taipei, Taiwan, 19–21 April 2024.

Abstract: The effective use of AI-powered ChatGPT in higher education highlights its potential as a knowledge acquisition tool, yet it brings to the fore the less-explored area of user information satisfaction (UIS), a gap addressing the development of the UIS model tailored to ChatGPT. In this foundational research grounded in UIS theory, a model was proposed based on critical factors to guide educational stakeholders in investigating issues such as plagiarism and ethical use. By analyzing responses from a diverse group of Indonesian users employed in higher education and using Structural Equation Modeling with Smart-PLS 4.0, we identified five key determinants: completeness, precision, timeliness, convenience, and format. The determinants affect user satisfaction, while traditionally emphasized factors such as accuracy and reliability do not significantly impact the academic utilization of ChatGPT. The results advocate for reliance on ChatGPT with limitations in regard to accuracy and suggest a change in the academic use of technology. The results also offer a perspective that blends theoretical innovation with practical application in educational settings.

Keywords: artificial intelligence; ChatGPT; user information satisfaction; higher education; accuracy

Citation: Fu, C.J.; Silalahi, A.D.K.; Shih, I.-T.; Phuong, D.T.T.; Eunike, I.J.; Jargalsaikhan, S. To Satisfy or Clarify: Enhancing User Information Satisfaction with AI-Powered ChatGPT. *Eng. Proc.* **2024**, *74*, 3. https://doi.org/10.3390/engproc2024074003

Academic Editors: Shu-Han Liao, Teen-Hang Meen and Cheng-Fu Yang

Published: 26 August 2024

1. Introduction

Since its emergence in the field of education in late 2022, AI-powered ChatGPT has drawn attention to its benefits and challenges. Studies have underscored risks, including plagiarism, misinformation [1], and ethical dilemmas [2], leading to hesitancy in its adoption in higher education. However, contrasting with these negative implications, there is evidence of ChatGPT's academic utility. As Roose [3] suggested, ChatGPT could be 'the teacher's best friend,' aiding in tasks such as creating outlines, sparking discussion ideas, and saving time on material preparation. This juxtaposition leads to the provisional view that ChatGPT, while potentially controversial, could be an indispensable, transformative AI tool in academia, bringing about what can be termed a 'Groundbreaking Performance Transformation' in future educational environments.

ChatGPT generates information in the form of text and images. ChatGPT is often considered a groundbreaking AI-powered tool in terms of user productivity, but this premise warrants further examination. This urgency arises as previous studies on ChatGPT have primarily focused on its benefits [4], risks [5], and academic integrity implications for users [6], among other aspects [7–9]. However, the information satisfaction generated by ChatGPT from a user's perspective has not yet been thoroughly evaluated. Therefore, to identify a neglected gap, a model introduced by Ives et al. [10] was used to measure User Information Satisfaction (UIS) related to this information system. We investigated UIS concerning the generative information from ChatGPT for academic purposes, too.

A UIS model was constructed for the information and systems of ChatGPT to determine seven measures, namely, completeness, precision, timeliness, convenience, format, accuracy, and reliability, in the UIS framework [10]. This study is the first to examine the UIS of ChatGPT since it was introduced to the market. The urgency of this research lies in the following: Users (consumers) need to attain satisfaction with the ChatGPT system, as measured by various factors. Additionally, a pragmatic evaluation of the current system reflects its sustainability and continued use from the perspectives of educational organization policies, the scholarly publishing environment, and other academic activities. The results of this study contribute to the development of a User Information Satisfaction (UIS) model for ChatGPT systems based on the seven analyzed factors and their impact on user satisfaction. For individual ChatGPT users, organizations, and governments, policies can be made based on the results.

2. Theoretical Background

2.1. UIS

UIS was introduced by Ives et al. [10] to evaluate information systems. Since its inception, numerous studies have been conducted to investigate users' levels of satisfaction with information systems across various sectors [11–13]. Notably, Ang and Soh [14] explored how UIS was measured in organizations, focusing on employee satisfaction for those without a computer studies background. This underscores the importance of UIS for information system users. Consequently, the applicability of the UIS concept can be extended to measure user satisfaction with respect to ChatGPT systems. Ives et al. [10] defined UIS for users as believing in the ability of the information system to meet their information requirements. UIS is a critical tool for evaluating the effectiveness of information systems used in organizations. Ives et al. [10] also emphasized the necessity of efforts to standardize UIS measurements for comparative studies for different systems and contexts. Therefore, applying UIS to the context of ChatGPT is crucial, given the lack of investigation of UIS from the perspective of ChatGPT users. Thus, it is necessary to explore how ChatGPT users perceive this system's ability to meet their information needs, thereby contributing valuable insights to the effectiveness of ChatGPT as an information tool.

2.2. Theoretical Framework

Previous studies have identified different UIS measures depending on the context and information systems (IS) under investigation. For example, Galletta and Lederer [15] identified 23 measures for assessing user satisfaction regarding the implementation and effectiveness of IS (Figure 1). Laumer et al. [11] identified four factors for measuring users' satisfaction with enterprise content management systems; they also conducted other diverse studies [10–12]. Owing to this research, the theoretical framework for measuring UIS is well established. However, there has been little measurement of UIS for AI-powered systems, including ChatGPT. Thus, we determined UIS measures for ChatGPT, providing information on OpenAI for users, developers, and companies whose operations involve the use of Chatbots. This attempt broadens the scope of UIS applications and contributes to the optimization of AI-powered systems in terms of meeting user needs. The developed measures can be used to understand how these technologies are tailored and improved, enhancing their utility and user satisfaction in various contexts.

Based on the concept of UIS defined in previous studies [4,10,11], we determined and tested seven measures for assessing the ChatGPT. These seven UIS measures were combined into a user satisfaction model. The UIS measures for ChatGPT include completeness, precision, timeliness, convenience, format, accuracy, and reliability. These measures were evaluated in terms of user satisfaction and organized within a conceptual research framework, as depicted in Figure 1. The result provides a holistic understanding of how users interact with and perceive the ChatGPT system. By analyzing these diverse measures, key areas of strength and potential improvement for ChatGPT were identified to enhance its effectiveness as a user-oriented tool. The results are expected to offer valuable insights into the optimization of ChatGPT and similar AI-powered systems.

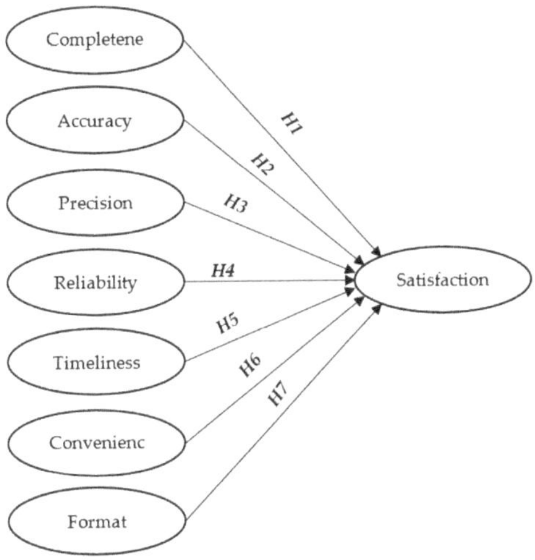

Figure 1. ChatGPT's UIS framework.

3. Hypotheses

ChatGPT UIS Measures and Satisfaction

We employed seven User Information Satisfaction (UIS) measures—completeness, accuracy, precision, reliability, timeliness, convenience, and format—to test user satisfaction. By doing so, we examined how each of these dimensions contributes to the overall satisfaction of users interacting with ChatGPT. This approach enables a detailed exploration of this system's efficacy and user experience, offering insights that can guide future enhancements and modifications to optimize ChatGPT for its users.

The *completeness* of ChatGPT's responses refers to its thoroughness and comprehensiveness in addressing user queries. Users value detailed and comprehensive answers, as they foster an understanding of a given subject [16]. The more complete a response provided by ChatGPT to its users, the higher the likelihood of user satisfaction, emphasizing the importance of depth and breadth in information delivery. Therefore, the following hypothesis was proposed.

H1. *The more complete the responses provided by ChatGPT, the higher the user satisfaction.*

Accuracy was conceptualized as the correctness and truthfulness of ChatGPT's responses. Accurate information is essential for users [4], particularly in decision-making. Thus, we posited a direct positive relationship between the accuracy of information provided and the level of user satisfaction, underlining the significance of providing correct and reliable answers to enhance user experience. Therefore, the following hypothesis was proposed.

H2. *The higher the accuracy of ChatGPT's responses, the greater the user satisfaction.*

Precision is related to the relevance and specificity with which ChatGPT responds to a user's inquiries. Users prefer targeted and relevant answers that address their specific concerns [17]. The more precise the information provided, the greater the user satisfaction, highlighting the value of tailor-made and context-specific responses. Therefore, the following hypothesis was proposed.

H3. *The precision of ChatGPT's responses in directly addressing the user's specific queries positively influences user satisfaction.*

Reliability refers to the consistency and dependability of ChatGPT's responses over time. Research on user interaction indicates that consistent performance builds user trust and satisfaction [18]. This underscores the importance of ChatGPT being able to maintain a stable and dependable output to keep users satisfied. Therefore, the following hypothesis was proposed.

H4. *The more reliable the information provided by ChatGPT, the higher the level of user satisfaction.*

Timeliness focuses on the speed of ChatGPT's responses. Quick and prompt replies have been posited to increase user satisfaction [19]. *Timeliness* is highly valued in the context of digital communication. Users often equate rapid responses with efficiency and effective service, thus enhancing their overall satisfaction with a tool. Therefore, the following hypothesis was proposed.

H5. *The greater the timeliness of ChatGPT, the greater the level of user satisfaction.*

Convenience in relation to using ChatGPT includes aspects such as ease of use and accessibility. We posited that convenience plays a significant role in user satisfaction. Studies on human–computer interaction have suggested that user-friendly and accessible tools significantly enhance user experience and satisfaction. This implies that the more convenient it is to interact with ChatGPT, the higher the level of user satisfaction. Therefore, the following hypothesis was proposed.

H6. *Greater convenience in interacting with ChatGPT will significantly boost user satisfaction.*

The format of ChatGPT's responses, including clarity, organization, and presentation, impacts user satisfaction. Well-structured and presented information aids comprehension and user satisfaction [20]. A user-friendly and well-organized response format positively influences the level of user satisfaction, as it facilitates easier understanding and interaction. Therefore, we proposed the following hypothesis.

H7. *The format in which ChatGPT presents its responses, if clear and well organized, positively impacts user satisfaction.*

4. Methodology

4.1. Measures

We adopted the UIS concept [10] as the foundational framework for developing this conceptual research structure. We used the seven UIS measures determined in previous studies, making modifications and adjustments specific to this study's purposes. This approach was necessary due to the absence of measures for evaluating the UIS of ChatGPT. We formulated 21 questions in four dimensions, modified from the work by Bhattacherjee [21]. For completeness, timeliness, and format, six items were adapted and refined from the work by Laumer et al. [11]. Accuracy was derived from Foroughi et al.'s work [4] and modified from the work by Ives et al. [10], including three items, namely, precision, reliability, and convenience, resulting in eight items. This adaptation ensured the measures were aligned with the unique characteristics and user interactions of ChatGPT, providing a robust and relevant evaluation of user satisfaction. Using this approach, a detailed and nuanced understanding of user satisfaction with respect to ChatGPT was acquired, contributing to the user experience research into AI-powered systems.

4.2. Data Collection

We adopted a quantitative methodology. A survey was designed for specific research participants. The data were gathered through an online survey based on a meticulously crafted questionnaire. This questionnaire comprised three parts. We asked for the consent of the participants, aligning with the study's use of purposive sampling. To be eligible, the respondents had to meet two key criteria: (a) they had to have used ChatGPT for over six months for academic purposes, and (b) they had to have a background in higher education, serving as faculty members, students (both graduate and undergraduate), or postdoctoral researchers. The second section of the questionnaire was created to collect sociodemographic data such as gender, age, type of university, and occupation. The third section was formulated to allow the respondents to answer specific questions. Using this approach, data were collected to accurately represent the experiences of ChatGPT users in academic environments and to understand how different demographic groups use and perceive ChatGPT.

The data were collected from August to November 2023 from a pool of 508 responses. In total, 73% of the respondents were males. Respondents who were 21 to 35 years old had the highest degree of ChatGPT usage (75%). Altogether, 57% graduated from public universities and 43% from private institutions. Undergraduate students constituted 39% of the participants, and 32% were graduate students (master's and doctoral candidates). Faculty members accounted for 15%, and 14% were postdoctoral researchers.

4.3. Data Analysis

We set up several stages for data analysis. To ensure validity and reliability, we conducted a Common Method Variance (CMV) test, employing Harman's Single-Factor method [22], tested using SPSS version 26. We conducted validity, reliability, and hypothesis analyses using Structural Equation Modeling and Smart-PLS 4.0 software. Outer Loadings (OLs), Composite Reliability (CR), Average Variance Extracted (AVE), and Variance Inflation Factor (VIF) were also analyzed [23]. Discriminant validity was tested using the Fornell–Larcker Criterion [24], the Heterotrait/Monotrait Ratio/HTMT [25], a Cross-Loadings Matrix [23], R-squared values [26], and model fit evaluation [23].

5. Results

5.1. CMV

Before data analysis, CMV was tested using Harman's Single-Factor test, in which all the measures were factored into a single dependent variable. If the total variance explained is below 50%, CMV is not considered a concern [22]. In total, 13.6% CMV was obtained without concern in this study. Thus, the credibility of the subsequent analysis was secured, ensuring the robustness and reliability of our data interpretation and results. This low CMV enhances the validity of this study, reinforcing the integrity of the research findings and their implications.

5.2. Validity and Reliability

Table 1 displays the results for validity and reliability, which were validated in this study.

Discriminant validity was tested to evaluate the efficacy of the model developed in this study. Three methods were employed, as illustrated in Tables 2 and 3. All diagonal and bolded values were greater than the intervariable correlation values. This suggested discriminant validity. Additionally, the HTMT values were below 0.90. These results confirm the distinctiveness of the factors of the model, ensuring that each measure captured a unique aspect of the phenomenon, which was crucial for ensuring the overall validity of the research findings.

Table 1. Convergent validity and reliability.

Constructs	OL	CA	CR	VIF	AVE
Accuracy	0.736–0.858	0.713	0.724	1.288–1.597	0.636
Completeness	0.735–0.964	0.790	0.936	1.385–1.385	0.734
Convenience	0.820–0.841	0.771	0.781	1.444–1.770	0.684
Format	0.870–0.871	0.781	0.681	1.314–1.363	0.758
Precision	0.792–0.850	0.736	0.655	1.044–1.317	0.526
Reliability	0.869–0.908	0.735	0.749	1.510–1.510	0.790
Satisfaction	0.797–0.832	0.822	0.822	1.678–1.913	0.652
Timeliness	0.860–0.889	0.709	0.699	1.392–1.392	0.765

Notes: The threshold for Outer Loadings (OLs) was >0.70; that for Cronbach's Alpha (CA) was 0.70; that for Composite Reliability (CR) was >0.70; that for Variance Inflation Factor (VIF) was <0.30; and that for Average Variance Extracted (AVE) was >0.50.

Table 2. Fornell–Larcker Criterion and HTMT.

Constructs	(1)	(2)	(3)	(4)	(5)	(6)	(7)	(8)
ACC (1)	**0.798**	*0.352*	*0.876*	*0.808*	*0.873*	*0.776*	*0.718*	*0.858*
CMP (2)	0.251	**0.857**	*0.277*	*0.449*	*0.655*	*0.374*	*0.176*	*0.282*
CVC (3)	0.652	0.210	**0.827**	*0.714*	*0.644*	*0.623*	*0.683*	*0.788*
FMT (4)	0.564	0.299	0.521	**0.871**	*0.875*	*0.598*	*0.784*	*0.691*
PRR (5)	0.685	0.315	0.664	0.525	**0.725**	*0.858*	*0.827*	*0.895*
RLB (6)	0.557	0.284	0.476	0.423	0.558	**0.889**	*0.537*	*0.249*
STS (7)	0.551	0.146	0.555	0.586	0.586	0.420	**0.808**	*0.682*
TML (8)	0.601	0.215	0.584	0.475	0.577	0.661	0.517	**0.875**

Notes: The diagonal bolded values are the square root of the AVE, which was used for Fornell–Larcker Criterion. The italic values indicate the HTMT, with a threshold of <0.90. ACC, accuracy; CMP, completeness; CVC, convenience; FMT, format; PRR, precision; RLB, reliability; STS, satisfaction; TML, timeliness.

Table 3. Cross-loadings matrix.

Items/Contructs	ACC	CMP	CVC	FMT	PRR	RLB	STS	TML
ACR.1	**0.795**	0.253	0.519	0.468	0.511	0.499	0.427	0.514
ACR.2	**0.858**	0.179	0.523	0.482	0.559	0.411	0.488	0.479
ACR.3	**0.736**	0.171	0.524	0.396	0.574	0.431	0.400	0.450
CMP.1	0.239	**0.964**	0.207	0.268	0.313	0.288	0.159	0.224
CMP.2	0.191	**0.735**	0.141	0.270	0.210	0.171	0.063	0.114
CNV.1	0.496	0.201	**0.820**	0.407	0.480	0.351	0.364	0.412
CNV.2	0.533	0.173	**0.841**	0.421	0.600	0.419	0.488	0.480
CNV.3	0.578	0.154	**0.820**	0.458	0.551	0.402	0.500	0.537
FMR.1	0.489	0.307	0.421	**0.870**	0.419	0.371	0.510	0.387
FMR.2	0.492	0.213	0.485	**0.871**	0.494	0.365	0.511	0.440
PRC.1	0.576	0.203	0.568	0.418	**0.850**	0.457	0.515	0.486
PRC.2	0.577	0.203	0.569	0.439	**0.838**	0.480	0.491	0.503
PRC.3	0.277	0.473	0.218	0.285	**0.792**	0.235	0.182	0.191
RLB.1	0.498	0.287	0.398	0.371	0.445	**0.869**	0.340	0.557
RLB.2	0.494	0.224	0.446	0.381	0.540	**0.908**	0.402	0.615
STS.1	0.438	0.093	0.441	0.489	0.456	0.295	**0.798**	0.364
STS.2	0.444	0.082	0.481	0.445	0.489	0.354	**0.832**	0.444
STS.3	0.459	0.151	0.421	0.493	0.446	0.361	**0.797**	0.410
STS.4	0.439	0.147	0.448	0.467	0.500	0.345	**0.802**	0.450
TML.1	0.525	0.202	0.523	0.413	0.502	0.591	0.427	**0.860**
TML.2	0.528	0.176	0.499	0.418	0.509	0.568	0.475	**0.889**

Discriminant validity was tested using the Cross-Loading Matrix method (Table 3). The correlation of each construct with its respective measurement items was greater than that with cross items. Thus, discriminant validity was confirmed in this study. The differentiation of the constructs ensured the reliability and accuracy of the measurement model, ensuring that each construct was distinctively and accurately captured in the research framework.

The model was tested using an evaluation of model fit and R-squared values. The SRMR value was 0.070, the Chi-Square value was 1631.471, and the NFI was 0.783, all of which fell within the threshold limits [23]. Subsequently, the R-squared value was assessed to determine the power of independent constructs for predicting the dependent constructs. An R-squared value of 0.581 was obtained, indicating that the seven ChatGPT UIS measures accounted for 58.1% of the variance in satisfaction. This meets the criteria set by Falk and Miller [26], as the R-squared value was above the 0.10 benchmark. These results demonstrate the model's good fit and underline the considerable explanatory power of the identified factors in determining user satisfaction with ChatGPT.

5.3. Hypothesis Testing

Table 4 and Figure 2 present a summary of the hypothesis testing. Accuracy ($\beta = 0.070$; $T = 1.247$) and reliability ($\beta = 0.016$; $T = 0.400$) were not significant predictors of satisfaction, leading to the rejection of hypotheses H2 and H4. Completeness ($\beta = 0.096$; $T = 2.863$), convenience ($\beta = 0.126$; $T = 2.192$), format ($\beta = 0.323$; $T = 5.115$), precision ($\beta = 0.245$; $T = 3.681$), and timeliness ($\beta = 0.138$; $T = 2.396$) significantly impacted satisfaction, supporting hypotheses H1, H3, H5, H6, and H7. Format and precision impacted satisfaction more than the other factors. These results highlight the varying degrees of influence of different UIS measures on user satisfaction, with several factors playing a more critical role than others in shaping user experience with respect to ChatGPT.

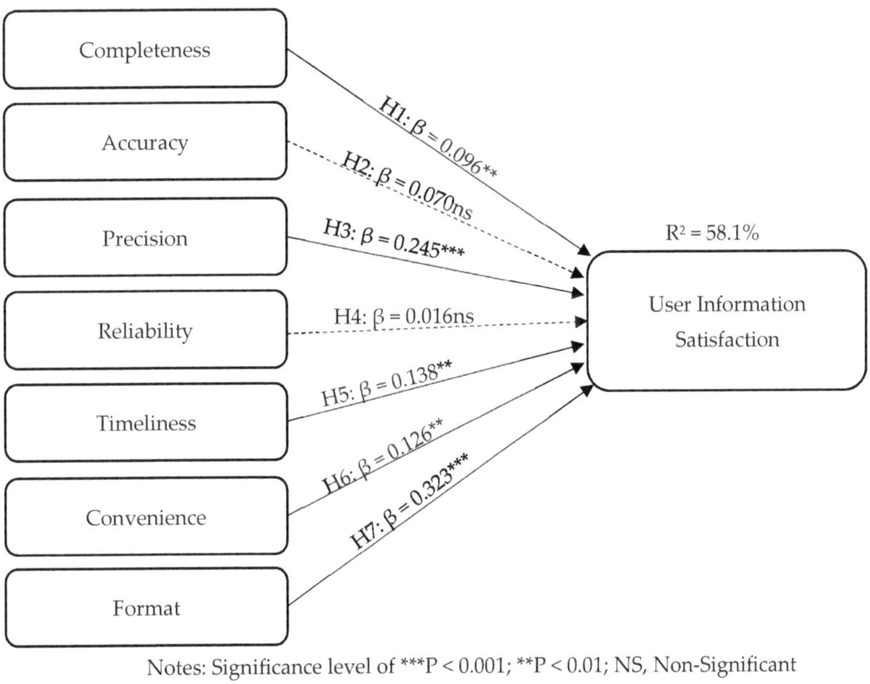

Figure 2. Hypothesis testing.

Table 4. Summary of hypothesis testing.

Hypothesis	β	T	Bootstrapping CI 97.5%		Decision
			Lower	Upper	
CMP → STS	0.096 **	2.863	0.168	0.040	Accept
AC → STS	0.070	1.247	0.037	0.182	Reject
PRC → STS	0.245 ***	3.681	0.117	0.378	Accept
RLB → STS	0.016	0.400	0.118	0.086	Reject
TML → STS	0.138 **	2.396	0.025	0.249	Accept
CVN → STS	0.126 **	2.192	0.014	0.239	Accept
FMT → STS	0.323 ***	5.115	0.202	0.444	Accept

Notes: AC, accuracy; CMP, completeness; CVN, convenience; FMT, format; PRC, precision; RLB, reliability; TML, timeliness; STS, satisfaction. Significance levels: *** $p < 0.001$; ** $p < 0.010$.

6. Discussion

We examined the UIS framework proposed by Ives et al. [10], which suggested that accuracy and reliability are essential for user satisfaction with respect to information systems. Contradicting this long-standing belief, the study's results revealed that these aspects did not significantly shape user satisfaction in the utilization of ChatGPT. This indicated that the parameters determining satisfaction are changing with advancements in generative AI technologies. This is contradictory to findings reported in previous studies [10]. Other dimensions including completeness, convenience, format, precision, and timeliness influenced users' satisfaction with ChatGPT. Users of ChatGPT valued the presentation and immediacy of information, not just its correctness or dependability. This underscores that with recent UIS theory adaptations, the changing landscape of user expectations is becoming more sophisticated [10,11].

7. Conclusions

Implication

The UIS framework was applied theoretically by examining the aspects of accuracy and reliability regarding user satisfaction as discussed by Ives et al. [10]. These factors did not significantly influence user satisfaction in the context of ChatGPT, pointing to a potential shift in the UIS paradigm as generative AI technology progresses. Such a result challenges and potentially redefines the established parameters of user satisfaction. The results of this study contribute to UIS by identifying the importance of completeness, convenience, format, precision, and timeliness. The evolving priorities of users were also redefined by advanced technology. The theoretical framework of UIS contributes attributes to the current digital interaction milieu and enhances our understanding of user satisfaction in regard to information systems.

The results of this study can be used to understand the application of ChatGPT in organizational and individual contexts. At an organizational level, the traditional emphasis on accuracy and reliability is changing, encouraging entities to recalibrate their focus toward completeness, convenience, format, precision, and timeliness in their information systems. Such a realignment leads to the creation of interfaces that are more attuned to user needs, potentially improving users' utilization of and satisfaction with AI-powered tools. This will result in the development of more intuitive and efficient systems, thereby enhancing the return on investment for AI technologies.

For those who regularly engage with AI programs such as ChatGPT, the results reported herein underscore the importance of mastering the features of this system that enhance its immediate utility. Understanding how to effectively navigate and extract value from AI interactions is crucial, suggesting that user education is mandatory in these aspects. As end-users become more adept at utilizing the streamlined and user-friendly features of such technologies, they can optimize efficiency and productivity, reaping the full benefits of the evolving digital tools at their disposal. This knowledge enables users to have realistic expectations and maximize the utility of AI in their work and learning environments, solidifying their role as competent navigators in the advancing technological landscape.

Despite its contributions, this study had limitations, such as a confined focus on ChatGPT while disregarding various other generative AI platforms. Furthermore, this study's reliance on self-reported measures of satisfaction introduced biases that hindered its ability to capture the nuanced reactions of users to AI interfaces. Further studies are necessary to include a broader range of AI tools and technologies in this field of research, thereby enriching the generalizability of the findings. Additionally, it is necessary to incorporate objective usage data to provide an understanding of user satisfaction and behavior and offer a holistic view of how individuals and organizations interact with AI systems. A longitudinal study must be conducted to assess users' satisfaction with AI over time as they become more accustomed to these technologies.

Author Contributions: Conceptualization, C.J.F. and A.D.K.S.; methodology, A.D.K.S. and I.-T.S.; software, A.D.K.S. and I.J.E.; validation, D.T.T.P., A.D.K.S., S.J. and I.J.E.; formal analysis, A.D.K.S.; investigation, I.J.E. and A.D.K.S.; resources, C.J.F. and A.D.K.S.; data curation, I.J.E., D.T.T.P. and S.J.; writing—original draft preparation, C.J.F., A.D.K.S. and I.-T.S.; writing—review and editing, A.D.K.S., I.-T.S., I.J.E., D.T.T.P. and S.J.; visualization, I.J.E. and S.J.; supervision, C.J.F., A.D.K.S. and I.-T.S.; project administration, A.D.K.S. All authors have read and agreed to the published version of the manuscript.

Funding: This research received no external funding.

Institutional Review Board Statement: Not applicable.

Informed Consent Statement: Not applicable.

Data Availability Statement: The data presented in this study are available on request from the corresponding author.

Conflicts of Interest: The authors declare no conflicts of interest.

References

1. Lund, B.D.; Wang, T.; Mannuru, N.R.; Nie, B.; Shimray, S.; Wang, Z. ChatGPT and a new academic reality: Artificial Intelligence-written research papers and the ethics of the large language models in scholarly publishing. *J. Assoc. Inf. Sci. Technol.* **2023**, *74*, 570–581. [CrossRef]
2. Bringula, R. What do academics have to say about ChatGPT? A text mining analytics on the discussions regarding ChatGPT on research writing. *AI Ethics* **2023**, 1–13. [CrossRef]
3. Roose, K. Don't Ban ChatGPT in Schools. Teach with It. 2023. Available online: https://www.nytimes.com/2023/01/12/technology/chatgpt-schools-teachers.html (accessed on 13 February 2024).
4. Foroughi, B.; Senali, M.G.; Iranmanesh, M.; Khanfar, A.; Ghobakhloo, M.; Annamalai, N.; Naghmeh-Abbaspour, B. Determinants of intention to use ChatGPT for educational purposes: Findings from PLS-SEM and fsQCA. *Int. J. Hum. Comput. Int.* **2023**, 1–20. [CrossRef]
5. Rivas, P.; Zhao, L. Marketing with chatgpt: Navigating the ethical terrain of gpt-based chatbot technology. *AI* **2023**, *4*, 375–384. [CrossRef]
6. Bin-Nashwan, S.A.; Sadallah, M.; Bouteraa, M. Use of ChatGPT in academia: Academic integrity hangs in the balance. *Technol. Soc.* **2023**, *75*, 102370. [CrossRef]
7. Dwivedi, Y.K.; Kshetri, N.; Hughes, L.; Slade, E.L.; Jeyaraj, A.; Kar, A.K.; Baabdullah, A.M.; Koohang, A.; Raghavan, V.; Ahuja, M.; et al. "So what if ChatGPT wrote it?" Multidisciplinary perspectives on opportunities, challenges and implications of generative conversational AI for research, practice and policy. *Int. J Inf. Manag.* **2023**, *71*, 102642. [CrossRef]
8. Baek, T.H.; Kim, M. Is ChatGPT scary good? How user motivations affect creepiness and trust in generative artificial intelligence. *Telemat. Inform.* **2023**, *83*, 102030. [CrossRef]
9. Kocoń, J.; Cichecki, I.; Kaszyca, O.; Kochanek, M.; Szydło, D.; Baran, J.; Bielaniewicz, J.; Gruza, M.; Janz, A.; Kanclerz, K.; et al. ChatGPT: Jack of all trades, master of none. *Inf. Fusion.* **2023**, *99*, 101861. [CrossRef]
10. Ives, B.; Olson, M.H.; Baroudi, J.J. The measurement of user information satisfaction. Commun. *ACM* **1983**, *26*, 785–793. [CrossRef]
11. Laumer, S.; Maier, C.; Weitzel, T. Information quality, user satisfaction, and the manifestation of workarounds: A qualitative and quantitative study of enterprise content management system users. *Eur. J. Inf. Syst.* **2017**, *26*, 333–360. [CrossRef]
12. Bai, B.; Law, R.; Wen, I. The impact of website quality on customer satisfaction and purchase intentions: Evidence from Chinese online visitors. *Int. J. Hosp. Manag.* **2008**, *27*, 391–402. [CrossRef]

13. Iivari, J.; Ervasti, I. User information satisfaction: IS implementability and effectiveness. *J. Inf. Manag.* **1994**, *27*, 205–220. [CrossRef]
14. Ang, J.; Soh, P.H. User information satisfaction, job satisfaction and computer background: An exploratory study. *J. Inf. Manag.* **1997**, *32*, 255–266. [CrossRef]
15. Galletta, D.F.; Lederer, A.L. Some cautions on the measurement of user information satisfaction. *Decis. Sci.* **1989**, *20*, 419–443. [CrossRef]
16. Gupta, S.; Motlagh, M.; Rhyner, J. The digitalization sustainability matrix: A participatory research tool for investigating digitainability. *Sustainability* **2020**, *12*, 9283. [CrossRef]
17. Reinecke, K.; Bernstein, A. Knowing what a user likes: A design science approach to interfaces that automatically adapt to culture. *MIS Q.* **2013**, *37*, 427–453. [CrossRef]
18. Chen, Y.; Zahedi, F.M.; Abbasi, A.; Dobolyi, D. Trust calibration of automated security IT artifacts: A multi-domain study of phishing-website detection tools. *Inf. Manag.* **2021**, *58*, 103394. [CrossRef]
19. Petter, S.; Fruhling, A. Evaluating the success of an emergency response medical information systemInt. *J. Med. Inform.* **2011**, *80*, 480–489. [CrossRef] [PubMed]
20. Park, S.; Zo, H.; Ciganek, A.P.; Lim, G.G. Examining success factors in the adoption of digital object identifier systems. *Electron. Commer. Res. Appl.* **2011**, *10*, 626–636. [CrossRef]
21. Bhattacherjee, A. Understanding information systems continuance: An expectation-confirmation model. *MIS Q.* **2001**, *25*, 351–370. [CrossRef]
22. Baumgartner, H.; Weijters, B.; Pieters, R. The biasing effect of common method variance: Some clarifications. *J. Acad. Mark. Sci.* **2021**, *49*, 221–235. [CrossRef]
23. Hair, J.; Hollingsworth, C.L.; Randolph, A.B.; Chong, A.Y.L. An updated and expanded assessment of PLS-SEM in information systems research. Ind. Manag. *Data Syst.* **2017**, *117*, 442–458. [CrossRef]
24. Fornell, C.; Larcker, D.F. Evaluating structural equation models with unobservable variables and measurement error. *J. Mark. Res.* **1981**, *18*, 39–50. [CrossRef]
25. Henseler, J.; Ringle, C.M.; Sarstedt, M. A new criterion for assessing discriminant validity in variance-based structural equation modeling. *J. Acad. Mark. Sci.* **2015**, *43*, 115–135. [CrossRef]
26. Falk, R.F.; Miller, N.B. *A Primer for Soft Modeling*; The University of Akron Press: Akron, OH, USA, 1992.

engineering proceedings

MDPI

Proceeding Paper

The Effect of Auditory Perceptual Training by Online Computer Software on English Pronunciation †

Ching-Wen (Felicia)

The Language Center, Chaoyang University of Technology, Taichung 412005, Taiwan;
feliciawang@o365.cyut.edu.tw

† Presented at the 2024 IEEE 4th International Conference on Electronic Communications, Internet of Things and Big Data, Taipei, Taiwan, 19–21 April 2024.

Abstract: Pronunciation is crucial to L2 learning. However, achieving speech proficiency is difficult. Class time constraints make demonstration–imitation pronunciation teaching methods less effective, even after repeated practice. Research suggests that pronunciation involves motor control, that auditory preparation enhances accuracy, and that learners produce more accurate pronunciation after perceiving accurate target sounds. This study proposes that the perception of accurate L2 target sounds will enhance pronunciation. To test this concept, the study employed online auditory training tasks for English learners enrolled at a private university in Taiwan. The results showed that auditory teaching results in positive learning outcomes.

Keywords: pronunciation; speech perception; speech production; perceptual training

Citation: Wang, C.-W. The Effect of Auditory Perceptual Training by Online Computer Software on English Pronunciation. *Eng. Proc.* **2024**, *74*, 4. https://doi.org/10.3390/engproc2024074004

Academic Editors: Shu-Han Liao, Teen-Hang Meen and Cheng-Fu Yang

Published: 26 August 2024

1. Introduction

Pronunciation courses in second language learning are often overlooked, partly due to teachers' lack of appropriate pronunciation training [1]. If second language learners do not receive proper pronunciation training from the beginning of their studies, they may learn the mispronunciation of words or to speak with a native language accent, which can affect a listener's comprehension of [2] and trust in a speaker [3]. Flege's [4] Speech Learning Model explains that if a learner's native language and second language have completely corresponding phonetics, there is no learning difficulty. However, when the native and second languages have similar but still different phonetics, the learning difficulty is greater than learning new elements.

Pronunciation teaching in classrooms is usually incidental, corrected only when errors occur during vocabulary or sentence reading. The systematic teaching of pronunciation as well as its formal inclusion in regular courses is often lacking. Furthermore, many pronunciation actions involve the control and coordination of muscles that are not easily observable, such as the mouth, nose, throat, and chest. Cognitive neuroscience research suggests that smoothly producing the action of speech requires activating the organs of speech and coordinating multiple perceptual channels (such as auditory, visual, body perception, etc.) and imitation functions [5,6].

To verify the hypothesis that auditory perception and pronunciation actions are complementary, this study developed a series of online listening tasks to train the auditory perception of low-achieving learners. The goal was to develop a teaching method for improving learners' pronunciation accuracy while demonstrating that understanding how students learn pronunciation will help teachers design effective pronunciation courses.

2. Literature Review

2.1. Motor Theory

Cognitive neuroscience regards verbal expression as a form of motor control. Guenther and Vladusich [7] suggest that to understand the action of speech it is necessary to comprehend all the brain regions involved in it. They integrated auditory and somatosensory perceptions with the brain's motor cortex, collectively called the speech–motor control system. This system encompasses all speech actions, from simple vocalizations to complex lexical items [8–10]. The internal forward model in motor control theory shows the relationship between the brain's motor commands and the effector organs [11]. For instance, when the brain issues a motor command, it simultaneously generates an efference copy to predict the result of the speech action. If the result differs from the efference copy, the brain reissues the command and corrects it. Hickok [12] proposed the Hierarchical State Feedback Control (HSFC) model which explains the general language production process and illustrates the importance of the auditory feedback system for pronunciation actions. It suggests that once speakers know what concept to express, they enter a coding stage to search for vocabulary, followed by the phonetic and auditory prediction stages. When the vocal cords emit a syllable, the auditory system feedbacks the phoneme to the speech action system. Auditory checking verifies the pronunciation accuracy of a target sound and predicts the expected phonetic result of the pronunciation action. If the predicted phonetic result differs from the actual result heard, the goal is not achieved, and auditory feedback must assist in correcting the pronunciation action. Thus, in the HSFC model, "predicted heard pronunciation" is the goal of speech action.

2.2. Auditory Perception Guiding Speech Action

Early experiments demonstrated the relationship between hearing and speech. Studies on motor learning and motor control showed how auditory perception influences speech actions. For example, the Lombard effect [13] indicates that people naturally increase their speech volume in noisy environments to confirm the content of their speech, as it is more difficult to hear their voice clearly in a loud environment. Houde and Jordan [14] had participants attempt to pronounce words containing the /ɛ/ sound (such as "peb") but played words with the /i/ sound (such as "peeb") through headphones. The results showed that participants adjusted their speech actions based on the sounds they heard, with the same phenomenon occurring even after substituting different vowels. These phenomena demonstrated that the brain uses auditory perception both to monitor and check the accuracy of speech actions.

2.3. Auditory Illusions in Everyday Life

Auditory illusions are perceptual illusions that often occur in real life. People interpret the events that occur in their environments based on their previous experiences and existing knowledge. This cognitive processing is common in vision or hearing [15]. Neuroscience researchers investigated the neural responses to continuous sound segments in the brain [16]. For example, when an octave of sound gradually rises from a low pitch to a high octave, the brain perceives the melody as continuously rising and never-ending under repeated playback. The brain does not perceive a decrease in scale. This phenomenon is known as the Shepard tone illusion. Deutsch [17] experimented with the words "no way" in a loop and asked the subjects to give feedback on what they heard. The results showed the subjects' word interpretations varied, such as "no brain", "no time", "runaway", etc. She called these variations phantom words and explained not only that knowledge, beliefs, and expectations influence what we hear but also that what we think we hear may not be what we do hear.

In addition, auditory illusions of entire sentences may occur. Warren [18] found that the brain's cognitive system tends to interpret unknown situations using known conditions. For example, when playing the sentence "The state governors met with their respective legislatures convening in the capital city" for subjects, he used a cough to cover the first /s/ sound in "legislatures", which produced "legi(cough)latures". However, the subjects did not notice the omission of the phoneme /s/ and could not even determine where in the sentence the cough had occurred. Scholars call this phenomenon phonemic restoration, which shows that our brains interpret what we hear based on our experiences and knowledge.

2.4. Native Language Interference in Second Language Pronunciation Accuracy

Regardless of whether a student is learning their native language or a second language, they need to go through the process of learning language production. However, during second language learning, a learner's native language may interfere with the operation of their auditory feedback mechanism. For example, since Japanese pronunciation does not include the English /r/ sound, when native speakers of Japanese hear the English syllable /ra/ they associate it with /la/, thereby not only confusing their auditory feedback but also leading to pronunciation errors. Thus, as prior research suggests, language experience affects speech perception [19]. In addition, if the brain's "predicted heard pronunciation" affects the accuracy of pronunciation, which the HSFC model implies, then how the auditory system stores phonetic data also becomes a key factor affecting how students learn speech production.

2.5. Auditory Identification Training Enhances Pronunciation Accuracy

Teachers often use their existing language experience as the basis for establishing and carrying out classroom pronunciation lessons. However, cognitive science suggests that training learners' listening ability should be the basis for training their pronunciation [20]. Alves and Luchini [20] trained the listening abilities of three groups of adult English learners from Argentina to determine the accuracy of their pronunciation development. The subjects in the first and second groups participated in all the listening training tasks. In addition, the second group received extra guidance on the target sound. However, the third group received no listening training at all. All three groups of subjects recorded their pronunciations of the target sounds before and after the listening training. The subjects also took a delayed test one month after the study to determine any longer-term effects of the training. The results showed that the pronunciation of the two groups of subjects who received the listening training improved significantly, and the learning effect continued for one month. In addition, the second group, which received extra guidance on the target sound, performed better than the groups that did not receive the extra guidance. The researchers inferred that listening training effectively improves learners' pronunciation accuracy. Therefore, their study encourages pronunciation teaching to enhance learners' awareness of target sound learning.

2.6. Summary

Researchers in the field of education have long been committed to improving teaching methods. On the other hand, scientists have been exploring the most effective methods of education from the perspective of learning, and inferring teaching methods from the outcomes of such studies. This study employed the latter approach by examining the situation of second language learners from not only the perspective of science but also through the establishment of a corresponding online learning platform and interactive online exercises that provide learners with a direction for self-study while also motivating their interest in learning. This collection of practice materials for second language learners, coupled with classroom listening and spelling activities to check learning output in real-time, lays out a foundation for teaching pronunciation to low-achieving freshmen.

3. Research Method

Low-achieving freshmen in the vocational education system often lack learning strategies and exposure to diverse interest-inducing teaching methods. These deficiencies make it more difficult to improve learning effectiveness. For example, even though pronunciation is fundamental to increasing second language vocabulary, particularly in phonetic languages, teaching curricula often overlook it because of a lack of effective and diverse teaching methods. This study aims to improve this situation by verifying a hypothesis based on cognitive science research that actively improving auditory perception can enhance pronunciation accuracy. Consequently, the targets in this study were freshmen enrolled in the vocational education system who had low English proficiency and practiced phonetic listening. Based on the preceding discussion, this study explored the impact of auditory perceptual training on learner pronunciation accuracy.

3.1. Participants

The research method in this study included implementing a curriculum developed for a basic English class of freshmen whose level of achievement in English was in the lowest 5% at a private university of technology in Taichung, Taiwan. The class consisted of about 45 students, including a few with reading or physical disabilities that excluded them from participating in this study. In general, these students' learning motivation was also low, partly because they had not been able to discover personally effective learning strategies. According to the university's statistics, each year about 5% of basic level students fail to pass the minimum English graduation threshold (CEFR A2) required by their departments.

3.2. Research Design and Procedure

The present research plan was to assist learners in pronunciation learning before and after each two-hour class by constructing an online training system. Figure 1 shows the procedure of the experiment by conducting the read-and-record English pronunciation pre-test in the second week of the semester before the formal course began. The participants took the same test in their final week of training. The pre-/post-tests did not include feedback. All the learners watched a 10-min rules of pronunciation video on the platform and performed listen-and-spell tasks using an alphabetical card set provided to each student. The in-class listen-and-spell activities consolidated their knowledge of the rules of pronunciation. Every day after the second week of class, the students performed either listen-and-identify or listen-and-record tasks, which helped them learn the rules of pronunciation. Each stage of the pronunciation rule training lasted for six days and the daily sessions for 10–15 min. After the third week, the first hour of class involved listen-and-spell exercises for guided pronunciation practice. The content of the remaining class hour included studies in local culture and teaching material from the class textbook.

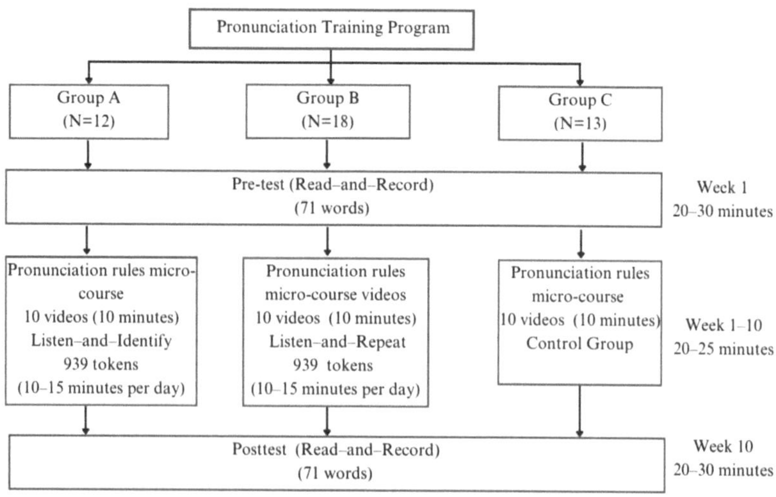

Figure 1. Research design and procedure.

The students began each online training session by watching a micro-course video devoted to the rule of pronunciation. After watching the video, the students listened to approximately 90 words that exemplified the day's pronunciation rules. Over the 10-week training period, the online system taught 939 vocabulary words, which the students used to complete the listen-and-identify or listen-and-repeat tasks. The students had already learned half of the words on the pre-test (old words). New words appeared on the post-test that the training sessions did not include. These unfamiliar words checked whether the training generalized learned sounds to new-word contexts. The group completing the listen-and-identify tasks received immediate feedback on their answers, while the group completing the listen-and-repeat (record) tasks received no feedback. The system recorded the learners' pronunciation performance (either their identifications or their recordings) and allowed the teacher to evaluate the effectiveness of the online pronunciation-learning process.

The study adopted an experimental teaching method to improve the learners' pronunciation accuracy. All three groups (A, B, and C) received ten online pronunciation micro-course videos, as well as listening- and spelling-teaching activities in class. The experimental Groups A and B received either the auditory perceptual training or the auditory perceptual training with recording, respectively. The control Group C only received the pronunciation micro-course videos and participated in the in-class listening- and spelling-teaching activities. The training method of Group B simulated a situation in which the students learned by themselves or spoke as soon as they heard the demonstration sound in class. However, for the analysis subjects, the students who completed the pre-test were involved in the training and the post-test, which left 12 students in Group A, 18 in Group B; and 13 in Group C.

3.3. Instruments and Scoring

The English pronunciation test content included common monosyllabic words of single vowels (such as a in 'bat'), diphthongs (such as a-e as in 'game'), simple consonants (such as d in 'did'), and compound consonants (such as -nk in 'pink'). The test platform displayed 71 vocabulary words, with the students recording their pronunciation of the vocabulary on the platform. All the recordings were manually scored; that is, real assessors judged all the English pronunciation tests by manually listening to them. If the judgment was that a recorded syllable matched its target sound, then it received 1 point; otherwise, it received 0 points. Each student's pre-test and post-test recordings were randomly presented, so the judging listener would not know whether the syllable was from a pre-test or a post-test recording file. Once the judges assessed all the recordings, the progress score was statistically analyzed and presented as a percentage. Paired-Samples T Tests validated the results of the pre- and post-tests for any significant improvement in pronunciation-learning performance.

4. Results

This study investigated whether listen-and-identify perceptual training achieves better pronunciation accuracy. Data analysis from the pre- and post-tests included the Paired-Samples T Tests to check for differences among the variables. After investigating the efficacy of the English pronunciation intervention training tasks (independent variables) on the post-test scores (dependent variable), the results of the Paired-Samples T Tests revealed significant improvement in all three groups. In Group A, the mean pre-test score was 38.3 (SD = 24.8), and the mean post-test score was 71.5 (SD = 28.4), $t(11) = -3.75$, $p = 0.003 < 0.05$, indicating a statistically significant enhancement in pronunciation ability. Similarly, in Group B, the mean pre-test score was 54.1 (SD = 25.3), and the mean post-test score was 76.8 (SD = 20.6), $t(17) = -3.85$, $p = 0.001 < 0.05$, demonstrating a significant improvement. Finally, in Group C, the mean pre-test score was 45.5 (SD = 24.4), and the mean post-test score was 73.1 (SD = 12.1), $t(12) = -4.01$, $p = 0.002 < 0.05$, also signifying significant advancement in English pronunciation. These findings underscore the positive impact of the pronunciation training program across the groups.

5. Discussion and Conclusions

The results of this study indicated that the training program effectively enhanced the participants' English pronunciation abilities. The motor theory posits that the motor system plays a crucial role in speech perception. The participants in Group A practiced listen-and-identify skills without speaking. A significant improvement in their post-test scores was achieved with training tasks that involved identifying words with the target sounds tuned to the students' perceptual representations. On the other hand, Group B practiced listen-and-repeat skills involving immediate reaction after listening to the target sounds. However, the procedure required the participants to listen before speaking and to accurately pronounce the target sounds. They had to maintain accurate auditory representations. Hence, Group B exemplified another form of perceptual training. Group C was the control group in the study. However, their test results showed significant improvement. One possible interpretation of this result is that the in-class listen-and-spell activities effectively contributed to their learning. Thus, even though Group C did not receive additional online training, visual aids nevertheless played a crucial role in their learning. The results of all three groups showed that the students engaged in perceptual training with every task. Auditory representation and speech had a close relationship. Designing a pronunciation course required training the learners to perceive the target sound accurately. While the common approach to teaching pronunciation is demonstration and repetition, the listen-and-identify approach is an effective alternative strategy that reinforces accurate pronunciation outcomes. The listen-and-spell activity also helped consolidate the learners' knowledge of the target sounds while enriching the learning enjoyment.

This study was preliminary research because the number of participants in the three groups was small, making it unfeasible to have a traditional control group because the teacher had to interact with all the students. Consequently, further research is necessary to verify and generalize the results of this study.

Funding: This research received no external funding.

Data Availability Statement: The original contributions presented in the study are included in the article, further inquiries can be directed to the corresponding author.

Conflicts of Interest: The author declares no conflicts of interest.

References

1. Camus-Oyarzun, P.A. The Effects of Pronunciation Instruction on the Production of Second Language Spanish: A Classroom Study. Ph.D. Thesis, Georgetown University, Washington, DC, USA, 2016.
2. Munro, M.J.; Derwing, T.M. Processing time, accent, and comprehensibility in the perception of native and foreign-accented speech. *Lang. Speech* **1995**, *38*, 289–306. [CrossRef] [PubMed]
3. Rubin, D.L.; Smith, K.A. Effects of accent, ethnicity, and lecture topic on undergraduates' perceptions of nonnative English-speaking teaching assistants. *Int. J. Intercult. Relat.* **1990**, *14*, 337–353. [CrossRef]
4. Flege, J.E. Second-language speech learning: Theory, findings and problems. In *Speech Perception and Linguistic Experience: Theoretical and Methodological Issues*; Strange, W., Ed.; York Press: Timonium, MD, USA, 1995.
5. Guenther, F.H. Speech sound acquisition, coarticulation, and rate effects in a neural network model of speech production. *Psychol. Rev.* **1995**, *102*, 594–621. [CrossRef] [PubMed]
6. Tremblay, S.; Shiller, D.M.; Ostry, D.J. Somatosensory basis of speech production. *Nature* **2003**, *423*, 866–869. [CrossRef] [PubMed]
7. Guenther, F.H.; Vladusich, T. A neural theory of speech acquisition and production. *J. Neurolinguistics* **2009**, *25*, 408–422. [CrossRef] [PubMed]
8. Fiez, J.A.; Petersen, S.E. Neuroimaging studies of word reading. *Proc. Natl. Acad. Sci. USA* **1998**, *95*, 914–921. [CrossRef] [PubMed]
9. Turkeltaub, P.E.; Eden, G.F.; Jones, K.M.; Zeffiro, T.A. Meta-analysis of the functional neuroanatomy of single-word reading: Method and validation. *NeuroImage* **2002**, *16*, 765–780. [CrossRef] [PubMed]
10. Argyropoulos, G.P.D. The cerebellum, internal models, and prediction in 'non-motor' aspects of language: A critical review. *Brain Lang.* **2016**, *161*, 4–17. [CrossRef] [PubMed]
11. Hickok, G. The architecture of speech production and the role of the phoneme in speech processing. *Lang. Cogn. Process.* **2014**, *29*, 2–20. [CrossRef] [PubMed]
12. Lane, H.; Tranel, B. The Lombard sign and the role of hearing in speech. *J. Speech Lang. Heart Res.* **1971**, *14*, 677–709. [CrossRef]
13. Houde, J.F.; Jordan, M.I. Sensorimotor adaptation in speech production. *Science* **1997**, *279*, 1213–1216. [CrossRef] [PubMed]

14. Hawkins, S. Phonological features, auditory objects, and illusions. *J. Phon.* **2010**, *38*, 60–89. [CrossRef]
15. Shimizu, Y.; Umeda, M.; Mano, H.; Aoki, I.; Higuchi, T.; Tanaka, C. Neuronal response to Shepard's tones. An auditory fMRI study using multifractal analysis. *Brain Res.* **2007**, *1186*, 113–123. [CrossRef] [PubMed]
16. Deutsch, D. Phantom Words. 2013. Available online: http://deutsch.ucsd.edu/psychology/pages.php?i=211 (accessed on 13 February 2017).
17. Warren, R.M. Perceptual restoration of missing speech sounds. *Science* **1970**, *167*, 392–393. [CrossRef] [PubMed]
18. Zhang, Y.; Kuhl, P.K.; Imada, T.; Kotani, M.; Tohkura, Y. Effects of language experience: Neural commitment to language-specific auditory patterns. *NeuroImage* **2005**, *26*, 703–720. [CrossRef] [PubMed]
19. Wang, Y.; Jongman, A.; Sereno, J.A. Acoustic and perceptual evaluation of Mandarin tone productions before and after perceptual training. *J. Acoust. Soc. Am.* **2003**, *113*, 1033–1043. [CrossRef] [PubMed]
20. Alves, U.K.F.; Luchini, P.L. Effects of perceptual training on the identification and production of word-initial voiceless stops by Argentinean learners of English. *Ilha Do Desterro* **2017**, *70*, 15–32. [CrossRef]

engineering proceedings

MDPI

Proceeding Paper

Performance of Green Industrial Estate: A Review †

Ikse Duma Alriansyach [1], Christiono Utomo [1,*], Yani Rahmawati [2] and Aqsha Aqsha [3]

1 Department of Civil Engineering, Institut Teknologi Sepuluh Nopember, Surabaya 60111, Indonesia; dumaalriansyach@gmail.com
2 Department of Architecture Engineering and Planning, Universitas Gadjah Mada, Yogyakarta 55281, Indonesia; yani.rahmawati@ugm.ac.id
3 Department of Chemical Engineering, Institut Teknologi Bandung, Bandung 40132, Indonesia; aqsha@che.itb.ac.id
* Correspondence: christiono@ce.its.ac.id
† Presented at the 2024 IEEE 4th International Conference on Electronic Communications, Internet of Things and Big Data, Taipei, Taiwan, 19–21 April 2024.

Abstract: Green industrial estates are implemented for sustainable development in the industrial sector. The industrial sector is a large consumer of energy and resources and produces pollutants. Environmentally friendly development in industrial estates is important in encouraging environmentally friendly production and ecological civilization as a strategic key to economic and social growth. This is an important basis for assessing the performance of green industrial estates. Research on green buildings in industrial estates has been conducted widely, including reviewing the performance of developing green industrial estates and using various methods. This research aims to determine research methods on the performance of green industrial estates using a literature review in reputable journals from 2014 to 2023. A mapping diagram was used to classify research types and data sources. The results showed that many researchers examined the performance of green industrial estates by reviewing environmental and economic aspects, and few researchers reviewed social aspects. Apart from these aspects, in reviewing the aspects of the performance of green industrial estate, researchers used modeling and case studies. The result of this research provides a reference for choosing the right method for assessing the performance of green industrial estates in future research.

Keywords: green; industrial estate; performance; research method

Citation: Alriansyach, I.D.; Utomo, C.; Rahmawati, Y.; Aqsha, A. Performance of Green Industrial Estate: A Review. *Eng. Proc.* **2024**, *74*, 5. https://doi.org/10.3390/engproc2024074005

Academic Editors: Shu-Han Liao, Teen-Hang Meen and Cheng-Fu Yang

Published: 27 August 2024

1. Introduction

Industrial estates are key factors of industrial production, manufacturing, and economic activity, areas with significant populations and trade associations. The number of global industrial estates is between 12,000 and 20,000, increasing construction in developed and developing countries [1]. One of the reasons for resource depletion and environmental degradation is that industrial estates are large consumers of energy and resources, and pollutant producers [2]. Industrial estates play an essential role in facilitating industrial sustainability and economic development. Green development is a model of economic transformation to improve people's welfare while preserving the environment and resources. Various problems associated with many industrial estates can occur, such as resource and energy consumption challenges and risks of high environmental impact [3]. Greening in industrial estates is related to Goal 9 of the Sustainable Development Goals (SDGs), which promotes inclusive and sustainable industrialization and encourages innovation while tackling climate change [4]. Sustainable development includes targeted infrastructure development nationally and regionally. This includes spatial planning, competition in investment incentives, the implementation of new construction projects, encouraging the regional use of buildings, and improving energy recovery processes [5]. For example, greening industrial estates in China is a way to explore sustainable development in the industrial sector. In addition, greening industrial estates creates collaborative and efficiency gains to provide a powerful tool for regional economic growth [6]. Energy infrastructure is shared in industrial estates to have a long service life to protect industrial estates from greenhouse gas emissions. Green industrialization requires infrastructure that is resilient, efficient, and sustainable [7].

Promoting green industrial estates is essential to reduce the impacts of policies and programs in their development. In evaluating the development, the performance of green development in industrial estates is evaluated. The performance is evaluated by determining how green industrial estates promote green innovation [8]. Many researchers assessed the performance of green industrial estates using various methods including surveys and case studies.

2. Background Knowledge

2.1. Green Industrial Estate

Notions such as green building and sustainable construction have emerged from the concept of sustainable development. Green buildings are a solution for the requirements of sustainable development in the construction industry. Characteristics of green buildings include energy and water efficiency, reduced consumption of natural resources, and improved health and the environment [9]. In sustainable development, the green building concept is an innovation [10]. Green buildings can be used to reduce the impact of global climate change in achieving energy efficiency, carbon reduction, and social responsibility [11]. Green development in the construction industry is closely related to urbanization and industrialization. Its features are adapted to the region, climate adaptation, building sustainability, and the surrounding environment. Green buildings are platforms for development under current resource and environmental constraints [12].

The green industrial zone is related to a shared philosophy of the people about how to enhance well-being, create employment and decent work opportunities, and maintain healthier global ecosystems. Green and environmentally friendly buildings slow global warming by changing the microclimate [13]. The green industrial estate promotes development in spatial planning, industrial development, energy utilization, resource utilization, infrastructure, ecological environment, operations, and management [6]. Industrial estates have played a key role in facilitating industrial sustainability and economic development in recent years. Green development in industrial estates is an important starting point in promoting green production and ecological civilization and a key strategic shaper for economic and social growth [3]. Industrial estates continue to grow rapidly being equipped with shared infrastructure with a long service life and limited greenhouse gas emissions. Greening industrialization requires efficient, tough, and sustainable infrastructure [7]. Local communities need to reduce waste and pollution, increase resource efficiency, and strive for sustainable development to increase economic benefits and the environmental quality of environmentally friendly industrial estates [14].

2.2. Performance of Green Industrial Estate

Several criteria are used in assessing the success and effectiveness of green industrial estates [6]. Green development efficiency is a criterion used to evaluate green development performance in industrial estates. When the environmental impact of a product from an industrial estate reduces, its economic value is increased. This shows how green efficiency is realized. Apart from factors that reduce environmental impacts and increase economic value, social impacts are difficult to measure though those are related to the performance of green development in industrial estates [15]. In evaluating the performance of green development in industrial estates, various points of view such as social justice, economic development, environmental risks, and resource efficiency are needed [16]. In Ref. [16], green industrial estates were evaluated from three perspectives: gross domestic product (GDP), environmental pollution, and resource consumption. Figure 1 shows the three aspects that represent the performance of industrial estates. It is important to evaluate the use of resources and environmental pressures from eco-industrial development in industrial estates. However, the complexity and difficulty of measuring resource flows make the evaluation difficult because environmentally friendly industrial estates change the resource flow [2].

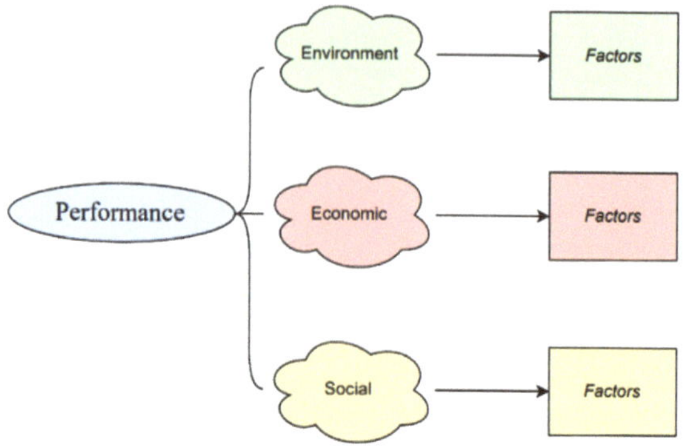

Figure 1. Aspects and factors of performance of green industrial estate.

2.2.1. Environment

Environmental pressure and increasing carbon emissions are challenges in an industrial estate. Reducing the resulting environmental impact can increase costs and encourage green efficiency. To achieve the goal of a green industrial estate preserving the environment, the following factors are used in the evaluation of the green industrial estate: economic growth, environmental preservation, climate change, and green development [6]. In worsening global environmental problems, green innovation helps reduce environmental pollution. Environmentally friendly industrial estates increase the economic benefits of a company while minimizing the environmental impact it produces [8].

2.2.2. Economy

In assessing the sustainability of the development of green industrial estates, various indicators are used. The application of industrial symbiosis is linked to economic aspects [15]. The benefits of green industrial estates include reduced waste disposal costs and reduced purchases of raw materials. The economic benefits are easy to measure [16]. Green industrial estates promote economic development [17]. The economic performance of an industrial estate is affected by economic fluctuation. Investments in research and continuous development in industrial estates increase economic resilience.

2.2.3. Society

In assessing sustainability, social aspects have been little discussed. An environmentally friendly industrial estate improves environmental, economic, and social performance in managing environmental and resource problems collaboratively. Social impacts from the development of green industrial estates are related to lifestyle and health in the vicinity of green industrial estates. However, assessing the performance of this social aspect requires appropriate evaluation because it is difficult to measure and assess its application [15].

3. Methodology

Previous Data

We reviewed the methods of previous research in analyzing green buildings in industrial estates. We analyzed articles from various quality journals on the performance of green in industrial estates. Related articles published from 2014 to 2023 were collected. Table 1 shows the list of journals and the SCImago Journal Rank (SJR) of articles from each journal.

Table 1. Selected journals in this study.

Journal Publications	SJR	Quartiles Category
Structural Change and Economic Dynamics	1.32	Q1 in Economics and Econometrics
Energy Strategy Reviews	2.06	Q1 in Energy
Nature Communications	5.11	Q1 in Biochemistry, Genetics, and Molecular Biology
Journal of Cleaner Production	1.98	Q1 in Renewable Energy, Sustainability, and the Environment
Journal of Environmental Management	1.67	Q1 in Environmental Engineering
Waste Management	1.74	Q1 in Waste Management and Disposal
Environmental Science and Pollution Research	0.94	Q1 in Environmental Chemistry
City and Environment Interactions	0.80	Q1 in Environmental Science
Sustainability	0.66	Q1 in Renewable Energy, Sustainability, and the Environment
Cleaner Engineering and Technology	0.77	Q1 in Environmental Engineering
Heliyon	0.60	Q1 in Multidisciplinary
Technological Forecasting and Social Change	2.64	Q1 in Management of Technology and Innovation
World Development	2.50	Q1 in Economics and Econometrics

4. Results and Discussion

The selected articles were used for performance analysis in green industrial estates. Table 2 shows the environmental factors of performance in the green industrial estate. Table 3 presents the economic factors, while Table 4 shows the social factors of the performance of green industrial estates in previous research.

Table 2. Environmental factors of performance.

No	Factors	Source
1	Investment in clean production	[2,6,14,16,18]
2	Developing the use of environmentally friendly energy	[2,3,6]
3	Reducing the rate of untreated industrial solid waste	[2,6,18,19]
4	Reducing carbon emissions	[1,6,7,15,20,21]
5	Increasing the exchange of products or materials	[2,22–24]
6	Comprehensive resource energy utilization	[2,3,20,21,24–28]
7	Technological innovation	[8,20,21]

Table 3. Economic factors of performance.

No	Factors	Source
1	Optimization of material and energy utilization at the lowest cost	[2,6]
2	Optimizing the use of public facilities	[2]
3	Value added per capita	[6,15,18]
4	Investment	[15]
5	Economic growth	[6,18]
6	Clean production audit	[2]
7	Utilization of waste resources	[1,2,19]
8	Comprehensive resource and energy utilization	[25]
9	Determining strategic locations to unite industry	[26]
10	Optimizing the flow of materials and waste	[22,24]
11	Industrial structure	[8,14,17]
12	Technological innovation	[17]
13	Planning and governance	[17]
14	Reducing the rate of untreated industrial solid waste	[19]

Table 4. Social factors of performance.

No	Factors	Source
1	Optimization of material and energy utilization at the lowest cost	[2,6]
2	Optimizing the use of public facilities	[2]
3	Satisfaction of residents	[15]
4	Contribution of the company's workforce	[15]
5	Environmental reporting	[15]

The factors related to the performance of green industrial estates were connected to the research methods. The type of research was divided into qualitative and quantitative and mixed quantitative–qualitative research. The quantitative method included modeling, surveys, questionnaires, interviews, and descriptive statistics. In contrast, the qualitative method included case studies and literature reviews.

To measure the performance of green industrial estates from the environmental aspect, modeling and case studies were used. Literature reviews, questionnaires, descriptive statistics, interviews, and surveys were also used. From the economic aspect, modeling and case study methods were widely used with literature reviews and descriptive statistics. From the social aspects, modeling, case studies, and literature reviews were employed (Figure 2).

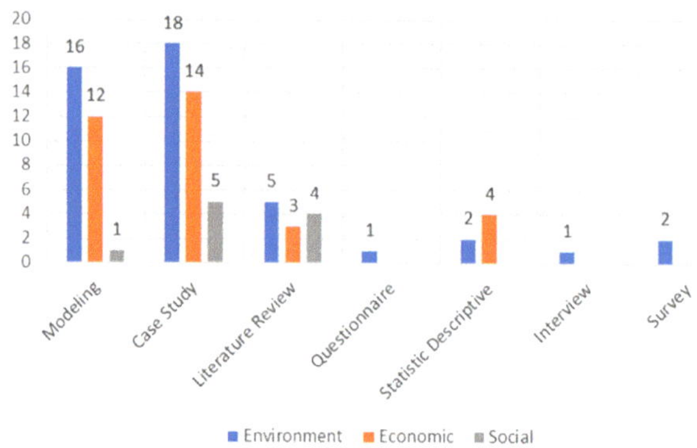

Figure 2. Method of factors of performance of green industrial estate.

5. Conclusions

We conducted a literature review on green industrial estate performance. The performance of green industrial estates was evaluated from the environmental, economic, and social aspects. For each aspect, criteria or factors were determined. Many researchers have reviewed environmental and economic aspects using modeling and case studies, whereas few researchers have reviewed the social aspects. In future research, appropriate methods should be used to evaluate the performance of green industrial estates.

Author Contributions: Conceptualization, I.D.A. and C.U.; methodology, I.D.A.; formal analysis, I.D.A.; investigation, Y.R.; resources, C.U.; writing—original draft preparation, I.D.A.; writing—review and editing, I.D.A., Y.R., A.A. and C.U.; supervision, C.U., Y.R. and A.A.; project administration, I.D.A.; funding acquisition, C.U., Y.R. and A.A. All authors have read and agreed to the published version of the manuscript.

Funding: The research have been funded by Program Riset Kolaborasi Indonesia (Skema A) 2023. Contract Number: 1660/PKS/ITS/2023.

Institutional Review Board Statement: Not applicable.

Informed Consent Statement: Not applicable.

Data Availability Statement: The data supporting the conclusions of this article will be made available by the authors on request.

Acknowledgments: The authors gratefully acknowledge financial support from the Institut Teknologi Sepuluh Nopember for this work, under the Capacity Development Program of Higher Education for Technology and Innovation Project Asian Development Bank Loan No 4110-INO.

Conflicts of Interest: The authors declare no conflicts of interest.

References

1. Yan, X.; Wang, L.; Fang, M.; Hu, J. How can industrial parks achieve carbon neutrality? Literature review and research prospect based on the citespace knowledge map. *Sustainability* **2023**, *15*, 372. [CrossRef]
2. Fan, Y.; Fang, C. Assessing environmental performance of eco-industrial development in industrial parks. *Waste Manag.* **2020**, *15*, 219–226. [CrossRef] [PubMed]
3. Lyu, Y.; Liu, Y.; Guo, Y.; Sang, J.; Tian, J.; Chen, L. Review of green development of Chinese industrial parks. *Energy Strategy Rev.* **2022**, *42*, 100867. [CrossRef]
4. United Nations. Sustainable Development. Available online: https://sdgs.un.org/goals (accessed on 11 July 2023).
5. Komarovska, A.; Ustinovichius, L.; Shevchenko, G.; Nazarko, L. Multicriteria evaluation of commercial industrial zone development. *Int. J. Strateg. Prop. Manag.* **2015**, *19*, 84–95. [CrossRef]
6. Yu, X. An assessment of the green development efficiency of industrial parks in China: Based on non-desired output and non-radial DEA model. *Struct. Chang. Econ. Dyn.* **2023**, *66*, 81–88. [CrossRef]
7. Guo, Y.; Tian, J.; Chen, L. Managing energy infrastructure to decarbonize industrial parks in China. *Nat. Commun.* **2020**, *11*, 1–9. [CrossRef] [PubMed]
8. Wu, Y.; Gao, X. Can the establishment of eco-industrial parks promote urban green innovation? Evidence from China. *J. Clean. Prod.* **2022**, *341*, 130855. [CrossRef]
9. Dwaikat, L.N.; Ali, K.N. The economic benefits of a green building—Evidence from Malaysia. *J. Build. Eng.* **2018**, *18*, 448–453. [CrossRef]
10. Meena, C.S.; Kumar, A.; Jain, S.; Ateeq, U.R.; Sachin, M.; Naveen, K.S.; Mohit, B.; Muhammad, S.; Elsayed, T. Eldin. Innovation in green building sector for sustainable future. *Energies* **2022**, *15*, 6631. [CrossRef]
11. Onuoha, I.J.; Aliagha, G.U.; Rahman, M.S.A. Modelling the effects of green building incentives and green building skills on supply factors affecting green commercial property investment. *Renew. Sustain. Energy Rev.* **2018**, *90*, 814–823. [CrossRef]
12. Zhu, J.; Cao, Y.; Zhai, J.; Zhao, X.; Zhao, Y.; Kang, S. Analysis on synergies and trade-offs in green building development: From the perspective of SDG 11. *Chin. J. Popul. Resour. Environ.* **2019**, *17*, 341–351. [CrossRef]
13. Utomo, C.; Astarini, S.D.; Rahmawati, F.; Setijanti, P.; Nurchayo, C.B. The influence of green building application on high-rise building life cycle cost and valuation in Indonesia. *Buildings* **2022**, *12*, 2180. [CrossRef]
14. Xu, F.; Xiang, N.; Tian, J.; Chen, L. 3Es-based optimization simulation approach to support the development of an eco-industrial park with planning towards sustainability: A case study in Wuhu, China. *J. Clean. Prod.* **2011**, *164*, 476–484. [CrossRef]
15. Valenzuela-venegas, G.; Salgado, J.C.; Diaz-Alvarado, F.A. Sustainability indicators for the assessment of eco-industrial parks: Classification and criteria for selection. *J. Clean. Prod.* **2016**, *133*, 99–116. [CrossRef]
16. Hou, D.; Li, G.; Chen, D.; Zhu, B.; Hu, S. Evaluation and analysis on the green development of China's industrial parks using the long-tail effect model. *J. Environ. Manag.* **2019**, *248*, 109288. [CrossRef]
17. Pan, S.C.; Hu, T.S.; You, X.; Chang, S.L. Characteristics and influencing factors of economic resilience in industrial parks. *Heliyon* **2023**, *9*, e14812. [CrossRef]
18. Tian, J.; Liu, W.; Lai, B.; Li, X.; Chen, L. Study of the performance of eco-industrial park development in China. *J. Clean. Prod.* **2014**, *64*, 486–494. [CrossRef]
19. Abu-Qdais, H.A.; Kurbatova, A.I. The role of eco-industrial parks in promoting circular economy in Rusia: A life cycle approach. *Sustainability* **2022**, *14*, 3893. [CrossRef]
20. Wang, Y.; Ren, H.; Dong, L.; Park, S.; Zhang, Y.; Xu, Y. Smart solutions shape for sustainable low-carbon future: A review on smart cities and industrial parks in China. *Technol. Forecast. Soc. Chang.* **2019**, *144*, 103–117. [CrossRef]
21. Zeng, D.Z.; Cheng, L.; Shi, L.; Luetkenhorst, W. China's green transformation through eco-industrial parks. *World Dev.* **2021**, *140*, 105249. [CrossRef]
22. Genc, O.; Kurt, A.; Yazan, D.M.; Erdis, E. Circular eco-industrial park design inspired by nature: An integrated non-linear optimization, location, and food web analysis. *J. Environ. Manag.* **2020**, *270*, 110866. [CrossRef]
23. Perrucci, D.V.; Aktas, C.B.; Sorentino, J.; Akanbi, H.; Curabba, J. A review of international eco-industrial parks for implementation success in the United States. *City Environ. Interact.* **2022**, *16*, 100086. [CrossRef]
24. Shah, I.H.; Dong, L.; Park, H.S. Tracking urban sustainability transition: An eco-efficiency analysis on eco-industrial development in Ulsan, Korea. *J. Clean. Prod.* **2020**, *262*, 121286. [CrossRef]
25. Gao, G.; Wang, S.; Xue, R.; Liu, D.; Huang, B.; Zhang, R. Eco-efficiency assessment of industrial parks in Central China: A slack-based data envelopment analysis. *Environ. Sci. Pollut. Res.* **2022**, *29*, 30410–30426. [CrossRef]

26. Nuhu, S.K.; Manan, Z.A.; Wan, A.S.R.; Reba, M.N. Integrated modelling approach for an eco-industrial park site selection. *J. Clean. Prod.* **2022**, *368*, 133141. [CrossRef]
27. Uusikartano, J.; Vayrynen, H.; Aarika-Stenroos, L. Public actors and their diverse roles in eco-industrial parks: A multiple-case study. *J. Clean. Prod.* **2021**, *296*, 126463. [CrossRef]
28. Kreiner, I.; Bressers, H.T.A.; Franco-Garcia, M.L. Challenges to implementing a sustainable strategic evaluation framework of industrial parks: Mexican case. *Clean. Eng. Technol.* **2023**, *13*, 100612. [CrossRef]

engineering proceedings

MDPI

Proceeding Paper

COVID-19 Data Analysis and Computation with Urban Structure Consideration †

Ryota Goto [1] and Ari Aharari [2,*]

1 Department of Applied Information Sciences, Graduate School of Engineering, SOJO University, Kumamoto 860-0082, Japan; g2311m05@m.sojo-u.ac.jp
2 Faculty of Computer and Information Sciences, SOJO University, Kumamoto 860-0082, Japan
* Correspondence: info@ahrary.org

† Presented at the 2024 IEEE 4th International Conference on Electronic Communications, Internet of Things and Big Data, Taipei, Taiwan, 19–21 April 2024.

Abstract: In early 2020, the outbreak of COVID-19 brought a global pandemic, challenging healthcare systems worldwide and prompting countries to implement various measures to contain the spread. These measures, while necessary, led to significant socioeconomic disruptions. One of the most pressing concerns was the strain on healthcare systems, which caused shortages of medical supplies, hospital beds, and healthcare personnel. This raised the prospect of a healthcare system collapse. Using data analysis, we studied how to understand the dynamics of COVID-19 transmission in the context of urban structures, focusing on preventing healthcare system collapse.

Keywords: COVID-19; data analysis; machine learning

1. Introduction

In early 2020, the outbreak of COVID-19 rapidly became a global pandemic, putting immense pressure on healthcare systems worldwide and leading to various containment measures being implemented by nations. While these measures were necessary to control the spread of the virus, they also caused significant disruptions to society. One of the most pressing issues was the strain on healthcare systems, which led to shortages of medical supplies, hospital beds, and healthcare personnel and increased the risk of system collapse. Two research studies have been conducted in this area. The first study, conducted by Sato et al., focused on the impact analysis of COVID-19 on hospital bed availability in Shiga Prefecture, Japan, using a mathematical infectious disease model. The second study was conducted by Hirata et al. to predict the spread and convergence of COVID-19 using deep learning techniques. Both studies analyzed related data and predicted COVID-19 effects without considering urban structures.

Urban areas in Japan are classified into diffuse and intensive urban areas. Diffuse urban areas refer to areas where the development of urban structures disperses from the central region to the surrounding areas. On the other hand, intensive urban areas refer to areas where urban structures develop intensively from the central region. In this study, we focused on Kumamoto Prefecture, Japan, which falls into the intensive urban category [1]. There is a risk of inadequate medical services due to a critical shortage in the medical field and the collapse of the healthcare system. The Japanese healthcare system will likely collapse when the hospital bed occupancy rate exceeds 50%. This rate is chosen based on the welfare index of infection status proposed by the Ministry of Health, Labor, and Welfare of Japan in 2020 [2]. The standard changes annually starting in 2020, and starting in 2022, a bed occupancy rate of 50% or less is considered appropriate.

In this research, we explored how COVID-19 spread within various urban structures and focused on maintaining the resilience of the healthcare system by keeping the bed oc-

Citation: Goto, R.; Aharari, A. COVID-19 Data Analysis and Computation with Urban Structure Consideration. *Eng. Proc.* **2024**, *74*, 6. https://doi.org/10.3390/engproc2024074006

Academic Editors: Shu-Han Liao, Teen-Hang Meen and Cheng-Fu Yang

Published: 27 August 2024

cupancy rate below 50%. This paper details the data collection from Kumamoto Prefecture, the data analysis, and the evaluation of two models.

2. Data Collections

In this research, we focused on intensive urban structure and collected all related data on Kumamoto Prefecture. Eight types of data were collected, including the number of infected individuals, hospitalized individuals, hospital beds, severely ill individuals, deaths, number of vaccinations, average temperatures, and changes in the mobility trends of visitors to specific locations (grocery stores, parks, etc.) over time. We collected two significant policies implemented in Japan.

The first was the declaration of a state of emergency [3]. This policy is based on the Law on Special Measures against the New Coronavirus, enacted on 13 March 2020. The prime minister declared the period and area where emergency measures could be used in the event of a nationwide and rapid spread of the virus, which could profoundly impact the lives of the people and the economy. The prefectural governor of the study area may request residents to refrain from leaving their homes and cooperate in other ways necessary to prevent the spread of the disease, except when necessary to maintain their livelihood. In addition, the governor may request or give instructions to close schools and restrict the use of facilities that attract large numbers of people, such as department stores and movie theaters, and may use land or buildings for the construction of temporary medical facilities when particularly necessary without the consent of the owners. The second policy is the Law on Priority Measures for the Prevention of the Spread of Disease [4]. Priority measures for the prevention of the spread of new coronavirus infection are region-specific efforts to prevent the spread of new coronavirus infection. The government publicly announces these measures for specific areas where the spread of infection is likely to have a significant impact on people's lives and the economy, and where there is a risk of disruption to the medical system and public health. Specific measures include restrictions on eating and drinking establishments, use of facilities, events, etc., as well as requests to go out, travel, and go to work.

2.1. *Infected Individuals, Hospitalizations, and Bed Capacities*

The number of infected individuals, hospitalized individuals, hospital beds, severely ill individuals, and fatalities were collected for this study. The data were compiled based on the data from the Health Information and Response System for Individuals Infected with New-type Coronavirus (HER-SYS) provided by the Ministry of Health, Labor, and Welfare [5–7]. The period of data collection was from 16 January 2020 to 8 May 2023.

2.2. *Vaccination Rate*

The vaccination rate for seven doses was collected. The data was compiled based on the Vaccination Record System (VRS) provided by Digital Agency [8] for 12 April 2021 to 16 November 2023.

2.3. *Average Temperature*

The average temperatures in Kumamoto Prefecture were collected from 9 May 2020 to 9 May 2023, and they were provided by the Japan Meteorological Agency [9].

2.4. *Mobility Changes*

The rate of change in mobility trends of visitors to specific locations (grocery stores, parks, etc.) from 1 January 2022 to 1 October 2022 was collected. Google's Community Mobility Report [10] was used to aggregate anonymous mobility data from Google Maps. The data showed how visitors to (or time spent at) places classified in each category changed compared to the base value for each day of the week. The details of the reference values and locations were as follows.

The base value was the median value by day of the week from 1 March 2020 to 2 June 2020 (5 weeks) in Kumamoto Prefecture (the period just before people's behavior changed in response to COVID-19). Study locations include grocery stores, parks, train stations, retail and entertainment (restaurants, cafes), residences, and workplaces.

3. Data Analysis

We visualized the data. Figure 1 displays the correlation between infected individuals and hospital bed occupancy rate. The result indicated a direct correlation, highlighting the critical influence of infection rates on the utilization of hospital resources. The bed occupancy rate exceeded 50% six times throughout the entire period.

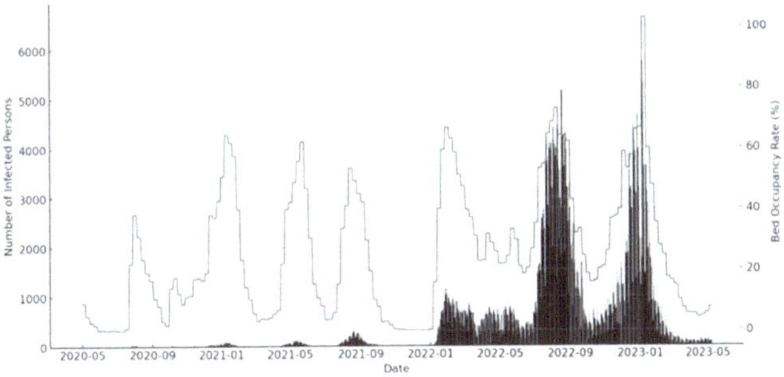

Figure 1. COVID-19 infected individuals and bed occupancy rate.

This finding is noteworthy given the current state of the world, where the COVID-19 pandemic has strained healthcare systems worldwide. It underscored the importance of taking measures to reduce the spread of the virus and ensure that hospital resources are available to those who need them the most. We plotted the vaccination rate from the first to the seventh dose over time (Figure 2). The data showed that up to the second dose, about 80% of the population was vaccinated. High vaccination rates are essential to curb the spread of the virus and reduce the burden on healthcare systems. However, there were still significant disparities in vaccination rates between different regions and demographic groups to achieve herd immunity.

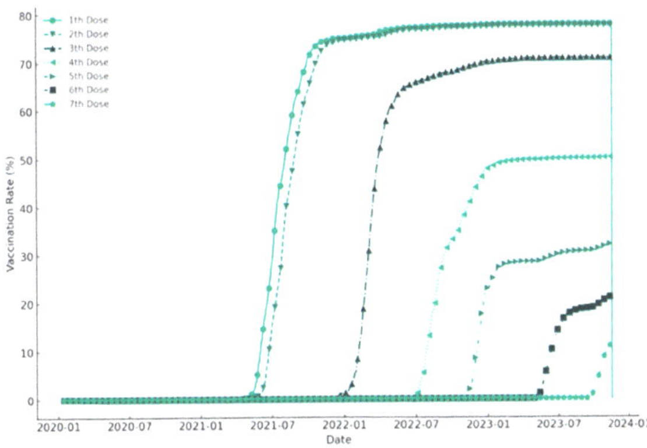

Figure 2. Vaccination rate over time.

We analyzed the relationship between mobility changes and average temperature. Increasing human movement affected the number of new infections. The data for average temperature and mobility changes is illustrated in Figure 3.

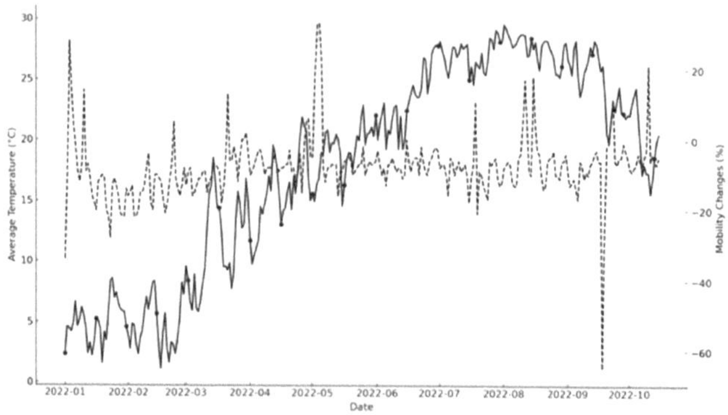

Figure 3. Average temperature and mobility change over time.

This finding highlights the importance of considering external factors that influence the spread of the virus such as mobility patterns and environmental conditions. It also emphasizes the need for targeted interventions that consider these external factors to curb the spread of the virus effectively. To better understand the data visualized above by focusing on the correlation between infected individuals and average temperature, we analyzed a linear trend, and the result suggested that higher temperatures were associated with higher reported infections (Figure 4). This reflected seasonal variations in virus transmission or testing behavior. The seasonal variation in virus transmission was more significant than expected. It also underscores the importance of considering external factors such as temperature when developing public health interventions to address the pandemic.

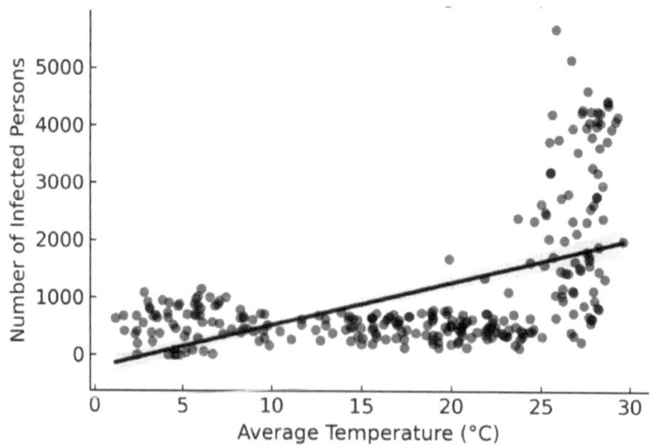

Figure 4. Correlation between infected individuals and average temperature.

We analyzed the correlation between infected individuals and vaccination rate (1st dose) as shown in Figure 5. The moderate positive correlation suggested that as the vaccination rate increased, so did the number of reported infections. This could be due to increased testing alongside vaccine rollout efforts or a reflection of peaks in reporting as vaccines became available. This finding highlights the need to be cautious when interpreting data related to vaccination rates and infection rates. While high vaccination rates are critical in curbing the spread of the virus, external factors such as testing behavior must be taken into account when interpreting these data.

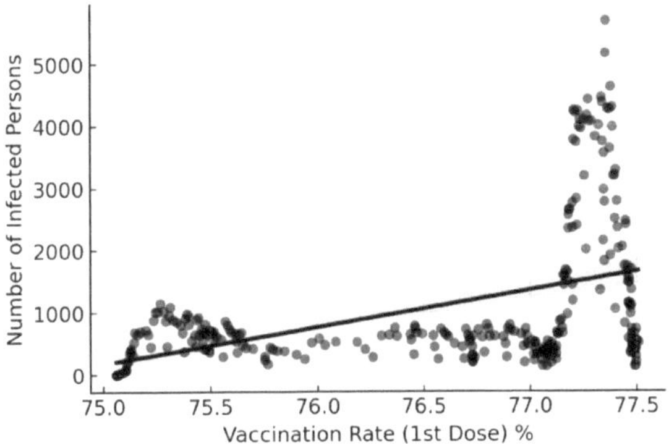

Figure 5. Correlation between infected individuals and vaccination rate (1st dose).

Finally, we investigated the correlation between residential mobility and infection (Figure 6). Higher residential stay percentages coincided with lockdown periods and were correlated with increased infection rates. The positive correlation was more visible, implying that the higher residential stay percentage (during lockdowns) was associated with more reported infections. This reflected the pattern of outbreaks leading to stricter homestay measures. This finding underscores the importance of targeted interventions and external factors such as mobility patterns to reduce the spread of the virus effectively. It also highlights the need for policymakers to balance lockdown measures' economic and public health impacts to address the pandemic effectively.

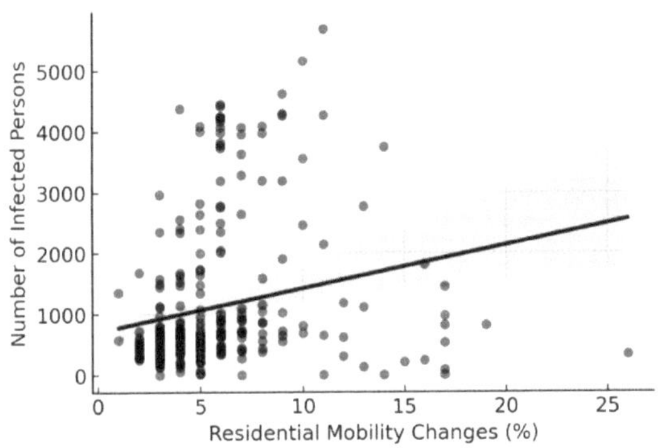

Figure 6. Correlation between infected individuals and mobility changes.

4. Model Development

We evaluated the effectiveness of the linear regression and Random Forest models in predicting hospital bed occupancy rates. The models were analyzed using various predictors, including mobility data, vaccination rates, weather conditions, and demographic factors. Performance metrics such as Mean Squared Error (MSE) and R-squared values are reported.

The four steps to evaluate the models included the following:

- Feature Selection: relevant features were selected based on the correlation and time series analysis conducted in the previous session;
- Data Preparation: the data were split into training and testing sets to validate the model's performance;
- Model Training: the model was trained on the training data;
- Model Evaluation: the model was evaluated using appropriate metrics such as R-squared and Mean Squared Error;

4.1. Linear Regression Model

We constructed a linear regression model to predict the bed occupancy rate and understand the direct linear relationships between the predictors, such as mobility changes, the number of infected individuals, weather, the response variable, and the bed occupancy rate. The model showed a mean square error (MSE) of 51.25. This value represents the average squared difference between the actual and predicted bed occupancy rates. A lower MSE indicates a better fit of the model to the data. Although the absolute number might seem high, it is more relevant when compared to the variance in bed occupancy rates. The R-squared (R^2) was 0.834. This metric indicates how well the features in the model explain the variability in bed occupancy rate. An R^2 of 0.834 suggested that the model explained approximately 83.4% of the variability in bed occupancy rate, which was good for complex real-world data.

Next, we visualized the linear regression model results to explore its performance and the nature of the errors. Figure 7 shows the result of checking the residuals (errors) distribution to indicate nonlinearity or heteroscedasticity. The residuals are scattered around the horizontal line at zero without apparent pattern or systematic deviation. This indicates that the model does not suffer from nonlinearities or heteroscedasticity (i.e., the variance of the residuals is constant across all levels of prediction). There are a few points further from the line, indicating several predictions with higher errors, which could be outliers or instances where the model assumptions fail.

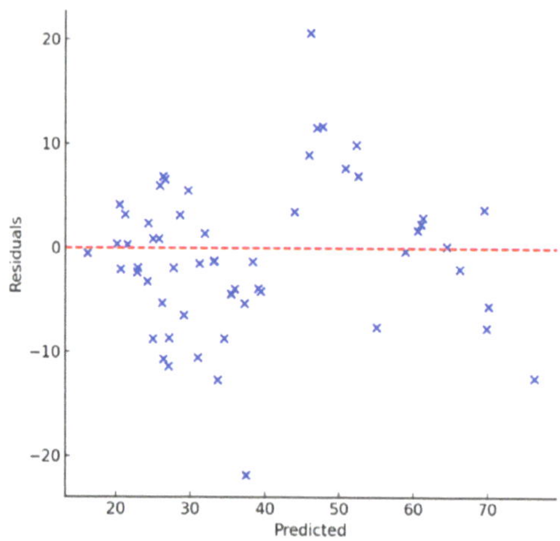

Figure 7. Analysis of model evaluation for residuals vs predicted.

Figure 8 shows the prediction results vs actual data to assess the model. The points are generally close to the diagonal line, showing that the predicted values are reasonably close to the actual values across the range. The model performed consistently across different values of the target variable with a slight deviation at higher actual values where the model underpredicted the occupancy rate. The linear regression model performed well given the complexity of the dataset and the relationships involved. However, models such as Random Forest can capture subtler interactions and nonlinearities not accounted for by linear regression.

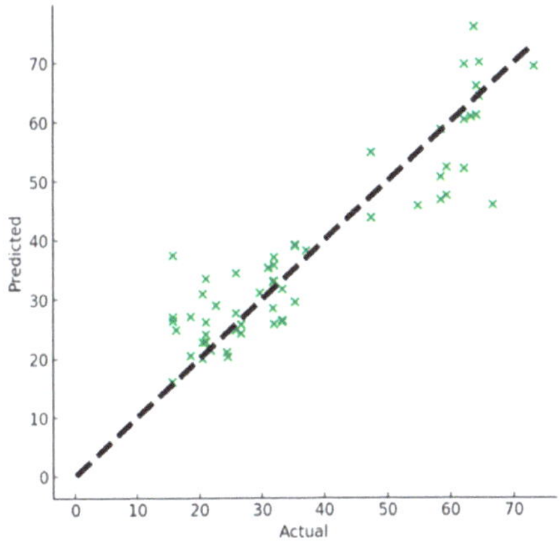

Figure 8. Analysis of model evaluation for predicted vs actual.

4.2. Random Forest Model

Random Forest is a robust ensemble method that performs well on complex datasets by effectively handling nonlinearities and feature interactions. The model showed an MSE of 48.02, indicating better results than the linear regression model. An R^2 of 0.844 suggested that the model explained approximately 84.4% of the variability in the bed occupancy rate, which is an improvement over the linear model. The residuals are randomly distributed around the zero line, suggesting that the Random Forest model does not exhibit systematic errors (Figure 9). No clear patterns indicate heteroscedasticity or nonlinearity. A few outliers exist where the model predictions deviate significantly from actual values due to unusual cases or noise in the data.

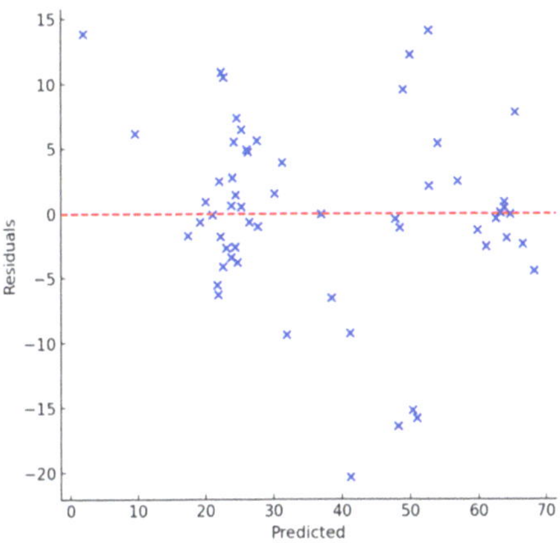

Figure 9. Analysis of model evaluation for residuals vs predicted.

The points closer to the diagonal line indicate better agreement between the predicted and actual values (Figure 10). The model was consistent across the range of bed occupancy rates. However, there were under or over-predictions at higher rates. The Random Forest model performed better than the linear regression model and effectively handled the data in this study.

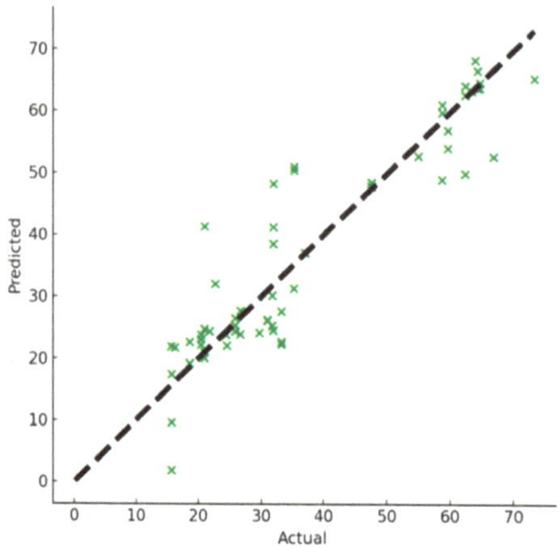

Figure 10. Analysis of model evaluation for predicted vs actual.

5. Conclusions

We conducted data analyses highlighting the importance of urban structures in managing the COVID-19 pandemic and preventing the collapse of healthcare systems. The findings suggested that a nuanced approach to pandemic preparedness and response is necessary with urban-specific strategies considering local conditions and infrastructure as crucial. The findings provide knowledge to safeguard public health and healthcare systems against pandemics in urban settings. We compared the effectiveness of two models, linear regression and Random Forest in predicting hospital bed occupancy rates. We evaluated the models using various predictors, such as mobility data, vaccination rates, weather conditions, and demographic factors. The Random Forest model showed an R^2 of 0.844, indicating that the model explained approximately 84.4% of the variability in the bed occupancy rate. This was a significant improvement over the linear model.

Author Contributions: Conceptualization, A.A.; methodology, R.G. and A.A.; software, A.A.; validation, R.G. and A.A.; formal analysis, R.G. and A.A.; data curation, R.G. and A.A.; writing—original draft preparation, R.G. and A.A.; writing—review and editing, A.A; visualization, R.G. and A.A.; supervision, A.A. All authors have read and agreed to the published version of the manuscript.

Funding: This research received no external funding.

Institutional Review Board Statement: Not applicable.

Informed Consent Statement: Not applicable.

Data Availability Statement: The secondary data that were used for analysis in this study are available from the corresponding author upon request.

Conflicts of Interest: The authors declare no conflicts of interest.

References

1. Ministry of Land, Infrastructure, Transport and Tourism. Compact Town Development Based on Public Transportation. Available online: https://www.mlit.go.jp/common/001095208.pdf (accessed on 17 March 2024).
2. "Indicators for Determining COVID-19 Level" such as Hospital Bed Usage Rate by Prefecture. Available online: https://www3.nhk.or.jp/news/special/coronavirus/level/ (accessed on 17 March 2024).
3. First State of Emergency Declaration. Available online: https://www3.nhk.or.jp/news/special/coronavirus/emergency/ (accessed on 17 March 2024).
4. What Are the Priority Measures to Prevent the Spread? Available online: https://www.kaonavi.jp/dictionary/manenboshitojyutensochi/ (accessed on 17 March 2024).
5. Ministry of Health, Labor and Welfare. New Coronavirus Infection Situation from Data. Available online: https://covid19.mhlw.go.jp/ (accessed on 17 March 2024).

6. Ministry of Health, Labor and Welfare. Survey on Medical Treatment Status, Number of Inpatient Beds, etc. Available online: https://www.mhlw.go.jp/stf/seisakunitsuite/newpage_00023.html (accessed on 17 March 2024).
7. Ministry of Health, Labor and Welfare. Press Release Materials Regarding the New Coronavirus Infection. Available online: https://www.mhlw.go.jp/stf/seisakunitsuite/bunya/0000121431_00438.html (accessed on 17 March 2024).
8. Digital Agency. New Coronavirus Vaccination Status. Available online: https://info.vrs.digital.go.jp/dashboard (accessed on 17 March 2024).
9. Japan Meteorological Agency. Historical Weather Data Resource. Available online: https://www.data.jma.go.jp/risk/obsdl/ (accessed on 17 March 2024).
10. Google. Community Mobility Reports. Available online: https://www.google.com/covid19/mobility// (accessed on 17 March 2024).

engineering proceedings

Proceeding Paper

Emotional Reactivity and Dysregulation and Problematic Internet Use on Twitter †

Esther Andangsari [1,*], Trisa Putri [1], Shavina Ghaisani [1], Moondore Ali [1], Greta Paramita [1] and Ade Kemala [2]

1 Psychology Department, Faculty of Humanities, Bina Nusantara University, Jakarta 11480, Indonesia; trisa.putri@binus.ac.id (T.P.); shavina.ghaisani@binus.ac.id (S.G.); mali@binus.edu (M.A.); greta@binus.ac.id (G.P.)
2 Data Science Program, School of Computer Science, Bina Nusantara University, Jakarta 11530, Indonesia; ade.kemala@binus.edu
* Correspondence: esther@binus.edu
† Presented at the 2024 IEEE 4th International Conference on Electronic Communications, Internet of Things and Big Data, Taipei, Taiwan, 19–21 April 2024.

Abstract: Social media users can experience Problematic Internet Use (PIU) in the form of psychological problems, such as loneliness, social anxiety, and depression. They tend to have antecedents in the form of emotional dysregulation and reactivity, making them easily respond to stimuli on social media that cause stress. This study aims to prove that emotional dysregulation and reactivity are precursors of PIU for social media users. With 307 Twitter users as the participants of this study, three proposed hypotheses were tested, and the results showed that emotional dysregulation causes PIU, with emotional reactivity as a mediator.

Keywords: emotion; emotional dysregulation; emotional reactivity; problematic internet use; Twitter; social media

Citation: Andangsari, E.; Putri, T.; Ghaisani, S.; Ali, M.; Paramita, G.; Kemala, A. Emotional Reactivity and Dysregulation and Problematic Internet Use on Twitter. *Eng. Proc.* **2024**, *74*, 7. https://doi.org/10.3390/engproc2024074007

Academic Editors: Shu-Han Liao, Teen-Hang Meen and Cheng-Fu Yang

Published: 27 August 2024

1. Introduction

The development of digital technology has increased the penetration rate of Internet usage in Indonesia by 1.17% compared to 2022 [1]. The COVID-19 pandemic had a positive impact, increasing Indonesian internet literacy in terms of productive and entertainment purposes. The data released by Asosiasi Penyelenggara Jasa Internet Indonesia (APJII, Indonesia Internet Service Provider Association) in 2023 showed that accessing social media was the main activity carried out by Internet users in Indonesia: 98.02% [1]. These data were also in line with the facts found in Ref. [2], showing that Indonesia is the fifth most Twitter-using country in the world.

The use of social media during the pandemic helped strengthen the mental health of users by making them pay attention to emotional regulation; however, on the other hand, social media dependence was associated with depression [3]. Problematic Internet Use (PIU) means an excessive use of social media that interferes with a person's mental health and can even result in negative behaviors, such as drug abuse, gambling [4], cyberbullying [5], and suicidal ideation and self-injury [6], during a student's academic life [7]. There are emotional reactions to Twitter posts that involve mutual aggression or hate speech [8], which has been researched in the context of Indonesia [9]. Emotional reactions to social media can indicate PIU [10] as users cannot manage their emotions [11–13].

This study aims to find empirical evidence on the role of emotional reactivity and dysregulation in predicting PIU among Twitter social media users. Twitter is a social media platform that has generated the most hate speech in Indonesia, from the Jakarta Governor Election in 2017 [14] to the Indonesian Presidential Election in 2019 [15]. Social discomfort was felt during this period due to fears of disintegration in Indonesia. The stimuli of such events were perceived by individuals or society as negative and resulted in emotional reactivity [16]. Emotional reactivity does not require an individual to have any emotional experience or reaction. An event that an individual has just experienced or observed can provoke an emotional reaction [16,17].

We observed that Twitter users wrote negative responses in their posts, showing their emotional reactivity on social media. The dimensions of emotional reactivity include sensitivity or reactivity, intensity, and persistence or perseveration [17,18], emphasizing the existence of emotional reactivity as an issue in social media activities. Twitter users who comment on a tweet present emotional sensitivity as they are vulnerable to being emotionally provoked by even simple stimuli. Furthermore, strong emotional reactions, such as outbursts of anger, presented in hateful words or negative sentences, are a sign of emotional intensity. Someone holding strong emotions and needing time to calm down indicates emotional persistence or perseverance. The consistency of emotional responses on Twitter from the 2017 Daerah Khusus Ibukota Jakarta governor election and the 2019 presidential election showed symptoms of emotional persistence among Twitter users in Indonesia. This raised the question of whether emotional reactivity, unidimensional and multidimensional, could predict PIU in Twitter users in Indonesia. Thus, we proposed the following hypotheses in this study (Figure 1).

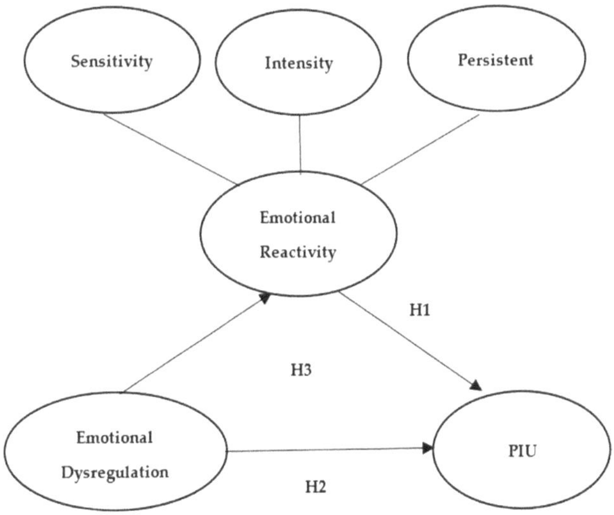

Figure 1. Relationships between variables and proposed hypotheses.

- H1: Individuals with high emotional reactivity (unidimensional) have significant PIU.

The inability to manage emotions is related to negative social media use behavior and results in PIU [10–12]; thus, this allows for the second hypothesis.

- H2: Individuals with high emotional dysregulation have PIU.

According to Herres et al. [19], people with high emotional reactivity have high emotional dysregulation. Emotional reactivity and dysregulation may lead to PIU. Emotional reactivity is a behavioral manifestation of emotional dysregulation in one's cognition. Therefore, emotional dysregulation impacts PIU through the mediation of emotional reactivity. Therefore, the third hypothesis was suggested for the relationship among the three variables.

- H3: Emotional dysregulation can significantly predict the onset of PIU through the mediation of emotional reactivity.

1.1. PIU

PIU is a problematic cognitive and behavioral maladaptive syndrome involving Internet use that negatively affects professional, social, and academic well-being [20,21]. It is assumed that PIU causes psychological problems, such as depression, loneliness, and anxiety. However, a meta-analysis showed that PIU is a consequence of psychological problems experienced by an individual [22,23]. This means that someone who experiences depression, loneliness, or anxiety has maladaptive cognition. Thus, the behavior of using the Internet becomes maladaptive. Thus, it is essential to understand that PIU is one of the mental disorders that someone in this digital era can experience [4,11]. PIU is considered a spectrum: individuals can be positioned on a spectrum ranging from very low PIU to very high PIU [24]. We used the PIU scale constructed by Caplan, which consisted of five dimensions in this study.

- Preference for Online Social Interaction (POSI): the tendency to interact with other people via the Internet because they feel safer and more comfortable.
- Mood regulation: the diversion of feelings or troubled moods by using the Internet as a means of escape.
- Cognitive preoccupation: obsessive thoughts about using the Internet even when offline.
- Compulsive Internet use: a condition where a person can no longer control their Internet use behavior. There is a tendency to use the Internet excessively without any clear purpose.
- Negative outcome: the impact experienced by individuals both personally and professionally as a result of Problematic Internet Use [21].

1.2. Emotional Reactivity

Emotional reactivity is an elicitation of a response relating to an external event or situation experienced by a person [16]. Individuals do not need previous experience for emotional reactivity to be triggered because emotional responses can emerge from just one specific stimulus. Emotional reactivity includes the sensitivity, intensity, and persistence of an emotion experienced by a person [19]. An individual with high emotional reactivity is likely to react to emotional stimuli or stressful situations [25]; thus, these individuals are associated with many mental health problems, from self-injury behavior and suicidal ideation to suicide attempts. Adolescents with high emotional reactivity are prone to interpersonal conflicts with friends or romantic relationships [26]. Emotional reactivity, in principle, is a conceptualized component in emotional regulation [27]. Emotional reactivity refers to direct emotional experiences relating to "good" and "bad" stimuli. Meanwhile, emotional regulation/dysregulation is an emotional process that is internally managed and is a contributing factor in certain mental disorders.

1.3. Emotional Dysregulation

Similar to emotional reactivity, emotional dysregulation is a potential factor in experiencing mental health disorders [13]. The concept of emotional dysregulation is a combination of traits such as sensitivity, intensity, and the deceleration of emotions back to baseline [28]. The conceptualization chosen in this study was based on previous research [29,30], which indicated that personality characteristics contribute to the appearance of individual posts on Twitter, including posts that can provoke emotional reactions in others. Emotional regulation/emotional dysregulation and emotional reactivity are two interrelated matters when discussing mental problems [31]. Psychological issues occur due to poor emotional dysregulation and reactivity. People with high emotional reactivity have high emotional dysregulation [18]; in other words, emotional dysregulation impacts a person's emotional reactivity. Individuals with anxiety have negative and poorly managed emotional patterns, causing poor emotional reactivity. This affects a person's psychological condition. Thus, in this study, we assumed that emotional dysregulation impacts PIU as a mental health disorder in the digital era.

2. Method

In total, 524 users were invited to this study. After elimination relating to the active use of Twitter for the last 3 months and accessible accounts, 307 participants remained. The participants were aged from 17 to 50 years old (M = 21.47; SD = 3.41), and 75.24% of them were females. The demographic data of the participants are shown in Table 1. Most participants lived outside Greater Jakarta (43.97%), which indicated that the participants were from many cities in Indonesia. Students accounted for 77.52% of the sample, which is in line with the data from APJII [1]. In total, 72.96% were active Twitter users, and 95.76% did not have jobs related to Twitter. The data showed a strong possibility of being exposed to hate speech and hoaxes.

Table 1. Demography of participants in this study (N = 307).

Item		Number	Ratio (%)
Residence location	Jakarta	88	28.66
	Bogor	12	3.91
	Depok	14	4.56
	Tangerang	44	14.33
	Bekasi	14	4.56
	Outside Greater Jakarta	135	43.97
Occupation	Student	238	77.52
	Private Employee	44	14.33
	Government Employee	4	1.30
	Entrepreneur	6	1.95
	Freelancer	2	0.65
	Housewife	3	0.98
	Others	10	3.26
Years of using Twitter	Less than 1 year	35	11.40
	1–3 years	48	15.64
	More than 3 years	224	72.96
Work on Twitter	Yes	13	4.24
	No	294	95.76

2.1. Procedure and Materials

All of the participants provided informed consent for ethical clearance purposes and stated their willingness to participate in this study. They were given instructions to fill out the three questionnaires and demographic data. PIU was measured using the Generalized Problematic Internet Use Scale 2 (GPIUS2) constructed by Caplan [21] and adapted to Bahasa Indonesia [32]. It consisted of 5 dimensions (POSI, mood regulation, cognitive preoccupation, compulsive Internet use, and negative outcome), and 15 items on a 7-point scale (1 = strongly disagree to 7 = strongly agree) were included in the dimensions. The internal consistency of GPIUS2 in the Bahasa Indonesia version in this study was $\alpha = 0.897$. Emotional reactivity was measured using the emotional reactivity scale (ERS) constructed by Nock et al. [17] and adapted to Bahasa Indonesia [9]. The ERS consisted of 21 items in 3 dimensions (emotional sensitivity, emotional intensity, and emotional persistence) on a 7-point scale from 1 = strongly disagree to 7 = strongly agree. The internal consistency of the ERS Bahasa Indonesia version in this study was $\alpha = 0.930$, and internal consistency for its dimensions ranged from $\alpha = 0.753$ to $\alpha = 0.891$. Emotional dysregulation was measured using the General Emotion Dysregulation Measure (GEDM) constructed by Linehan [33], modified by Newhill et al. [34], and adapted to Bahasa Indonesia. The GEDM consisted of 13 items in 3 dimensions (emotional sensitivity, emotional response, and slow return to baseline) on a 5-point scale from 1 = very weak to 5 = very strong. The internal consistency of GEDM in the Bahasa Indonesia version was $\alpha = 0.917$.

2.2. Data Analysis

The data were analyzed using linear regression statistics for H1 and H2 and mediation analysis for H3. The data were analyzed using JASP 0.17.1.0 version. Demographic data were presented with descriptive statistics.

3. Results and Discussion

The descriptive score is shown in Table 2. We calculated PIU as a single score, emotional reactivity in unidimensional and multidimensional scores, and emotional dysregulation as a unidimensional score.

Table 2. Scores of each dimension.

Dimension	Mean	Standard Deviation (SD)	Minimum	Maximum
PIU	67.10	18.90	22.00	113.00
Emotional reactivity	66.82	16.77	26.00	105.00
Emotional reactivity—sensitivity	31.37	9.10	10.00	50.00
Emotional reactivity—intensity	23.13	5.65	8.00	35.00
Emotional reactivity—persistence	12.32	3.74	4.00	20.00
Emotional dysregulation	40.01	11.05	14.00	65.000

Based on the regression analysis results (Table 3), hypothesis H1 was supported ($R^2 = 0.21$, F(77.014, 1)), indicating that emotional reactivity played a significant role in predicting PIU. Emotional reactivity had an effect of 46% on PIU. The participants with a high score on emotional reactivity had a strong spectrum of PIU ($R^2 = 0.22$, F(28.958, 3)). Emotional persistence had an effect of 25.1% on PIU. Twitter users had a slow response to return to their emotional baseline after reacting to the emotional stimuli on Twitter. H2 was also supported ($R^2 = 0.16$, F(56.49, 1)), and emotional dysregulation had a 40% effect on PIU. The results showed a strong effect of emotional dysregulation on PIU, meaning that Twitter users with high emotional dysregulation were higher on the spectrum for PIU.

Table 3. Results of regression analysis.

	Sum of Square	Degree of Freedom	F	Significance
PIU on emotional reactivity (ER)	21,431.12	1	77.014	$p < 0.001$
PIU on sensitivity, intensity, persistence	24,358.39	3	28.958	$p < 0.001$
PIU on emotional dysregulation (ED)	17,081.73	1	56.49	$p < 0.001$
	R	**R^2**	**Adjusted R^2**	**root mean square error**
PIU on emotional reactivity (ER)	0.46	0.21	0.21	16.84
PIU on sensitivity, intensity, persistence	0.47	0.22	0.22	16.75
PIU on emotional dysregulation (ED)	0.40	0.16	0.15	17.39
	Standardized (β)	**t-value**	**Significance**	
PIU on emotional reactivity (ER)	0.457	8.982	$p < 0.001$	
PIU on sensitivity	0.223	2.470	$p > 0.001$	
PIU on intensity	0.055	0.614	$p > 0.001$	
PIU on persistence	0.251	3.742	$p < 0.001$	
PIU on emotional dysregulation (ED)	0.395	7.516	$p < 0.001$	

H3 was supported in this study. Thus, emotional reactivity was a significant mediator in predicting PIU on emotional dysregulation. The result of the H3 test is shown in Table 4 and Figure 2. PIU had no significant effect on emotional dysregulation, which is in line with previous research [13].

Table 4. Mediation effect of emotional reactivity, supporting H3.

Measurement	Estimate	Standard Error	z-Value	Significance
Direct effect: PIU on emotional dysregulation	<−0.001	0.01	−0.10	$p > 0.001$
Indirect effect: emotional dysregulation → emotional reactivity → PIU	0.04	0.01	4.49	$p < 0.001$
Total effect: PIU on emotional dysregulation	0.04	0.004	7.54	$p < 0.001$
Path Coefficient	**Estimate**	**Standard Error**	**z-Value**	**Significance**
PIU on emotional reactivity	0.47	0.10	4.53	$p < 0.001$
PIU on emotional dysregulation	<−0.001	0.01	−0.10	$p > 0.001$
Emotional reactivity on emotional dysregulation	0.08	0.003	30.89	$p < 0.001$

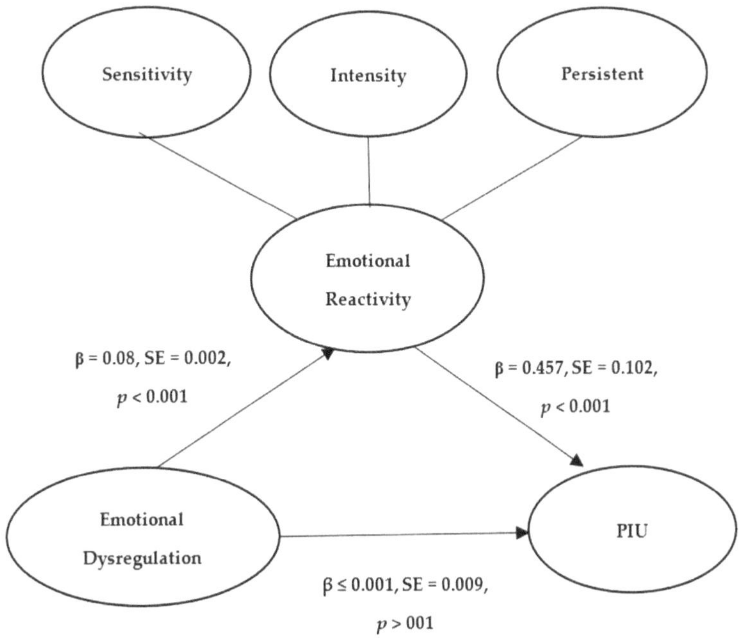

Figure 2. Mediation effect of emotional reactivity.

The path coefficients indicated that emotional reactivity played an important role in predicting PIU. Emotional dysregulation was a precursor of emotional reactivity. When it is difficult for Twitter users to manage their emotions, it is easy for them to respond emotionally to the stimuli they receive [19,25]. The findings from the path coefficient showed the role of emotional reactivity in predicting PIU [10]. Emotional dysregulation alone did not play a significant role in predicting PIU owing to the unique behavior of Twitter users. Instead, emotional dysregulation affects sensitivity, intensity, and slow response [28]. Twitter users seem to be easily provoked emotionally when interacting with social media. They can manage their emotions but easily react emotionally or have strong emotional reactivity. The results of PIU regression on the dimensions of emotional reactivity (Table 4) revealed that the participants were slow in returning to their baseline when experiencing negative emotions. They were provoked emotionally, not because of their sensitivity to stimuli, but because of difficulty returning to their emotional baseline or because of strong emotional persistence. Thus, emotional dysregulation is associated with PIU through emotional reactivity as a mediator. Emotional reactivity manifests the difficulty for Twitter users to return to the baseline of their emotional reactions.

4. Conclusions

Emotional reactivity is a mediator of the relationship between PIU and emotional dysregulation. For Twitter users, emotional dysregulation can be used to predict PIU through emotional reactivity. Such results show the importance of being selective about posts on Twitter. Social media, as a product of digital technology, provides benefits but may cause mental problems due to carelessness. Social media users need to recognize their emotional responses. The more they realize their weakness in managing their emotions, the easier it is for them to control their emotional responses, and the better they can select posts on social media. Sometimes, it is recommended to pause social media activities. Social media users can be active on social media when emotional conditions return to their baseline. In this study, we surveyed normal users. Subsequent research is needed to examine users with mental problems to develop an early warning system for emotional reactivity on social media that can alert users relating to their mental status.

Author Contributions: Conceptualization, E.A. and M.A.; methodology, E.A., T.P., S.G., M.A., G.P. and A.K.; validation, E.A., T.P., S.G. and M.A.; formal analysis, E.A., T.P., S.G. and M.A.; investigation, T.P., S.G., M.A., G.P. and A.K.; resources, E.A., T.P., S.G., M.A., G.P. and A.K.; data curation, E.A., T.P., S.G., M.A., G.P. and A.K.; writing—original draft preparation, E.A., T.P., S.G. and M.A.; writing—review and editing, E.A.; visualization, E.A.; supervision, E.A.; funding acquisition, M.A. All authors have read and agreed to the published version of the manuscript.

Funding: This research was funded by an International Research Grant from BINA NUSANTARA UNIVERSITY No: 029/VRRTT/III/2023. The APC was funded by the authors themselves.

Institutional Review Board Statement: The authors have been registered ethical consideration to the Bina Nusantara University ethical committee for the publication ethic. However, the committee still sent for ethical approval. For this reason, the authors passed the preregistration to the Open Science Framework (OSF) via link https://osf.io/k3rup.

Informed Consent Statement: Informed consent was obtained from all subjects involved in this study.

Data Availability Statement: Data in this study was registered on Mendeley Data as Andangsari, Esther Widhi; Putri, Trisa; Ghaisani, Shavina; Ali, Moondore Madalina; Paramitha, Greta Vidya; Kemala, Ade Putera (2024), "Problematic Internet Use (PIU), Emotional Dysregulation, and Emotional Reactivity of Twitter Users" see Problematic Internet Use (PIU), Emotional Dysregulation, and Emotional Reactivity of Twitter Users—Mendeley Data.

Conflicts of Interest: The authors declare no conflicts of interest. The funders had no role in the design of the study, in the collection, analyses, or interpretation of data, in the writing of the manuscript, or in the decision to publish the results.

References

1. Asosiasi Penyelenggara Jasa Internet Indonesia. Available online: https://apjii.or.id/berita/d/survei-apjii-pengguna-internet-di-indonesia-tembus-215-juta-orang (accessed on 31 July 2024).
2. Data Indonesia. Available online: https://dataindonesia.id/internet/detail/indonesia-masuk-negara-paling-banyak-main-twitter-pada-awal-2023 (accessed on 31 July 2024).
3. Yang, Y.; Liu, K.; Li, S.; Shu, M. Social media activities, emotion regulation strategies, and their interactions on people's mental health in COVID-19 pandemic. *Int. J. Environ. Res. Public Health* **2020**, *17*, 8931. [CrossRef] [PubMed]
4. Tullett-Prado, D.; Stavropoulos, V.; Gomez, R.; Doley, J. Social media use and abuse: Different profiles of users and their associations with addictive behaviours. *Addict. Behav. Rep.* **2022**, *17*, 100479. [CrossRef] [PubMed]
5. Rębisz, S.; Jasińska-Maciążek, A.; Grygiel, P.; Dolata, R. Psycho-Social Correlates of Cyberbullying among Polish Adolescents. *Int. J. Environ. Res. Public Health* **2023**, *20*, 5521. [CrossRef]
6. Andangsari, E.W.; Djunaidi, A.; Fitriana, E.; Harding, D. Loneliness and Problematic Internet Use (PIU) as Causes of Academic Procrastination. *Int. J. Soc. Sci. Stud.* **2018**, *6*, 113–122. [CrossRef]
7. Liu, M.; Xiao, J.; Kamper-DeMarco, K.E.; Fu, Z. Problematic internet use and suicidality and self-injurious behaviors in adolescents: Effects of negative affectivity and social support. *J. Affect. Disord.* **2023**, *325*, 289–296. [CrossRef] [PubMed]

8. Arce-García, S.; Díaz-Campo, J.; Cambronero-Saiz, B. Online hate speech and emotions on Twitter: A case study of Greta Thunberg at the UN Climate Change Conference COP25 in 2019. *Soc. Netw. Anal. Min.* **2023**, *13*, 48. [CrossRef]
9. Sari, T.I.; Ardilla, Z.N.; Hayatin, N.; Maskat, R. Abusive comment identification on Indonesian social media data using hybrid deep learning. *IAES Int. J. Artif. Intell.* **2022**, *11*, 895–904. [CrossRef]
10. Andangsari, E.W.; Dhowi, B.; Djunaidi, A.; Fitriani, E.; Harding, D. Problematic Internet Use (PIU): The role of emotional factors on social media activities. In Proceedings of the 2nd International Conference on Informatics and Computing, ICIC 2017, Jayapura, Indonesia, 1–3 November 2017. [CrossRef]
11. Russo, A.; Santoro, G.; Schimmenti, A. Interpersonal Guilt and Problematic Online Behaviors: The Mediating Role of Emotion Dysregulation. *Clin. Neuropsychiatry* **2022**, *19*, 236–247. [CrossRef]
12. Gioia, F.; Rega, V.; Boursier, V. Problematic internet use and emotional dysregulation among young people: A literature review. *Eur. J. Public Health* **2022**, *32*, 41–54. [CrossRef]
13. Casale, S.; Caplan, S.E.; Fioravanti, G. Positive metacognitions about Internet use: The mediating role in the relationship between emotional dysregulation and problematic use. *Addict. Behav.* **2016**, *59*, 84–88. [CrossRef]
14. Juditha, C. Hatespeech in Online media: Jakarta on Election 2017. *J. Penelit. Komun. Opini Publik* **2017**, *21*, 223284.
15. Nurul, F.A.; Nurhadi, N.; Pranawa, S. Konflik dan Ujaran Kebencian di Twitter. *Jupiis J. Pendidik. Ilmu-Ilmu Sos.* **2020**, *12*, 132. [CrossRef]
16. Thompson, R.J.; Mata, J.; Jaeggi, S.M.; Buschkuehl, M.; Jonides, J.; Gotlib, I.H. The everyday emotional experience of adults with major depressive disorder: Examining emotional instability, inertia, and reactivity. *J. Abnorm. Psychol.* **2012**, *121*, 819–829. [CrossRef]
17. Ripper, C.A.; Boyes, M.E.; Clarke, P.J.F.; Hasking, P.A. Emotional reactivity, intensity, and perseveration: Independent dimensions of trait affect and associations with depression, anxiety, and stress symptoms. *Pers. Individ. Dif.* **2018**, *121*, 93–99. [CrossRef]
18. Nock, M.K.; Wedig, M.M.; Holmberg, E.B.; Hooley, J.M. The Emotion Reactivity Scale: Development, Evaluation, and Relation to Self-Injurious Thoughts and Behaviors. *Behav. Ther.* **2008**, *39*, 107–116. [CrossRef]
19. Herres, J.; Caporino, N.E.; Cummings, C.M.; Kendall, P.C. Emotional reactivity to daily events in youth with anxiety disorders. *Anxiety Stress Coping* **2018**, *31*, 387–401. [CrossRef]
20. Davis, R.A. Cognitive-behavioral model of pathological Internet use. *Comput. Human Behav.* **2001**, *17*, 187–195. [CrossRef]
21. Caplan, S.E. Computers in Human Behavior Theory and measurement of generalized problematic Internet use: A two-step approach. *Comput. Hum. Behav.* **2010**, *26*, 1089–1097. [CrossRef]
22. Song, H.; Zmyslinski-Seelig, A.; Kim, J.; Drent, A.; Victor, A.; Omori, K.; Allen, K. Does Facebook make you lonely?: A meta analysis. *Comput. Hum. Behav.* **2014**, *36*, 446–452. [CrossRef]
23. Caplan, S.E. Problematic Internet use and psychosocial well-being: Development of a theory-based cognitive-behavioral measurement instrument. *Comput. Hum. Behav.* **2002**, *18*, 553–575. [CrossRef]
24. Griffiths, M.D.; Kuss, D.J.; Billieux, J.; Pontes, H.M. The evolution of Internet addiction: A global perspective. *Addict. Behav.* **2016**, *53*, 193–195. [CrossRef]
25. Shapero, B.G.; Farabaugh, A.; Terechina, O.; DeCross, S.; Cheung, J.C.; Fava, M.; Holt, D.J. Understanding the effects of emotional reactivity on depression and suicidal thoughts and behaviors: Moderating effects of childhood adversity and resilience. *J. Affect. Disord.* **2018**, *245*, 419–427. [CrossRef]
26. Cook, E.C.; Blair, B.L.; Buehler, C. Individual Differences in Adolescents' Emotional Reactivity across Relationship Contexts. *J. Youth Adolesc.* **2018**, *47*, 290–305. [CrossRef] [PubMed]
27. Becerra, R.; Campitelli, G. Emotional Reactivity: Critical Analysis and Proposal of a New Scale. *Int. J. Appl. Psychol.* **2013**, *3*, 161–168.
28. Arrivillaga, C.; Hallauer, C.J.; Montag, C.; Elhai, J.D. Emotion dysregulation factors associated with problematic smartphone use severity: The mediating role of fear of missing out. *Addict. Behav.* **2023**, *143*, 107708. [CrossRef]
29. Ong, V.; Rahmanto, A.D.S.; Williem; Suhartono, D.; Nugroho, A.E.; Andangsari, E.W.; Suprayogi, M.N. Personality prediction based on Twitter information in Bahasa Indonesia. In Proceedings of the 2017 Federated Conference on Computer Science and Information Systems (FedCSIS), Prague, Czech Republic, 3–6 September 2017. [CrossRef]
30. Adi, G.Y.N.N.; Harley, M.; Ong, V.; Suhartono, D.; Andangsari, E.W. Automatic personality recognition in Bahasa Indonesia: A semi-supervised approach. *ICIC Express Lett.* **2019**, *13*, 797–805.
31. Gross, J.J.; Jazaieri, H. Emotion Regulation, and Psychopathology. *Clin. Psychol. Sci.* **2014**, *2*, 387–401. [CrossRef]
32. Andangsari, E.W.; Dhowi, B. Two Typology Types of Loneliness and Problematic Internet Use (PIU): An Evidence of Indonesian Measurement. *Adv. Sci. Lett.* **2016**, *22*, 1711–1714. [CrossRef]
33. Lineha, M.M. *Cognitive-Behavioral Treatment of Borderline Personality Disorder*; The Guilford Press: New York, NY, USA, 1993.
34. Newhill, C.E.; Bell, M.M.; Eack, S.M.; Mulvey, E.P. Confirmatory Factor Analysis of the Emotion Dysregulation Measure. *J. Soc. Soc. Work Res.* **2010**, *1*, 159–168. [CrossRef]

engineering proceedings

MDPI

Proceeding Paper

Strategy of Phytoremediation for Sustainable Use of Arsenic-Rich Farmland †

Chang-Chao Chen [1], Min-Siou Lin [1], Pei-Cheng Cheng [2], Chin-Yuan Huang [3,*] and Shu-Fen Cheng [3,*]

1 Institute of Biochemical Technology, Chaoyang University of Technology, Taichung 41349, Taiwan; ccc145508@gmail.com (C.-C.C.); minsiou.lin@gmail.com (M.-S.L.)
2 Institute of Environmental Engineering, National Sun Yat-Sen University, 70 Lienhai Rd., Kaohsiung 80424, Taiwan; eric62795@gmail.com
3 Department of Environmental Engineering and Management, Chaoyang University of Technology, Tai-chung 41349, Taiwan
* Correspondence: sanada.r88686@msa.hinet.net (C.-Y.H.); shufen@cyut.edu.tw (S.-F.C.)
† Presented at the 2024 IEEE 4th International Conference on Electronic Communications, Internet of Things and Big Data, Taipei, Taiwan, 19–21 April 2024.

Abstract: Arsenic-rich groundwater causes arsenic accumulation in arable soils for irrigation. For such arsenic-contaminated farmland, phytoremediation is a feasible method in terms of cost and maintenance of soil. We studied arsenic-rich farmland planted with maize, *Rotala rotundifolia*, and the arsenic super-accumulating plant *Pteris vittata* and explored the arsenic absorption capacity of these plants to assess the effect of phytoremediation on arsenic-contaminated farmland. The arsenic removal by *Pteris vittata* was about 200 mg/m^2 y. It would take about 90 years to reduce the soil arsenic below the regulatory standard of 60 mg/kg using *Pteris vittata*. Planting maize removed about 25.5 mg/m^2 y of arsenic, and the arsenic concentration of the maize kernels was less than 0.2 mg/kg on a dry basis. It was below the standards of the animal food and human consumption limit. *Pteris vittata* needs to be planted first to rapidly reduce the bioavailable arsenic concentration in the soil. Subsequent planting of maize for remediating the soil while producing corn enables the sustainable production and utilization of farmland.

Keywords: phytoremediation; arsenic; farmland; phytoattenuation; maize

Citation: Chen, C.-C.; Lin, M.-S.; Cheng, P.-C.; Huang, C.-Y.; Cheng, S.-F. Strategy of Phytoremediation for Sustainable Use of Arsenic-Rich Farmland. *Eng. Proc.* **2024**, *74*, 8. https://doi.org/10.3390/engproc2024074008

Academic Editors: Shu-Han Liao, Teen-Hang Meen and Cheng-Fu Yang

Published: 27 August 2024

1. Introduction

Affected by geological factors, countries such as India, Bangladesh, Cambodia, China, Vietnam, Myanmar, the United States, Mexico, and Argentina are facing the problem of arsenic-rich groundwater [1–3]. Many areas in Taiwan such as Langyang Plain, Guandu Plain, Yunjianan Plain, and Pingtung Plain face the problem of arsenic-rich groundwater [4]. *Oryza sativa* is the most important food crop in Taiwan. In farmland with arsenic-rich groundwater, the soil accumulates arsenic due to long-term irrigation.

Long-term consumption of an arsenic-rich diet leads to chronic arsenic poisoning such as abnormal skin pigmentation, keratinization, skin cancer, and visceral cancer. In Taiwan, there have been cases of black foot disease caused by drinking arsenic-rich groundwater. The WHO recommends a limit of 10 µg/L for arsenic in drinking water [5]. In Taiwan, the edible limit of inorganic arsenic in rice is 0.35 mg/kg for brown rice and 0.2 mg/kg for white rice [6]. The total arsenic of other cereal crops is regulated, and the edible limit standard is 1.0 mg/kg (fresh weight). In order to prevent food crops from being rich in arsenic, many countries have established arsenic control standards for agricultural soils. The regulated value for rice fields in Japan is 15 mg/kg, and the farmland soil control standard is 60 mg/kg in Taiwan.

In Taiwan, there are many farmlands where the arsenic concentration exceeds the soil control standard due to groundwater irrigation. Physical or chemical technology, such as soil washing and soil solidification, costs considerably and destroys the characteristics of the soil. Phytoremediation does not destroy the productive properties of soil and is an ecologically and economically viable technology to remove contaminants. The techniques of phytoremediation include phytoextraction, phytostabilization, phytodegradation, phytoevaporation, and promotion of microbial decomposition in the rhizosphere. For arsenic-contaminated soils, phytoextraction is the most commonly used technique for phytoremediation. Through plant growth and metabolism, the arsenic in the soil is absorbed and accumulated in the plant. Then, through plant harvesting, the arsenic is removed [7]. The properties of plants as a phytoextractor include the following: (1) high tolerance to heavy metals, (2) high enough accumulation capacity for heavy metals and ease of harvesting, (3) accumulation of large amounts of biomass in contaminated soil, and (4) rapid root growth [8–11].

Pteris vittata L. also called Centipede Grass, is a certified arsenic-accumulating plant and has been used for the phytoremediation of polluted soils [12–17]. *Pteris vittata* L. grows on soils with arsenic content as high as 1500 mg/kg, and the accumulated arsenic concentration in leaves can reach 2500–22,630 mg/kg (dry basis). In non-arsenic-contaminated soil, arsenic accumulates up to 744 mg/kg in the above ground tissues of *Pteris vittata*, which is much higher than the arsenic content of general plants (<10 mg/kg) [12]. When the initial total arsenic concentration in the soil was about 63.9 mg/kg, the arsenic content in the soil decreased by 5 mg/kg after 7 months, and the arsenic reduction rate reached 7.84% [18]. In experiments of planting *Pteris vittata* L. in the southwest of England, the total arsenic concentration in the soil was 471 mg/kg, and the concentration of arsenic in the feather leaves was 4371 mg/kg. However, the biomass yield of *Pteris vittata* L. is low, with a yield of about 0.76 Mg/ha [15]. Kertulis-Tartar et al. [19] tested *Pteris vittata* L. in Florida with a mass yield of approximately 1.3 Mg/ha. Liu et al. [20] carried out a planting experiment of *Pteris vittata* L., and the aboveground biomass was lower than 2 Mg/ha. Excessive arsenic concentration in the soil inhibited the physiological activities of *Pteris vittata* L., reduced biomass yield, and caused a slow removal rate of arsenic from soil [21].

Arsenic is in a pentavalent form in aerated soil. The concentration of pentavalent arsenic in soil solution is very low (<1 μM) due to the strong adsorption of iron, manganese, and aluminum (hydroxide) oxides in soil and therefore reduces the bioavailability of arsenic in soil [22]. In anaerobic soils, arsenic is mainly in the trivalent form [23]. Soil immersed in water limits the transmission of oxygen, and due to the metabolism of facultative and anaerobic bacteria in the soil a reducing environment is created, resulting in the reductive dissolution of iron oxides and the release of arsenic into the soil solution. Aquatic environments enhance the bioavailability of arsenic in soil [24]. A variety of aquatic plants such as water hyacinths have a high absorption capacity for arsenic in water so can be used for arsenic removal in water [25]. Chen et al. pointed out that cattail had a strong tolerance to antimony and arsenic in slag, and the annual transfer amount of arsenic to cattail was 31.46 mg/m^2; however, more than 98% of arsenic was accumulated in the root of cattail [26,27]. Lin et al. [28] studied the arsenic content of rice plants in the arsenic-rich area of the Guandu Plain in Taiwan. The average arsenic concentrations in roots, stems, and leaves of rice were 98.7, 3.49, and 0.074 mg/kg (dry weight), respectively. The arsenic content in the roots of rice accounted for about 96.8% of the whole plant, and that of the stems and leaves accounted for 3.1 and 0.1%. The cumulative concentration of arsenic in aquatic plants in roots was higher than that of stem and leaf. *Rotala rotundifolia* is an aquatic plant native to Taiwan. The studies pointed out that *Rotala rotundifolia* had a high translocation ability for arsenic, and the arsenic concentration in the stem and leaves reached 7822 mg/kg (dry weight). The lack of a translocation barrier in the root leads to a high accumulation concentration of arsenic in the stem and leaves [29].

Phytoremediation is the friendliest remediation technology for heavy metal contamination in farmland, but it is limited by the long time requirement. Even if hyperaccumulator plants are used, it often takes decades, hundreds of years, or even thousands of years to reduce the concentration of heavy metals in the soil through plant extraction to meet regulatory standards [30,31], making it difficult to promote phytoremediation technology. Therefore, phytoremediation must be sustainable and feasible only when the crops planted have a stable economic base. Meers et al. [32] put forward the concept of "Phytoattenuation", arguing that the ability of plants to extract heavy metals must not be the main screening condition for the development of phytoattenuation. Matching with proper agronomic management, by planting crops to produce hygienic, safe, and economical products while the effect of soil pollution reduction is gradually achieved, makes phytoremediation sustainable and applicable. Mi et al. planted *Pteris vittata* L. and maize in soil with an arsenic content of 103.8 mg/kg. The accumulative arsenic concentration of *Pteris vittata* L. was 169.33–204.26 mg/kg, and that of maize stalk was 41.60–55.48 mg/kg [33,34]. Although the cumulative concentration of arsenic in maize is low, it has a high biomass yield with economic benefits. Cheng et al. planted maize on lead-contaminated farmland, producing 93.37 Mg/ha per year (in dry mass). If it is used as bioenergy, it produces 1545 GJ per hectare per year, which is equivalent to the combustion energy of 74 Mg of raw coal. An additional, about 25 Mg of feed corn could be produced per hectare per year [35].

An arsenic-contaminated farmland in Taiwan was selected for this study, growing the arsenic super-accumulator plant *Pteris vittata* L., the aquatic plant *Rotala rotundifolia*, and the food crop maize. The arsenic removal amount and economic benefits of three crops were compared, and the most feasible phytoremediation strategy for arsenic-contaminated farmland was determined.

2. Materials and Methods

2.1. Experiment Site

The farmland for the field experiment was located at No. 533, Ximenkou Section, Changhua City, Taiwan, the coordinates are X:201682, Y:2661575. Soil arsenic was accumulated from the long-term use of arsenic-rich groundwater for irrigation. Arsenic concentration decreased with the distance from the water inlet. The arsenic concentration in the topsoil was measured with a hand-held XRF on a 1 × 1 m grid before the experiment. For planting experiments, three soil arsenic concentration ranges were selected: a high-concentration area of more than 100 mg/kg, a medium-concentration area of 60–80 mg/kg, and a low-concentration area of below 40 mg/kg. After removing the weeds in each block, a rotary yak was used for stirring to make the soil arsenic concentration evenly distributed.

2.2. Soil Properties

Trial crops included *Pteris vittata* L., *Zea mays* L., and *Rotala rotundifolia*. Each plant was planted in three blocks in three concentration ranges, and the area of each block was 2 × 2 m. Each block was divided into four grids, and the soil in the center of the four grids was taken and mixed into a soil sample. The soil properties were analyzed, including soil texture, pH (the weight ratio of soil and reagent water was 1:1 mixed and stirred, and the supernatant liquid was taken for pH electrode analysis after standing still), organic matter content (Walkley–Black wet oxidation method and potassium dichromate titration method), soil conductivity (saturated soil paste extraction method), and total arsenic (decomposed organic acids with hydrogen peroxide, extracted with 9.6 M hydrochloric acid, and then reduced to arsine). Bioavailable arsenic concentration was analyzed using a 0.1 N hydrochloric acid extraction method and the sequential extraction method described by Wenzel et al. (2001). The dissolved fraction (F1) and the exchangeable fraction (F2) of Wenzel sequential extraction methods were extracted with 0.05 M $(NH_4)H_2PO_4$ and 0.05 M $NH_4H_2PO_4$, respectively [36]. The extracts were analyzed quantitatively by an Inductively Coupled Plasma Optical Emission Spectrometer (ICP-OES, Thermo CAP 6300, ThermoFisher, Waltham, MA, USA).

2.3. Planting Experiment

Pteris vittata L. were bred using spores. Then, seedlings with a height of about 10 cm were transplanted with a row spacing of 40 × 30 cm. Five plants were planted in each row and each experimental block had 4 rows (Figure 1a). Plants were collected after 9 months, in winter, when the plants began to wither, and the quality of each plant was measured. Three samples were randomly taken from each block and were separated into the aboveground tissues and the underground tissues, of which the arsenic content of the plants was measured. For maize, Tainan No. 24 hard corn was selected for the planting test. The seeds were germinated to about 3 cm before transplanting, being planted with a row spacing of 30 × 20 cm, 6 rows in each block, 8 plants in each row were planted (Figure 1b). The height and biomass of corn were measured when it was mature; about 120 days after planting. Three samples were randomly taken from each block, and the biomass and arsenic content of each part of the plant were measured by separating them into roots, stems, leaves, bract leaves, cobs, and kernels. *Rotala rotundifolia* was planted by cuttings. The stems of the plants were 5–8 cm long and with 3–4 stems in each clump, of which the row spacing is 25 cm × 20 cm. *Rotala rotundifolia* is an amphibious plant. In the planting period, the soil surface was kept flooded with a water depth of greater than 5 cm (Figure 1c). Three samples were randomly taken from each block 3 and 6 months after planting and were separated into aboveground and underground tissues to measure the arsenic content. Plants were harvested to measure the biomass after 6 months. The rhizosphere soil was taken from the three plants when they were harvested to analyze the bioavailable arsenic content.

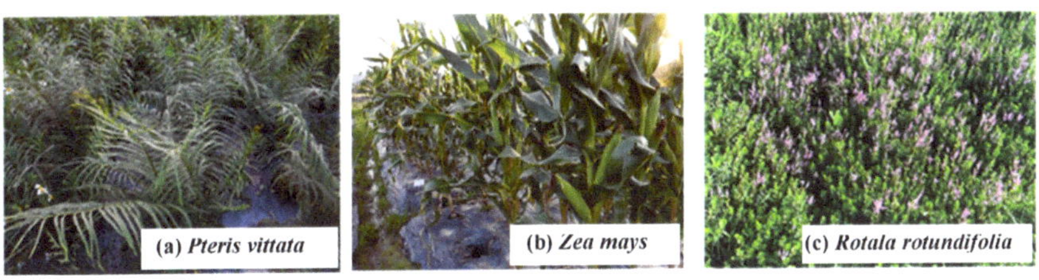

Figure 1. Field planting of test plants. (**a**) *Pteris vittata* L.; (**b**) *Zea mays* L.; and (**c**) *Rotala rotundifolia*.

3. Results

3.1. Soil Properties and Arsenic Concentration

The results of the soil characteristics analysis in the field test are shown in Table 1. The soil texture was sandy loam, with pH ranging from 6.58 to 6.81. The conductivity was 162 to 269 μS/cm, and the organic matter content was 3.06 to 3.22%. The total arsenic concentration of the soil in the high-concentration area (H) was between 102.2 and 108.7 mg/kg, with an average of 105.5 ± 3.3 mg/kg, In the medium-concentration area (M), the concentration was between 61.1 and 79.3 mg/kg, with an average concentration of 68.9 ± 9.4 mg/kg. The concentration in the low-concentration area (L) was between 28.8 to 38.7 mg/kg, and the average concentration was 34.1 ± 5.0 mg/kg. As for the concentration of bioavailable arsenic in the soil, which was extracted with 0.1 M HCl, it averaged 0.64 mg/kg in low-concentration soil; 0.72 mg/kg in medium-concentration soil; and 1.61 mg/kg in high-concentration soil. F1 and F2 of the Wenzel sequence extraction method represented the bioavailability. In the low-concentration soil the arsenic concentration was 5.4 mg/kg; in the medium-concentration soil it was 11.1 mg/kg; and in the high-concentration soil it was 21.0 mg/kg.

Table 1. Soil properties.

Properties		Unit	L	M	H
As concentration		mg/kg	34.1 ± 5.0	68.9 ± 9.4	105.5 ± 3.3
pH		-	6.58	6.61	6.81
Conductivity		μS/cm	245	162	269
Organic matter		%	3.23	3.22	3.06
Bioavailable As concentration	0.1 M HCl	mg/kg	0.64	0.72	1.61
	Wenzel F1 + F2	mg/kg	5.4	11.1	21.0

L: low As-concentration soil; M: medium As-concentration soil; H: high As-concentration soil; and Wenzel F1 + F2: the total As concentration of the dissolved fraction (F1) and the exchangeable fraction (F2) of the Wenzel sequence extraction method.

3.2. *Pteris vittata* L.

After breeding *Pteris vittata* L. with spores, it was transplanted to the field when it grew to about 10 cm. After 9 months of growth, winter had arrived and the plants began to wither; the plants were harvested and separated into the aerial tissues and the underground tissues (rhizome and adventitious roots). After air-drying at 70 °C, the plant biomass was measured (Table 2). The average weight of each plant in the high-concentration area was 108.4 ± 31.7 g; it was 135.1 ± 28.3 g in the medium-concentration area and 156.0 ± 45.7 g in the low-concentration area. Although there were no statistically significant differences (Fisher's protected least significant difference test, LSD test, at $p < 0.05$), the average biomass decreased with increasing soil arsenic concentrations.

Table 2. The average biomass and arsenic removal amount of *Pteris vittata* L. 9 months after planting.

Soil Type	Average Biomass (g Per Plant, Dry Basis)			As Removal Amount (mg)	
	Underground	Aboveground	Total	Per Plant	Per m^2
PL	20.4 ± 8.6	135.6 ± 29.6	156.0	7.63	63.61
PM	14.7 ± 5.7	120.4 ± 34.1	135.1	14.27	118.93
PH	17.2 ± 4.9	91.2 ± 29.1	108.4	24.20	201.68

PL: low As-concentration soil; PM: medium As-concentration soil; and PH: high As-concentration soil.

The arsenic content of the plants was measured at 3 and 9 months after planting and the results are shown in Figure 2. When *Pteris vittata* L. had grown for three months, the average arsenic concentrations in the underground tissues and shoots that were in the low-concentration area were 8.3 and 54.9 mg/kg; they were 54.6 and 101.5 mg/kg in the medium-concentration area and 62.2 and 164.4 mg/kg in the high-concentration area. After 9 months of growth, the average arsenic concentration in the underground tissues of *Pteris vittata* L. in the low-concentration area increased to 58.16 mg/kg, and the average arsenic concentration in the shoots was 47.5 mg/kg. The average concentrations of arsenic in the underground tissues and shoots in the medium-concentration area were 117.4 and 104.2 mg/kg, and they were 169.0 and 233.5 mg/kg in the high-concentration area. The analysis results showed that the average arsenic concentration in the underground tissues and shoots of *Pteris vittata* L. increased with increasing soil arsenic content. After 3 months, the arsenic content in the underground tissues of *Pteris vittata* L. continued to accumulate, but there were no significant differences in the accumulation of arsenic concentration in the shoots (at $p < 0.05$ by LSD test). Harvesting of aboveground tissues every 3 months after planting is therefore recommended.

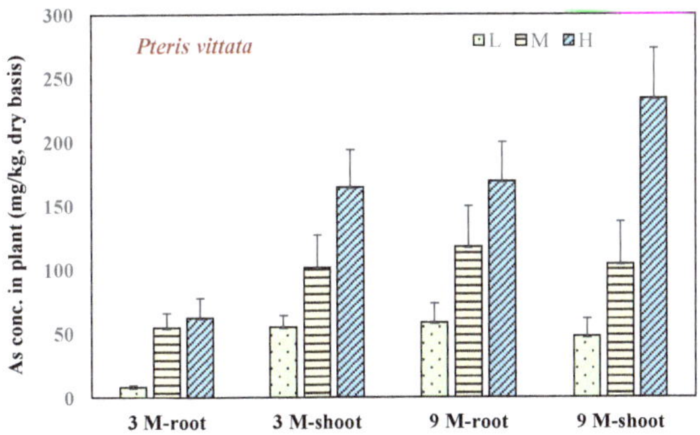

Figure 2. Arsenic concentrations in *Pteris vittata* L. 3 M: 3 months after planting; 6 M: 6 months after planting; root: the underground tissues; and shoot: the aerial tissues.

3.3. *Zea mays* L.

For corn, in various soil arsenic concentration test areas, the plant height and growth (total biomass) were measured when the plants were mature. The statistical results are shown in Table 3. The average height of plants in the high-concentration area was 224.1 ± 21.1 cm; in the medium-concentration area was 218.0 ± 29.4 cm; and in the low-concentration area was 217.0 ± 39.1 cm. As for the average growth of each plant, it was 530.8 ± 43.7 g in the high-concentration area; 510.7 ± 88.5 g in the medium-concentration area; and 538.7 ± 108.1 g in the low-concentration area. The proportion of biomass (dry basis) of each part of the maize plants was similar in different experimental areas. On average, roots accounted for 11.3%; stems accounted for 25%; leaves accounted for 11.2%; husks accounted for 11.9%; the corn cobs accounted for 11.6%; and corn kernels accounted for 28.4%. The average yield of corn kernels per plant in the high-concentration area was 143.4 ± 46.3 g; it was 127.4 ± 51.2 g in the medium-concentration area and 178.8 ± 57.0 g in the low-concentration area. The results of the LSD test (at $p < 0.05$) showed that within the range of soil arsenic concentration of 28.8–108.7 mg/kg (in this study), there were no significant differences in corn plant height, growth, and corn kernel yield among the experimental groups, indicating that the soil arsenic concentration did not inhibit the growth of maize within this range. The analysis results of arsenic concentration in various parts of the maize from various concentration areas are shown in Figure 3. The concentration distribution of arsenic in maize plants was highest in roots, with an average of 3.330–4.673 mg/kg, followed by leaves with an average of 1.252–1.519 mg/kg; stems and bracts had similar concentrations, with an average of 0.307–0.47 mg/kg and corn kernel concentration was the lowest, where the average dry basis arsenic concentration was between 0.083 and 0.162 mg/kg. The fresh weight concentration should be less than 1.0 mg/kg, which is in line with the human consumption limit standard stipulated in Taiwan. The average arsenic content in roots, stems, and leaves increased with the higher soil arsenic concentration. However, there was no consistent trend in bract leaves, corn cobs, and corn kernels.

Table 3. Average biomass and arsenic removal amount of *Zea mays* L.

Soil Type	Average Biomass (g Per Plant, Dry Basis)							As Removal Amount (mg)	
	Root	Stem	Leaf	B.Leaf	Cob	Kernel	Total	Per Plant	Per m^2
ZL	60.4	121.3	61.0	58.0	59.2	178.8	538.7	0.36	6.05
ZM	59.0	134.3	58.4	67.9	63.7	127.4	510.7	0.43	7.09
ZH	58.7	148.6	57.0	62.5	60.7	143.4	530.8	0.49	8.16

ZL: low As-concentration soil; ZM: medium As-concentration soil; and ZH: high As-concentration soil.

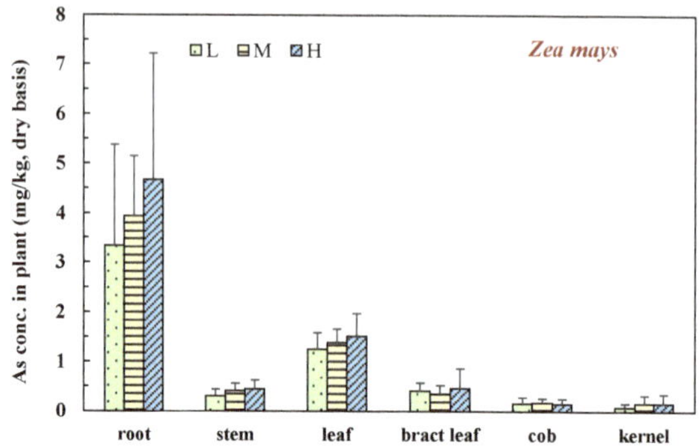

Figure 3. Arsenic concentrations in various tissues of *Zea mays* L.

3.4. *Rotala rotundifolia*

Rotala rotundifolia were harvested 6 months after planting. The dry biomass yield per m^2 was 138.8 mg in the low-concentration area; 175.6 mg in the medium-concentration area; and 188.9 mg in the high-concentration area (Table 4). The higher the soil arsenic concentration was the more the biomass increased. The biomass of *Rotala rotundifolia* was mainly distributed in the shoots, accounting for about 97.2%.

Table 4. Average biomass and arsenic removal amount of *Rotala rotundifolia*.

Soil Type	Average Biomass (g/m^2, Dry Basis)			As Removal Amount (mg/m^2)		
	Root	Shoot	Total	Root	Shoot	Total
GL	3.9 ± 0.3	134.9 ± 23.0	138.8	1.144	7.732	8.877
GM	3.4 ± 0.4	172.2 ± 13.1	175.6	0.225	0.969	1.194
GH	7.1 ± 1.3	181.8 ± 39.8	188.9	0.302	0.680	0.982

GL: low As-concentration soil; GM: medium As-concentration soil; and GH: high As-concentration soil.

Figure 4 shows the arsenic concentration on a dry basis of *Rotala rotundifolia* 3 months and 6 months after planting. After 3 months of growth, the average arsenic concentration in the root of *Rotala rotundifolia* in the low-concentration group was 15.93 mg/kg; in the medium-concentration group it was 3.59 mg/kg and in the high-concentration group it was 7.26 mg/kg. After 6 months of growth, the concentration of arsenic in the roots of each experimental group increased significantly. The average arsenic concentration in the roots of the low-concentration group was the highest at 293.42 mg/kg. As for the medium-concentration group, it was 66.15 mg/kg, and for the high-concentration group it was 42.52 mg/kg. The results showed that the root arsenic concentration decreased with the increase in soil arsenic concentration. The average arsenic concentration in the stem and leaves 3 months after planting was 12.84 mg/kg in the low-concentration group, 5.60 mg/kg in the medium-concentration group, and 1.73 mg/kg in the high-concentration group. The average arsenic concentration in stems and leaves six months after planting was 57.32 mg/kg in the low-concentration group, 5.63 mg/kg in the medium-concentration group, and 3.74 mg/kg in the high-concentration group. The arsenic concentration in stems and leaves was the same as that in roots but decreased with the increase in soil arsenic concentration, and only the low-concentration experimental group showed a significant increase in arsenic concentration at six months after planting compared with three months. In addition, the increase of arsenic concentration in the stem and leaves of the medium- and high-concentration experimental groups was limited. The experiment results showed that a high arsenic concentration in the soil will inhibit the absorption of arsenic by *Rotala rotundifolia*.

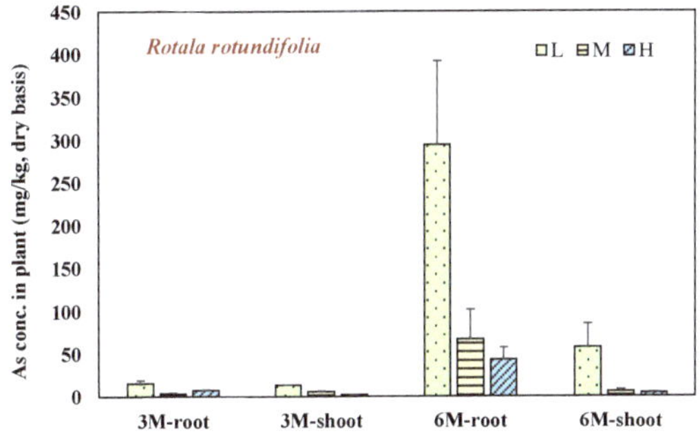

Figure 4. Arsenic concentrations in *Rotala rotundifolia*. 3 M: 3 months after planting; 6 M: 6 months after planting; root: the underground tissues; and shoot: the aerial tissues.

3.5. Changes in the Bioavailable Arsenic Concentration in the Soil

We analyzed the changes in bioavailable arsenic concentrations in rhizosphere soils before and after the planting of three plants. The results of the 0.1 N hydrochloric acid extraction method and F1 and F2 of the Wenzel sequential extraction method are shown in Figure 5. Before planting, the average concentration of bioavailable arsenic in the low-concentration soil was 0.64 mg/kg. After planting, the bioavailable arsenic concentration in the rhizosphere soil of *Pteris vittata* L. was reduced by about 53%; that of maize was reduced by 52% and a 33% reduction was observed by planting *Rotala rotundifolia*. The average concentration of bioavailable arsenic in medium-concentration soil before planting was 0.72 mg/kg. The concentration decreased by 51% after planting *Pteris vittata* L., 26% after planting corn, and 31% after planting *Rotala rotundifolia*. The average concentration of bioavailable arsenic in high-concentration soil before planting was 1.53 mg/kg. The average concentration decreased by 38% after planting *Pteris vittata* L.; 29% after planting corn; and 25% after planting *Rotala rotundifolia*. The bioavailable arsenic concentration decreased the most after the planting of *Pteris vittata* L., and the higher the soil arsenic concentration, the lower the reduction rate.

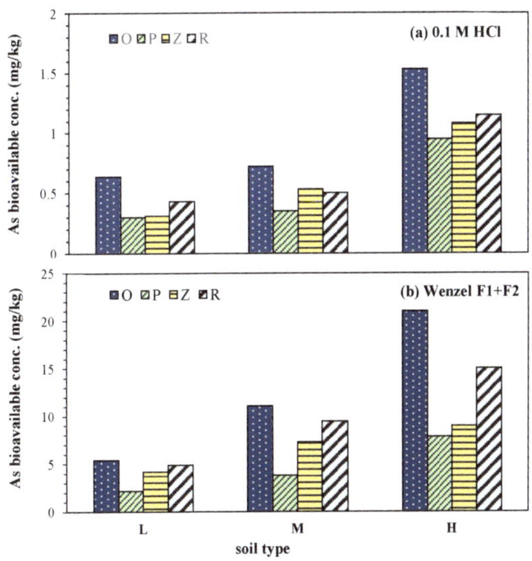

Figure 5. Changes in bioavailable arsenic concentrations in rhizosphere soils before and after planting these three plants.

The analysis results of the Wenzel sequence extraction method [24] are shown in Figure 5b. The total concentration of the soluble fraction and the exchangeable fraction before planting was 5.4 mg/kg in low-concentration soil, 11.1 mg/kg in medium-concentration soil, and 21.0 mg/kg in high-concentration soil. After planting, the bioavailable arsenic concentration was reduced, and the planting of *Pteris vittata* L. caused the highest reduction, reducing by 60–66%. The bioavailable arsenic showed a 23% to 57% reduction after planting corn and a 10% to 28% decrease after planting *Rotala rotundifolia*, which was the least of the three.

4. Discussion

The average biomass of the underground tissues of *Pteris vittata* L. accounted for 13% while shoots accounted for 87% of total biomass. The raw mass of the underground tissues and shoots of *Pteris vittata* L. was multiplied by the arsenic content (Table 2). On average, in the low-concentration area, 7.633 mg of arsenic was absorbed by each plant of *Pteris vittata* L.; in the medium-concentration area, 14.271 mg was absorbed and in the high-concentration area, 24.201 mg was absorbed. If the planting density is 40 × 30 cm, 63.6–201.68 mg of arsenic was removed per square meter over 9 months. About 13% of the plants were distributed in the underground tissues and about 87% were distributed in the shoots. If only the shoots are harvested, about 53.72–177.46 mg/m^2 of arsenic could be removed.

The weight of arsenic absorbed by each plant of maize was calculated by multiplying the average biomass of each part of the maize by the arsenic concentration. The arsenic content was removed by planting corn based on a planting density with a row spacing of 30 × 20 cm shown in Table 3. In the high-concentration area, 8.163 mg/m^2 of arsenic could be removed; in the medium-concentration area, 7.086 mg/m^2 was removed, and in the low-concentration area, 6.052 mg/m^2 was removed. The average corn planting period is about 120 days per round, and three rounds are planted per year. In one year, about 25.5 mg/m^2 of arsenic could be removed in a high-concentration area, 21.56 mg/m^2 could be removed in a medium-concentration area, and 18.2 mg/m^2 of arsenic could be removed in a low-concentration area.

The amounts of arsenic that could be removed by planting *Rotala rotundifolia* were shown in Table 4. After 6 months of planting, the amount of arsenic removed was between 0.982 mg/m^2 and 8.877 mg/m^2, and the highest amount of arsenic removed was in the low-concentration test group. On average, about 80% of the arsenic was contained in the plant shoots of *Rotala rotundifolia*. If the aboveground tissues were harvested once every 6 months after planting, the amount of arsenic that could be removed each time would be between 0.680 and 7.732 mg/m^2. Assuming that the stems and leaves that grow after the first harvest will have the same arsenic absorption capacity, harvesting twice a year could remove up to 1.36–15.5 mg/m^2 of arsenic per year.

The arsenic concentration in the high-concentration soil was about 105.5 mg/kg, and approximately 200 mg/m^2 of arsenic could be removed in 1 year by planting *Pteris vittata* L. The soil density was calculated as 1300 kg/m^3, and the thickness of the remediation soil was calculated as 30 cm of topsoil. It was estimated that it would take at least about 90 years to reduce the soil arsenic concentration from 105.5 mg/kg to below the regulatory standard of 60 mg/kg by planting *Pteris vittata* L. *Pteris vittata* L. has no economic value, and it is not feasible to grow it for 90 years without production income.

Planting corn in high-concentration areas could remove about 25.5 mg/m^2 of arsenic in one year; although the removal rate of corn is only one-eighth of the fern, the arsenic concentration of corn kernels was less than 0.2 mg/kg (dry basis). This not only meets the animal feed standard, but also meets the human consumption limit standard of 1.0 mg/kg (fresh weight concentration), which has production benefits. In addition, other parts of these plants, such as roots, stems, and leaves, had high biomass and could be used as biomass fuel. Maize is dry-farmed and requires less irrigation water during the growth process, which slows down the accumulation rate of arsenic in the soil.

The annual removal of arsenic from planting *Rotala rotundifolia* was about 15.5 mg/m^2, which was lower than that of corn. Since it is an aquatic plant, a large amount of water is necessary in the planting process. If groundwater is used for irrigation, it may cause a higher concentration of arsenic to accumulate in the soil. Therefore, using *Rotala rotundifolia* for phytoremediation was not feasible.

Pteris vittata L. can rapidly reduce bioavailable arsenic in the soil. In the early stage of phytoremediation of arsenic-contaminated soils, *Pteris vittata* L. can be planted for the first 2–3 years to reduce the bioavailable arsenic concentration in the soil. Then, *Zea mays* L. can be planted. *Zea mays* L. is dry-farmed, so there is no need to irrigate a lot during growth. A small amount of arsenic can be removed through the high mass of *Zea mays* L. plants, preventing the continuous accumulation of arsenic in the soil. The concentration of arsenic in kernels can be lower than the limit for human consumption. It can be used as animal feed and human consumption with economic benefits.

5. Conclusions

Arsenic-contaminated farmland was remediated by phytoremediation with the application of the arsenic super-accumulator plant, *Pteris vittata* L.; however, the time required to reach the regulatory standard of 60 mg/kg is long. If there is no production for a long time, the remediation cannot be continued. Less water is required during the growth of maize, which slows down the accumulation of arsenic in the soil from irrigation with groundwater. Although the concentration of arsenic accumulated in maize plants was low, the amount of arsenic removed was considerable due to the high biomass of the maize plants. The content of arsenic in corn kernels was lower than the limit for human consumption, which allows for economic value. Maize can be used as a remediation crop on arsenic-contaminated farmland. Phytoremediation and production at the same time make the land use sustainable.

Author Contributions: Conceptualization, S.-F.C. and C.-C.C.; methodology, C.-C.C. and C.-Y.H.; experiment analysis, M.-S.L. and P.-C.C.; writing—original draft preparation, C.-C.C.; writing—review and editing, S.-F.C. and C.-Y.H. All authors have read and agreed to the published version of the manuscript.

Funding: This research received no external funding.

Institutional Review Board Statement: Not applicable.

Informed Consent Statement: Not applicable.

Data Availability Statement: The original contributions presented in the study are included in the article, further inquiries can be directed to the corresponding author.

Conflicts of Interest: The authors declare no conflicts of interest.

References

1. Smith, A.H.; Lingas, E.O.; Rahman, M. Contamination of drinking-water by arsenic Bangladesh: A public health emergency. *Bull. World Health Organ.* **2000**, *78*, 1093–1103.
2. Mandal, B.K.; Suzuki, K.T. Arsenic round the world: A review. *Talanta* **2002**, *58*, 201–235. [CrossRef]
3. Abedi, T.; Mojiri, A. Arsenic uptake and accumulation mechanisms in rice species. *Plants* **2020**, *9*, 129. [CrossRef]
4. Liu, C.W.; Wu, M.Z. Geochemical, mineralogical and statistical characteristics of arsenic in groundwater of the Lanyang Plain, Taiwan. *J. Hydrol.* **2019**, *577*, 123975. [CrossRef]
5. World Health Organization. Arsenic. Geneva 2018. WHO Fact Sheet. Available online: https://www.who.int/en/news-room/fact-sheets/detail/arsenic (accessed on 18 April 2024).
6. Taiwan FDA. Sanitation Standard for Contaminants and Toxins in Food. 2021. Available online: https://law.moj.gov.tw/ENG/LawClass/LawAll.aspx?pcode=L0040138 (accessed on 18 April 2024).
7. Dradrach, A.; Karczewska, A.; Szopka, K. Arsenic uptake by two tolerant grass species: *Holcus lanatus* and *Agrostis capillaris* growing in soils contaminated by historical mining. *Plants* **2020**, *9*, 980. [CrossRef]
8. Alkorta, I.; Hernandez-Allica, J.; Becerril, J.M.; Amezaga, I.; Albizu, I.; Onaindia, M.; Garbisu, C. Chelate-enhanced phytoremediation of soils polluted with heavy metals. *Rev. Environ. Sci. Bio-Technol.* **2004**, *3*, 55–70. [CrossRef]
9. Yang, X.; Feng, Y.; He, Z.; Stoffella, P.J. Molecular mechanisms of heavy metal hyperaccumulation and phytoremediation. *J. Trace Elem. Med. Biol.* **2005**, *18*, 339–353. [CrossRef] [PubMed]

10. Santos, F.S.; Hernandez-Allica, J.; Becerril, J.M.; Amaral-Sobrinho, N.; Mazur, N.; Garbisu, C. Chelate-induced phytoextraction of metal polluted soils with *Brachiaria decumbens*. *Chemosphere* **2006**, *65*, 43–50. [CrossRef] [PubMed]
11. Gajić, G.; Djurdjević, L.; Kostić, O.; Jarić, S.; Stevanović, B.; Mitrović, M.; Pavlović, P. Phytoremediation potential, photosynthetic and antioxidant response to arsenic-induced stress of *Dactylis glomerata* L. sown on fly ash deposits. *Plants* **2020**, *9*, 657. [CrossRef]
12. Ma, L.Q.; Komar, K.M.; Tu, C.; Zhang, W. A fern that hyperaccumulates arsenic. *Nature* **2001**, *409*, 579. [CrossRef]
13. Srivastava1, M.; Santos, J.; Srivastava, P.; Ma, L.Q. Comparison of arsenic accumulation in 18 fern species and four *Pteris vittata* accessions. *Bioresour. Technol.* **2010**, *101*, 2691–2699. [CrossRef]
14. Jiang, Y.; Lei, M.; Duanc, L.; Longhurst, P. Integrating phytoremediation with biomass valorisation and critical element recovery: A UK contaminated land perspective. *Biomass Bioenergy* **2015**, *83*, 328–339. [CrossRef]
15. Fayiga, A.O.; Saha, U.K. Arsenic hyperaccumulating fern: Implications for remediation of arsenic contaminated soils. *Geoderma* **2016**, *284*, 132–143. [CrossRef]
16. Cantamessa, S.; Massa, N.; Gamalero, E.; Berta, G. Phytoremediation of a highly arsenic polluted site, using *Pteris vittata* L. and arbuscular mycorrhizal fungi. *Plants* **2020**, *9*, 1211. [CrossRef] [PubMed]
17. Zemanová, V.; Pavlíková, D.; Hnilička, F.; Pavlík, M. Arsenic toxicity-induced physiological and metabolic changes in the shoots of *Pteris cretica* and *Spinacia oleracea*. *Plants* **2021**, *10*, 2009. [CrossRef] [PubMed]
18. Chen, T.B.; Zhang, B.C.; Huang, Z.C.; Liu, Y.R.; Zheng, Y.M.; Lei, M.; Liao, X.Y.; Piao, S.J. Geographical distribution and characteristics of habitat of As-hyperaccumulator *Pteris vittata* L. in China. *Geogr. Res.* **2005**, *24*, 825–833.
19. Kertulis-Tartar, G.M.; Ma, L.Q.; Tu, C.; Chirenje, T. Phytoremediation of an arsenic-contaminated site using *Pteris vittata* L.: A two-year study. *Int. J. Phytoremediation* **2006**, *8*, 311–322. [CrossRef]
20. Liu, Y.R.; Chen, T.B.; Huang, Z.C.; Liao, X.Y. As hyperaccumulation of *Pteris vittata* L. as influenced by As concentrations in soils of contaminated fields. *Environ. Sci.* **2005**, *26*, 181–186.
21. Faizan, M.; Sehar, S.; Rajput, V.D.; Faraz, A.; Afzal, S.; Minkina, T.; Sushkova, S.; Adil, M.F.; Yu, F.; Alatar, A.A.; et al. Modulation of cellular redox status and antioxidant defense system after synergistic application of zinc oxide nanoparticles and salicylic acid in rice (*Oryza sativa*) plant under arsenic stress. *Plants* **2021**, *10*, 2254. [CrossRef]
22. Fitz, W.J.; Wenzel, W.W. Arsenic transformation in the soil-rhizosphere-plant system: Fundamentals and potential application to phytoremediation. *J. Biotechnol.* **2002**, *99*, 259–278. [CrossRef]
23. Takahashi, Y.; Minamikawa, R.; Hattori, K.H. Arsenic behavior in paddy fields during the cycle of flooded and non-flooded periods. *Environ. Sci. Technol.* **2004**, *38*, 1038–1044. [CrossRef] [PubMed]
24. Inskeep, W.P.; McDermott, T.R.; Fendorf, S. *Arsenic (V)/(III) Cycling in Soils and Natural Waters: Chemical and Microbiological Processes, Environmental Chemistry of Arsenic*; Marcel Dekker: New York, NY, USA, 2001.
25. Alvarado, S.; Guédez, M.; Lué-Merú, M.P.; Nelson, G.; Alvaro, A.; Jesús, A.C.; Gyula, Z. Arsenic removal from waters by bioremediation with the aquatic plants Water Hyacinth (*Eichhornia crassipes*) and Lesser Duckweed (*Lemna minor*). *Bioresour. Technol.* **2008**, *99*, 8436–8844. [CrossRef] [PubMed]
26. Chen, J.F.; Wu, P.; Zhang, M.; Zhang, C.P.; Han, Z.W. Accumulation characteristics of Sb and As in cattail growing in antimony mine tailings. *Chin. J. Ecol.* **2015**, *34*, 2645–2649.
27. Chen, T.; Bao, N.Y.; Du, C.X.; Wang, Y.; Liu, Y.G. Effects of exogenous phosphorus input on growth and arsenic accumulation in *Typha angustifolia* L. contaminated by arsenic. *J. South. Agric.* **2020**, *51*, 2104–2112.
28. Lin, S.C.; Zhao, F.J.; Huang, W.D.; Shyu, G.S.; Yao, P.H.; Chang, T.K. The relationship between arsenic species in paddy soils and arsenic content of rice tissues at Guandu plain. *J. Taiwan Agric. Eng.* **2008**, *54*, 60–70.
29. Marbaniang, D.; Chaturvedi, S.S. Laboratory study of arsenic uptake and phytoremediation potential of three aquatic macrophytes of meghalaya, India. *Int. J. Sci. Technol. Res.* **2014**, *3*, 47–53.
30. Brunettia, G.; Farrag, K.; Rovirae, P.S.; Nigrof, F.; Senesia, N. Greenhouse and field studies on Cr, Cu, Pb and Zn phytoextraction by *Brassica napus* from contaminated soils in the Apulia region, Southern Italy. *Geoderma* **2011**, *160*, 517–523. [CrossRef]
31. Wittersa, N.; Mendelsohnb, R.; Van Passela, S.; Van Slyckenc, S.; Weyensa, N.; Schreursa, E.; Meersc, E.; Tackc, F.; Vanheusdena, B.; Vangronsveld, J. Phytoremediation, a sustainable remediation technology? II: Economic assessment of CO_2 abatement through the use of phytoremediation crops for renewable energy production. *Biomass Bioenergy* **2012**, *39*, 470–477. [CrossRef]
32. Meers, E.; Slycken, S.V.; Adriaenseb, K.; Ruttens, A.; Vangronsveld, J.; Laing, G.D.; Witters, N.; Thewys, T.; Tack, F.M.G. The use of bio-energy crops (*Zea mays*) for 'phytoattenuation' of heavy metals on moderately contaminated soils: A field experiment. *Chemosphere* **2010**, *78*, 35–41. [CrossRef]
33. Mi, Y.H.; Lei, M.; Li, Q.W.; Chen, L.; Du, L.J.; Deng, X.X.; Yang, X.K.; Zhang, W.B. Phytoremediation and human health risk of farmland polluted by heavy metal in Southern Yunnan Mining Area. *Ecol. Environ.* **2016**, *25*, 864–871.
34. Lukacova, Z.; Svubova, R.; Selvekova, P.; Hensel, K. The effect of plasma activated water on Maize (*Zea mays* L.) under arsenic stress. *Plants* **2021**, *10*, 1899. [CrossRef] [PubMed]

35. Cheng, S.S.; Huang, C.Y.; Lin, Y.C.; Lin, S.C.; Chen, K.L. Phytoremediation of lead using corn in contaminated agricultural land—An in situ study and benefit assessment. *Ecotoxicol. Environ. Saf.* **2015**, *111*, 72–77. [CrossRef] [PubMed]
36. Wenzel, W.W.; Kirchbaumer, N.; Prohaska, T.; Stingeder, G.; Lombi, E.; Adriano, D.C. Arsenic fractionation in soils using an improved sequential extraction procedure. *Anal. Chim. Acta* **2001**, *436*, 309–323. [CrossRef]

engineering proceedings

Proceeding Paper

Information Technology-Integrated Curriculum and Distance Learning During COVID-19 Pandemic in Preschool †

Yu-Fang Huang and Poh-Hwa Liang *

Department of Early Childhood Development and Education, Chaoyang University of Technology, Taichung 413310, Taiwan; yufang19990519@gmail.com
* Correspondence: phliang@cyut.edu.tw

† Presented at the 2024 IEEE 4th International Conference on Electronic Communications, Internet of Things and Big Data, Taipei, Taiwan, 19–21 April 2024.

Abstract: This study aims to investigate how preschool teachers integrated information technology into the curriculum before the pandemic and implemented distance education during the pandemic in Taiwan. We used a qualitative research method in which four preschool teachers and four parents participated. The following research results are presented: (1) preschool teachers' implementation of the information technology-integrated curriculum before the pandemic, (2) preschool teachers' implementation of distance education during the pandemic, and (3) parents' views on the implementation of the information technology-integrated curriculum and distance learning.

Keywords: distance learning; information technology integrated curriculum; preschool curriculum

Citation: Huang, Y.-F.; Liang, P.-H. Information Technology-Integrated Curriculum and Distance Learning During COVID-19 Pandemic in Preschool. *Eng. Proc.* **2024**, *74*, 9. https://doi.org/10.3390/engproc2024074009

Academic Editors: Shu-Han Liao, Teen-Hang Meen and Cheng-Fu Yang

Published: 27 August 2024

1. Introduction

With the rapid development of information technology, teachers leverage information technology and media to assist in preparing teaching materials, collecting resources before classes, and exploring learning opportunities with children. During the global COVID-19 pandemic, in-person teaching was impractical, necessitating a shift to distance learning. To curb the spread of the COVID-19 pandemic in schools, the Ministry of Education in Taiwan recommended preventive leave from educational institutions [1]. They advised implementing measures such as suspending physical classes and transitioning to distance learning, following the recommendations of the Central Pandemic Command Center for Severe Special Infectious Pneumonia. The Ministry also formulated the "Implementation Standards for Adjusting Teaching Methods on Campus in Response to the Severe Special Infectious Pneumonia (COVID-19) Pandemic" to ensure that students maintain their right to learn during these challenging times [2].

We investigated the activities related to the information technology-integrated curriculum before the pandemic and those that teachers designed for distance education in preschools during the pandemic. Additionally, we explored parents' views on the implementation of the information technology-integrated curriculum and distance education in preschools. We researched (1) how preschool teachers implemented the information technology-integrated curriculum before the pandemic, (2) what challenges preschool teachers faced regarding implementing the information technology-integrated curriculum, and (3) what parents' views and roles were regarding the curriculum and distance learning.

2. Information Technology-Integrated Curriculum, Distance Learning, and Teachers' Roles in Preschool

The National Association for the Education of Young Children (NAEYC) and Fred Rogers Center published a position statement, addressing that technology can provide young children with opportunities for cognitive, social, emotional, physical, and language development. The statement emphasizes the appropriate use of technology and interactive media in the classroom to enhance and expand children's learning experiences [3]. Integrating information technology and media into teaching activities fosters a positive attitude toward children's learning. Integrating information technology into learning activities enhances children's social skills and supports their collaboration in learning [4].

Distance learning involves the use of information technology and media for conducting teaching activities, with teaching and learning occurring in different settings [5]. The implementation methods of distance learning include: (1) Synchronous learning: Teachers and students are online simultaneously, allowing for real-time interaction; (2) Asynchronous learning: Teachers upload teaching materials, videos, and others to the online platform in advance, allowing students to access them at their convenience without the need to be online simultaneously with teachers; and (3) Blended (Hybrid) learning: This teaching mode combines synchronous and asynchronous learning activities [1,6–8].

3. Parents' Views on Curriculum and Distance Learning for Young Children

Parents' positive views of the integration of information technology and media into teaching activities support the implementation of information technology integration in teaching at the preschool level [9]. On the contrary, several parents prefer traditional teaching and cannot fully accept the information technology-integrated curriculum [10]. Parents' views on distance learning vary. Several parents believe that it can enhance learning when properly arranged and used [11]. Conversely, it was believed that distance learning may have adverse effects on the physical and psychological development of young children [12,13]. Distance learning is a concern for children's development because most parents are in dual-income families in Taiwan. Parents have their jobs and cannot assist their children in learning. Since preschool children cannot learn independently, it is not appropriate to use distance learning at the early childhood stage [14].

4. Method

We conducted interviews in the qualitative research methodology. Semi-structured interviews with guided and open-ended questions were performed. Through these interviews, preschool teachers implemented the information technology-integrated curriculum and distance learning, while parents shared their perspectives on these aspects. Before the interviews, we predetermined the interview outline based on the research questions. The interviews were carried out with open-ended questions. The content of the interviews was adjusted for the order and quantity of questions in real time, ensuring that the researchers could gather valuable and objectively reasonable information.

4.1. Participants

We invited four preschool teachers and four parents to participate, and the teachers' backgrounds are illustrated in Table 1. Two teachers were from public preschools, while the others were from private preschools. Additionally, the parents of children enrolled in these preschools were interviewed, and their background information is illustrated in Table 2.

Table 1. Teachers' backgrounds.

Code	Education Level	Teaching Experience	Type of Preschool	Type of Distance Learning
T1	College	10 years	private	asynchronous learning
T2	College	6 years	private	blended (hybrid) learning
T3	Master	5 years	public	asynchronous learning
T4	Master	25 years	public	asynchronous learning

Table 2. Parents' backgrounds.

Code	Education Level	Children's Age	Children's Teacher	Main Facilitator
P1	College	5 years old	T1	Mother
P2	Junior College	4 years old	T2	Mother
P3	College	6 years old	T3	Mother
P4	Master	5 years old	T4	Mother

4.2. Data Analysis and Verification

The collected data were coded as a verbatim manuscript in open, axial, and selective coding for subsequent data analysis [15]. In open coding, factors influencing the implementation of distance learning were explored for teachers, children, parents, and the environment. After analyzing and classifying the content, general categories were described. In axial coding, we analyzed the data to identify correlations according to the categories of open coding. We classified the data according to the research questions. The factors influencing the implementation of distance teaching in preschools were divided into four levels: teacher level, child level, parent level, and environmental level. Relevant factors were subdivided into categories, such as information technology and media equipment, and teaching course activity design at the teacher level. In selective coding, we analyzed the data based on the results of open coding and axial coding in each category. Data were compared to present the context and significance of the research questions.

In order to ensure the credibility and accuracy of the research data, we reviewed detailed records of information, expert inspection, participant verification, and peer verification. These methods were employed to enhance the reliability of this research and ensure the accuracy, authenticity, and completeness of the research data.

5. Results

We analyzed the results from the following three aspects: (1) preschool teachers' implementation of the information technology-integrated curriculum before the pandemic, (2) preschool teachers' implementation of distance education during the pandemic, (3) parents' views on the implementation of the information technology-integrated curriculum and distance learning.

5.1. Implementation of the Information Technology-Integrated Curriculum Before the Pandemic

The implementation of the information technology-integrated curriculum before the pandemic was carried out in three phases: teaching preparation (pre-activity), teaching process (during activity), and post-teaching. In the preparation phase, teachers created teaching resources. In the teaching process, they used technology to support activities, complement and enhance children's learning experiences, record their progress, provide interactive teaching activities, and offer information technology and media resources for learning corners. In the post-teaching phase, integrated learning activities and learning assessments took place. The three phases of implementation for the four teachers are presented in Table 3.

Teachers regarded their role in implementing information technology integration into teaching as a facilitator, guide, demonstrator, observer, evaluator, information integrator (scaffold), and presenter. The challenges for teachers in the curriculum activities included their ability to use technologies, the availability of information technology equipment resources, and factors related to the teaching environment.

Table 3. Three phases of the information technology-integrated curriculum before the pandemic.

Phases of Implementation	Teaching Activities	T1	T2	T3	T4
Teaching Preparation	create teaching resources		◎		◎
Teaching Process	support activities	◎		◎	◎
	complement and enhance children's learning experiences	◎			◎
	record children's progress	◎		◎	
	provide interactive teaching activities	◎		◎	
	offer information technology and media resources for learning corners		◎	◎	◎
Post-Teaching	integrate learning activities				◎
	assess children's learning			◎	

Note. ◎ Indicates teachers' implementation of information-integrated activities.

5.2. Implementation of the Information Technology-Integrated Curriculum During the Pandemic

During the pandemic, teaching in preschools changed to remote teaching, encompassing asynchronous learning and blended (hybrid) learning. Distance learning content is categorized into asynchronous course content (covering teaching activities across the six major learning areas, special courses, and teaching material resource packs) and synchronous course content (involving thematic learning activities, learning corners, children's song teaching, interactive games, and group discussions). The contents of distance learning are presented in Table 4.

Table 4. Contents of distance learning.

Type of Distance Learning	Teacher	Asynchronous Course Content			Synchronous Course Content
		Teaching Activities Across the Six Major Learning Areas	Special Courses	Teaching Material Resource Packs	Thematic Learning Activities, Learning Corners, and Group Discussions
Asynchronous learning	T1	◎	◎		
	T3	◎			
	T4	◎			
Blended (Hybrid) learning	T2	◎		◎	◎

Note. ◎ Indicates teachers' implementation of distance learning.

Teachers play various roles in distance learning activities, acting as behind-the-scenes curriculum developers, messengers, demonstrators, facilitators, and caregivers. Among the four teachers mentioned, the factors influencing their implementation of distance learning are categorized into teacher-level, child-level, parent-level, and environmental-level. Teacher-level influencing factors included information technology and media equipment considerations, and the design of teaching curriculum activities. At the child level, factors influencing teachers' implementation of distance learning activities involved children's learning situations, their inability to independently use information technology and media tools, and their interaction with peers. Influencing factors at the parent level encompassed parents' factors, the presence of other family members, and information technology equipment at home. Environmental factors included considerations such as the exclusion of young children's play areas at home or other locations.

5.3. Parents' Views on the Curriculum and Distance Learning

Positive parental views on the curriculum in preschools encompassed appropriate time management, the use of suitable information technology and media, and teaching activities to support teachers. Parental perspectives on the implementation of distance learning in preschools involved considerations of appropriate timing and activity scheduling, the suitability of asynchronous learning in preschool settings, and the complementary role of technology in the physical curriculum. A negative view included less appropriate synchronous teaching in preschools and appropriate physical courses for children. In distance learning activities, parents took on the roles of companions, teaching assistants, observers, recorders of children's learning outcomes, and time controllers (Table 5). Challenges of remote learning for parents included the need to assist with the implementation of remote learning activities, the time-intensive nature of supporting young children, the increased educational responsibilities, and the potential impact on other family members.

Table 5. Parents' roles in children's distance learning.

Parents' Roles	P1	P2	P3	P4
companions	◎			
teaching assistants		◎	◎	◎
observers		◎		
recorders of children's learning outcomes	◎		◎	◎
time controllers				◎

Note. ◎ Indicates the roles that parents take on in their children's distance learning.

6. Discussion and Conclusions

The research results showed that most teachers focused on operating information technology and media tools in the implementation of integration in each phase and provided children with fewer opportunities to freely explore information technology and media in their learning. However, several teachers evaluated whether the information technology and media tools as well as the content of learning activities were appropriate. They adjusted the content for subsequent courses if the activities did not meet the learning objectives designed by teachers. Such an approach complies with the recommendations provided by NAEYC and Fred Rogers Center [3].

Parents believed that the integration of information technology into teaching helped teachers implement courses. With the assistance of information technology and media, teachers provided children with more diverse and enriched learning content. Parents believed that the integration of information technology into the curriculum motivated children, enhanced their interest in learning, and improved their learning outcomes. The finding is consistent with the previous study showing that parents supported the implementation of the curriculum of the preschool [9].

However, the results indicated differences between the information technology-integrated curriculum and distance education during the COVID-19 period. For instance, when information technology is integrated into the curriculum, teachers use tools to record children's learning activities through photos or videos. In contrast, in distance learning activities, teachers found it challenging to capture these moments themselves. Therefore, teachers cooperated with parents to record children's learning and asked them to transmit it back to teachers through information technology and media. If parents do not accompany their children in distance learning or fail to transmit the learning outcome back to teachers, it becomes difficult for teachers to understand the learning situation of children in distance education. Parents believed that the curriculum was more appropriate for children in preschools for physical teaching. No matter whether teachers implement synchronous or asynchronous teaching, it is difficult for them to grasp the learning situation of each child. In addition, children's spoken language development is affected by distance education. This result is similar to previous studies in that parents believed that it was less appropriate for young children to regard distance learning because they cared for the development and learning of their children [11,14].

Author Contributions: Both authors contributed equally to this work. All authors have read and agreed to the published version of the manuscript.

Funding: This research received no external funding.

Institutional Review Board Statement: Not applicable.

Informed Consent Statement: Informed consent was obtained from all subjects involved in the study.

Data Availability Statement: The data presented in this study are available on request from the corresponding author.

Conflicts of Interest: The authors declare no conflict of interest.

References

1. Ministry of Education. *National Reference Guidelines for Online Learning at Home for Students in Senior High Schools and Below*; (enacted on 21 June 2021, revised on 10 May 2022). Available online: https://elearning.cloud.edu.tw/onlinelearning/file_download/%E5%85%A8%E5%9C%8B%E9%AB%98%E7%B4%9A%E4%B8%AD%E7%AD%89%E4%BB%A5%E4%B8%8B%E5%AD%B8%E6%A0%A1%E5%AD%B8%E7%94%9F%E5%B1%85%E5%AE%B6%E7%B7%9A%E4%B8%8A%E5%AD%B8%E7%BF%92%E5%8F%83%E8%80%83%E6%8C%87%E5%BC%95(%E4%BF%AE%E6%AD%A33%E7%89%88-%E6%AD%A3%E5%BC%8F).pdf (accessed on 1 December 2022).
2. Ministry of Education. Implementation Standards for Campus Adjustments to Teaching Methods in Response to the "Severe Special Infectious Pneumonia" (COVID-19) Pandemic. (announced on 19 February 2020, revised on 28 May 2022). 2022. Available online: https://cpd.moe.gov.tw/page_two.php?id=34015 (accessed on 8 December 2022).
3. NAEYC & Fred Rogers Center. Technology and Interactive Media as Tools in Early Childhood Programs Serving Children from Birth through Age 8. 2012. Available online: http://www.naeyc.org/files/naeyc/file/positions/PS_technology_WEB2.pdf (accessed on 15 August 2022).
4. Hyun, E. A study of 5-to 6-year-old children's peer dynamics and dialectical learning in a computer-based technology-rich classroom environment. *Comput. Educ.* **2005**, *44*, 69–91. [CrossRef]
5. Moore, M.G.; Kearsley, G. *Distance Education: A Systems View of Online Learning*, 3rd ed.; Wadsworth: Belmont, MA, USA, 2012.
6. Sun, A.; Chen, X. Online education and its effective practice: A research review. *J. Inf. Technol. Educ. Res.* **2016**, *15*, 157–190. [CrossRef] [PubMed]
7. *International Association for K-12 Online Learning, The Online Learning Definitions Project*; International Association for K-12 Online Learning (iNACOL): Vienna, Austria, 2011.
8. Smaldino, S.E.; Lowther, D.L.; Russell, J.D.; Mims, C. *Instructional Technology and Media for Learning*, 9th ed.; Pearson Merrill/Prentice Hall: Hoboken, NJ, USA, 2008.
9. Gjelaj, M.; Buza, K.; Shatri, K.; Zabeli, N. Digital technologies in early childhood: Attitudes and practices of parents and teachers in Kosovo. *Int. J. Instr.* **2020**, *13*, 165–184. [CrossRef]
10. Zhu, S.; Yang, H.H.; MacLeod, J.; Shi, Y.; Wu, D. Parents' and students' attitudes toward tablet integration in schools. *Int. Rev. Res. Open Distrib. Learn.* **2018**, *19*, 222–241. [CrossRef]
11. Fontenelle-Tereshchuk, D. Homeschooling' and the COVID-19 crisis: The insights of parents on curriculum and remote learning. *Interchange* **2021**, *52*, 167–191. [CrossRef] [PubMed]
12. Ben-Amram, M.; Davidovitch, N. School and home as study spaces: Attitudes of preschool educators, parents, and students to e-learning during the COVID-19 period: The case of Israel. *Int. J. Educ. Methodol.* **2021**, *7*, 717–731. [CrossRef]
13. Lau, E.Y.; Lee, K. Parents' views on children's distance learning and screen time during COVID-19 class suspension in Hong Kong. *Early Educ. Dev.* **2021**, *32*, 863–880. [CrossRef]
14. Stites, M.L.; Sonneschein, S.; Galczyk, S.H. Preschool parents' views of distance learning during COVID-19. *Early Educ. Dev.* **2021**, *32*, 923–939. [CrossRef]
15. Corbin, J.; Strauss, A. *Basics of Qualitative Research: Techniques and Procedures for Developing Grounded Theory*, 3rd ed.; SAGE: Newbury Park, CA, USA, 2008.

engineering proceedings

MDPI

Proceeding Paper

Two Faces of Grassland: A Comparative Study on the Impact of Tourism Development Model on Grassland Environment †

Jing Wang and Shu-Chen Tsai *

Department of Environmental Design, College of Arts and Design, Jimei University, Xiamen 361021, China; wangjing@jmu.edu.cn

* Correspondence: tsaishuchen@jmu.edu.cn

† Presented at the 2024 IEEE 4th International Conference on Electronic Communications, Internet of Things and Big Data, Taipei, Taiwan, 19–21 April 2024.

Abstract: With the boom in outdoor recreational activities in Inner Mongolia, grassland protection has become significant, but the impact of different tourism models on the grassland environment has received little attention. The purpose of this study was to explain the impact of different tourism development models on the grassland environment from a local perspective through small-scale case studies. We took two types of grasslands as objects: the scenic grassland led by developers and the natural grassland led by herdsmen. The study results showed the following: (1) there are four types of tourism development models in the research area; (2) three factors that affect model development are physical geography, seasonality, and policy; and (3) herders emphasized the risks of grassland under climate change. Finally, the main factor that divides the grassland into two appearances is the formalization of tourism content. The concentration of livestock impacts the tourism model. The optimized tourism model was small-scale grassland ecotourism, which best integrated culture and development potential.

Keywords: case study; local perspective; cultural landscape; ecotourism; Inner Mongolia

Citation: Wang, J.; Tsai, S.-C. Two Faces of Grassland: A Comparative Study on the Impact of Tourism Development Model on Grassland Environment. *Eng. Proc.* **2024**, *74*, 10. https://doi.org/10.3390/engproc2024074010

Academic Editors: Shu-Han Liao, Teen-Hang Meen and Cheng-Fu Yang

Published: 27 August 2024

1. Introduction

In the definition of cultural landscape, grassland and its human ecosystem have become valuable world heritage [1]. Grassland is one of the most iconic, flagship, and commercialized tourism products in Mongolia, and the combination of grassland, nomads, cattle, sheep, and yurts is an attractive cultural landscape [2]. The Mongolian grassland has a long history. It is an important cultural belt bridging Europe and Asia and also a geographical area that regulates the climate in the north and south of Mongolia. The nomadic life of the horse-riding nomads on the Mongolian grasslands has a history of nearly 5,000 years. The drying of the grasslands caused by climate warming and the development of horse-riding technology are important in the formation of nomadic culture [3,4]. The interaction between horse-riding nomads and settled civilizations has promoted historical evolution. However, due to the lack of written records of nomads, most descriptions are made from the perspective of settled civilization. For example, the historian Sima Chian (109 to 91 BC) of the Han dynasty wrote "Historical Records" and the biography of the Xiongnu (means horse-riding nomads) records that they migrated in search of water and grass, did not build permanent castles, and did not engage in farming [5].

The foreign cultures described by historians have exaggerated the legends and imaginations of horse-riding nomads. Thousands of years of accumulated curiosity have made settled civilizations want to explore the mystery of nomads. Therefore, nomads have become a tourist attraction for settled societies.

According to statistics, the number of foreign tourists entering Inner Mongolia has increased every year since 1999, and by 2019, it exceeded 1.85 million, which was five times more than the number in 1999 (Figure 1). In the first five days of China's Golden Week in 2023, Inner Mongolia received 14.5343 million domestic tourists, 1.29 times more than that of the same period in 2019, and tourism revenue reached 9.933 billion yuan (RMB), 1.12 times that of 2019 [6].

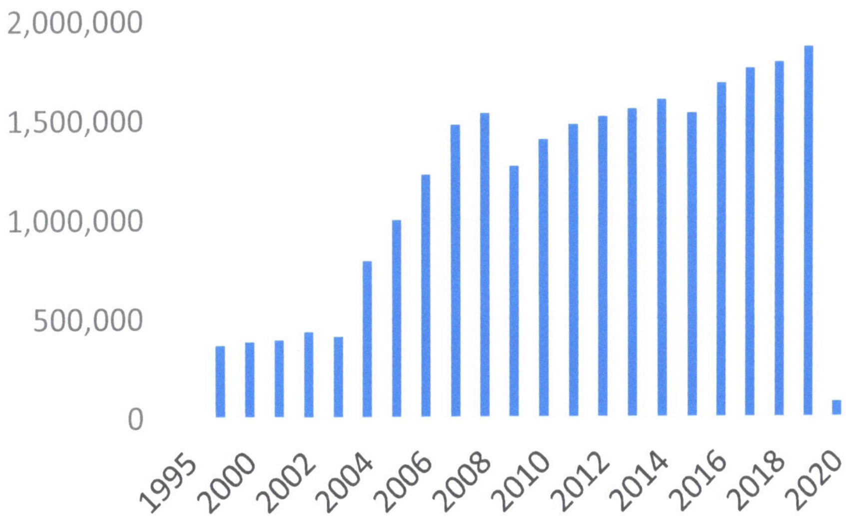

Figure 1. Number of inbound foreigners (including foreign Chinese) tourists (person-time).

Overgrazing is an early cause of grassland decline [7]. However, the development of tourism in Inner Mongolia's grasslands had already made social and environmental impacts in 1999 [8]. Factors such as climate and socioeconomic structure have caused ecosystem degradation [9,10]. Research has pointed out that there is an imbalance between tourism demand and tourism destination protection [11]. The spatial correlation effect of tourism eco-efficiency in Inner Mongolia decreased from 2009 to 2019, and the differences among cities were large, indicating that spatial heterogeneity contains important influencing factors [12]. In particular, grassland has high ecological environmental vulnerability, and the spatiotemporal concentration of grassland tourism may exacerbate the vulnerability of grassland ecology [13]. Although the number of studies on grassland ecology in Inner Mongolia has grown exponentially in the past thirty years, effective strategies have still not been proposed to protect biodiversity, ecosystem functions and ecosystem services [9].

This study used CiteSpace to analyze research topics (Figure 2). Bibliometric analysis of publications from 2015 to 2023 was conducted in the Web of Science, a core social science database with indices of the subject "Inner Mongolia" and "steppes" (on 29 November 2023). Through manual search, we found 439 papers involving "Inner Mongolia", "steppes", "ecotourism", "cultural landscape", "case study", and "local perspective". Frequently appearing keywords were "climate change", "ecosystem services", "vegetation", "management", "impacts", and "dynamics". Most of the research focused on grassland ecology and ecological protection and the development models to promote tourism performance [14,15]. A few studies have proposed the topic of using ecotourism to deal with environmental protection based on the conditions of over-exploitation, environmental imbalance, and pollution [11,16,17].

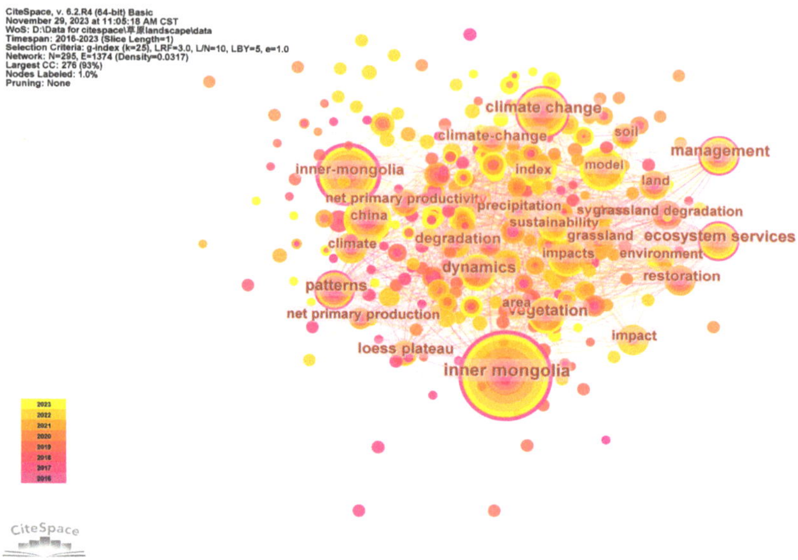

Figure 2. Analysis of related topics related to this study.

Previous large-scale spatial studies on Inner Mongolia pointed out the overall problems, strategies of grasslands, and the environmental decline of grasslands. Different types of grassland development models inevitably affect changes in the grassland environment. All previous research results show the perspective of development and policy, although several studies proposed local participation [14,17]. However, there are no studies that have discussed the development of the grassland environment from the perspective of local herdsmen. The current discussion of tourism development in Inner Mongolia lacks the voices of local herdsmen. Herdsmen are the main users and managers of grasslands, and environmental issues in grasslands need to be dealt with from local perspectives. Therefore, the purpose of this study was to explain the impact of different tourism development models on the grassland environment from the perspective of herders.

2. Methodology

2.1. Method and Materials

The research methods used in this study included case study, text analysis and geospatial information analysis. Through purposive sampling, the Xilingele League, which has rich grassland resources and was developed earlier, and the Baotou City Darhan Muminggan United Banner (hereinafter referred to as Damao Banner), which has relatively slow development and degraded grassland, were selected as the research area. In-depth interviews were conducted to collect the experiences and opinions of local herders, local residents and tourists on tourism development, a total of five samples (Table 1). The interview was conducted from October 2023 to December 2023. In-depth interview data were used for text analysis, and the analysis results were used to explain the pattern and impact of grassland tourism development. Arc MAP 10.2 was used as a spatial data analysis tool. The main data included the 2000 grassland resource map and the 2005 soil type map. In this study, in-depth interviews with local herders, tourists and others were conducted to obtain text materials. The reliability and validity of this study are verified by three kinds of data: oral verbatim draft, literature, and spatial data.

Table 1. Summary and Coding of Interview Samples.

No.	Code	Background and Interview Summary
1	M-1 (Ages 35)	He is Mongolian and lives in the Xilingele League. His family has always been engaged in animal husbandry, and his main job now is also herding and selling horses, cattle and sheep. Most of his family and friends around him are still engaged in animal husbandry. There are also a few friends who are engaged in family-run tourism. He describes the climate as the main reason why the grassland ecosystem is difficult to recover. In recent years, there has been less precipitation, which has made it difficult for the grasslands to recover. He has a positive attitude toward the development of tourism, which he believes can be a good driver of the economy. However, he is skeptical that tourism can promote the ecological recovery of grasslands. As for the comparison between the tourism industry run by herdsmen and the tourist attractions invested by developers, he thinks that the family-oriented ones are closer to the herdsmen's life and the food quality is higher, while the scenic ones have a more beautiful environment and better facilities, but they are not close enough to the life of the Mongolian people.
2	F-1 (Ages 25)	She is a local of Inner Mongolia but not a traditional nomad living in an urban area. She has traveled to different grassland sites. She thinks the main reason why the grassland environment is difficult to recover is overgrazing on the one hand and climate problems on the other. The grassland she traveled to is in Damao Banner, and she believes that the grassland in Damao Banner is severely degraded compared to the Xilingele League. The main reasons are: 1. Damao Banner's geographic location is not as favorable as Xilingele's, and Xilingele's pasture attributes belong to the meadow grassland, with more rainfall and rivers and lakes; and 2. Damao Banner's demand for mutton is great, and Damao's mutton has a greater reputation, so it is more dependent on grazing, and the overgrazing situation is even more serious; in the comparison between herders' self-owned tourism industry and the tourist attractions invested by the developers, she similarly thinks that the scenic spots are better equipped, and the environment is more beautiful. In the comparison between herder-owned tourism and developer-invested tourist attractions, she also thinks that the scenic spots are well-equipped and have more beautiful environments, but the quality of the food is better.
3	M-2 (Ages 65+)	He is a native of Erdos, Inner Mongolia, and is almost 70 years old. His ancestors relied on grazing for their livelihood. He believes that the most important factor affecting the grassland ecology is the climate. However, with the implementation of national policies such as the ban on grazing, the grassland ecology has improved to a large extent. For the grassland development of tourism, his attitude is that it will not destroy the ecology but also will not improve. He believes that only herders around large tourist attractions have the possibility of developing tourism because tourists are not willing to choose to go to more remote areas. Regarding the different types of tourism development, he believes that government-led large-scale tourist attractions are better because they have better facilities and a more beautiful environment, while family-oriented tourist areas such as the Shepherd's House do not have all the facilities and have fewer choices of activities to enjoy. As for the transmission of culture, he does not think that scenic programs will make the authenticity of culture lost. He said that people of the older generation are very grateful to the state; it is the state's policy to make people's lives better, and the environment has become better.
4	F-2 (Ages 33)	She is from Hohhot and has only been to the Ordos Grassland in August 2023. They chose to take a self-driving tour and visited the large scenic spots in Ordos. The attractions were chosen because of their proximity and the reputation of the scenic spots. The infrastructure in the scenic area is very good, and there are many experience programs, such as horseback riding, archery, sheep feeding, go-karting, skating and so on, but she thinks the most interesting thing is to take the children to contact with nature and take a lot of pictures of the children, which is very memorable. Although she did not witness any uncivilized behavior of tourists, she still thinks that the influx of tourists into grassland tourism for the grassland ecology will certainly have a negative impact.

Table 1. *Cont.*

No.	Code	Background and Interview Summary
5	F-3 (Ages 57)	She is a native of Henan Province and came to Baotou, Inner Mongolia, for business in 1998 and has lived in Baotou for over 20 years. She has been to many neighboring attractions. One of her deepest impressions is that in August 2003, she was invited by a friend to go to the grassland of Damao Banner, the hometown of the Little Sisters of the Grassland Heroes, Longmei and Yurong. She recalled that at that time, the grassland of Damao Banner was a piece of dry grass; they went to the local herdsman's house as a guest, listened to the story of Longmei and Yurong, and ate a lot of grassland food in the yurt. She has since traveled to many grasslands for fun. In 2018, Chunkun Mountain in Guyang County had a beautiful landscape with large swaths of green and grass growing so tall that it was soothing to look at and want to live there. She has also traveled to many grasslands for fun. She believes that the most important thing in grassland ecology is rainfall; without rain, grass in the grassland cannot grow.

Note: The age of the interviewees is the year according to the interview time. Based on the research ethics, the reporter uses the code name instead. Code F means female, and M means male.

2.2. Study Area

Xilingele League is located in the eastern part of the Inner Mongolia Autonomous Region between 110°50′–119°58′ east longitude and 41°30′–46°45′ north latitude. Xilingele is a Mongolian word meaning river [gele] on a ridge [xilin]. Meanwhile, it is one of the few well-preserved areas of the Inner Mongolia grassland region. The ecological environment of the Xilingele League is fragile, and the population is densely distributed. It is the area with the most tense relationship between man and land in the entire Mongolian Plateau [18]. The other case, Damao Banner, is located in the west of the Inner Mongolia Autonomous Region, with geographical coordinates between 09°16′–111°25′ E and 41°20′–42°40′ N. It covers seven towns with a total population of 120,000 [19]. Damao Banner is a border banner with Mongolians as the main body, Han as the majority, multi-ethnic groups living together, and mainly pastoralists (Figure 3).

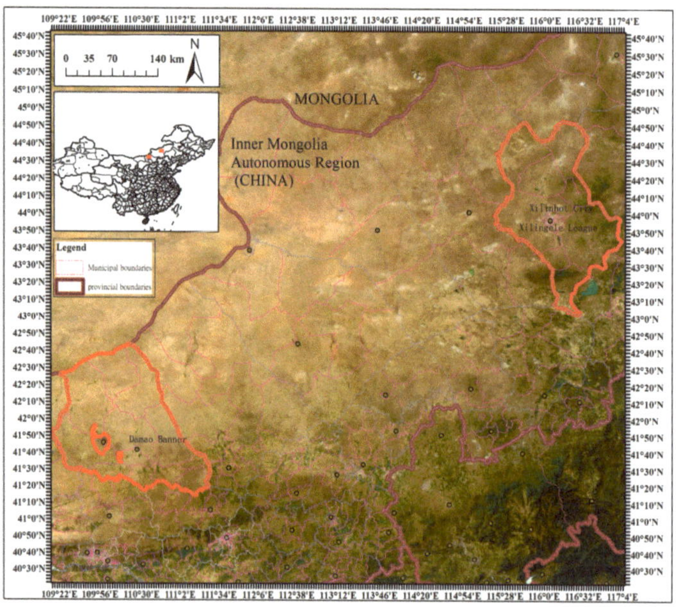

Figure 3. Study area.

3. Results

3.1. Grassland Tourism Development Model

3.1.1. Overview of Tourism Development in the Two Study Areas

Damao Banner is an artificial grassland with poor natural conditions. Herders are restricted by their economic conditions. Several herders operate grassland tourism without investing in facilities and projects. Therefore, the tourism types that can be developed are based on their conditions. However, tourists can experience the most primitive herders' life. This type of tourism development is characterized by high cultural quality and low economic capacity. The geographical conditions of Xilingele show better natural landscapes and historical monuments, which are most suitable for the development of tourism, such as Xilingele Jiuqu Bay and Xilingele Duolun Lake scenic area. However, these areas have often been discovered by people with "insightful" and "investment capabilities" and have been developed into relatively large-scale tourism development zones or national scenic areas with government approval. Their investment is increasing, their infrastructure is better, and tourists stay in hotels or semi-Mongolian yurts (made of bricks). This type of tourism development is characterized by high economic capital and low cultural quality.

3.1.2. Tourism Development Model

Through the text analysis of interviews, the development models of grassland tourism in the study area were divided into the following four models: Complete family tourism (the main income of the family comes from tourists), half pastoral/tourism (half of the family's income comes from tourists), developers investment and national scenic area. The four different tourism development models depend on the source of income and the grassland tourism activities they can provide to tourists (Table 2).

Table 2. Tourism Models and Corresponding Activities.

Model / Theme	Complete Family Tourism	Developer Investment	National Scenic Area	
Natural scenic sightseeing	√	√	√	√
Cultural heritage sightseeing	×	×	~	√
Nomadic traditional activities	~	~	√	√
Traditional nomadic culture	√	√	√	√
Non-traditional excursions	~	~	√	√
Mongolian cuisine	√	√	√	√
Accommodations	~	~	√	√

Note: supply or not. Yes: √; no: ×; conditional: ~.

Tourism activities in the grassland include natural scenery sightseeing (grassland scenery, rivers and lakes, etc.), cultural heritage sightseeing (palaces, temples, etc.), Nomadic traditional activities (such as Naadam Conference, bonfire parties, song and dance performances, etc.), experiencing traditional nomadic culture (horseback riding, archery, etc.) Wrestling, etc.), non-traditional activities (grass skiing, driving karts, jeeps, etc.), tasting Mongolian cuisine (grilled meat, roasted whole lamb, tripe meat, kumiss, etc.), and accommodation (hotel or yurt-like).

3.2. Factors Affecting Grassland Tourism Development Model

3.2.1. Physical Geographical Factors

Physical geographical conditions affect the differences in grassland tourism development, especially hydrology and soil factors (Table 3).

Table 3. Physical Geographical Factors of Two Study Areas.

Geo. Factor	Xilingele League	Damao Banner
Topography	The terrain slopes from southeast to northwest, and the terrain is mainly plains and low mountains and hills. Covers a lava tableland and has a relatively flat topography.	It is high in the south and low in the north, tilting from southwest to northeast. Hills and low mountain basins are staggered in distribution. The south is a hilly area; there are low mountains in the central and western parts, and the north is a plateau and platform.
Climate	temperate semi-arid climatic region. The climate is characterized by the alternation of dry summers and cold winters.	Mid-temperate semi-arid continental climate
Hydrology	high moisture and high temperature; The mean annual precipitation is between 250 and 350 mm. Without major rivers, the surface water system is poorly developed. Most of the lakes and ponds are salty or alkaline. Wells are a major watersource for people and domestic animals.	The average annual precipitation is 255.6 mm.
Soil (Figure 4)	soil type in this region is chestnut, an alkaline soil with low organic matter content (less than 4%), poor fertility, and a marked calcic horizon. Other soils include chernozem, meadow, and saline types.	The soil is mainly chestnut soil and brown soil, showing obvious zonal distribution, while meadow soil, fluvo-aquic soil, saline soil and stony soil are non-zonal soils.
Ecological (Figure 5)	Temperate typical grassland ecosystem	Temperate desert grassland ecosystem and temperate typical grassland ecosystem.

Note: The data are cited from [10,19].

The Xilingele League belongs temperate typical grassland ecosystem. In most years, up to 80% of the total precipitation falls from May to September, coinciding with the peak temperatures. This coincidence of high moisture and temperature favors the growth of plants; otherwise, accumulated snow is important for winter water use and for the regrowth of plants in spring [10]. High temperatures and abundant rainfall are conducive to plant growth, attracting tourists with the vast natural landscape of green grassland:

> *"Our place in Xilingele is originally a prairie area, so you have to grasp the mountains and rivers."* (Table 1, M-1).

The geographical location of Damao Banner is between a temperate desert grassland ecosystem and a temperate typical grassland ecosystem. Beginning in 1975, the Grassland Research Institute attempted to establish artificial grasslands in Damao Banner on the Wulanchabu Plateau. In the course of nine years, this project resulted in the creation of 807 hectares of artificial grassland [20]. Artificial grassland has ecological and economic functions. It regulates the climate and functions for grazing. Damao Banner has little rainfall and diverse soil types.

Although the conditions are not suitable for grassland growth, the saline-alkali soil contains trace elements, and the free-range sheep must find scarce grass and water sources in the saline-alkali land. Their tender meat attracts tourists. A tourism model of sharing meals with herdsmen was developed.

> *"I went to some herdsmen's houses and their roasted mutton was so delicious that you could eat it with your hands."* (Table 1, F-1).

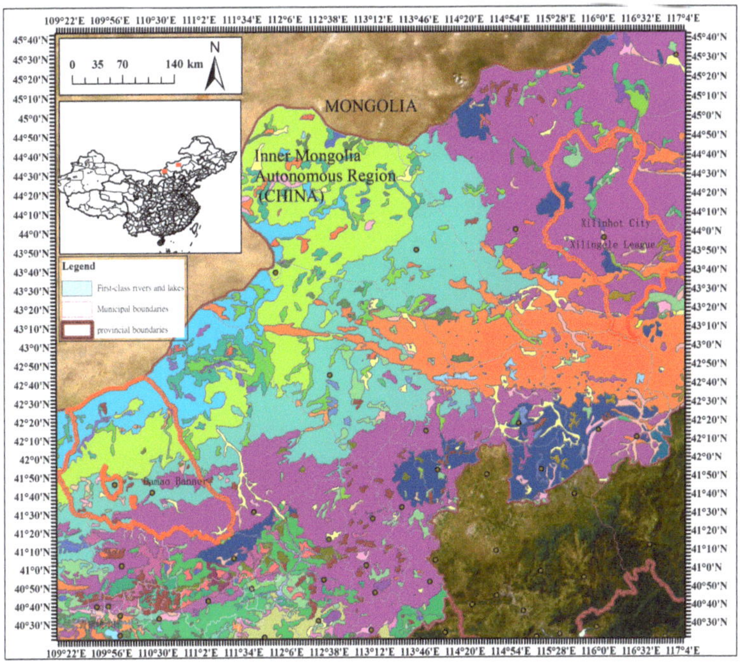

Figure 4. Soil type of study area.

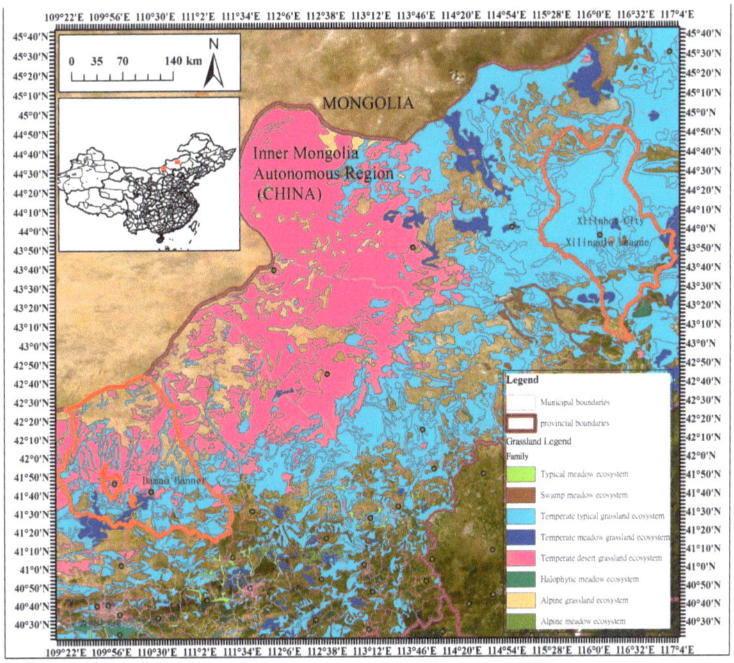

Figure 5. Grassland type of study area.

3.2.2. Seasonal Factors

Due to the cyclical characteristics of pasture growth, grassland tourism has two peak periods. The first peak is mostly concentrated between June and September when the grassland is at the end of the regreening period (returning to green, which refers to the transplantation of plant seedlings. After overwintering, it changes from yellow to green and resumes growth for a period of time), the grassland is the greenest, and the scenery is the most beautiful. From July to September, students have summer vacation, and most travel platforms and developers promote packages, so a large number of tourists enter Inner Mongolia during this period.

The second peak period is concentrated in the winter from December to February of the following year. The grassland is covered with snow. The other seasons of these two peak tourism periods are the greening period and the yellowing period of the grassland (Table 4). The prohibition of grazing during the greening period is a tacit agreement between herders and grasslands.

Table 4. Seasonal Characteristics of Grassland Tourism.

Month	4	5	6	7	8	9	10	11	12	1	2	3
Peak season for Grassland tourism												
Regreening period												
Withering period												
Grazing prohibited period												

"The Grazing prohibited period is from April 1st to July 1st every year" (Table 1, M-2).

3.2.3. Policy Factors

In 2005, China promulgated the Measures for the Balanced Management of Grassland and Livestock as a law that focuses on maintaining a virtuous cycle in the grassland ecosystem, effectively improving the ecological environment of the grassland, restoring the grassland to a certain extent, and alleviating the excessive demands of the livestock industry on the grassland.

> *"Yes, give subsidies! The so-called April 1st to July 1st is the Turn Green period of the grassland"* (Table 1, M-2).

However, the implementation of the grazing ban policy, grass-livestock balance and other policies have also reduced the family income of herdsmen, prompting families whose main income is livestock to find new sources of income. As a result, half-grazing and half-tourism have been formed, or the entire family is fully engaged in the tourism business:

> *"We often go to herdsmen's homes. The herdsmen's grasslands are their own grasslands or other people's grasslands (contracted). What he set up was nothing special, just a few yurts, a camel and a horse, and we went archery, horseback riding, and camel riding."* (Table 1, M-2).

The other is to benefit from the strong support and policy guarantees of the government. The government provides strong support for the development of grassland tourism. Capital investment from enterprises or developers has enabled the rapid development of grassland tourism.

3.3. Grassland Tourism Development and Protection: Pastoralists' Perspectives

Herdsmen have been sensitive to the climate change of drought and lack of rain in recent years, especially the delayed greening of grasslands. The livestock industry in the two study areas is the most direct bearer of changes in the grassland environment.

"In particular, grassland is not the same as humanistic architecture, which always be there, but grassland pays great attention to the months. It may be that the rain falls later this year, so it will become green later." (Table 1, F-1)

Although the development of grassland tourism has greatly promoted tourism income, it has not greatly promoted the restoration of the grassland environment for the following reasons:

1. *The area of grassland used for tourism development is limited, and even if it is protected, it is only protected in a very limited environment, with little effect* (Table 1, M-1).
2. *There is no causal relationship between the development of grassland tourism and environmental protection because developers only choose areas with beautiful environments and prosperous pastures to develop tourism rather than selecting grasslands with severe desertification for the purpose of restoring the grassland environment* (Table 1, F-1).
3. *The grassland environment is greatly affected by rain and temperature. In recent years, with the continuous decrease in rainfall, it has been difficult for the grassland to turn green* (Table 1, F-1).
4. *Developers' business behavior is aimed at seeking economic benefits. Therefore, if the quality of the grassland environment is not directly linked to the developers' economic benefits, they will not pay for it* (Table 1, M-1).

4. Discussion

4.1. "Formalization" Causing Differentiation in Grassland Tourism Development

Under the influence of "globalization", standardized consumer culture disappears or is homogenized into local traditional culture and is also replaced with regional identity and traditions [21]. The different cultures on the grasslands are the focus of contemporary tourism. However, tourism with sightseeing as the center stage caters to the needs of tourists [22]. At present, most tourists visit famous tourist attractions. Whether these tourist venues or routes led by developers display or sell local culture, they package the cultural festivals, historical sites and even daily lives of nomads in situations and images. Maximizing profits is the goal of every developer. They select projects with more economic value to retain, while those that are not cost-effective must be discarded. On the other hand, not all local customs can be consistent with tourism planning. Tourism practitioners need to consider tourists' perceptions and experiences. Therefore, local culture is often presented to tourists with a stage effect through certain artistic processing. The performances after artistic processing make the traditional culture of nomadic people more colorful, but at the same time, it also loses its authenticity. The total of the package itinerary may become a bitter nothingness [23].

However, there are also people who "do not take the usual path." They visit traditional herders' homes, see the beautiful scenery of the grasslands, eat the most traditional Mongolian meals, and experience the cultural life and production methods of the nomadic people. Conversations with local people who have experienced different values and generate more thoughts showed the following. *"I think it's still the kind that hasn't developed yet, and it might be closer, because once it develops, it will have some very formal things."* (Table 1, F-1)

"Visiting herdsmen's homes", a tourism concept, is different from the exquisite beauty of developers and the development model of grassland tourism. "No development" and "no formalization" may become the most authentic aspect of grassland tourism.

4.2. Impact of Grassland Tourism Model on Environment

The development of tourism can preserve the culture or relics that are about to disappear, but the commercialization of culture causes the culture to lose its intrinsic meaning and weaken the importance of culture to the local people [24]. The developer's investment encourages the package of the commercialized tourism model, which directly affects the selection and refinement of traditional culture in line with the preferences of the wider public but causes unforeseen environmental problems. For example, horse-riding activity causes conflicts between the physiological characteristics of horses and the demand of the tourism business [17]. Pollution by waste and the disappearance of animals on the grasslands are observed by herdsmen. It is impossible to distinguish which tourism model has caused it, but the influx of tourists changes the grassland environment.

> *"There are no trash cans or garbage recycling on the grassland. It just decomposes naturally and no one handles it at all."* (Table 1, F-1)

> *"You see, for example, there may still be wolves in Xilingele, but now there are basically none in Damao Banner, and it is no longer suitable for them to survive."* (Table 1, F-1)

Because the herders lack the knowledge and skills to develop ecotourism, they do not understand their own value and the role they should play. This study holds that guiding herders to develop small-scale family tourism mode can not only help herders increase their income and promote the spread of grassland culture but also disperse the phenomenon of a large number of tourists concentrated in time and space in scenic spots, thus promoting the sustainable development of grassland ecological environment.

4.3. Optimizing Development Model

The development of tourism has undoubtedly promoted the development of the grassland economy. Scenic spot sightseeing, cultural experiences, accommodation, food, specialties and related cultural and creative products all promote economic circulation. Tourists have started a series of consumption in traveling. However, herdsmen want to develop the economy in a suitable way and still rely on the development of animal husbandry to obtain income. How to guide herders for appropriate grassland development with more benefits is an important issue. The development of small-scale grassland ecotourism closer to the lifestyle of nomadic people is the direction to optimize the grassland tourism model with great development potential.

5. Conclusions

From the perspective of herdsmen and tourists, this paper discusses how to promote the sustainable development of grassland through tourism. It is found that terrain, climate, hydrology, soil and ecology have caused the two appearances of grassland ecological environment and tourism mode. The results show that herdsmen have a positive attitude toward the economic benefits of developing grassland tourism but do not recognize that tourism will promote grassland ecological protection. At present, the existing grassland tourism modes are mainly large-scale commercial tourism dominated by developers and small-scale original pristine tourism dominated by herdsmen families. Now, the grassland tourism model must be optimized. Developers need to mitigate commercialization, promote grassland culture to a greater extent, reproduce grassland production and lifestyle, and provide tourists with a richer experience. Developers and herdsmen should pay more attention to the ecological protection of grasslands. Only in this way can we better promote the sustainable development of grassland culture, economy and ecology. This study highlights the protective effect of small-scale ecotourism on the grassland environment, which can not only make up for the defects of homogenization of tourist attractions by developers but also promote the restoration and protection of grassland.

Author Contributions: Conceptualization, S.-C.T.; methodology, S.-C.T.; software, S.-C.T. and J.W.; validation, S.-C.T. and J.W.; formal analysis, J.W. and S.-C.T.; investigation, J.W.; resources, J.W. and S.-C.T.; data curation, J.W. and S.-C.T.; writing—original draft preparation, J.W.; writing—review and editing, S.-C.T.; visualization, S.-C.T.; supervision, S.-C.T. All authors have read and agreed to the published version of the manuscript.

Funding: This research was funded by the scientific research start-up fund of Jimei University, China, grant number Q202214.

Institutional Review Board Statement: This study was approved by the Science and Technology Ethics Committee at Jimei University (JMU202307039). No harm was caused to the participants during the study.

Informed Consent Statement: Informed consent was obtained from all subjects involved in the study.

Data Availability Statement: The data of this study are available from the corresponding author upon reasonable request.

Acknowledgments: The study benefited from all respondents, including herders, tourists, etc. Thanks to everyone who worked on this study. All deficiencies in the article are the responsibility of the authors.

Conflicts of Interest: The authors declare no conflicts of interest.

References

1. UNESCO. Cultural Landscapes in the 21st Century: Tourism and Economics. In Proceedings of the Forum UNESCO 10th International Seminar, University of Newcastle, Upon Tyne, UK, 11–16 April 2005.
2. Buckley, R.; Ollenburg, C.; Zhong, L. Cultural landscape in Mongolian tourism. *Ann. Tour. Res.* **2008**, *35*, 47–61. [CrossRef]
3. Tsai, W. *From Marco Polo to Macartney: Inner Asia and China since the Mongol Era*; Gūsa Press: New Taipei City, Taiwan, 2020.
4. Hayashi, T. *The Birth of Steppe Kingship: Scythia and the Huns, the Civilization of Early Nomadic Countries*; Gūsa Press: New Taipei City, Taiwan, 2019.
5. Sima, C. Xiongnu records. In *Historical Records*; Chung Hwa Book Company (Hong Kong) Limited: Hong Kong, China, 2011.
6. Yang, C.-A. China's Golden Week: Inner Mongolia's Revenue Increases Sixfold This Year. *Business Times*, 10 June 2023.
7. Jiang, Y. Investigation of herbage resources and collection of materials on typical regions of the tropical, subtropical and temperate grasslands of China. *Compil. Sci. Results* **1988**, *3*, 1–5.
8. Wei, Z.; Yang, J.; Han, G. The Management of Rangeland for Tourism. *Inn. Mong. Grassl. Ind.* **1999**, *3*, 34–37. (In Chinese)
9. Wu, J.; Zhang, Q.; Li, A.; Liang, C. Historical landscape dynamics of Inner Mongolia: Patterns, drivers, and impacts. *Landsc. Ecol.* **2015**, *30*, 1579–1598. [CrossRef]
10. Wu, J.G.; OL, L. The Xilingol grassland. In *Grasslands and Grassland Sciences in Northern China*; National Research Council, Ed.; National Academy Press: Washington, DC, USA, 1992; pp. 67–84.
11. Dong, J.; Xing, Z.; Song, Z.; Bao, T. Research on the Role of Ecotourism from the Perspective of Ecological Civilization. *Fresenius Environ. Bull.* **2021**, *30*, 3291–3297.
12. Wang, Y.; Wu, X. The spatial pattern and influencing factors of tourism eco-efficiency in Inner Mongolia, China. *Front. Public Health* **2022**, *10*, 1072959. [CrossRef] [PubMed]
13. Liu, L. Some thoughts on the development of grassland tourism. *J. Inn. Mong. Univ. Financ. Econ.* **2005**, *3*, 92–95. (In Chinese)
14. Wang, Y.; Zhang, Y. Discussion on the Sustainable Development of Rural Tourism in Inner Mongolia: Based on the Perspective of Rural Tourism Development. *Stud. Sociol. Sci.* **2016**, *7*, 51–60.
15. Zhong, L.-S.; Niu, Y.-F.; Liu, J.-M.; Chen, T. Development of Grassland Tourism Resource in Inner Mongolia Autonomous Region. *J. Arid. Land Resour. Environ.* **2005**, *19*, 105–110. (In Chinese)
16. Wang, Y.; Zhang, P. (Eds.) An ecotourism perspective: The development of tourism industry in Inner Mongolia. In Proceedings of the International Conference on Manufacture Engineering and Environment Engineering (MEEE), Hong Kong, China, 3–5 July 2013.
17. Li, L.; Dong, Y.; Zhang, T.; Wang, H.; Li, H.; Li, A. Environmental and social outcomes of ecotourism in the dry rangelands of China. *J. Ecotourism* **2023**, *22*, 430–450. [CrossRef]
18. Tong, B.; Bao, Y.; Yang, B.; A, R. The Evolvement Characteristics and Mechanism of Settlement System in Xilingol Pastoral Area. *Sci. Geogr. Sin.* **2018**, *38*, 410–418. [CrossRef]
19. Chang, H.; Yang, W.; Shi, L.; Liu, Y.-H.; Qiu, X.; Yi, F.-Y.; Sun, H.-L. Spatial and temporal changes of carbon sequestration and soil conservation based on land-use in the farming pastoral ecotone of north China. *J. Agric. Resour. Environ.* **2021**, 484–493. [CrossRef]
20. Dong, J. Huangmohua caoyuan jianli rengong caodi zhonghexing fengcan jishu [Integrated Techniques for Establishing Artificial Grasslands in Desertified Grasslands]. *Keyan Chengguo Huibian* **1988**, *3*, 22–26.
21. Schiller, H.I. Communication And Cultural Domination. *Int. J. Politics* **1975**, *5*, 1–127.
22. MacCannell, D. Staged Authenticity: Arrangements of Social Space in Tourist Settings. *Am. J. Sociol.* **1973**, *79*, 589–603. [CrossRef]
23. MacCannell, D. Why it Never Really was About Authenticity. *Society* **2008**, *45*, 334–337. [CrossRef]
24. Greenwood, D. Culture by the Pound: An Anthropological Perspective on Tourism as Cultural Commoditization. In *Tourists and Tourism: A Reader*; Gmelch, S., Ed.; Waveland Press: Long Grove, IL, USA, 2004.

engineering proceedings

Proceeding Paper

Mandarin Learners' Use Perceptions of AI-Based Native Speaker Online Discussion Forums †

Jureynolds

Chinese Department, Bina Nusantara University, Jakarta 11480, Indonesia; jureynolds@binus.edu

† Presented at the 2024 IEEE 4th International Conference on Electronic Communications, Internet of Things and Big Data, Taipei, Taiwan, 19–21 April 2024.

Abstract: Current developments in language learning technology can connect native speakers to an artificial intelligence (AI)-based discussion forum for foreign language learning; HiNative is an application that answers the problems of foreign language learners by providing a discussion forum with answers that AI and native speakers double-check. This research was conducted on 56 respondents. In this study, portability, application usability, and interaction with native speakers were examined. The data obtained from the questionnaire were analyzed using a qualitative descriptive method. Mandarin learners responded positively to the portability of the HiNative application. Connections between native speakers assisted by AI increase the motivation of Mandarin language learners.

Keywords: AI-based apps; native; perceptions

Citation: Jureynolds. Mandarin Learners' Use Perceptions of AI-Based Native Speaker Online Discussion Forums. *Eng. Proc.* **2024**, 74, 11. https://doi.org/10.3390/engproc2024074011

Academic Editors: Shu-Han Liao, Teen-Hang Meen and Cheng-Fu Yang

Published: 27 August 2024

1. Introduction

Learning a foreign language is a manageable challenge, thanks to the help of increasigly sophisticated technology. Mobile assisted language learning (MALL), a mobile-based language learning approach, has simplified language learning by allowing individuals to learn anytime and anywhere. It is supported by easy access to information in transition between mobile devices [1].

One of the foreign languages that is increasingly popular to learn is Mandarin, which has become popular in various parts of the world. Along with this increasing interest, there are many Mandarin learning applications such as HelloChinese, ChineseSkill, Duolingo, and many other related apps. The existing types of applications provide material in various categories, such as structured lessons, games, flashcards, and learning videos [2]. Language learning assisted by mobile apps positively impacts learner autonomy [3]. However, language learning requires direct interaction with other people, especially native speakers. They can provide an understanding of the language so that native speakers become a source of "truth" [4]. However, the objectives of foreign language learning must be adjusted so that the learner becomes part of the learning [5].

In this context, the role of technology becomes significant in enabling students to take part in foreign language learning with native speakers. The application focused on in this research is HiNative, which is based on a model of online questions and answers and discussions on a discussion forum platform. The app allows interaction between foreign language learners (askers) and native speakers of the language (answerers). HiNative apps give askers the freedom to ask questions related to the target language, while answerers can respond using their language and provide examples to support their explanations.

Based on this background, Mandarin learners' perceptions of using the HiNative application were analyzed in this research. This online discussion forum utilizes AI technology and a "human touch" from native speakers.

2. Literature Review

2.1. MALL and AI

MALL is a language learning app for mobile devices. It integrates various language learning activities and prioritizes personal learning. The app is appropriate for students to learn anywhere and anytime [6]. Reciprocal learning can also be carried out using mobile devices in MALL, because it can accommodate collaborative learning between students through mobile device connectivity [7]. Language learning can be more comprehensive with multiple functions [8]. Integrating AI with MALL can revolutionize language learning, making it more personalized and enabling real-time language practice.

AI is used in language learning such as chatbots, virtual reality platforms, and personalized learning management systems to increase effective learning and learner satisfaction and motivation [9–11]. The use of AI in language learning activities improves the instruction and acquisition of language [12,13]. However, the effectiveness of language learning supported by AI depends on the involvement of teachers and students, and the role of AI in learning has received attention in research [14,15].

2.2. HiNative App for Foreign Language Learning

The HiNative application is known as an application that connects two groups of users, language learners and native speakers, using a question-and-answer method between the two groups [16,17]. HiNative supports the foreign language learning process, especially in aspects such as vocabulary learning, sentence structure, pronunciation, and the target language's culture [18–20].

3. Material and Methods

A descriptive qualitative analysis approach was used to determine Mandarin learners' perceptions of HiNative apps. The participants were 56 students majoring in Mandarin at a university in Indonesia. The participants in this research were accustomed to using the discussion forum. They used the HiNative apps intensively for a week and filled out a questionnaire. The questionnaire was created based on the technology acceptance model (TAM) framework and using a five-point Likert scale. TAM is a theoretical framework used in information systems to test the attitudes and behavior of mobile app users. The questionnaire items were formulated in three aspects: usability (PEOU), interaction (PU), and portability (PO). The usability aspect focused on a user-friendly interface and straightforward interaction, leading to a positive perception of ease of use. The interaction aspect focused on participants' communication with native speakers through existing mobile apps, supporting language skills and cultural understanding. Portability referred to the ease of access obtained, influenced by the mobile apps' ease of use and usefulness.

4. Results

4.1. Usability

Usability consisted of five items regarding mobile app usability when learning Mandarin (Table 1, Figure 1).

Table 1. Usability aspect.

Code	Items	Mean
Q1	HiNative is easy to use on my mobile phone	4.64
Q2	The features of HiNative make it easier to solve problems	4.34
Q3	The existing features make me understand the use of vocabulary/grammar	4.07
Q4	HiNative allows me to use Mandarin naturally	4.21
Q5	HiNative overall helped me in learning Mandarin	4.50
	Usability aspect perception	4.35

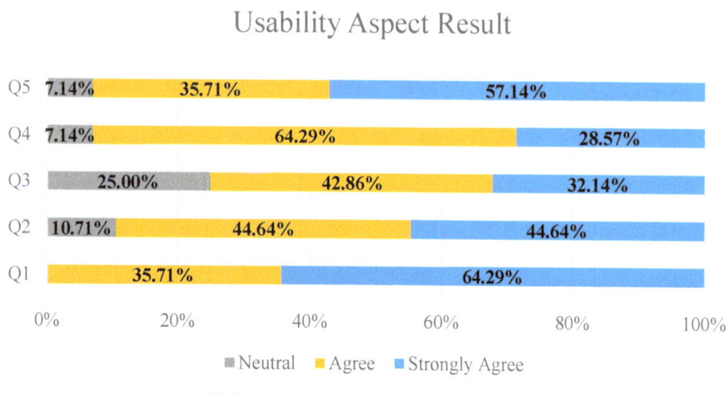

Figure 1. Usability of HiNative app.

After using the HiNative apps for one week, all participants agreed the HiNative apps were easy to use. The ease of access using the smartphone aligned with the perception of HiNative to solve problems encountered when learning Mandarin. In total, 44.64% of participants agreed with this statement, and 10.71% had a neutral opinion. The average score for this statement reached 4.34 (Table 1). This indicates that HiNative apps, which have a natural corpus, can be used to learn vocabulary/grammar in conversations. Massive numbers of learner corpora increase awareness about second language grammar [21] so that students can create their own learner corpora with near-natural corpora based on explanations and communication from native speakers in HiNative apps.

Of the features of the HiNative apps, all participants agreed that the functions in the HiNative apps helped them understand the use of Mandarin vocabulary/grammar. The useful knowledge was provided in the Q&A feature and discussion forum from native speakers using AI technology in the chatbot. In total, 75% agreed that HiNative enabled them to use Mandarin fluently, and 25.00% of the participants had a neutral opinion regarding this statement. Using HiNative apps, the user becomes a "silent reader," so that language practice is "imitation" without modifications according to the context of the speaker. Imitation is critical in foreign language learning because it is a cognitive construct of pronunciation, collocation of words, sentence sequences, and grammar [22]. However, imitation does not enhance language skills if it avoids conversational situations, motivation, and learning strategies [23].

Among all respondents, 93% strongly agreed that HiNative Apps helped them learn Mandarin. The relevant items in the questionnaire scored higher than 4, which indicated that they agreed that HiNative is an easy app for learning Mandarin.

4.2. Interaction

This aspect consisted of four items about perceptions of the interactions between participants and native speakers in HiNative apps (Table 2, Figure 2).

Communication between participants and native speakers is a form of learning material comprising voice recordings, example sentences, and explanations from the Q&A sessions. Among participants, 89% agreed that voice recordings provided by native speakers helped them with Mandarin pronunciation, 82% agreed that the examples of sentences and their usage provided by native speakers helped them understand Mandarin sentence structures, 14.29% had a neutral opinion, and 3.57% disagreed. The participants in discussion forums can become "silent viewers" who only see the presentation or answers from native speakers without being involved in two-way communication. In total, 86% agreed that communication with native speakers improved Mandarin language skills, and 14.29% had a neutral opinion. Overall, 89% of the participants agreed that communication with native speakers increased motivation and interest in learning Mandarin. Their perceptions of the interaction were high, with an average score over 4. All participants agreed that HiNative apps supported language skills and cultural understanding. Compared with usability, interaction scored lower, reflecting that language learning relies on direct spoken and written interaction, and active participation in two-way communication is crucial. Interactive approaches in second language learning help learners by providing opportunities, situations, and processes conducive to development, such as input, negotiation, output, feedback, and attention [24]. Interactional feedback also positively impacts second language acquisition learners [25].

Table 2. Interaction.

Code	Items	Mean
Q1	Voice recordings provided by native speakers help me improve my Mandarin pronunciation	4.32
Q2	The examples given by native speakers help me to understand Mandarin sentence structures	4.07
Q3	Communication with native speakers helps me improve my Mandarin skills	4.25
Q4	Communication with native speakers increases my interest and motivation to learn Mandarin	4.32
	Interaction aspect perception	4.24

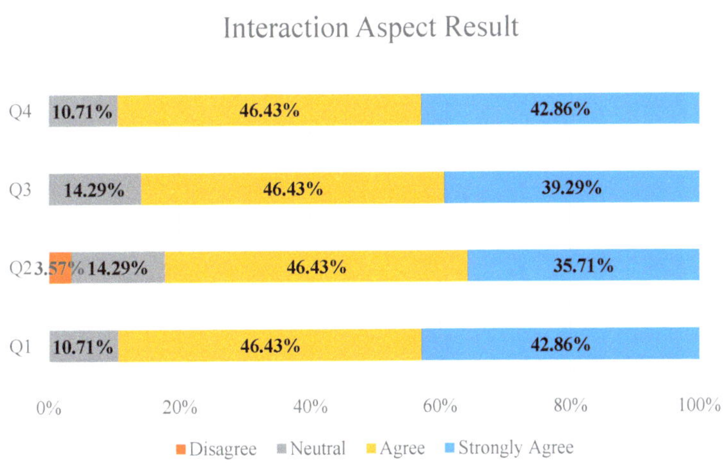

Figure 2. Interaction of HiNative app.

4.3. Portability

This aspect consisted of three items (Table 3, Figure 3).

Table 3. Portability aspect.

Code	Items	Mean
Q1	HiNative apps can be used anywhere and any time	4.71
Q2	I use HiNative apps in out-of-class learning	4.39
Q3	HiNative apps can be accessed with different electronic devices	4.39
	Portability aspect perception	4.50

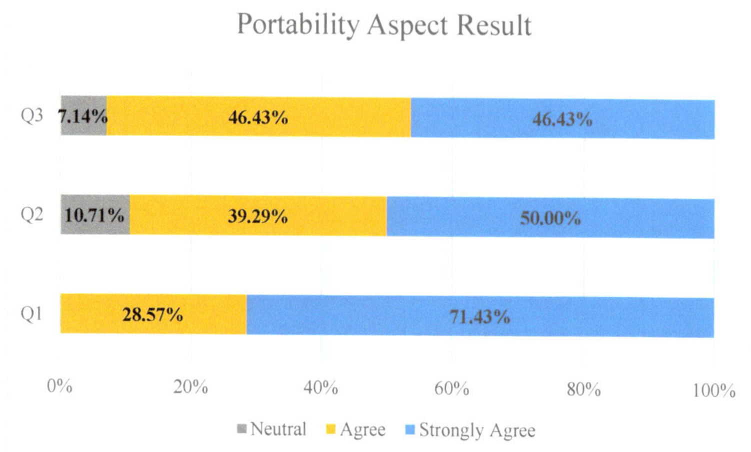

Figure 3. Portability of HiNative app.

Mobile apps are created for users to use anywhere and any time. All participants agreed that HiNative apps can be used anywhere and any time. Regarding its use in learning outside the classroom, 89 agreed that the HiNative app adopts the MALL principle for learning Mandarin, integrating various language learning activities and prioritizing personal learning [26]. In total, 10.71% had a neutral opinion because MALL learning is also related to the learner's intrinsic motivation, namely the initiative to learn independently. MALL learning does require internet access. Apart from smartphones, tablet computers are often used. In this study, 89 of the participants agreed they could access it using electronic devices. This encouraged students to access learning via devices other than smartphones. Their perceptions of portability showed that the HiNative app has the characteristics of mobile learning and portability and can be used anywhere at any time to support the Mandarin language learning process. The average score for portability was the highest (4.50), indicating ease of access, which was influenced by the ease of use and usability brought by the HiNative apps.

5. Conclusions

Student perceptions regarding the use of HiNative apps as an AI-based native speaker online discussion forum for learning Mandarin were examined. The participants responded positively to the use of this application in learning Mandarin. The HiNative app for learning Mandarin helped students improve their Mandarin language skills. They communicated with native speakers, which increased their motivation and interest in learning Mandarin.

Funding: This research received no external funding.

Institutional Review Board Statement: Ethical review and approval were waived for this study because the participants were voluntarily involved. It is because it is a journey for their personalized learning-supported tools.

Informed Consent Statement: Patient consent was waived for this study because the participants were voluntarily involved.

Data Availability Statement: The original contributions presented in the study are included in the article, further inquiries can be directed to the corresponding author.

Conflicts of Interest: The author declares no conflict of interest.

References

1. Şen, N.S. A Critical Review on the Mobile Assisted Language Learning with a Focus on Empirical Studies. *J. Learn. Teach. Digit. Age* **2021**, *6*, 117–126.
2. Chuang, H.Y. Mobile Assisted Language Learning APPs for the Chinese Classroom. *J. Technol. Chin. Lang. Teach.* **2016**, *7*, 113–119.
3. Zieni, H.A. The Effect of Mobile Learning on Learner Autonomy: A Suggested Measurement Tool to Assess the Development of Learner Autonomy. *J. AsiaTEFL* **2019**, *16*, 1020–1031. [CrossRef]
4. Alghazo, S.; Zidan, M. Native-Speakerism and Professional Teacher Identity in L2 Pronunciation Learning. *Indonesian J. Appl. Linguist.* **2019**, *9*, 241–251. [CrossRef]
5. Andreou, G. The Native Speaker Ideal in Foreign Language Teaching. *Electron. J. Foreign Lang. Teach.* **2009**, *6*, 200–208.
6. Gholami, J.; Azarmi, G. An Introduction to Mobile Assisted Language Learning. *Int. J. Manag. IT Eng.* **2012**, *2*, 1–9.
7. Kukulska-Hulme, A.; Shield, L. An Overview of Mobile Assisted Language Learning: From Content Delivery to Supported Collaboration and Interaction. *ReCALL* **2008**, *20*, 271–289. [CrossRef]
8. Yang, J. Mobile Assisted Language Learning: Review of the Recent Applications of Emerging Mobile Technologies. *Engl. Lang. Teach.* **2013**, *6*, 19–25. [CrossRef]
9. Haristiani, N. AI (AI) Chatbot as Language Learning Medium: An Inquiry. *J. Phys. Conf. Ser.* **2019**, *1387*, 012020. [CrossRef]
10. Chen, X.; Zou, D.; Cheng, G.; Xie, H. AI-Assisted Personalized Language Learning: Systematic Review and Co-Citation Analysis. In Proceedings of the 2021 International Conference on Advanced Learning Technologies (ICALT), Tartu, Estonia, 12–15 July 2021; pp. 241–245. [CrossRef]
11. Ma, L. An Immersive Context Teaching Method for College English Based on AI and Machine Learning in Virtual Reality Technology. *Mob. Inf. Syst.* **2021**, *2021*, 2637439. [CrossRef]
12. Ali, Z. AI (AI): A Review of Its Uses in Language Teaching and Learning. *IOP Conf. Ser. Mater. Sci. Eng.* **2020**, *769*, 012043. [CrossRef]
13. Yanhua, Z. The Application of AI in Foreign Language Teaching. In Proceedings of the 2020 International Conference on AI and Education (ICAIE), Tianjin, China, 26–28 June 2020; pp. 40–42. [CrossRef]
14. Yang, H.; Kyun, S. The Current Research Trend of AI in Language Learning: A Systematic Empirical Literature Review from an Activity Theory Perspective. *Australas. J. Educ. Technol.* **2022**, *38*, 180–210. [CrossRef]
15. Liang, J.-C.; Hwang, G.-J.; Chen, M.-R.A.; Darmawansah, D. Roles and Research Foci of AI in Language Education: An Integrated Bibliographic Analysis and Systematic Review Approach. *Interact. Learn. Environ.* **2023**, *31*, 4270–4296. [CrossRef]
16. Nishioka, H. Learning Languages and Culture Using HiNative. *Compass* **2020**, *13*, 1–7. [CrossRef]
17. Nushi, M.; Izadi, T.; Jozagian, M. HiNative: A Global Q&A Platform to Learn Language and Culture. *Issues Trends Learn. Technol.* **2023**, *10*. [CrossRef]
18. Kasrani, I.M.; Vasoya, M.M.; Shivakumar, A.; Pei, Y. A Mobile Cloud Computing Based Independent Language Learning System with Automatic Intelligibility Assessment and Instant Feedback. In Proceedings of the International Conference on Mobile Learning, Lisbon, Portugal, 14–16 April 2018.
19. Sarnovska, N. Use of Mobile Applications in English Language Researching by Students of Higher Educational Establishments. ΛΟΓΟΣ. *Art Sci. Mind* **2019**, *8*, 105–107. [CrossRef]
20. Pavlenko, O.O.; Bondar, O.Y.; Yon, B.G.; Kwangoon, C.; Tymchenko-Mikhailidi, N.S.; Kassim, D.A. The Enhancement of a Foreign Language Competence: Free Online Resources, Mobile Apps, and Other Opportunities. *CTE Workshop Proc.* **2019**, *6*, 279–293. [CrossRef]
21. Francis, G. Grammar Teaching in Schools: What Should Teachers Be Aware Of? *Lang. Aware.* **1994**, *3*, 221–236. [CrossRef]
22. Xiang-Liu, J. The Cognitive Foundation of Imitation and Its Implication to Foreign Language Teaching. *J. Hengyang Norm. Univ.* **2006**. [CrossRef]
23. Baltzer, A. Om Imitation i Tilegnelse Af Modersmål Og Fremmedsprog. *Nord. Psykol.* **1973**, *25*, 113–121. [CrossRef]
24. Mackey, A.; Goo, J. Interaction Approach in Second Language Acquisition. In *The Encyclopedia of Applied Linguistics*; Wiley: Hoboken, NJ, USA, 2012.
25. Mackey, A. Feedback, Noticing and Instructed Second Language Learning. *Appl. Linguist.* **2006**, *27*, 405–430. [CrossRef]
26. Palalas, A. Mobile-Assisted Language Learning: Designing for Your Students. In *Second Language Teaching and Learning with Technology: Views of Emergent Researchers*; Thouësny, S., Bradley, L., Eds.; Research-publishing.net: Dublin, Ireland, 2011; pp. 71–94. [CrossRef]

engineering proceedings

Proceeding Paper

Bitcoin Cycle through Markov Regime-Switching Model †

Yi-Chun Shih, Wen-Tsung Huang * and Pao-Peng Hsu

Department of Insurance and Finance Management, Chaoyang University of Technology, Taichung 413310, Taiwan; ycshih@cyut.edu.tw (Y.-C.S.); penghp@cyut.edu.tw (P.-P.H.)
* Correspondence: wthuang@cyut.edu.tw
† Presented at the 2024 IEEE 4th International Conference on Electronic Communications, Internet of Things and Big Data, Taipei, Taiwan, 19–21 April 2024.

Abstract: We analyzed Bitcoin's cyclical patterns used by the Markov regime-switching model and explored the impacts of inflation and the US Dollar Index on Bitcoin's cyclicality. The results showed Bitcoin's cyclical pattern, the effects of the US dollar index and VIX on Bitcoin's cyclical pattern, and how the US dollar index and VIX affect BTC's structural changes in Bitcoin.

Keywords: Markov regime-switching model; bitcoin; structural changes

1. Introduction

Bitcoin is a new digital money and payment tool that allows traders to transact without the intervention of financial intermediaries. Due to the accelerated application and development of blockchain, the price of Bitcoin hit an all-time high of USD 66,974 in November 2021. However, the price of Bitcoin declined by 50% three months later. This exemplifies the high volatility of Bitcoin, which is affected by its unusually high returns. This volatility engendered the Bitcoin bubble from 2017 to 2018 and early 2021. In November 2018, Bitcoin's price fell by 54% in one month. Furthermore, Bitcoin's price fell by 14% in three weeks in January 2021 [1,2]. At the end of 2022, Bitcoin prices crashed due to the collapse of Terra/Luna and the bankruptcy of FTX. These events highlight the importance of cryptocurrency options as a dependable means of hedging price risks.

Since Bitcoin is a virtual currency without intrinsic value, many studies have been conducted to find out the factors that affect the price of Bitcoin. Choi and Shin [3] provide systematic evidence demonstrating the relationship between inflation, uncertainty, and Bitcoin and gold prices. In the study, factors such as the S&P 500, VIX, and policy uncertainty were taken into account. The VIX and the dollar affect the price of Bitcoin [4–6]. VIX is regarded as a factor affecting the Bitcoin price mainly because of Bitcoin's hedging effect [7]. Most studies regard the US dollar as a factor in Bitcoin prices, mainly because of the competition between physical and virtual currency [6].

Figure 1 illustrates that the US dollar index rises with interest rates. Figure 2 demonstrates that since 2021, Bitcoin's price has fallen, whereas the US dollar index has risen. Such changes have influenced the competition between cryptocurrencies and traditional currencies in the monetary policy of the US Federal Reserve. During periods of high inflation, demand increases for immediate payments, and consumers may prefer traditional currencies over cryptocurrencies, thereby strengthening the US dollar. Additionally, rising interest rates favor the US dollar; one disadvantage of Bitcoin is that it does not generate interest income.

All economic activities undergo periods of recession, depression, recovery, and prosperity, resulting in a cyclical phenomenon [8]. Although Bitcoin has no intrinsic value, investors' behavior patterns cause Bitcoin prices to be cyclical [9]. Therefore, discussions of Bitcoin price cyclical patterns are essential topics for investors and risk averters. Using the Markov-switching (MS) model, we characterized nonlinearity according to individual economic variables [10–12] and found the cyclical pattern of Bitcoin. In addition, the US

Citation: Shih, Y.-C.; Huang, W.-T.; Hsu, P.-P. Bitcoin Cycle through Markov Regime-Switching Model. *Eng. Proc.* **2024**, *74*, 12. https://doi.org/10.3390/engproc2024074012

Academic Editors: Shu-Han Liao, Teen-Hang Meen and Cheng-Fu Yang

Published: 27 August 2024

dollar index and VIX were used to explore the impact of these two factors on the Bitcoin price cyclical pattern and whether they would drive the structural change of Bitcoin.

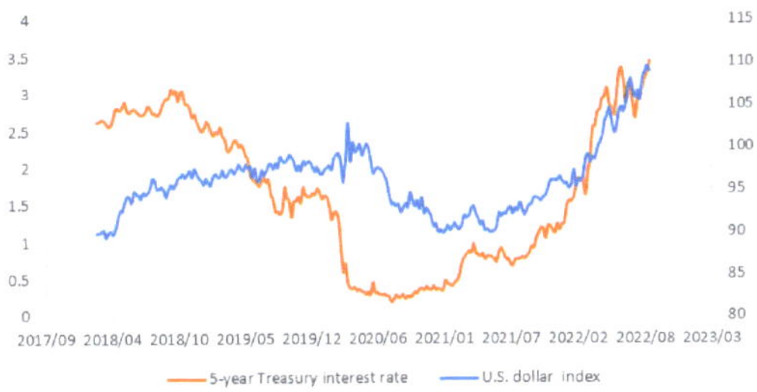

Figure 1. Weekly price trends of the US dollar index and 5-year Treasury interest rate.

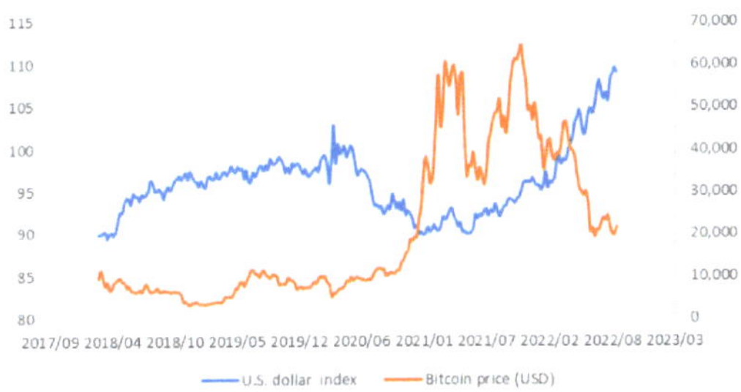

Figure 2. Weekly price trends of the US dollar index and Bitcoin price.

The rest of this paper is organized as follows. Section 2 describes the data and MS model. Section 3 presents empirical results. The conclusion is presented in the final section.

2. Statistical Methodology and Data Description

2.1. MS Model

Consider the MS model given by

$$y_t - u_{S_t} = \varphi_1\left(y_{t-1} - u_{S_{t-1}}\right) + \varphi_2\left(y_{t-2} - u_{S_{t-2}}\right) + \ldots + \varphi_q\left(y_{t-q} - u_{S_{t-q}}\right) + e_t \quad (1)$$

where φ_i is the coefficient on the autoregressive term; S_t is the unobserved state of the Bitcoin (BTC) cycle: $e_t \sim i.i.d.N\left(0, \sigma_{S_t}^2\right)$. u_{S_t} and σ_{S_t} are the state-dependent conditional mean and standard derivation of y_t, respectively, and q is the lag length of the autoregressive specification.

The BTC cycle follows a two-state Markov chain. $S_t = 1$ and $S_t = 2$ represent high growth (HG) and low growth (LG), respectively. A two-state Markov process with a fixed transition probability matrix is provided as follows:

$$p(S_t = j \mid S_{t-1} = j) = p_{jj},\ p(S_t = i \mid S_{t-1} = i) = p_{ji}, \forall i, j = 1, 2 \quad (2)$$

where $p_{11} + p_{12} = p_{21} + p_{22} = 1$. The stochastic process S_t is a stationary process when $0 < p_{ii} < 1$ and $\forall i = 1, 2$. Following Hamilton's (1989) suggestion, we used the smoothed probability to determine whether the BTC was in state one or state two, as well as to determine the turning point of the BTC cycle.

2.2. Data Description

The data used in this study were related to the following variables: Bitcoin (BTC), the US dollar index (US), and the Chicago Board Options Exchange's Volatility Index (VIX). The

BTC, US, and VIX data were collected from January 2018 to September 2022. In addition, to highlight the effects of US and VIX on the BTC cyclical pattern, we regarded only BTC in the MS model as Model I. VIX and BTC were contained in the MS model as Model II. US and BTC were contained in the MS model as a Model III. Three variables, VIX, US, and BTC, are considered in the MS model as Model IV.

3. Results and Discussion

Figure 3 shows the long–short cycle of BTC, with the blue line representing the bull market and the orange line representing the bear market. For the models, $\sigma_1 < \sigma_2$, and μ_2 was 0.091 (Table 1). Even in the bear market, the price of Bitcoin was still in an upward trend. The duration of Model I in Table 1 was 40.357 in the bull market and 8.409 in the bear market, indicating that Bitcoin will be in the bull market most of the time from 2018 to 2022. In addition, the coefficients of X_{VIX} and X_{US} in Model II and Model III were negative, indicating that the rise of VIX and US caused BTC to fall, and the effect of USD against Bitcoin impacted that of VIX on Bitcoin. The bear market duration affected Model III more than Model I. However, the same phenomenon appeared in the bull market, indicating that adding the dollar factor causes Bitcoin's cycle to change from a short cycle to a longer cycle.

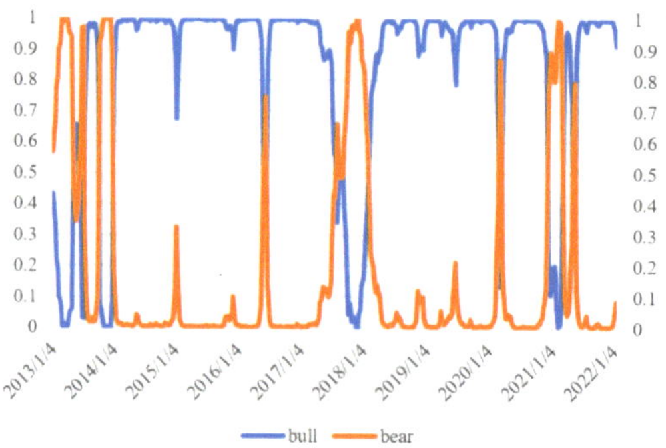

Figure 3. Smoothing probability of HG and LG for BTC.

Table 1. Estimation results of three models.

Model I		**Model II**		**Model III**		**Model IV**	
σ_1	0.007	σ_1	0.007	σ_1	0.007	σ_1	0.007
σ_2	0.053	σ_2	0.053	σ_2	0.053	σ_2	0.053
u_1	0.010	x_{VIX}	−0.061	x_{US}	−0.654	x_{VIX}	−0.063
u_2	0.091	u_1	0.010	u_1	0.010	x_{US}	−0.753
p_{11}	0.975	u_2	0.101	u_2	0.091	u_1	0.010
p_{12}	0.119	p_{11}	0.975	p_{11}	0.979	u_2	0.102
p_{21}	0.025	p_{12}	0.128	p_{12}	0.103	p_{11}	0.982
p_{22}	0.881	p_{21}	0.025	p_{21}	0.021	p_{12}	0.098
		p_{22}	0.872	p_{22}	0.897	p_{21}	0.018
						p_{22}	0.902
Duration							
p_{11}	40.357		39.508		47.970		54.595
p_{22}	8.409		7.843		9.701		10.212

Figure 4 shows the cyclical patterns of VIX, US, and BTC. The gray line is for US, the blue line represents BTC, and the orange line is for VIX. As shown in Figure 2, VIX affected the structural transformation of BTC from 2016 to 2020, but in 2021, the US affected the structural transformation of BTC. VIX significantly impacted BTC during the epidemic, especially in early 2020. However, in early 2021, the U.S. Federal Reserve's monetary policy impacted the global financial market and strengthened the US's structural transformation of BTC. This result is in line with expectations.

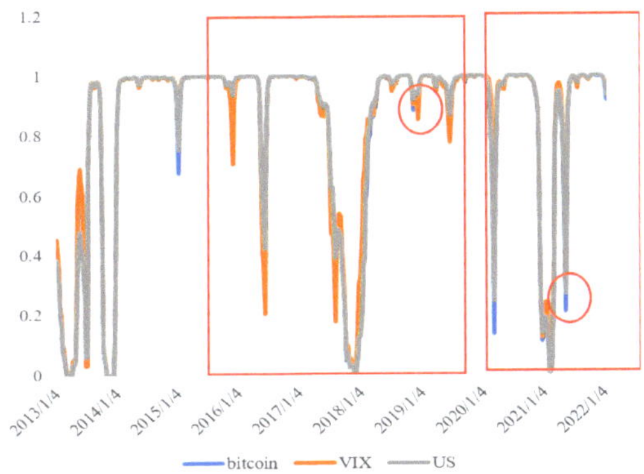

Figure 4. Smoothing probability of HG and LG regimes for VIX, US, and BTC.

4. Conclusions

We applied an MS model to examine the cyclical patterns of US, VIX, and BTC. The results revealed BTC's cyclical pattern, the effects of the US and VIX on BTC's cyclical pattern, and how the US and VIX affected the structural transformation of BTC.

Author Contributions: Conceptualization, P.-P.H., W.-T.H. and Y.-C.S.; methodology, P.-P.H. and W.-T.H.; validation, P.-P.H. and W.-T.H.; formal analysis, P.-P.H.; resources, P.-P.H.; data curation, Y.-C.S.; writing—original draft preparation, P.-P.H.; writing—review and editing, W.-T.H.; visualization, W.-T.H.; supervision, P.-P.H. and W.-T.H.; project administration, W.-T.H. All authors have read and agreed to the published version of the manuscript.

Funding: This research received no external funding.

Institutional Review Board Statement: Not applicable.

Informed Consent Statement: Not applicable.

Data Availability Statement: The data supporting this study's findings are available from the corresponding author upon reasonable request.

Acknowledgments: We would like to thank His Chang for her helpful assistance regarding the data resource.

Conflicts of Interest: The authors declare no conflicts of interest.

References

1. Cross, J.L.; Hou, C.; Trinh, K. Returns, volatility and the cryptocurrency bubble of 2017–18. *Econ. Model.* **2021**, *104*, 105643. [CrossRef]
2. Dong, F.; Xu, Z.; Zhang, Y. Bubbly Bitcoin. *Econ. Theory* **2021**, *74*, 973–1015. [CrossRef]
3. Choi, S.; Shin, J. Bitcoin: An inflation hedge but not a safe haven. *Financ. Res. Lett.* **2022**, *46*, 102379. [CrossRef] [PubMed]
4. Zhu, Y.; Dickinson, D.; Li, J. Analysis on the influence factors of Bitcoin's price based on VEC model. *Financ. Innov.* **2017**, *3*, 3. [CrossRef]
5. Blau, B.M.; Griffith, T.G.; Whitby, R.J. Inflation and Bitcoin: A descriptive time-series analysis. *Econ. Lett.* **2021**, *203*, 109848. [CrossRef]
6. Hsu, P.-P.; Chen, Y.-H.C.; Wang, C.-H. Currency or commodity competition? Bitcoin price trends in the post-pandemic era. *Int. J. Appl. Econ. Financ. Account.* **2023**, *15*, 61–70. [CrossRef]
7. Chen, C.; Liu, L.; Zhao, N. Fear Sentiment, Uncertainty, and Bitcoin Price Dynamics: The Case of COVID-19. *Emerg. Mark. Financ. Trade* **2020**, *56*, 2298–2309. [CrossRef]
8. Burns, A.F.; Mitchell, W.C. *Measuring Business Cycles*; Columbia University Press (for NBER): New York, NY, USA, 1946.

9. Wang, J.; Ma, F.; Bouri, E.; Guo, Y. Which factors drive Bitcoin volatility: Macroeconomic, technical, or both? *J. Forecast.* **2022**, *42*, 970–988. [CrossRef]
10. Hamilton, J.D. A New Approach to the Economic Analysis of Nonstationary Time Series and the Business Cycle. *Econometrica* **1989**, *57*, 357–384. [CrossRef]
11. Mérida, A.; Golpe, A.A. Tourism-Led Growth Revisited for Spain: Causality, Business Cycles and Structural Breaks. *Int. J. Tour. Res.* **2014**, *18*, 39–51. [CrossRef]
12. Hsu, P.-P. Examination of Taiwan's travel and tourism market cycle through a two-period Markov regime-switching model. *Tour. Manag.* **2017**, *63*, 201–208. [CrossRef]

engineering proceedings

Proceeding Paper

Benefits of Improving Urban Park Playground Facilities through Inclusive Design Concept Using Computer Software †

Jung-Hua Wu, Sheng-Jung Ou, Wei-Chieh Yeh and Huang-Liang Lee *

Department of Architecture, College Design, Chaoyang University of Technology, Taichung 413310, Taiwan; vincent7963@gmail.com (J.-H.W.); sjou@cyut.edu.tw (S.-J.O.); jasonbufet@gmail.com (W.-C.Y.)

* Correspondence: hlli@cyut.edu.tw

† Presented at the 2024 IEEE 4th International Conference on Electronic Communications, Internet of Things and Big Data, Taipei, Taiwan, 19–21 April 2024.

Abstract: For inclusive design, we conducted the Taichung Melody Project to enhance the urban park's children's playground in terms of inclusivity and user-friendliness. The post-occupancy evaluation was used for Sanxin Park to analyze the improvement effect and the satisfaction degree with the park facilities, park sensory, and park management. The purpose of park use directly impacted sensory satisfaction and management satisfaction. The research results can be used as a reference for future key projects of park playground improvement.

Keywords: inclusive design; children's playground; barrier-free environment; post occupancy evaluation; Taichung Melody

Citation: Wu, J.-H.; Ou, S.-J.; Yeh, W.-C.; Lee, H.-L. Benefits of Improving Urban Park Playground Facilities through Inclusive Design Concept Using Computer Software. *Eng. Proc.* **2024**, *74*, 13. https://doi.org/10.3390/engproc2024074013

Academic Editors: Shu-Han Liao, Teen-Hang Meen and Cheng-Fu Yang

Published: 28 August 2024

1. Introduction

As urban forests, parks function as a place for leisure and disaster prevention. Since 2019, the Taichung City Government has promoted the "Taichung Melody Project" to promote a better lifestyles, provide a healthy living environment, promote friendliness, and improve the safety of children. We explored the results of Sanxin Park renovation through a satisfaction survey regarding the facilities, sensory aspects, and management of the park. Based on the results, we provide suggestions for the "Taichung Melody Project".

2. Literature Review and Methods

2.1. Literature Review

2.1.1. Inclusive Playground

The "Inclusive Playground" refers to a barrier-free environment with a diverse and friendly atmosphere, and spacious, safe, interactive, interesting, and comfortable characteristics (Construction Bureau of Taichung City Government, 2018) [1]. Such a park considers the demands of different user groups including children. The facilities of a park and a playground must meet the needs of the users, who participate in a wide range of activities regardless of their ability (Lin and Chen, 2022; Huang, 2020) [2–4]. The park environment needs to be developed to foster friendliness as the population structure in Taiwan is changing. Park facilities and park management need to meet the needs of children with different physical and mental conditions to to participate in activities through an inclusive design method.

2.1.2. Barrier-Free Environment Design (BD)

The concept of BD advocates that people with disabilities can live as ordinary people without any differences. The United Nations also advocated for the concept of "Normalization" at a conference in 1963, and published "The Convention on the Rights of Persons with Disabilities" in 1975. At the same time, the International Organization for Standardization

(ISO) also introduced the design guideline "A General Normative Series for Thinking about the Needs of People with Disabilities" (Tseng, 1996) [5] to facilitate the creation of a friendly barrier-free environment. The idea of "Normalization" has since expanded from Europe to the United States and the whole world (Tseng, 1996) [5]. The barrier-free norms and concepts in Taiwan have been revised and enhanced year by year. The concept of friendliness has been applied in the design of substantive space units in combination with the theory of universal design and the implementation of school education.

2.1.3. Post-Occupancy Evaluation (POE)

POE originated in the United States and the United Kingdom as an indicator of quality improvement, satisfaction, and importance of a space originally designed by a government or private person (Huang, 2000) [6]. Chen (1993) proposed that POE was a widely used in surveying users, managers, or persons of interest from a completed event to learn about the use of facilities and the relationship between people and the environment and to review the original plan, design, and construction details [7]. Rabinowitz and White (1988) pointed out that relevant facilities began to be evaluated using the criteria from a systematic, objective, and rigorous perspective after it was put into use [8]. The POE model was used in this study to investigate users' satisfaction with the facilities, sensory aspects, and management of the park playground concerned after its improvement.

2.2. Research Methods

We explored the post-occupancy satisfaction of park users with the facilities, sensory aspects, and management of Taichung Sanxin Park. The research structure is shown in Figure 1.

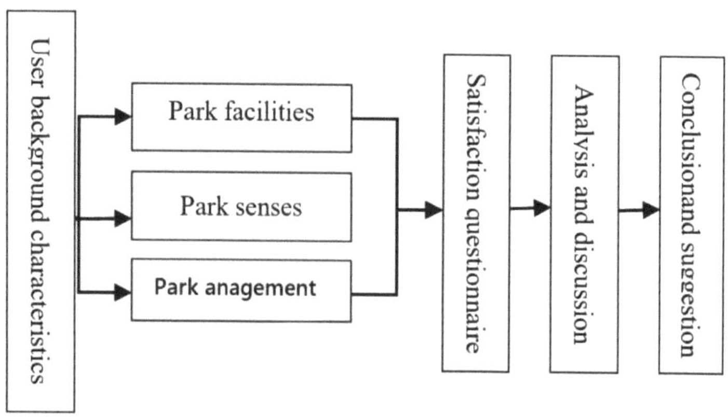

Figure 1. Research structure of this study.

The research structure, motivation, and objectives were established based on a literature review. The following research hypotheses were proposed.

H0. *User background has insignificant impacts on the perception of park facilities, park sensory attributes, and park management.*

H1. *User background has significant impacts on the perception of park facilities, park sensory attributes, and park management.*

A questionnaire survey was used as the main tool in this study to collect data. The five-point Likert scale was used, ranging from 1 (very dissatisfied) to 5 (very satisfied), using an anonymous method. The questionnaires were distributed in Sanxin Park from 6 to 8 April 2022, taking Sanxin Park users as the subjects. In total, 105 questionnaires were distributed. The 105 completed questionnaires were collected, out of which 5 were discarded and 100 were analyzed. Statistical analysis was performed using SPSS 27 for descriptive statistics and ANOVA. Gender, education, occupation, living area, frequency of use of the park, purpose of use of the park, and other demographic characteristics and statuses were analyzed as the background information. ANOVA was used to analyze and compare the results on the satisfaction of park facilities, park sensory attributes, and park management to examine differences between the different backgrounds of users.

3. Case Description

Sanxin Park is located in Xitun District, Taichung City, and did not meet the standards of BD before construction. The playground facilities were improved for environmental reasons and for the needs of children aged 6–16 years old with various physical and mental conditions under the concept of inclusiveness and friendliness. It became the first park playground for children in wheelchairs to play on the Slide and Swing in Taichung City after improvement. The play space with the hill-shaped slide of the barrier-free ramps also provided children of all ages to play.

3.1. Space Overview

The area of Sanxin Park is 10,713 m^2; the improved playground area is 385 m^2. An integrated game set was offered before the improvement, but it did not conform to the provisions of the new playground regulations, and the surrounding moving lines without footpath series were not in line with the barrier-free regulations (Figure 2). Therefore, the game facility and barrier-free space were improved to meet the requirements of relevant regulations. Better achievements and benefits could be achieved after improvement, as well as inclusiveness and friendliness.

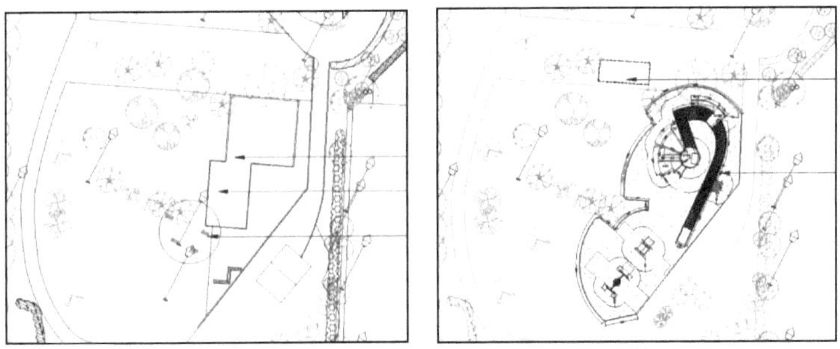

(**a**) (**b**)

Figure 2. Park design before (**a**) and after (**b**) renovation.

3.2. Countermeasures for Space Renovation

The original integrated game set did not conform to the new regulations, and the utilization rate was low. Therefore, a volcano-shaped game set was built, which included a slide, climbing space, and other functions. Moreover, barrier-free standard ramps were set up for children in wheelchairs to be able to play on the slide. A game for children under the age of 6 years old was provided, and a rocking horse facility was added. One wheelchair swing and one bird's nest swing were built, providing wheelchair users with a swing (Figure 3).

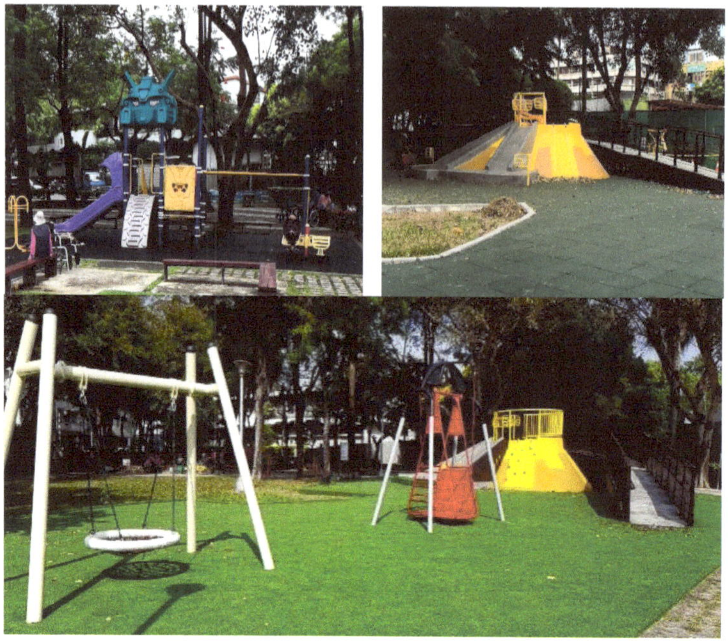

Figure 3. Drawing of current state of playground after renovation.

4. Discussion

4.1. Demographics and Behavior of Users

Descriptive statistics are shown in Table 1. Briefly, 53% of the users were males and 47% were females. In total, 74% did not have a bachelor's degree, and 26% of the respondents were employed. A hidden sampling bias was negligible. In total, 67% of the users were residents, 66% of the users visited the park frequently, among whom 39% visited Sanxin Park two to four times a week, and 27% visited the park every day. Furthermore, 33% dropped by and stayed in the park alone, and 23% visited the park for parent–child activities. The main users of Sanxin Park were residents and working people, and 66% visited the park frequently. Most users used the park for parent–child activities, leisure, and exercise. Sanxin Park had enhanced environmental accessibility and satisfaction after its improvement. The content of the questionnaire comprised codes: code A for park facilities, B for park sensory attributes, and C for park management and other project satisfaction metrics.

Table 1. Descriptive statistics.

	Frequency/Percentage			**Frequency/Percentage**		
Gender	Male	53	53.0	Female	47	47.0
Educational background	Bachelor's degree	17	17.0	PhD	1	1.0
	Master's degree	8	8.0	Other	74	74.0
Occupational identity	In employment	26	26.0	Retiree	37	37.0
	Unemployed	11	11.0	Household management	26	26.0
Nearby residents	Yes	67	67.0	No, and they did not work nearby	20	20.0
	No, but they all worked nearby	13	13.0			

Table 1. *Cont.*

	Frequency/Percentage			Frequency/Percentage		
Frequency of visiting Sanxin Park	Every day	27	27.0	Once a week for holidays	7	7.0
	2–4 times a week	39	39.0	Rarely or the first time	27	27.0
Main purpose of visiting Sanxin Park	Stroll	7	7.0	Parent–child activities	23	23.0
	Rest and enjoyed the scenery	18	18.0	Dropping by and staying	33	33.0
	Exercise	18	18.0	Others	1	1.0

4.2. Park Facility Satisfaction

The survey results on user satisfaction with the facility are shown in Table 2. Nearly 80% of the users were satisfied with the park facilities, and approximately 20% of the users had neutral opinions. Two users and three users were very dissatisfied with the wheelchair swing and bird's nest swing in the facilities, respectively. According to the variance test (Table 3), occupation, distance from visitors' homes, and the purpose of park use were factors affecting satisfaction with the facility.

Table 2. Satisfaction with facility.

	Very Satisfied	Satisfied	Fair	Dissatisfied	Very Dissatisfied
A1. What is your overall satisfaction with the improvement of Sanxin Park?	28	51	20	1	0
A2. How satisfied are you with newly the built volcano-shaped game set in Sanxin Park?	28	48	20	4	0
A3. How satisfied are you with the rocking horse game set in Sanxin Park?	27	51	21	1	0
A4. How satisfied are you with the newly built wheelchair swing in Sanxin Park?	25	49	21	3	2
A5. How satisfied are you with the newly built bird's nest swing in Sanxin Park?	26	46	21	4	3

Table 3. Variation test results on satisfaction with Sanxin Park.

	Gender			Educational Background			Occupation		
	Degree of Freedom	F Value	Significance	Degree of Freedom	F Value	Significance	Degree of Freedom	F Value	Significance
A1	1	0.002	0.960	4	2.093	0.088	3	5.923	0.001
A2	1	0.556	0.458	4	2.308	0.064	3	4.491	0.005
A3	1	0.095	0.758	4	0.888	0.474	3	4.523	0.005
A4	1	1.197	0.277	4	0.904	0.465	3	4.731	0.004
A5	1	0.592	0.443	4	1.246	0.297	3	4.361	0.006
B1	1	10.137	0.289	4	1.417	0.234	3	7.104	0.000
B2	1	0.869	0.353	4	1.857	0.124	3	7.614	0.000

Table 3. *Cont.*

	Gender			Educational Background			Occupation		
	Degree of Freedom	F Value	Significance	Degree of Freedom	F Value	Significance	Degree of Freedom	F Value	Significance
B3	1	0.869	0.353	4	1.437	0.228	3	7.614	0.000
B4	1	0.783	0.378	4	0.895	0.470	3	8.298	0.000
B5	1	1.845	0.177	4	3.039	0.021	3	6.077	0.001
C1	1	0.001	0.970	4	1.740	0.148	3	3.627	0.016
C2	1	0.037	0.848	4	1.754	0.145	3	3.766	0.013
C3	1	1.898	0.171	4	1.200	0.316	3	4.936	0.003
C4	1	20.035	0.157	4	0.689	0.601	3	3.620	0.016
C5	1	20.439	0.122	4	1.963	0.106	3	2.390	0.073
	Nearby residents			Use frequency			Purpose of park use		

For the sensory attributes of the park, 80% of the users were satisfied with the game sets in the park, approximately 20% of the users held neutral opinions, and only five users were satisfied with the safety of the game sets. One user was very dissatisfied with the overall experience, fun, stimulation, and challenges provided by park (Table 4). According to the variance test (Table 3), occupation, nearby residents, and the purpose of park use were significant factors influencing satisfaction with the sensory attributes of the park. The use frequency was significant in influencing satisfaction with the game sets in the park.

Table 4. Satisfaction with sensory attributes.

	Very Satisfied	Satisfied	Fair	Dissatisfied	Very Dissatisfied
B1. What is your overall satisfaction with the game sets in Sanxin Park?	25	52	22	0	1
B2. How satisfied are you with the fun of the game sets in Sanxin Park?	24	53	22	0	1
B3. How satisfied are you with the stimulation provided by the game sets in Sanxin Park?	24	53	22	0	1
B4. How satisfied are you with the challenge provided by the game sets in Sanxin Park?	24	52	22	1	1
B5. How satisfied are you with the safety of the game sets in Sanxin Park?	24	50	19	2	5

4.3. Satisfaction with Park Management

In total, 80% of the users were satisfied with park management, approximately 50% of the users held neutral opinions, and nearly 10% of the users had barrier-free space in the park. One user was very dissatisfied with the proportion of green space and the game sets available in the park (Table 5). Occupation, among the demographic, characteristics was a significant factor influencing satisfaction with the management of the park. However, it was an insignificant factor influencing satisfaction with the barrier-free space of the park. The proportion of nearby residents to the green space of the park, the availability of game sets, and the barrier-free space were significant influences on satisfaction. Frequency of use was significant in terms of satisfaction with the proportion of green space in the park. The purpose of park use was a significant influencing factor, but understanding of Taichung Melody was insignificant.

Table 5. Satisfaction with management.

	Very Satisfied	Satisfied	Fair	Dissatisfied	Very Dissatisfied
C1. Do you know about "Taichung Melody"?	23	28	47	2	0
C2. How satisfied are you with the "Taichung Melody"?	23	28	49	0	0
C3. How satisfied are you with the proportion of green space in Sanxin Park?	23	32	40	4	1
C4. How satisfied are you with the richness of the game sets in Sanxin Park?	23	38	37	1	1
C5. How satisfied are you with the barrier-free space in Sanxin Park?	21	31	33	6	9

5. Conclusions and Suggestion

In this study, more than 80% of the users were satisfied in the post-occupancy evaluation of the improved facilities, indicating that the park facilities had been improved to meet the needs of the users. Two users were very dissatisfied with the wheelchair swing and three users were very dissatisfied with the bird's nest swing. The lack of accessibility of these two facilities might lead to poor user experience. Nearly 80% of the users were satisfied with the overall experience of the game sets in the park, indicating that the improved park met the sensory needs of the users. Five users were very dissatisfied with the safety of the game sets. The buffer space of the game sets might be insufficient, resulting in poor user experience. Nearly 50% of the users were satisfied with park management, while nearly 10% of the users were very dissatisfied with the barrier-free space in the park; they suggested that the accessibility and safety measures of the playground need to be improved. In addition, the users were not serious about the "Taichung Melody Project", indicating that the public relations department also provided insufficient publicity and promotion. The users of Sanxin Park were mostly parents and children. Therefore, the park needs to have facilities with increased accessibility and that safety measures need to ensure greater protection to avoid user injuries. The public relations department needs to focus on the promotion efforts for Taichung Melody so that more people in the community can understand the objectives of the plan.

Author Contributions: Writing—review and editing, J.-H.W.; methodology, S.-J.O.; software, W.-C.Y.; validation, H.-L.L. All authors have read and agreed to the published version of the manuscript.

Funding: This research received no external funding.

Institutional Review Board Statement: Not applicable.

Informed Consent Statement: Not applicable.

Data Availability Statement: Data are contained within the article.

Conflicts of Interest: The authors declare no conflict of interest.

References

1. Construction Bureau of Taichung City Government. *Taichung Melody Manuals*; Construction Bureau of Taichung City Government: Taichung, Taiwan, 2018.
2. Lin, P.-M. *Environmental Attribute, Place Attachment and Satisfaction for Inclusive Park—A Case Study on "Chiayi Culture Park"*; Department of Leisure and Recreation College of Applied Arts and Sciences, National Formosa University: Yunlin County, Taiwan, 2022.
3. Chen, Y.-L. Post Occupancy Evaluation of Melody Inclusive Park in Taichung City. Master's Thesis, Department of Landscape Architecture Tunghai University, Taichung, Taiwan, 2022.
4. Huang, H.-C. *A Study of Service Experience Quality and Satisfaction of Park's Inclusive Playgrounds—Evidence from Shude Inclusive Playground in Taipei City*; National Taiwan University of Science and Technology Department of Design: Taipei, Taiwan, 2020.
5. Tzeng, S.-Y. A Comparison of Barrier Free Norms in Taiwan And Overseas Counteies. *J. Archit.* **1996**, *18*, 1–16.
6. Huang, S.-M. *The Study on the Building of School-Building School Essays of Huang, Shyh-Meng*; Building Information Quarterly Magazine: Taipei, Taiwan, 2000.
7. Chen, K.-L. *University Library Building and Post-Occupancy Evaluation-Case Study of Chung Yuan Christian University Library*; Jet Pacific Press: Taichung, Taiwan, 1993.
8. Preiser, W.F.E.; Rabinowitz, H.Z.; White, E.T. *Post-Occupancy Evaluation*; Van Nostrand Reinhold: New York, NY, USA, 1988.

engineering proceedings

Proceeding Paper

Framework for Optimizing the Operation and Maintenance of Bridges †

Areej AlBanwan

Energy and Building Research Center, Sustainability and Reliability of Infrastructure Program, Kuwait Institute for Scientific Research, P.O. Box 24885 Safat, Kuwait City 13109, Kuwait; abanwan@kisr.edu.kw

† Presented at the 2024 IEEE 4th International Conference on Electronic Communications, Internet of Things and Big Data, Taipei, Taiwan, 19–21 April 2024.

Abstract: Ensuring the safety and reliability of bridges through the implementation of cost-effective asset management strategies is crucial for sustaining a resilient transportation infrastructure network. Thus, the utilization of structural health monitoring (SHM) was investigated to enhance the operation and maintenance of bridges, with a focus on best practices and strategic implementation. Specifically, this study aimed to explore methods that leverage SHM to enhance bridge-asset management practices. The existing literature on bridge asset management was used as a foundation for identifying the value of SHM in bridge operation and maintenance. While the general literature on SHM and asset management is extensive, very few studies effectively linked these two domains. By conducting a comprehensive review of relevant studies and successful integration cases, the results of this study offered the appropriate application of SHM in bridge asset management. The processes observed were then integrated into a strategic framework, serving as a practical guide for managers seeking to implement SHM effectively in bridge asset management, particularly during the operation and maintenance phase of the bridge lifecycle.

Keywords: bridges; operation; maintenance; asset management; structural health monitoring; framework

1. Introduction

Bridges are vital components of a nation's infrastructure, and proper asset management is crucial to ensuring continued functionality, safety, and longevity. Optimal asset management is challenging, as the costs of these activities in a lifecycle must be minimized, while ensuring that the performance and reliability of the infrastructure related to the asset's condition, serviceability, safety, and capacity are adequately addressed. Traditional bridge management often relies on periodic visual inspections and maintenance schedules. However, these methods may not adequately capture the dynamic condition of a bridge. To address this limitation, structural health monitoring (SHM) has emerged as a promising solution that provides real-time data about a bridge's structural condition, enabling proactive and data-driven decision-making in asset management. SHM leverages sensor technology to continuously monitor the structural health of a bridge and provide real-time data for condition assessment. In this study, the literature was reviewed to see if the SHM technology can be employed successfully to manage infrastructure assets, specifically bridges and road bridges. The best practices of organizations that manage bridge assets during the operations and maintenance phase of the asset lifecycle are used to develop a framework of strategic bridge asset management processes to effectively integrate structural health monitoring into this critical phase of the asset lifecycle.

Citation: AlBanwan, A. Framework for Optimizing the Operation and Maintenance of Bridges. *Eng. Proc.* **2024**, *74*, 14. https://doi.org/10.3390/engproc2024074014

Academic Editors: Shu-Han Liao, Teen-Hang Meen and Cheng-Fu Yang

Published: 27 August 2024

2. Literature Review

2.1. Overview of Asset Management

Asset management is used to ensure that an asset, such as a bridge, operates to enhance the asset's life, optimizes maintenance and management costs, and meets present and long-term needs [1]. An asset management system, also referred to as an asset management framework, encompasses a set of interrelated elements designed to establish asset management policies, objectives, and processes, with the overarching goal of successfully achieving those objectives. [2]. Numerous asset management frameworks exist, each presenting distinctive methodologies to optimize the management of assets. Asset managers are encouraged to evaluate and adopt the most suitable approach based on the unique nature and context of their assets [3].

A fundamental commonality across all asset management systems is the concept of the asset lifecycle. This lifecycle encompasses all the stages an asset undergoes, from its inception to its eventual end-of-life [3]. Bridge asset management processes are integral components, seamlessly integrated into the four key phases that define the asset's lifecycle:

- Planning;
- Acquisition and procurement;
- Operation and maintenance;
- Disposal and decommission.

The initial planning phase involves defining strategic objectives and goals for the asset. Asset management processes within this phase determine the asset's intended purpose, long-term goals, and the allocation of resources. Asset management processes in the acquisition and procurement stage select the most appropriate assets, ensuring quality and compliance with the standards and optimizing the procurement and construction processes [4]. Once an asset is operational, the focus shifts to its ongoing operation and maintenance. Asset management processes in this phase are centered on the day-to-day management of the asset to ensure optimal performance. This includes preventive and corrective maintenance, as well as monitoring and adapting to changing needs and conditions [4]. The disposal and decommission phase marks the end of an asset's lifecycle, during which assets are decommissioned, dismantled, or disposed of.

2.2. Core and Advanced Asset Management

The International Infrastructure Management Manual (IIMM) differentiates between core and advanced asset management practices to cater to organizations with varying levels of complexity and maturity in their asset management processes [5]. Core asset management ensures basic maintenance and compliance but may not fully leverage data-driven decision making or advanced technology. Advanced asset management involves a proactive, data-intensive, and strategic approach to asset management, often leveraging cutting-edge technologies and predictive analytics to optimize asset performance and enhance decision making. According to audits undertaken by the US Government Accountability Office (USGAO) and the New Zealand Office of the Auditor General (NZOAG), data gaps exist in existing asset management practices, hindering the development of advanced asset management practices [6,7].

2.3. Overview of SHM

SHM requires the strategic installation of sensors at critical locations in a structure to assess its overall structural health [8]. It involves measuring a structure's operating and loading environment, along with its critical responses, to detect and evaluate signs of operational, serviceability, or safety issues, such as malfunctions or abnormalities [9]. The application of SHM extends to asset assessment, providing an immediate understanding of a structure's health, monitoring the progression of structural deterioration, and expanding the safe operating range of structures [10]. According to the Imperial College London, damage detection methods vary depending on the SHM system's intended use [11]. The damage assessment scale comprises four levels:

- Damage detection;
- Damage localization;
- Damage characterization (based on size and severity);
- Prognosis and estimation of the remaining useful life.

Each level of damage assessment requires a different number and location of transducers. In SHM, transducers are frequently integrated into sensors to capture data on the structural behavior of a given structure by converting physical quantities, including strain, pressure, temperature, or displacement, into electrical signals that are easily measured and analyzed. Early identification of problems through damage detection prevents severe damage, allowing for the strategic scheduling of maintenance tasks and avoiding unnecessary inspections. These objectives summarize the primary goals of structural health monitoring [8].

2.4. *Value Assessment of SHM Systems*

Before deploying an SHM system, it is crucial to assess its potential value. Nepomuceno et al. [12] developed an approach for assessing the value of an SHM system for a bridge before deployment. This assessment considers factors such as the bridge's importance, condition, and expected service life. By evaluating the potential value of an SHM system, bridge owners and managers can make informed decisions regarding its implementation.

2.5. *Applications of SHM in Bridge Asset Management*

Various authors have effectively integrated SHM into bridge-asset management systems during the operation and maintenance phase of their assets' lifecycle. Figueiredo et al. [13] used SHM to make informed decisions about bridge maintenance, repair, and rehabilitation, validating their approach with real-world bridge data. Ni and Wong [14] designed an integrated SHM and maintenance management system for sea-crossing viaduct bridges, optimizing maintenance based on criticality and vulnerability. Seo et al. [15] conducted a summary review of SHM applications for highway bridges, highlighting the benefits of SHM in detecting and monitoring structural deterioration, assessing the remaining service life, and guiding maintenance decisions. Phares [16] developed a bridge asset management system that leveraged SHM to extend service life and reduce costs, rendering it economically justifiable. Dubbs [17] demonstrated the value of SHM integration by illustrating its ability to provide actionable information in areas such as maintenance work orders, operations, public safety, structural safety, and security, ultimately paving the way for an advanced asset management system.

2.6. *Condition-Based, Predictive, and Preventive Maintenance*

Flanigan et al. [18] proposed a reliability-based framework for linking long-term monitoring data to condition ratings. This framework adopted reliability analysis techniques to assess the condition of bridges based on the collected monitoring data, thus enabling condition-based maintenance (CBM). By quantitatively linking monitoring data to condition ratings, bridge owners and managers can prioritize maintenance and allocate resources effectively only when asset conditions dictate its necessity. Predictive maintenance modeling contributes to the future network-wide management of bridges. Stevens et al. [19] reviewed various approaches in bridge predictive maintenance modeling and outlined the challenges in their adaptation. In these models, data from SHM systems were used to predict the future performance and deterioration of bridges, enabling proactive maintenance strategies. While SHM is often associated with predictive maintenance, it also supports preventive maintenance by creating condition thresholds or triggers that determine when inspection maintenance activities must be carried out. These thresholds are based on observed data patterns and allow maintenance teams to address minor issues before they escalate.

2.7. Risk and Criticality in Data Collection

Bush et al. [20] developed a data collection and monitoring strategy for the asset management of road bridges. In this approach, bridges within a network were classified into one of three data collection categories: core, intermediate, or advanced. The classification considered the risk profile and the criticality of each bridge in the network, and a simple scoring scheme was proposed. Depending on a bridge's criticality level and risk, its data collection technique was shifted from core, to intermediate, to advanced. Correspondingly, the bridge is moved towards higher levels of data collection that involve collecting more detailed and reliable data. The higher data collection categories rely on proactive and planned integration of SHM systems for asset management. By providing a flexible approach to data collection, the bridge asset manager can tailor the strategy to align with local network requirements, risk tolerance, and budget, thereby ensuring the cost efficiency of strategy implementation.

3. Proposed Framework

A bridge asset management framework that effectively integrates structural health monitoring techniques into the operation and maintenance phase of the asset lifecycle is illustrated in Figure 1. This framework encompasses the following key activities and processes: value assessment, criticality assessment, risk assessment, asset management strategy, performance monitoring and condition assessment, and maintenance optimization.

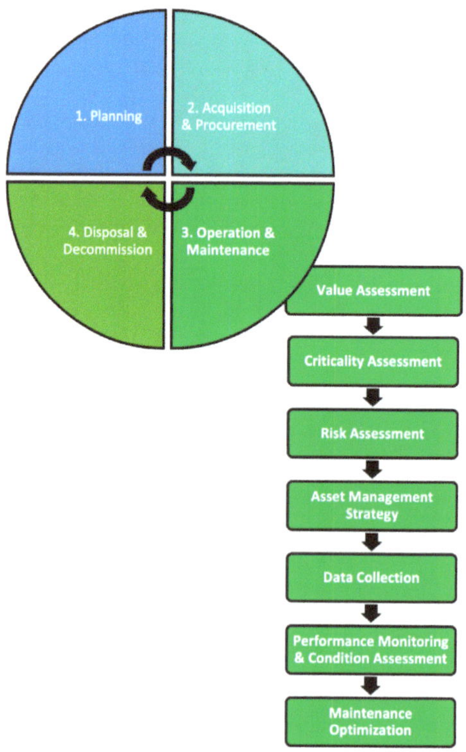

Figure 1. SHM-integrated bridge asset management framework.

3.1. Value Assessment

Objectively determine the state of the bridge after a visual inspection has deemed it structurally inadequate. Assess the value of implementing an SHM system for the bridge by evaluating factors such as the bridge's significance within the network, current condition, and expected service life. This initial assessment will help determine whether SHM is warranted for the specific bridge.

3.2. Criticality Assessment

Perform a criticality assessment to determine the importance of each bridge within the network. Criticality is often based on factors such as the bridge's role in the transportation network and its potential impact on public safety.

3.3. Risk Assessment

Assess the potential risks associated with the observed structural anomalies, taking into account factors such as traffic load, weather conditions, and material properties. Assign the level of risk to each observed anomaly based on its potential impact on safety and structural integrity. This assessment helps prioritize bridges for more detailed monitoring and maintenance efforts.

3.4. Asset Management Strategy

Align the asset management strategy with the specific needs of the bridge to ensure that the chosen strategy is tailored to the bridge's unique characteristics. Evaluate the need for advanced asset management based on the bridge's condition, demand, and importance within the network. Apply a simple asset management approach for low-risk and low-criticality bridges and advanced asset management for high-risk and high-criticality bridges.

3.5. Data Collection

Classify bridges within a network into one of three data collection categories (core, intermediate, or advanced) by considering the risk profile and criticality of each bridge within the classification. Core bridges require less frequent visual inspections and limited, usually reactive SHM. Intermediate and advanced bridges will require more frequent visual inspections and proactive, planned integration of SHM systems accordingly.

3.6. Performance Monitoring and Condition Assessment

With the data collection and monitoring strategy in place, establish a performance monitoring and condition assessment program that links SHM data to condition ratings. This is essential in ensuring that the collected SHM-based monitoring data are leveraged to evaluate the condition of bridges and enable condition-based maintenance.

3.7. Maintenance Optimization

Based on the condition assessment, maintenance and repair activities are optimized to balance the cost of repairs and the preservation of the bridge's structural integrity. This includes scheduling repairs when necessary, allocating resources efficiently, and reducing network interruption. For bridges in a relatively healthy condition, a predictive maintenance approach is suitable, using real-time monitoring and data analysis to efficiently anticipate and address emerging issues and avoid unnecessary maintenance work. For bridges with identified structural issues, vulnerabilities, or a higher risk profile, preventive maintenance is appropriate, employing scheduled, routine maintenance to prevent potential problems. This data-driven approach ensures that maintenance efforts are focused on critical areas of the bridge, thereby extending its service life.

4. Conclusions

This study provides a foundation for adopting SHM in bridge asset management, emphasizing the potential benefits of this technology in managing bridge assets. The presented framework offers a data-driven and proactive approach for enhancing bridge asset management processes during the operation and maintenance phase of the bridge lifecycle.

This framework ensures that the assessment of value, criticality, and risks guides the data collection strategy, enabling targeted SHM implementation, optimal resource allocation, and effective condition-based maintenance strategies, tailored to each bridge within a network. Similarly, the asset management strategy guides the data collection strategy, ensuring the necessary data are available to implement the required asset management approach. By implementing this framework, stakeholders involved in bridge asset management can be better equipped to use SHM to make informed decisions regarding operation, maintenance, repair, and rehabilitation.

Shaping the future of bridge asset management via SHM remains imperative. Future research needs to validate the framework's effectiveness and adaptability for the unique characteristics of different bridge structures. Additionally, the development of standardized guidelines and best practices for SHM integration must be an ongoing priority, enabling bridge authorities and asset managers to make well-informed decisions. In summary, enhancing bridge asset management through SHM is a dynamic and ever-evolving field, with the potential to transform how we monitor, maintain, and extend the life of critical infrastructure. The framework presented in this study represents a significant step toward more efficient, data-driven, and proactive bridge asset management.

Funding: This research received no external funding.

Institutional Review Board Statement: Not applicable.

Informed Consent Statement: Not applicable.

Data Availability Statement: All the data used in the experiment have been made available in the present article.

Acknowledgments: The author wishes to acknowledge the numerous authors whose work formed the basis of this literature review. Their insights and contributions were invaluable in shaping the strategic framework of this research.

Conflicts of Interest: The author declares no conflicts of interest.

References

1. Kim, J.R.; Chae, M.J.; Park, J.W.; Lee, G.; Cho, M.Y. Review of Wireless Sensors for Road and Bridge Asset Management. In Proceedings of the 2010 Construction Research Congress, Banff, AB, Canada, 8 May 2010.
2. *ISO55000*; Asset Management—Overview, Principles and Terminology. BSI Standards: London, UK, 2014.
3. The Institute of Asset Management. *The Pathway to Excellence in Asset Management: IAM Maturity Scale and Guidance*; IAM: London, UK, 2022.
4. Too, E.G. A Framework for Strategic Infrastructure Asset Management. In *Definitions, Concepts and Scope of Engineering Asset Management*; Amadi-Echendu, J., Brown, K., Willett, R., Mathew, J., Eds.; Springer: London, UK, 2010; Volume 1, pp. 31–62. [CrossRef]
5. Institute of Public Works Engineering Australia. *International Infrastructure Management Manual*, 4th ed.; National Asset Management Steering (NAMS) Group: Wellington, New Zealand, 2011.
6. US Government Accountability Office. *Highway Bridge Program: Clearer Goals and Performance Measures Needed for a More Focused and Sustainable Program*; US Government Accountability Office: Washington, DC, USA, 2008.
7. New Zealand Office of the Auditor General. *New Zealand Transport Agency: Information and Planning for Maintaining and Renewing the State Highway Network*; New Zealand Office of the Auditor General: Wellington, New Zealand, 2010.
8. Güemes, A.; Fernandez-Lopez, A.; Pozo, A.R.; Sierra-Pérez, J. Structural Health Monitoring for Advanced Composite Structures: A Review. *J. Compos. Sci.* **2020**, *4*, 13. [CrossRef]
9. Li, J.; Hao, H. A Review of Recent Research Advances on Structural Health Monitoring in Western Australia. *Struct. Monit. Maint.* **2016**, *3*, 33–49. [CrossRef]
10. Vanderzee, P.J.; Wingate, F.B. Structural Health Monitoring for Bridges. In *Infrastructure Reporting and Asset Management*; Adjo Amekudzi, A., McNeil, S., Eds.; American Society of Civil Engineers: Reston, VA, USA, 2008; pp. 178–182. [CrossRef]
11. Imperial College London. Available online: https://www.imperial.ac.uk/structural-integrity-health-monitoring/research/life-cycle-assessment-of-complex-structures/structural-health-monitoring (accessed on 1 November 2023).
12. Nepomuceno, D.T.; Vardanega, P.J.; Tryfonas, T.; Pregnolato, M.; Bennetts, J.; Webb, G.; Foster, A.; Augustine, L.; Holland, M. SHM Deployments for Two Bridge Structures: Assessing Potential Value. In Proceedings of the Eleventh International Conference on Bridge Maintenance, Safety and Management (IABMAS 2022), Barcelona, Spain, 11–15 July 2022.

13. Figueiredo, E.; Radu, L.; Park, G.; Farrar, C. Integration of SHM into bridge management systems: Case study-Z24 bridge. In *Structural Health Monitoring 2011: Condition-Based Maintenance and Intelligent Structures, Proceedings of the 8th International Workshop on Structural Health Monitoring, Stanford, CA, USA, 13–15 September 2011*; Stanford University: Stanford, CA, USA, 2011; Volume 1, pp. 725–732.
14. Ni, Y.Q.; Wong, K. Integrating Bridge Structural Health Monitoring and Condition-Based Maintenance Management. In Proceedings of the Workshop on Civil Structural Health Monitoring (CSHM-4), Berlin, Germany, 6–8 November 2012; Volume 18.
15. Seo, J.; Hu, J.W.; Lee, J. Summary Review of Structural Health Monitoring Applications for Highway Bridges. *J. Perform. Constr. Facil.* **2015**, *30*, 04015072. [CrossRef]
16. Lu, P.; Phares, B. *Integration of Structural Health Monitoring (SHM) into Multilayer Statewide Bridge Maintenance and Management Practices—SHM-Facilitated Condition Based Maintenance (SHM-CBM) Prioritization System*; Midwest Transportation Center, Bridge Engineering Center Iowa State University: Ames, IA, USA, 2018.
17. Dubbs, N.C. Expanding the Case for Structural Health Monitoring: A Focus on Its Role in Maintenance and Operations and Asset Management Systems. In Proceedings of the Structures Congress 2018, Fort Worth, TX, USA, 19–21 April 2018. [CrossRef]
18. Flanigan, K.A.; Lynch, J.P.; Ettouney, M. Quantitatively Linking Long-Term Monitoring Data to Condition Ratings through a Reliability-Based Framework. *Struct. Health Monit.* **2020**, *20*, 2376–2395. [CrossRef]
19. Stevens, N.; Lydon, M.; Marshall, A.H.; Taylor, S. Identification of Bridge Key Performance Indicators Using Survival Analysis for Future Network-Wide Structural Health Monitoring. *Sensors* **2020**, *20*, 6894. [CrossRef]
20. Bush, S.; Omenzetter, P.; Henning, T.; McCarten, P. A Risk and Criticality-Based Approach to Bridge Performance Data Collection and Monitoring. *Struct. Infrastruct. Eng.* **2013**, *9*, 329–339. [CrossRef]

engineering proceedings

Proceeding Paper

The Influence of Nudges on Workers' Safety Behavior in the Construction Industry †

Tzu-Lien Tzou [1], Pin-Chan Lee [2,*] and Tzu-Ping Lo [3]

[1] Occupational Safety and Health Administration, Ministry of Labor, New Taipei City 24219, Taiwan; ttzou2232@osha.gov.tw
[2] Taiwan Construction Occupational Safety and Health Promotion Association, New Taipei City 234635, Taiwan
[3] Yuejin Integration Tech, Ltd., New Taipei City 234635, Taiwan; kinolu9@gmail.com
* Correspondence: pinchan.lee@gmail.com
† Presented at the 2024 IEEE 4th International Conference on Electronic Communications, Internet of Things and Big Data, Taipei, Taiwan, 19–21 April 2024.

Abstract: The nudge theory has been applied to improve safety behavior in various industries. We implemented the nudge theory in the construction industry to improve worker safety. Nudges for construction safety were grouped into three categories and used in a project. The application of nudges improved workers' safety behavior, particularly in highlighting control measures. The background analysis results reveal that the implementation of nudges did not vary by gender, nationality, or age, demonstrating its high universality. The results of this study offer a reference for stakeholders in the construction industry who are aiming to bolster worker safety.

Keywords: construction safety; nudge theory; workers' safety behavior

Citation: Tzou, T.-L.; Lee, P.-C.; Lo, T.-P. The Influence of Nudges on Workers' Safety Behavior in the Construction Industry. *Eng. Proc.* **2024**, *74*, 15. https://doi.org/10.3390/engproc2024074015

Academic Editors: Shu-Han Liao, Teen-Hang Meen and Cheng-Fu Yang

Published: 27 August 2024

1. Introduction

Construction engineering, characterized by labor-intensive processes, diverse machinery, and complex interfaces, is considered a high-risk workplace. According to relevant studies in the literature [1,2], unsafe behavior is the primary cause of accidents in the construction industry. Therefore, it is crucial to enhance workers' safety behavior and reduce occupational accidents. There are laws, regulations, standards, and other mandates to secure workers' safety behavior, but these mandates are top-down commands. To encourage workers to voluntarily change their behaviors, the nudge theory can be used as an emerging and effective method [3].

The nudge theory, rooted in behavioral economics and psychology, employs ingenious design to assist individuals in making correct decisions. The nudge theory has been applied to improve safety behavior in various industries. Although its application in the construction industry is in its infancy, it has already shown impressive results. However, nudge measures must possess practical and easily promotable characteristics to effectively change safety behavior [4].

Therefore, we categorized construction safety nudges into Alerting Potential Hazards, Highlighting Control Measures, And Promoting Health Care and proposed practical nudges through collaborative discussions with construction safety experts. We established the nudge measure scale and the worker safety behavior scale and used them in a project to verify the effect of using nudges. Recommendations were made for strategies to implement the nudge theory based on research results.

2. Literature Review

2.1. Nudge Theory

The nudge theory was proposed by Thaler and Sunstein [5], originating from behavioral economics and psychology. Through ingenious design, it assists people in making robust decisions. The UK announced the establishment of the 'Nudge Unit', composed of scientists, psychologists, and policy experts, to apply the nudge theory to government policy implementation to enhance execution capability and service efficiency and yielded high cost-effectiveness for the UK.

Improving workers' safety behavior is an essential research topic regarding the nudge theory. Prabowo and Syaifullah [3] believe that unsafe behavior is the most critical factor leading to occupational accidents, and nudges are emerging and effective in eliminating or reducing unsafe behavior. Lindhout and Reniers [4] regard the nudge theory as an effective safety management tool capable of influencing workers' behavior and compliance. They organized nine design principles of nudges based on the literature review and believed that more practical and easily promotable nudges effectively change safety behavior. Szaszi et al. [6] investigated the effectiveness of the nudge theory as a safety behavior intervention measure. They found that the nudge theory, as an intervention, is low-cost and easy to implement and effectively influences the target group to unconsciously perform specific behaviors.

The nudge theory has been applied to improve safety behavior in various industries. Although its application in the construction industry has just begun, it has already shown astonishing results. The Royal Dutch Shell's Southbank office refurbishment project is a well-known case. The results of the nudges were clear: the levels of unsafe behaviors while working at height were reduced by 82% and by 93% for material movements in just 12 weeks [7]. The project also won the International Safety Award with Merit from the British Safety Council and the Health, Safety & Wellbeing Initiative of the Year award at the Association for Project Safety's National CDM Awards 2018.

Prabowo and Syaifullah [3] believe that nudges are effective in eliminating or reducing unsafe behavior in the construction industry. They explored the example of increasing the usage of personal protective equipment (PPE). They posted workers' hearing test results with and without PPE on the bulletin board as nudges. The pre-test and post-test comparisons showed that the nudges were gentle and effective interventions to eliminate workers' unsafe behavior. They also believed that nudges must be integrated into risk management and occupational safety and health management systems to improve organizational safety culture. Talabi et al. [8] believe that safety design and nudges must be implemented together, with safety design being used to eliminate construction risks while promoting nudges to reduce workers' unsafe behavior and reduce occupational accidents. Talabi et al. [9] considered nudges as effective safety interventions to enhance workers' safety behavior; they claimed that nudges must not be regarded directly as control measures but as reinforcements of control measures. Digital technology is gradually becoming a medium for nudges. Nioi et al. [10] used a mobile app to push information, such as UV radiation, sun safety, dietary health, and daily UV index, in the workers' area as nudges.

The nudge theory has been successfully applied to improve construction workers' safety behavior. Through development, digital technology has also become an essential medium for nudges. Moreover, the literature shows that practical and feasible nudging measures effectively changed safety behavior.

2.2. Safety Behavior

Many studies demonstrated that improved workers' safety behavior effectively reduced the occurrence of occupational accidents in construction. In ref. [11], safety behavior activities were implemented in two construction sites, each with approximately 200 workers, mainly from Bangladesh, China, Singapore, and Thailand. An online safety behavior tracking system was established to support the activities. The results show that through safety behavior activities and online tracking systems, continuous improvement in construction site safety was achieved. In a large construction site in Iran, the effectiveness of safety behavior was verified [12]. The results show that the safety index of the experimental group was significantly higher than that of the control group. Safety behavior activities at two construction sites in Singapore showed that the overall safety scores of the two projects were improved after implementing safety behavior activities [13]. In a construction site in Hong Kong, the impact of managerial behavior on workers' safety behavior was investigated [14]. The results show that managerial behavior affected the effectiveness and sustainability of workers' safety behavior, thereby improving the safety performance of the construction industry.

In addition to the effectiveness of safety behavior, the indicators of workers' safety behavior in the construction industry are also important. Chouudhry proposed using PPE; housekeeping; access to heights, plant, and equipment; and scaffold-type worker safety behavior indicators as interventions [15]. With these interventions, safety behavior significantly increased, and frontline worker safety was improved. Li et al. [1] proposed four categories and 10 unsafe behavior indicators, including falls, collisions, traffic accidents, and a lack of sensor detection. They analyzed the changes in indicator data to evaluate the safety performance of construction projects. The research results show that the safety index improved after promoting safety behavior activities, and this index is used in the construction industry. Guo et al. [16] established effective safety behavior indicators for Singapore tunnel engineering, including lifting operations, excavation, high-altitude operations, work platforms and passages, handling, hot work, factories and equipment, traffic management, personal protective equipment, and nine other categories. Ting et al. [17], based on previous studies, made adjustments according to actual application feedback, proposing four categories of safety behavior indicators: working environment, tools and equipment, body movement, and personal protective equipment. These indicators were applied to 19 engineering projects for over 10 years. The overall Total Recordable Case Rate (TRCR) significantly decreased after promoting safety behavior. The safety behavior indicators proposed by Ting et al. showed reliability and validity [18,19].

3. Methodology

3.1. Research Objective

We proposed practical construction safety nudges and investigated whether these nudges affected workers' safety behavior. We also explored whether different background conditions, such as gender, nationality, age, and position, result in variations in safety behavior performance.

3.2. Nudges for Construction Safety

Practicality and ease of promotion are key success factors for nudges [4]. Therefore, through collective discussions among safety experts, we categorized construction safety nudges into three classes: Alerting Potential Hazards, Highlighting Control Measures, and Promoting Health Care. To date, many practical nudges have been proposed (Table 1).

Table 1. Construction safety nudges.

Alerting Potential Hazards: Setting up warning slogans, signs, signals, etc., to alert workers to potential hazards.		
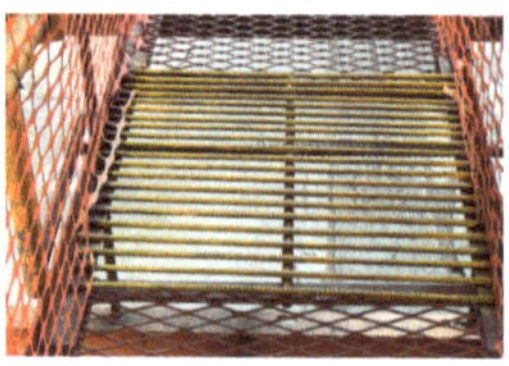	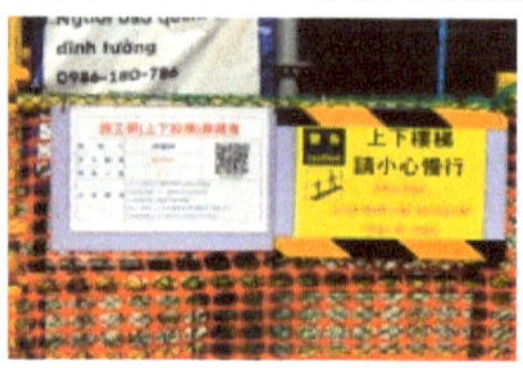	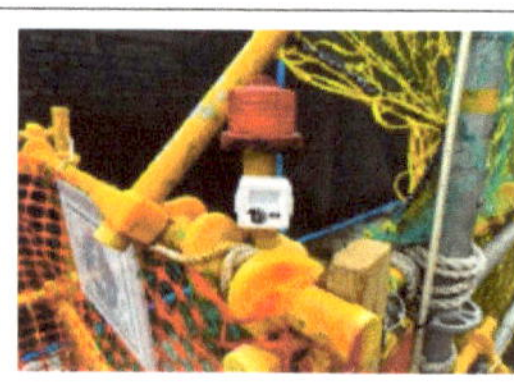
Paint safety passage rebar to prevent falls.	Add glow stickers by slogans for visibility.	Use sensor alerts for hazards.

Table 1. *Cont.*

<table>
<tr><td>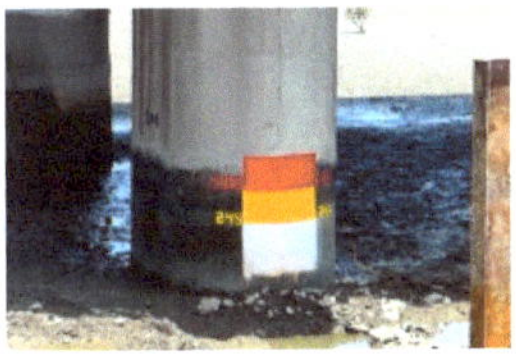
Mark pier levels against drowning.</td><td>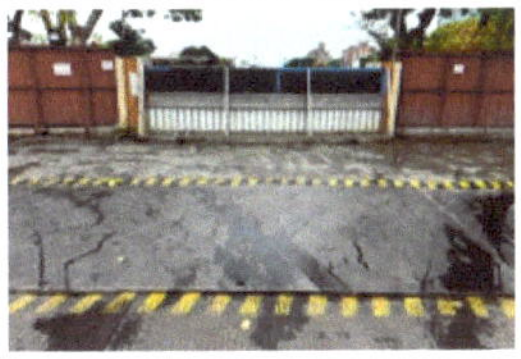
Install lines at platform road for alerts.</td><td>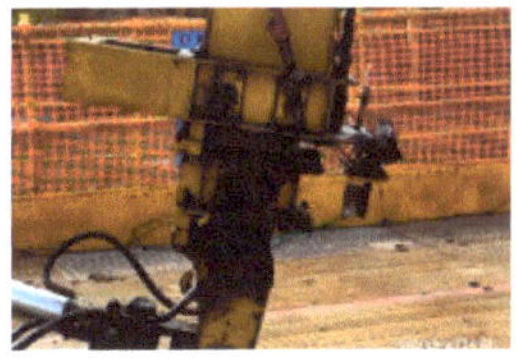
Add cameras in blind spots for collision warnings.</td></tr>
<tr><td colspan="3">Highlighting Control Measures: Enhance controls with added design for effectiveness.</td></tr>
<tr><td>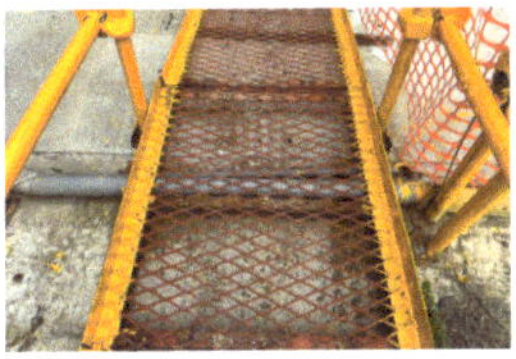
Use mesh on bridges for safety.</td><td>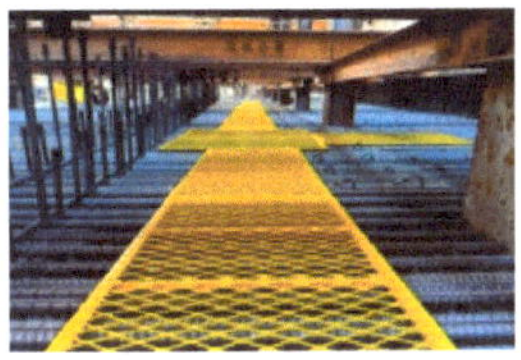
Lay mesh on rebar to prevent falls.</td><td>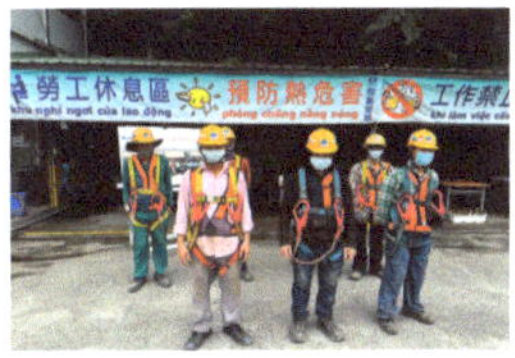
Paint belt hooks for compliance checks.</td></tr>
<tr><td>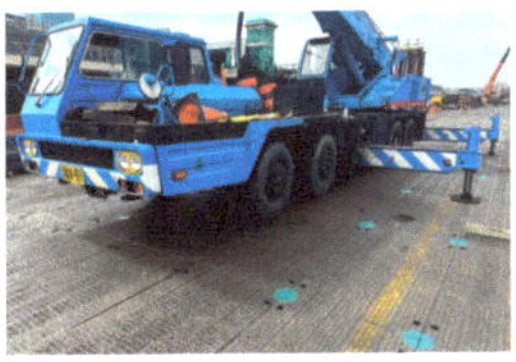
Paint crane supports for collapse prevention.</td><td>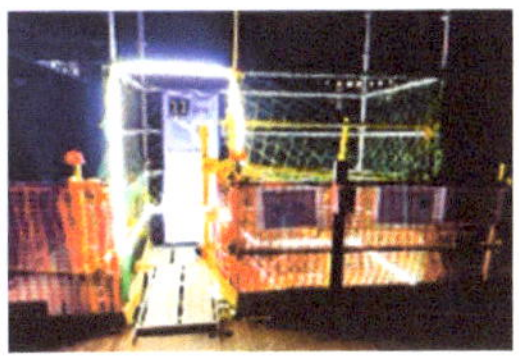
Install LED lights for nighttime construction safety.</td><td>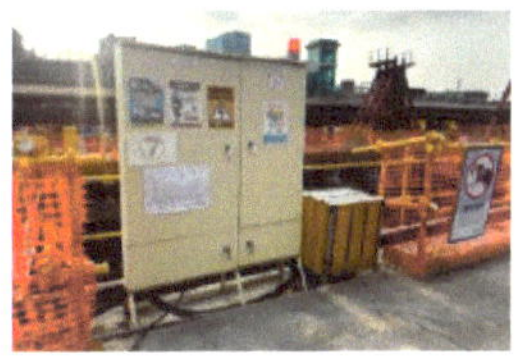
Post warning lights on electric boxes to prevent shock.</td></tr>
<tr><td colspan="3">Promoting Health Care: Various nudges concerned with the physical and mental health of workers.</td></tr>
<tr><td>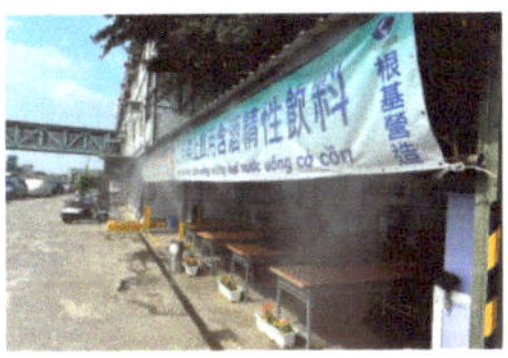
Use smart mist system for thermal stress prevention.</td><td>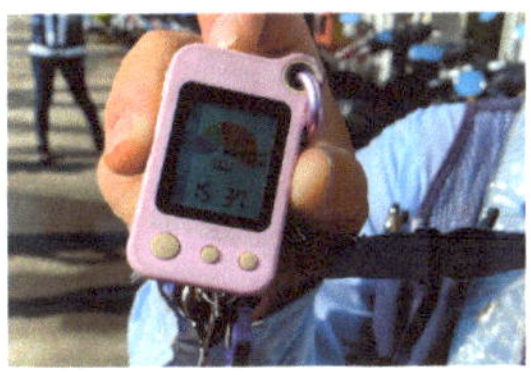
Give supervisors heat index detectors for break reminders.</td><td>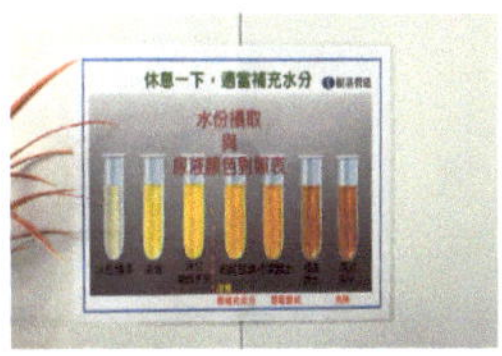
Post urine charts in restrooms for hydration reminders.</td></tr>
<tr><td>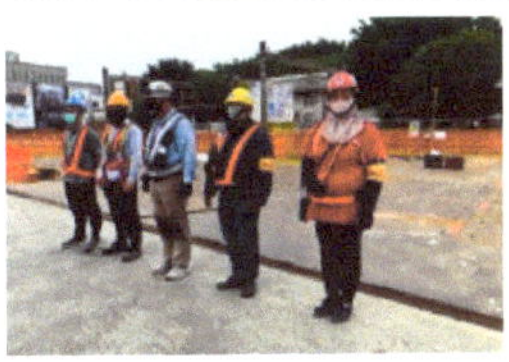
Color-code helmets for worker types.</td><td>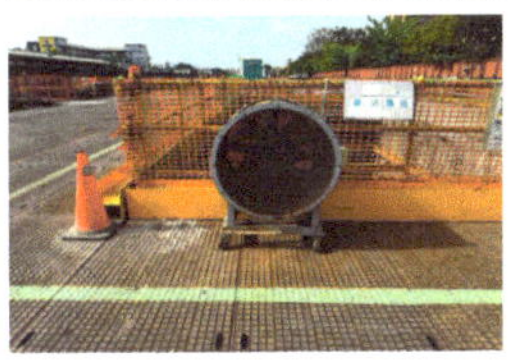
Install fans for heat safety.</td><td>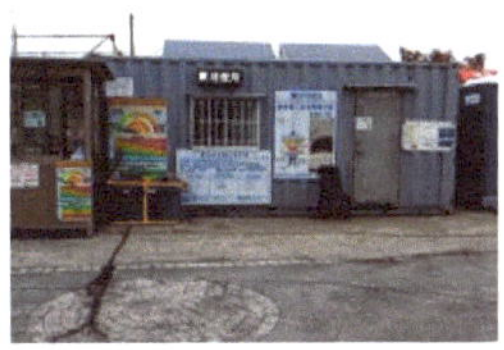
Set up solar rest area for workers.</td></tr>
</table>

3.3. *Nudge Measure Scale and Worker Safety Behavior Scale*

The nudge measure scale and the worker safety behavior scale were designed using a five-point scale, where 1 represents 'strongly disagree', 2 represents 'disagree', 3 represents 'neutral', 4 represents 'agree', and 5 represents 'strongly agree'. After a discussion with experts, the nudge measure scale was defined as shown in Table 2, including the labels X1 (Alerting Potential Hazards), X2 (Highlighting Control Measures), and X3 (Promoting Health Care).

Table 2. Nudge measure scale.

X1 Alerting Potential Hazards
X1.1 Visibility of the location of the hazard
X1.2 Awareness of the type of hazard
X1.3 Understanding of the potential impact of the hazard
X2 Highlighting Control Measures
X2.1 Awareness of control measures
X2.2 Recognition of the key protection aspects
X2.3 Understanding of the usage of control measures
X3 Promoting Health Care
X3.1 Awareness of health care measures
X3.2 Understanding of the purpose of health care measures
X3.3 Ability to remind oneself to pay attention to health status

The worker safety behavior scale demonstrated practicality and effectiveness in [17]. Therefore, we adjusted the worker safety behavior scale (Table 3), using labels including Y1 (working environment), Y2 (tools and equipment), Y3 (activity procedure), and Y4 (personal protective equipment).

Table 3. Worker safety behavior scale.

Y1 Working Environment
Y1.1 Notice the Condition of the Surfaces
Y1.2 Notice Extreme Temperature/Stress Exposure
Y1.3 Ensure Appropriate Lighting
Y1.4 Observe Signs and Barriers
Y1.5 Store Materials in Order
Y1.6 Segregate Garbage or Waste in Place
Y2 Tools and Equipment
Y2.1 Select the Correct Tools/Equipment
Y2.2 Inspect the Conditions of Tools/Equipment Before Use
Y2.3 Use Tools/Equipment Correctly
Y2.4 Operate Machines/Vehicles Well
Y3 Activity Procedure
Y3.1 Avoid Dangerous Areas
Y3.2 Stay Away from Hot Work Fire
Y3.3 Avoid Taking Shortcuts
Y3.4 Proceed and Operate with Care
Y3.5 Be Aware of Moving/Rotating Machines
Y3.6 Notice Proper Body Posture
Y3.7 Use Ladders Properly

Table 3. *Cont.*

Y3.8 Clime with Right Body Movement
Y3.9 Communicate Proactively
Y4 Personal Protective Equipment
Y4.1 Select the Correct PPE for the Job
Y4.2 Inspect the Condition of PPE Before Use
Y4.3 Use PPE Correctly

3.4. Statistical Analysis

We conducted descriptive statistics to illustrate the background information of the respondents and used t-tests or an ANOVA to examine differences in worker safety behavior scores based on different backgrounds (such as gender, nationality, age, and position). A correlation coefficient analysis was used for nudges (X1 to X3) to test multicollinearity issues. Subsequently, a regression analysis was conducted to explore the relationship between nudges and workers' safety behavior (Y1 to Y4), examining their explanatory power and statistical significance. Finally, a correlation coefficient analysis was also applied to workers' safety behavior to test its correlation.

4. Results and Discussions

4.1. Background Analysis

We selected a project located in Tainan to investigate the changes in workers' safety behavior after the implementation of nudges. A total of 81 valid questionnaires were collected. The demographics of the respondents were as follows:

1. Seventy-nine males and two females;
2. Eleven Taiwanese people and seventy foreign nationals;
3. Four respondents aged 20–30 years old, eighteen respondents aged 30–40 years old, forty-five respondents aged 40–50 years old, twelve respondents aged 50–60 years old, and two people over 60 years old;
4. Seventy-four workers and seven managers.

Although most of the questionnaires were answered by workers regarding the impact of the nudges on their safety behavior, several were filled out by managers, reflecting their observations on whether the workers' safety behavior was affected.

4.2. Workers' Safety Behavior

The average value of workers' safety behavior (Y) was 4.56, with the average value for working environment (Y1) being 4.55, the average value for tools and equipment (Y2) being 4.57, the average value for activity procedure (Y3) being 4.57, and the average value for personal protective equipment (Y4) being 4.56. These indicated that the implementation of nudges on the construction site enhanced workers' safety behavior. The top four highest-scoring items included Use PPE Correctly (Y4.3), Proceed and Operate with Care (Y3.4), Store Materials in Order (Y1.5), and Operate Machines/Vehicles Well (Y2.4). For example, adding conspicuous markings to personal protective equipment (such as spray painting safety belt hooks) as a nudge guided workers to unconsciously use PPE correctly, as shown in Figure 1.

In workers' safety behavior, the Pearson correlation coefficients for Y1 to Y4 were calculated, and a Bonferroni correction with a threshold was set at 0.05. The results revealed a significant correlation between working environment (Y1) and activity procedures (Y3) ($r = 0.50$), and also between tools and equipment (Y2) and activity procedures (Y3) ($r = 0.39$). Figure 2a illustrates the establishment of a cross-bridge passage using a diamond lattice grid as a nudge. Such a nudge affected the Notice the Condition of the Surfaces (Y1.1) and Avoid Taking Shortcuts (Y3.3) items. Figure 2b shows the posting of an electrical map on a temporary electrical box as a nudge. This nudge influenced the Inspect the Conditions of Tools/Equipment Before Use (Y2.2) and Proceed and Operate with Care (Y3.4) items.

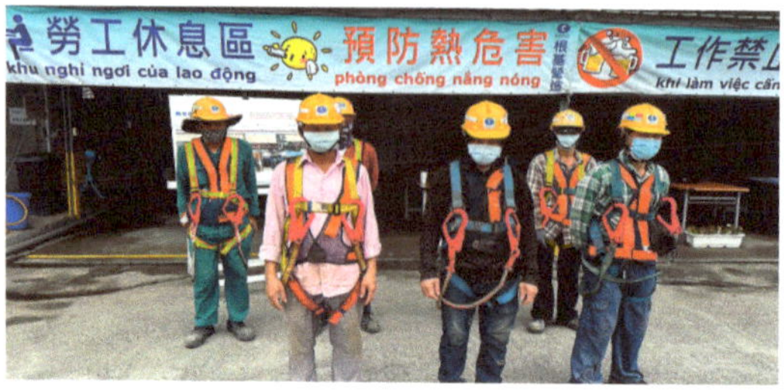

Figure 1. Spray painting safety belt hooks as nudges.

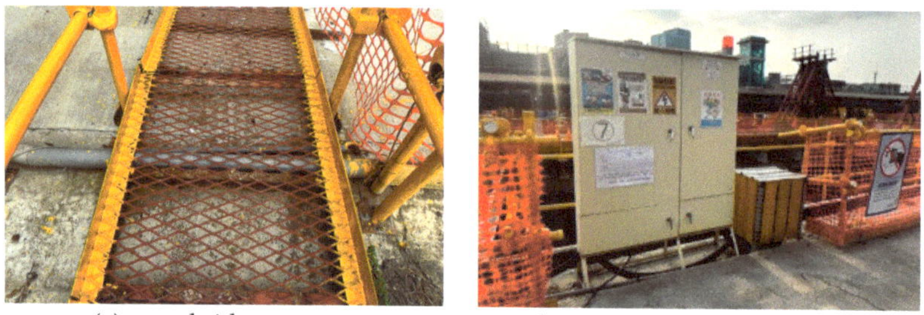

(**a**) cross-bridge passage (**b**) posting of an electrical map

Figure 2. Examples of nudges.

T-tests or an ANOVA were used to test workers' safety behavior based on different backgrounds (gender, nationality, age, and position). The results indicate that only different positions exhibited significant differences, while other backgrounds showed no significant differences in the performance of workers' safety behavior. The nudges had universality and can be applied to most construction sites. In terms of different positions, the worker safety behavior scores determined by on-site managers (4.73) were higher than the self-evaluated scores by the workers (4.55). This result may be due to the on-site managers having a better understanding of the purpose and usage of the nudges, resulting in higher observed scores. Therefore, it is necessary to enhance the promotion of various nudges to workers to improve their safety behavior.

4.3. Regression Analysis

A correlation coefficient analysis was conducted for the nudges (X1, X2, and X3). The correlation coefficient between X1 and X2 was 0.327, that between X1 and X3 was 0.387, and that between X2 and X3 was 0.372. The correlations among the variables were not high, indicating that the issue of multicollinearity among the independent variables was not severe, and the regression analysis results could be relatively trusted. The regression analysis result regarding the nudges (X1, X2, X3) and workers' safety behavior (Y) is shown in Equation (1).

$$Y = 1.8374 + 0.2111X1 + 0.2193X2 + 0.1688X3 \quad (1)$$

The coefficient of X1 is 0.2193, with a p-value of less than 0.001, indicating a statistically significant positive correlation between X1 and Y, and the same applies to X2 and X3. The R-squared value is 0.591, demonstrating reasonable explanatory power. According to Equation (1), the influence of nudges was in the order of Highlighting Control Measures (X2), Alerting Potential Hazards (X1), and Promoting Health Care (X3). Thus, construction sites may prioritize nudges that highlight control measures as they have the greatest impact on workers' safety behavior.

The statistical analysis results are summarized in Figure 3, showing that the implementation of nudges can indeed enhance workers' safety behavior, with the Highlighting Control Measures (X2) item having the greatest impact. The most effective items included Use PPE Correctly (Y4.3), Proceed and Operate with Care (Y3.4), Store Materials in Order (Y1.5), and Operate Machines/Vehicles Well (Y2.4).

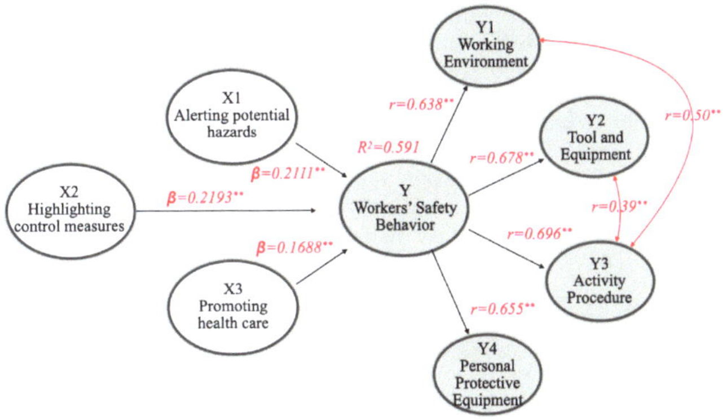

Figure 3. Influence of nudges on workers' safety behavior.

5. Conclusions

Based on a literature review, we posited that construction safety nudges enhanced workers' safety behavior, thereby reducing the occurrence of occupational accidents. Therefore, through expert discussions, the nudges were categorized into three types, namely Alerting Potential Hazards, Highlighting Control Measures, and Promoting Health Care, and many practical nudges were proposed. Additionally, we developed scales for nudge measures and workers' safety behavior as measurement tools. The results from the investigation and analysis indicate that nudges improved workers' safety behavior, with the Highlighting Control Measures being the most influential nudge. Construction sites may prioritize implementation from this category. The nudge measures proposed in this study are characterized by their practicality and high cost-effectiveness. They were given feedback from the construction industry for universality. Although we focused on a single construction site, construction safety nudges need to be promoted nationwide. More extensive survey data are needed to validate the research hypotheses. Once a large amount of data are collected, structural equation modeling can be employed for further analysis.

Author Contributions: Writing—original draft preparation, P.-C.L. and T.-P.L.; writing—review, T.-L.T. All authors have read and agreed to the published version of the manuscript.

Funding: This research received no external funding.

Institutional Review Board Statement: Not applicable.

Informed Consent Statement: Not applicable.

Data Availability Statement: Data are contained within the article.

Acknowledgments: This study extends its gratitude to the Occupational Safety and Health Administration of the Ministry of Labor for their support, as well as to the Taiwan Construction Industry Occupational Safety and Health Promotion Association and Kedge Construction Co., Ltd. for providing the test construction site and valuable suggestions.

Conflicts of Interest: Author Tzu-Ping Lo was employed by the company Yuejin Integration Tech, Ltd. The remaining authors declare that the research was conducted in the absence of any commercial or financial relationships that could be construed as a potential conflict of interest.

References

1. Li, H.; Hsu, S.C.; Gray, M.; Huang, T. Proactive behavior-based safety management for construction safety improvement. *Saf. Sci.* **2015**, *75*, 107–117. [CrossRef]
2. He, C.; McCabe, B.; Jia, G.; Sun, J. Effects of safety climate and safety behavior on safety outcomes between supervisors and construction workers. *J. Constr. Eng. Manag.* **2020**, *146*, 04019092. [CrossRef]
3. Prabowo, A.; Syaifullah, D.H. Eliminating Unsafe Behaviour Through the Implementation of Nudge Theory in Indonesian Industry. In Proceedings of the Second Asia Pacific International Conference on Industrial Engineering and Operations Management, Surakarta, Indonesia, 14–16 September 2021.
4. Lindhout, P.; Reniers, G. What about nudges in the process industry? Exploring a new safety management tool. *J. Loss Prev. Process Ind.* **2017**, *50*, 243–256. [CrossRef]
5. Thaler, R.H.; Sunstein, C.R. *Nudge: Improving Decisions about Health, Wealth, and Happiness*; Yale University Press: New Haven, CT, USA, 2008.
6. Szaszi, B.; Palinkas, A.; Palfi, B.; Szollosi, A.; Aczel, B. A systematic scoping review of the choice architecture movement: Toward understanding when and why nudges work. *J. Behav. Decis. Mak.* **2018**, *31*, 355–366. [CrossRef]
7. Overbury. Pink Walls Prevent Falls in An Award-Winning H&S Study. 2018. Available online: https://www.overbury.com/knowledge/news/h-s-study-pink-walls (accessed on 27 May 2024).
8. Talabi, B.O.; Edum-Fotwe, F.T.; Gibb, A.G.F. Construction actor safety behaviour: Antecedents, current thinking and directions. In Proceedings of the ARCOM Doctoral Workshop: Health, Safety and Wellbeing, University of Edinburgh, Edinburgh, UK, 11 February 2015; pp. 9–20.
9. Talabi, B.O.; Gibb, A.G.F.; Edum-Fotwe, F.T. Behaviour-based safety (BBS): A construction industry's perspective. In Proceedings of the CIB W099 Benefitting Workers and Society through Inherently Safe(r) Construction, Belfast, Ireland, 9–11 September 2015; pp. 181–190.
10. Nioi, A.; Wendelboe-Nelson, C.; Cowan, S.; Cherrie, M.; Rashid, S.; Cowie, H.; Davis, A.; Ritchie, P.; Lansdown, T.C.; Cherrie, J.W. Nudging construction workers towards better sun-safety behaviour: Summary of the evidence for practitioners. *Policy Pract. Health Saf.* **2020**, *18*, 25–33. [CrossRef]
11. Zhang, M.; Fang, D. A continuous Behavior-Based Safety strategy for persistent safety improvement in construction industry. *Autom. Constr.* **2013**, *34*, 101–107. [CrossRef]
12. Oostakhan, M.; Mofidi, A.; Talab, A.D. Behavior-Based Safety approach at a large construction site in Iran. *Iran. Rehabil. J.* **2012**, *10*, 21–25.
13. Fang, D.; Wu, H. Development of a Safety Culture Interaction (SCI) model for construction projects. *Saf. Sci.* **2013**, *57*, 138–149. [CrossRef]
14. Zhang, P.; Li, N.; Fang, D.; Wu, H. Supervisor-focused Behavior-Based Safety method for the construction industry: Case study in Hong Kong. *J. Constr. Eng. Manag.* **2017**, *143*, 05017009. [CrossRef]
15. Choudhry, R.M. Behavior-based safety on construction sites: A case study. *Accid. Anal. Prev.* **2014**, *70*, 14–23. [CrossRef] [PubMed]
16. Guo, B.H.; Goh, Y.M.; Wong, K.L.X. A system dynamics view of a behavior-based safety program in the construction industry. *Saf. Sci.* **2018**, *104*, 202–215. [CrossRef]
17. Ting, H.I.; Lee, P.C.; Chen, P.C.; Chang, L.M. An adjusted behavior-based safety program with the observation by front-line workers for mitigating construction accident rate. *J. Chin. Inst. Eng.* **2020**, *43*, 37–46. [CrossRef]
18. Lee, P.C.; Wei, J.; Ting, H.I.; Lo, T.P.; Long, D.; Chang, L.M. Dynamic analysis of construction safety risk and visual tracking of key factors based on behavior-based safety and building information modeling. *KSCE J. Civ. Eng.* **2019**, *23*, 4155–4167. [CrossRef]
19. Chen, Q.; Long, D.; Yang, C.; Xu, H. Knowledge Graph Improved Dynamic Risk Analysis Method for Behavior-Based Safety Management on a Construction Site. *J. Manag. Eng.* **2023**, *39*, 04023023. [CrossRef]

engineering proceedings

MDPI

Proceeding Paper

Contractor Perceptions of Off-Site Modular Construction in Kuwait: An Investigation of Current Practices †

Areej AlBanwan *, Nourah AlMutawaa and Abdullah AlFoudari

Energy and Building Research Center, Sustainability and Reliability of Infrastructure Program, Kuwait Institute for Scientific Research, P.O. Box 24885 Safat, Kuwait City 13109, Kuwait; nmutawaa@kisr.edu.kw (N.A.); afoudari@kisr.edu.kw (A.A.)

* Correspondence: abanwan@kisr.edu.kw

† Presented at the 2024 IEEE 4th International Conference on Electronic Communications, Internet of Things and Big Data, Taipei, Taiwan, 19–21 April 2024.

Abstract: Kuwait faces a pressing challenge in expanding its existing buildings to meet growing demands. The rising popularity of modular construction systems, with their off-site construction approach, offers promising solutions. In this research, we explored the characteristics of Kuwait's modular construction industry, including clients' awareness levels, preferences, and key motivations for adopting modular construction over the traditional construction approach. This research addressed a critical gap in the current literature by providing an outlook on Kuwait's modular construction industry, which has been notably absent in existing literature. Valuable insights gained through questionnaire surveys distributed to industry contractors highlighted the off-site construction methods used, the sectors they serve, and the key advantages of using modular construction in Kuwait. These findings contribute to researching unexplored aspects of modular construction in Kuwait. They also provide stakeholders with valuable insights, enabling them to make well-informed decisions for their construction projects.

Keywords: modular construction; prefabrication; off-site construction; contractor perception; Kuwait

Citation: AlBanwan, A.; AlMutawaa, N.; AlFoudari, A. Contractor Perceptions of Off-Site Modular Construction in Kuwait: An Investigation of Current Practices. *Eng. Proc.* **2024**, *74*, 16. https://doi.org/10.3390/engproc2024074016

Academic Editors: Shu-Han Liao, Teen-Hang Meen and Cheng-Fu Yang

Published: 27 August 2024

1. Introduction

Like many rapidly developing countries, Kuwait faces a substantial challenge in expanding its existing infrastructure to meet the demands of a growing population. With urbanization on the rise and a pressing need for housing and infrastructure development, the construction industry is under constant pressure to deliver efficient, cost-effective, and sustainable solutions [1]. Consequently, the rising popularity of off-site modular construction for expanding residential buildings in Kuwait has drawn attention requiring a potential solution to these challenges. Thus, we explored the current state of the off-site modular construction industry in Kuwait, focusing on contractor perceptions and their role in shaping the industry's development. Modular construction, characterized by its off-site assembly of prefabricated components, is becoming prominent on a global scale due to its potential to enhance construction efficiency, reduce costs, and minimize environmental impact. In the modular construction approach compared with traditional on-site construction, most building components are fabricated and assembled at the construction site [2]. Modular construction systems allow various building elements to be manufactured in a controlled factory environment, transported to the construction site and rapidly assembled [3]. These benefits are particularly pertinent in Kuwait, where rapid construction is crucial to the increasing demand for building expansions while prioritizing both quality and cost-effectiveness. In this study, we addressed a significant gap in the current literature as there is limited information available on the off-site modular construction industry in Kuwait. While more research has been done on modular construction globally, Kuwait's specific conditions and practices remain largely unexplored.

2. Literature Review

2.1. Key Definitions and Principles

In recent years, the adoption of off-site and modular construction techniques has significantly increased, primarily due to the advantages of modularization and prefabrication, which improve efficiency, reduce time, minimize cost, and enhance the quality of construction projects [4]. The terms "off-site construction", "modular construction", and "prefabrication" are interconnected due to their shared goal of improving the efficiency and quality of construction projects. While they have distinct features, they often overlap and complement each other in various ways:

- Off-site construction encompasses a range of techniques to move construction activities away from the construction site. Buildings and the majority or all of their primary components are manufactured and pre-assembled, or partially assembled, in the factory. This pre-assembly includes attaching fixtures, wiring, plumbing, and other necessary elements. This means that the components, elements, or modules are ready for installation once they arrive at the construction site [5];
- Modular construction is a subset of off-site construction that involves fabricating pre-designed building units or 'modules' at an off-site location, which are then transported to the construction site as components and assembled to complete buildings or structures. This construction method capitalizes on modularization and breaks down a larger system, structure, or project into smaller, self-contained modules or components [6];
- Prefabrication involves manufacturing building components at a distance from the final location, often in a factory, before they are transported to the construction site for assembly. These prefabricated elements include wall panels, roof trusses, and plumbing systems. While prefabricated components may be used in modular construction, prefabrication is not limited to off-site work. It involves the production of pre-manufactured elements assembled on-site, which is also a part of traditional construction methods [7].

In summary, off-site construction involves manufacturing components away from the construction site. Modular construction is a specific type of off-site construction focusing on pre-designed modules for assembly, and prefabricated construction encompasses a wide range of prefabricated building elements used in various construction methods in both on-site and off-site approaches.

2.2. Modular Construction Industry

Off-site modular construction can be used for either permanent or temporary building structures. Permanent modular construction (PMC) involves the use of prefabricated modules to construct permanent buildings, such as residential and commercial buildings [6]. On the other hand, temporary modular construction (TMC), or relocatable buildings, involves the use of prefabricated modules to construct temporary buildings that can be relocated, such as disaster relief housing, clinics, medical facilities, and temporary residential or commercial spaces [6].

The modular construction industry comprises manufacturers, manufacturer-directors, and dealers. Manufacturers produce modules for general contractors or modular dealers. Manufacturer-direct entities, on the other hand, cater to general contractors and dealers but also engage directly with property owners to offer modular solutions, often assuming the role of a general contractor [8]. Both manufacturers and manufacturer-directing organizations may have specializations focusing on specific building types, such as residential or commercial, and may serve the relocatable or permanent construction markets.

Modules are fabricated from various materials, including wood framing, cold-formed steel framing, hot-rolled steel, concrete, or a blend of materials [8]. Not all manufacturers engage in the production of modules across all these materials. Instead, manufacturers often specialize in a specific type of construction to optimize their factory operations and efficiencies. The selection of module materials is typically dictated by the project's specific needs, site-related factors, and budget considerations, making it a contingent decision by project stakeholders [8]. Notably, in Kuwait, wood is excluded as a construction material due to its inability to withstand the country's high temperatures, which often exceed 50 °C in the summer.

Off-site modular construction offers a range of advantages that cater to specific market sectors that particularly require speed of construction, cost-efficiency, and minimal disruption of the building process. This approach finds significant applications in various sectors, including residential buildings, mixed residential and commercial structures, private and social housing, hotels, military accommodations, health sector facilities, and educational institutions. Moreover, modular construction is also well-suited for rooftop extensions on existing buildings and the addition of new balconies and lifts to enhance the functionality of established structures. The diverse applications of modular construction make it an attractive choice for meeting the unique demands of different market segments while ensuring rapid and cost-effective project delivery [9].

2.3. Classification of Off-Site Construction Methods

Different types of off-site construction can be classified based on the degree of prefabrication. Five sub-categories are described in this approach, as shown in Figure 1 [10]. This classification ranges from component (the lowest level of prefabrication) to panel, volume, hybrid, and complete building (the highest degree of prefabrication This classification highlights the versatility of prefabrication methods in construction as follows:

- Prefabricated components include individual building elements and parts that are produced in a factory setting. These components can include beams, columns, windows, or smaller sections of walls and floors [9];
- Panelized construction involves the prefabrication of linear or flat, two-dimensional panels, used mainly for structural frames and walls. These are often prefinished with their insulation and boarding attached before being transported to the construction site and assembled to form the expanded building structure [9];
- Volumetric construction involves the prefabrication of fully completed, three-dimensional modules, which are then transported to the site for installation to create significant sections of the building [9];
- Hybrid construction combines various elements, including linear components, panels, and modules, to create a mixed-construction system. This method blends different prefabrication techniques to achieve a customized and efficient building solution that leverages the strengths of each element used [9];
- Complete building systems involve the assembly of modular components into fully finished structures before they are delivered to the construction site. In this method, the building or structure is essentially prefabricated to a high degree of completion in a factory setting, and it arrives at the site ready for installation and immediate use [9].

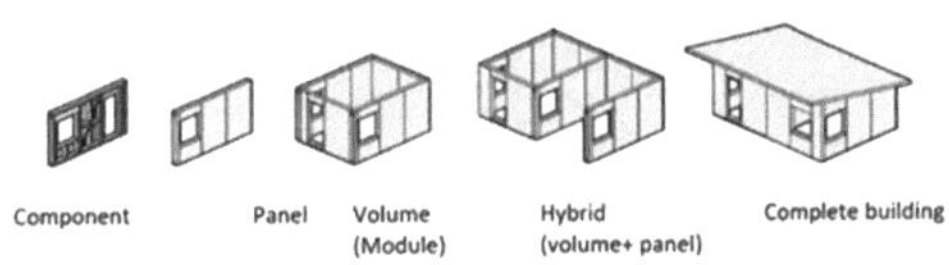

Figure 1. Off-site construction methods based on degree of prefabrication [10].

In summary, panelized construction is more suitable for smaller expansions or renovations, offering greater design flexibility and customization options. Volumetric construction is more suitable for larger expansions, allowing for rapid assembly and reduced on-site labor. Hybrid construction can offer the benefits of both panelized and volumetric methods, making it versatile and suitable for a wide range of project types. Complete building systems are characterized by exceptional efficiency, quality, and speed, making them suitable for applications such as modular homes or portable structures. Overall, off-site construction offers a flexible and efficient way to expand existing buildings, and these methods provide a range of modularization options for achieving this goal.

2.4. Advantages and Disadvantages of Modular Construction

One of the main advantages of modular construction is its speed, which is up to 50% faster than traditional construction methods [11]. This accelerated construction pace is accompanied by better quality control, as the modules are constructed in a controlled factory environment, reducing the risk of errors and defects. Moreover, as components are prefabricated off-site, the reduction in on-site installation processes increases installation efficiency and simultaneously enhances working conditions and productivity [12]. This approach also significantly reduces the need for on-site labor, which results in reduced labor expenses and enhances overall project cost-effectiveness. Similarly, the modular construction approach reduces waste, noise, and dust on site, minimizing the impacts on the community while simultaneously improving the environmental quality [4]. Since most project activities are completed off-site, modular construction minimizes the disruptions to ongoing activities, making it particularly beneficial for expanding existing buildings where occupants need to continue their activities without significant interruptions.

While modular construction offers numerous advantages, it has challenges and limitations. One significant challenge pertains to transportation logistics, particularly for larger components or modules. Transporting oversized modules to the construction site requires specialized equipment and can cause delays, incur extra costs, and add complexity to the construction process [13]. Therefore, careful planning with explicit scope and design details is required before the start of the project. Furthermore, resizing or reshaping modules on the construction site is challenging. Additionally, modular construction may not be suitable for all types of buildings, particularly high-rises or structures in areas prone to strong seismic activity [4]. While off-site construction offers cost savings compared to traditional on-site methods, it necessitates the establishment of a fabrication plant, which leads to increased capital expenses [14]. Furthermore, the non-acceptance of this construction technology by the general and sometimes professional public are disadvantages of modular construction [15].

3. Methodology

To achieve the research objectives, a literature review was conducted to gather relevant information for the development of a structured questionnaire. The questionnaire was divided into two main sections. The first section was designed to gather information regarding respondents and organizational profiles. The second section was designed to gather insights into Kuwait's industry characteristics by exploring topics such as client awareness, the type of modular construction adopted, the sectors where off-site construction was implemented, the types of off-site construction offered by contracting companies, and the key advantages driving the adoption of off-site modular construction in Kuwait. Printed questionnaires were distributed to contracting companies involved in off-site and modular construction across various sectors in Kuwait. A total of 18 surveys from 6 different companies were analyzed, and a descriptive approach was used to evaluate, sort, and present the information gathered. The data has been presented using columns and pie charts. These visual representations were chosen because they effectively illustrate the distribution and proportions of the responses, making it easier to identify patterns and trends within the data.

4. Results and Discussion

4.1. Respondent and Organization Profile

In the initial section of the survey, respondents were asked about their professional roles, organization type, industry experience, and the types of projects their organizations had undertaken to understand the diverse landscape of the surveyed companies. The most prevalent job title among respondents was "Engineer", constituting 50% of the responses, followed by "Architect" and "Manager", each representing 22.2%. An additional 5.6% of respondents belonged to the category of "Other", which included company owners, as illustrated in Figure 2. In the analysis of organization types, 61.1% of respondents identified as general contractors, and 38.9% identified as sub/specialty contractors, as outlined in Figure 3.

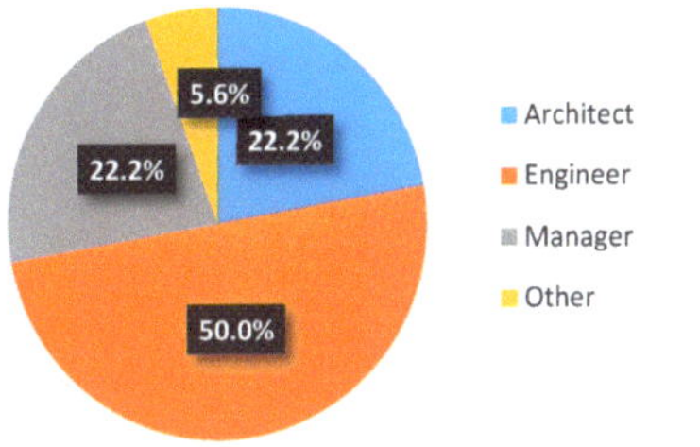

Figure 2. Professional background of respondents.

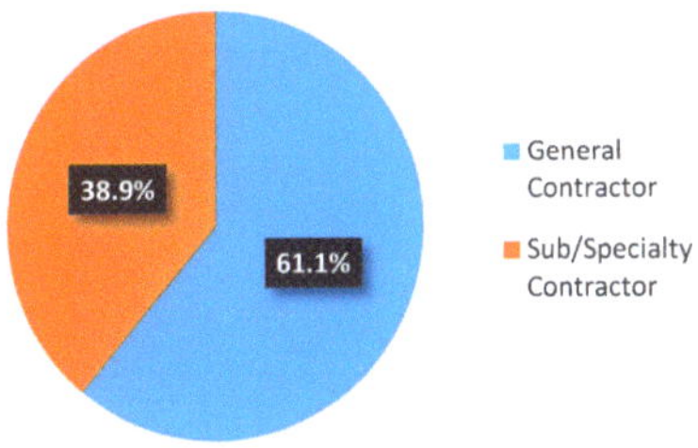

Figure 3. Type of organization of respondents.

In terms of industry experience, a majority (61.1%) of respondents were affiliated with companies that have been operating for 10–20 years, followed by 22.2% of respondents who worked in companies with over 20 years of experience, and 16.7% were associated with companies operating for 5–10 years. Notably, none of the surveyed companies reported operating for less than 5 years, as depicted in Figure 4. When examining project experience, a substantial portion of the respondents (77.8%) represented companies that had been involved in more than 20 projects featuring modular components. A smaller fraction (16.7%) had undertaken 5–10 projects, and the least represented group of respondents (5.6%) reported company involvement in 10–20 modular construction projects, as depicted in Figure 5.

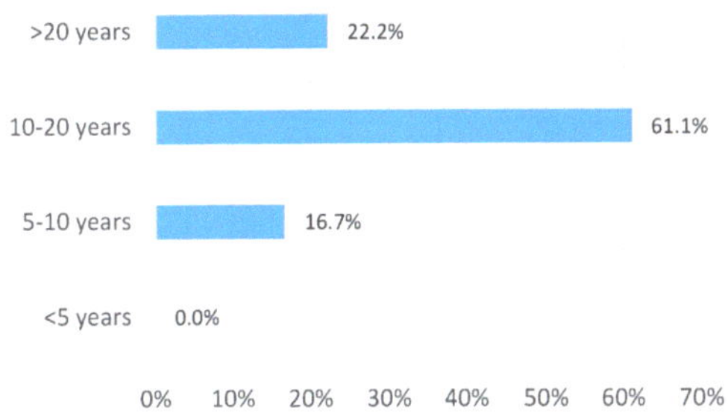

Figure 4. Years of operation in the construction industry.

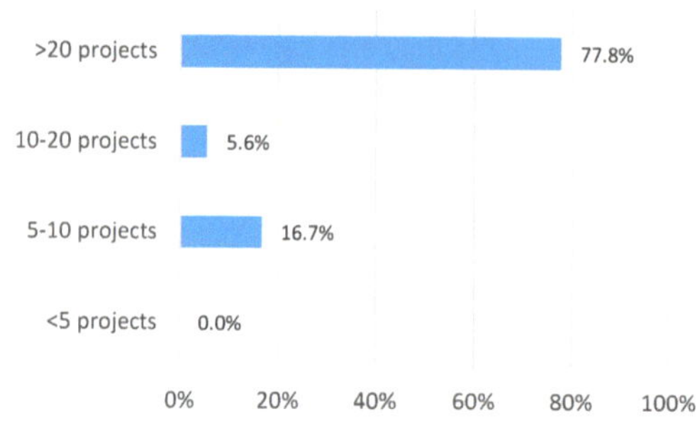

Figure 5. Number of off-site modular construction projects executed.

The respondents were further questioned about the types of projects undertaken by their companies to identify the sectors served by modular construction firms in Kuwait. Based on the findings, a significant majority (45.6%) of respondents' companies were equally involved in residential and commercial building projects, followed by medical building projects (6.7%), institutional building projects (1.1%), and other projects (1.1%), including chalets, as illustrated in Figure 6.

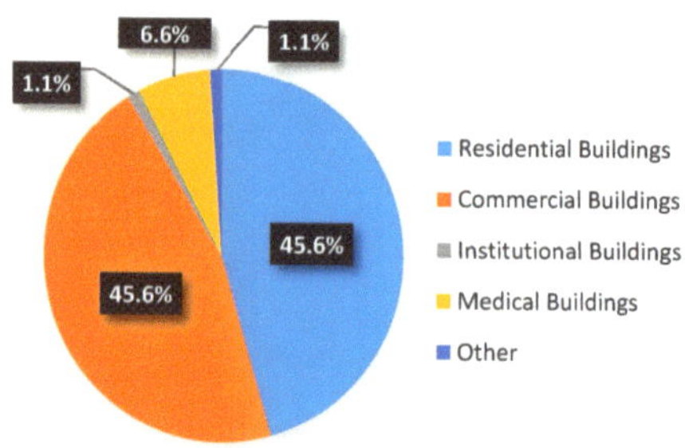

Figure 6. Types of off-site modular construction projects carried out by respondents' companies.

4.2. Client Awareness of Modular Construction

In the second segment of the questionnaire, respondents were directed to provide insights on clients' awareness of modular construction as a building construction method. The findings revealed a notably low level of client awareness of modular construction, with 83.3% of respondents stating a lack of awareness among their customer base, and only 16.7% of respondents found some awareness among their customer base, as shown in Figure 7.

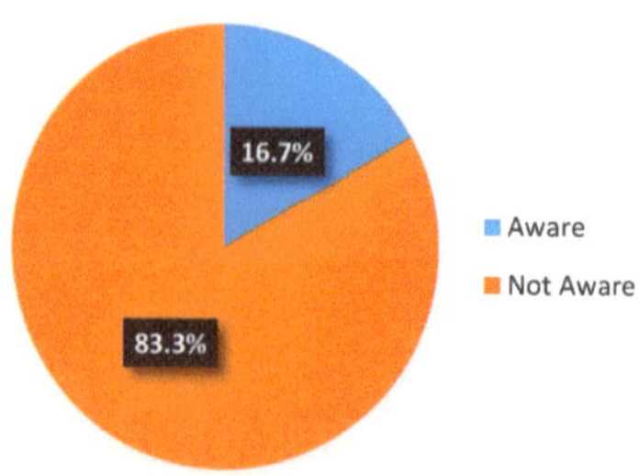

Figure 7. Client awareness level as perceived by contractors.

4.3. Type of Modular Construction

Figure 8 indicates the type of modular construction method adopted by the surveyed respondents according to client demand. According to the results, most respondents (66.7%) adopted permanent modular construction. In comparison, 33.3% adopted temporary/relocatable modular construction, indicating client preference for permanent applications in modular construction.

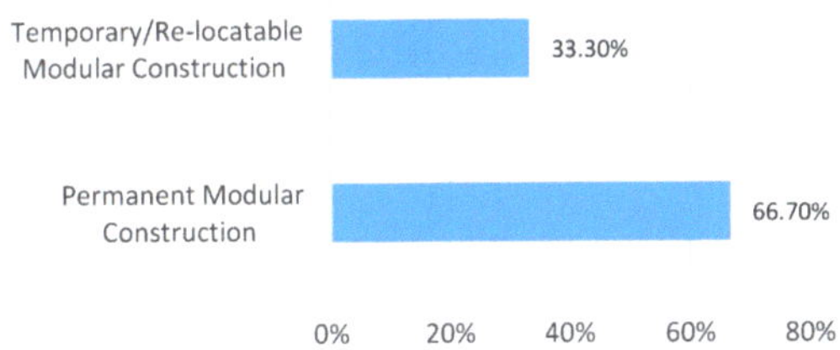

Figure 8. Type of modular construction adopted by respondents' companies.

4.4. Client Preferences and Motivations

We delved into the types of clients that request off-site modular construction and the key advantages motivating clients to adopt this construction method in Kuwait. The responses to the questionnaire survey were analyzed to identify respondent preferences and priorities. By assessing the frequency and ranking of the selected options, a total score was computed to establish the average rank for each option. Figure 9 depicts client demand for off-site modular construction across various sectors, as perceived by the surveyed respondents. The findings revealed a hierarchical preference with residential clients securing the top rank, followed by commercial, medical, institutional, and other clients (such as chalet and farm owners). The residential demand suggested a robust market for modular construction within the residential sector.

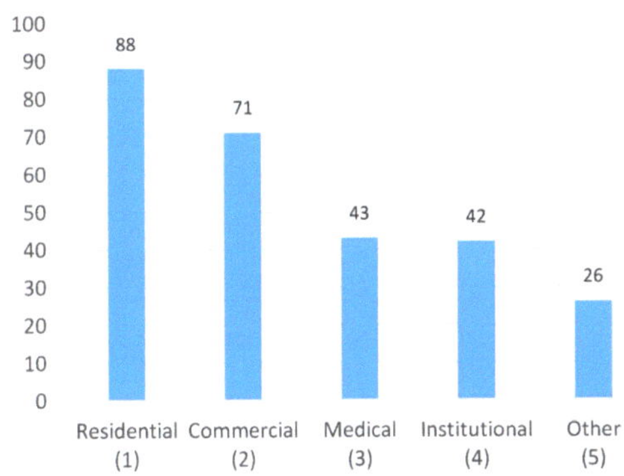

Figure 9. Client-driven ranking of sectors utilizing modular construction.

Figure 10 illustrates the key advantages influencing clients to opt for off-site modular construction. Notably, shorter construction time emerged as the top-ranked factor, followed closely by the considerations of minimized waste and noise during execution. The third-ranking position was contended between shorter material supply time and reduced costs. These insights from respondents showed the intricacies of client decision-making processes, offering a clearer understanding of the factors influencing client adoption of off-site modular construction methods in Kuwait.

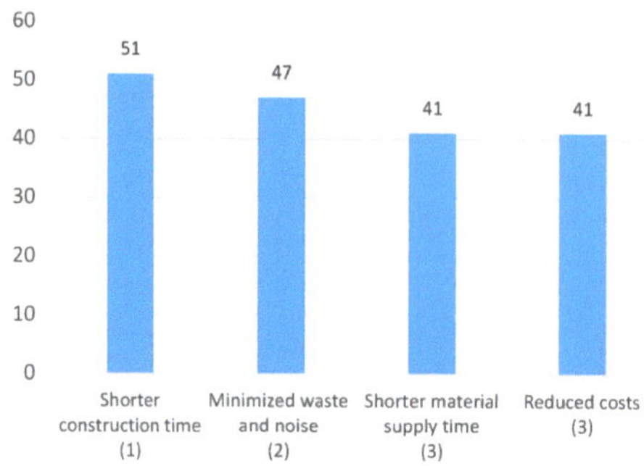

Figure 10. Client-driven ranking of key advantages influencing modular construction adoption.

4.5. *Off-Site Construction Methods*

Diverse off-site construction methods can be classified based on the degree of prefabrication, as demonstrated in Figure 1. During the survey, respondents were asked about the off-site construction options offered by their organizations. The results revealed a close but distinct hierarchy in the prevalence of these options, as depicted in Figure 11. Notably, 83.3% of respondents identified panelized construction as the most prevalent type of off-site construction offered by Kuwaiti contracting firms. Following closely behind, hybrid construction was provided by 77.8% of the respondents' companies, prefabricated components offered by 72.2%, and lastly, volumetric construction, while slightly less common, was provided by 66.7% of the companies of the respondents. These results indicated the prevalence of off-site construction practices of the surveyed contracting companies in Kuwait and highlighted the spectrum of options available to stakeholders.

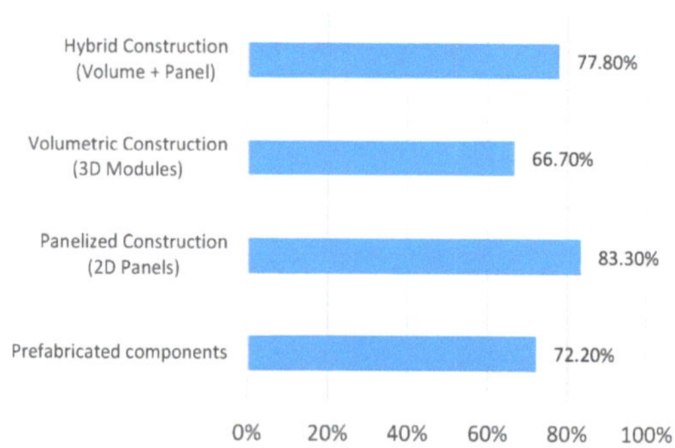

Figure 11. Types of off-site construction provided by contractors in Kuwait.

5. Conclusions

This research provided a fundamental overview of the state of off-site modular construction in Kuwait, focusing on the perceptions of contractors. It also addressed a significant gap in the existing literature by exploring the off-site construction landscape in Kuwait, including industry characteristics, the modular construction methods employed, the sectors served, and the key advantages offered. The findings underscored the prevalence of specific off-site construction methods, with panelized construction emerging as the most widely employed type, followed closely by hybrid construction, prefabricated components, and volumetric construction. A low level of client awareness regarding modular construction as a construction method was found, with most respondents indicating a lack of awareness among their customer base. Despite this, there is a clear demand for off-site modular construction in various sectors in Kuwait, with residential buildings taking the lead, followed by commercial buildings, medical buildings, and institutional buildings. The motivations behind clients adopting modular construction were explored, with a significant percentage indicating a preference for permanent use over temporary applications. The key advantages influencing client adoption of this construction technology included shorter construction time, minimized waste and noise during execution, and reduced costs, respectively.

As a pathway for future investigation, more in-depth research is needed on the materials employed for modular construction in Kuwait, with a focus on the technical factors influencing its selection, such as cost, time, and overall quality. Additionally, evaluating the existing regulations and exploring the drivers and barriers to implementing off-site modular construction in Kuwait is essential for a more detailed understanding of the industry's dynamics. Adopting a qualitative approach through interviews with industry experts, policymakers, and key stakeholders would offer deeper insights and perspectives on these multifaceted aspects and play a crucial role in fostering the efficient adoption of modular construction practices in Kuwait.

Author Contributions: Conceptualization, A.A. (Areej AlBanwan) and N.A.; methodology, A.A. (Areej AlBanwan); validation, A.A. (Abdullah AlFoudari); formal analysis, N.A. and A.A. (Abdullah AlFoudari); investigation, N.A.; resources, A.A. (Abdullah AlFoudari); data curation, A.A. (Areej AlBanwan); writing—original draft preparation, A.A. (Areej AlBanwan); writing—review and editing, N.A. and A.A. (Abdullah AlFoudari); visualization, N.A.; supervision, A.A. (Abdullah AlFoudari); project administration, A.A. (Areej AlBanwan) All authors have read and agreed to the published version of the manuscript.

Funding: This research received no external funding.

Institutional Review Board Statement: Not applicable.

Informed Consent Statement: Not applicable.

Data Availability Statement: All the data used in the experiment has been made available in the present article.

Acknowledgments: The authors wish to acknowledge the invaluable contribution of the contractors who participated in this study, without whom this research would not have been possible.

Conflicts of Interest: The authors declare no conflicts of interest.

References

1. Alghais, N. Developing Urban Models to Address Population Growth Impacts and Assisting with Future Urban Planning in Kuwait and Other Arabian Gulf Countries. Ph.D. Dissertation, School of Earth and Environmental Sciences, The University of Queensland, Brisbane, Australia, 19 October 2018. [CrossRef]
2. Chen, C. Advantages and barriers of modular construction method in constructing buildings. *Smart Infrastruct. Constr.* **2023**, *176*, 75–84. [CrossRef]
3. Goodier, C.; Gibb, A. Future opportunities for off-site in the UK. *Constr. Manag. Econ.* **2007**, *25*, 585–595. [CrossRef]
4. Salama, T.; Moselhi, O.; Al-Hussein, M. Overview of the Characteristics of the Modular Industry and Barriers to Its Increased Market Share. *Int. J. Ind. Constr.* **2021**, *2*, 30–53. [CrossRef]
5. National Institute of Building Sciences. Available online: https://www.nibs.org/oscc (accessed on 1 November 2023).
6. Modular Building Institute. *Permanent Modular Construction 2022 Annual Report*; Modular Building Institute: Charlottesville, VA, USA, 2022.
7. Serrats, M. *PreFab Houses DesignSource*; Harper Design International: New York, NY, USA, 2012.
8. Whole Building Design Guide. Available online: https://www.wbdg.org/resources/site-and-modular-construction-explained (accessed on 1 November 2023).
9. Lawson, M.; Ogden, R.; Goodier, C. *Design in Modular Construction*; CRC Press: London, UK, 2019.
10. Moradibistouni, M.; Gjerde, M. Potential for Prefabrication to Enhance the New Zealand Construction Industry. In *Back to the Future: The Next 50 Years: Proceedings of the 51st International Conference of the Architectural Science Association, Wellington, New Zealand, 29 November–2 December 2017*; Victoria University of Wellington: Wellington, New Zealand, 2017.
11. Modular Building Institute. Available online: http://www.modular.org/what-is-modular-construction (accessed on 2 November 2023).
12. Pasquire, C.; Connolly, G.E. Leaner construction through off-site manufacturing. In Proceedings of the IGLC-10, Gramado, Brazil, 8 August 2002.

13. Karthik, S.; Sharareh, K.; Behzad, R. Modular Construction vs. Traditional Construction: Advantages and Limitations: A Comparative Study. In Proceedings of the Creative Construction e-Conference, Opatija, Croatia, 28 June–1 July 2020. [CrossRef]
14. Ferdous, W.; Bai, Y.; Ngo, T.D.; Manalo, A.; Mendis, P. New advancements, challenges and opportunities of multi-storey modular buildings—A state-of-the-art review. *Eng. Struct.* **2019**, *183*, 883–893. [CrossRef]
15. Hořínková, D. Advantages and Disadvantages of Modular Construction, including Environmental Impacts. *Mater. Sci. Eng.* **2021**, *1203*, 032002. [CrossRef]

engineering proceedings

Proceeding Paper

Impacts of Architectural Sights on Anxiety Relief in a High-Density City †

Yung-Chia Chiu [1,2,*], Ming-Chyuan Ho [3], Jui-Che Tu [4] and Yi-Jhen Jhuang [2]

1 School of Design, National Yunlin University of Science and Technology, Douliu 643, Taiwan
2 Department of MICE Marketing & Event Management, Shu-Te University, Kaohsiung 824, Taiwan; s21111168@stu.edu.tw
3 Department of Industrial Design, National Yunlin University of Science and Technology, Douliu 643, Taiwan; homc@yuntech.edu.tw
4 Department of Creative Design, National Yunlin University of Science and Technology, Douliu 643, Taiwan; tujc@yuntech.edu.tw
* Correspondence: mk04271@gmail.com; Tel.: +886-918208680
† Presented at the 2024 IEEE 4th International Conference on Electronic Communications, Internet of Things and Big Data, Taipei, Taiwan, 19–21 April 2024.

Abstract: Due to rapid urbanization, high-density cities have become a dominant human habitat, and sustainable urban development has become a key concept in urban governance. Thus, it is important to understand the impact of visual elements in urban architecture on stress to make accurate and practical planning and strategies for healthy and sustainable living environments. We examined the designs and features of building facades that alleviate stress and identified measuring metrics for stress relief in viewers. We selected 20 Taiwanese-style public buildings for the examination. To understand the relationship between architecture and stress relief, 70 participants were interviewed in a semi-structured method after showing images of the 20 buildings. We used the semantic differential method and a 7-point image scale to rate stress relief from various architectural styles. The participants found the use of multiple materials or lighting in public buildings interesting but not stress-relieving. A greater amount of cooler and heavier materials made of iron in the building exterior increased stress. This finding offers insights into planning and developing sustainable and psychologically supportive urban environments.

Keywords: stress-relief architecture; public building; sustainable development; affective atmospheres; building forms

Citation: Chiu, Y.-C.; Ho, M.-C.; Tu, J.-C.; Jhuang, Y.-J. Impacts of Architectural Sights on Anxiety Relief in a High-Density City. *Eng. Proc.* **2024**, *74*, 17. https://doi.org/10.3390/engproc2024074017

Academic Editors: Shu-Han Liao, Teen-Hang Meen and Cheng-Fu Yang

Published: 28 August 2024

1. Introduction

City planners and society increasingly recognize the importance of the ecosystem in sustainable urban development. Spaces require services related to the ecosystem for recreation, aesthetics, and spiritual experiences [1]. Therefore, it is essential to evaluate the aesthetic elements that impact the delivery of cultural ecosystem services in architecture. These factors are distinct from others as they demand on-site experience and directly affect human well-being [2].

Stress Reduction Theory (SRT) is a theory of environmental psychology that explains the relationship between environmental exposure and mental stress [3]. High-density cities have become dominant in urban habitats worldwide due to rapid urbanization over the past decade. Research suggests that high-density urban landscapes are more oppressive than low- or medium-density urban landscapes [4]. In this study, we examined the public buildings in Taiwan, focusing on stress relief and perceived safety. In this research, office workers from high-stress groups were interviewed after work to find (1) what public building features citizens like, (2) if the preference is consistent in different visitor needs (e.g., overall preference, stress relief, and perceived safety), (3) if diverse materials and building envelopes are important factors influencing user preferences, and (4) if importance varies based on different needs, such as stress relief and perceived safety. Different preferences are expected for public buildings related to different needs. Thus, we hypothesized that a variety of materials and building facades are important influencing factors depending on citizen needs.

2. Quality of Life and City Sustainability

2.1. Correlation between High-Density Cities and Mental Stress

In urban development, quality of life is defined in three dimensions. The first dimension relates to personal aspects, such as overall happiness and satisfaction with the city. Therefore, individuals hope to fulfill their physiological needs such as drinking, eating, and sleeping, as well as obtain necessities such as housing and adequate income. Therefore, we examined the collective dimension of an individual's social and economic position in the community [5,6]. This dimension refers to a sense of belonging to society, which is positively or negatively related to an individual's social circumstances [7]. Additionally, the material dimension is defined as goods and services in sufficient quality and quantity [8]. Access to goods and services of sufficient quantity and quality enables individuals to meet their needs, including transportation, health, education, leisure, and culture [9]. This discussion will cover the city's offerings.

Ulrich et al. [10] proposed SRT and argued that natural environments reduce mental stress while artificial environments induce it. Although this theory has been referred to by researchers, its application was controversial in artificial environments, with most focusing on natural environments or materials. The theory suggests that urban density is positively correlated with mental stress. In urban areas, individuals are frequently exposed to buildings, which substantially impacts their mental well-being.

Architecture is crucial in populated cities and contributes to depression [11]. Although many studies have examined the effect of natural elements in cities on citizen stress, none have yet explored the potential correlation between artificial elements in cities and mental stress. According to Asgarzadeh et al. [12,13], individuals essentially have a form of negative psychological stress. Crowded environments can weaken people's self-control, leading to mental stress [14,15].

2.2. Quality of Life and Architectural Development

The definition of quality of life in an urban environment varies depending on the country, region, and the physical and social circumstances of an individual [3]. Although such statements often refer to residents' satisfaction with their city, the assessment methods can vary. Researchers use qualitative methods and scales to measure personal perceptions and satisfaction. Quantitative methods are also used with indicators such as wealth, affordability, health, quality, and safety of access to services. Urban quality of life indices derived from these methods differ according to measures of an individual's ability to survive and thrive as a result of the economic, social, and urban solutions provided by the city [3]. The quality of life is greatly influenced by the quality of the city. Therefore, it is important to ensure that cities are well-organized and designed to promote the well-being of citizens. Cluttered cities can exacerbate psychological stress among residents.

At the socioeconomic level, studies attribute the quality of life in urban environments to the provision of an economic, social, and urban framework that is conducive to human activities. Tan et al. [16] have suggested that the quality of urban life improves with changes in social development, which increases opportunities for high-paying jobs or changes and enables individuals to afford or pursue better housing and other facilities, thereby improving their quality of life [17]. Interest in post-work quality of life is growing. Thus, after-work classes and yoga practices for relaxation are increasing. Additionally, cultural, spiritual, and community attachment are important in determining the quality of urban life. Local traditions and architecture enhance the vitality of urban life and increase personal satisfaction [3]. Simultaneously, a strong sense of community attachment enhances social cohesion and resilience to maintain urban sustainability and quality of life [3]. This, in turn, affects the competition and comparison of urban architectural appearance. Ultimately, a livable city depends not only on economic factors but also on the mental well-being of its residents, better access to various social services such as hospitals and doctors, and a generally well-educated population [3]. Therefore, under such circumstances, the improvement in the urban environment becomes even more important.

2.3. Visual Complexity of Buildings

The term 'message' has different meanings depending on the context [18]. In the case of buildings in the city, changes in appearance convey the design concept. In neuroscience, the term is often used to refer to stimulus encoding, decision making, and memory storage. In an urban context, what citizens see can be interpreted as a form of messaging, such as the appearance of buildings and crowded streets (Figure 1). This can lead to psychological stress for individuals. The brain receives messages from multiple sensory channels to process stimuli. The key challenge is to capture people's attention with only relevant information. Objectivity must be maintained, and subjective judgment must be excluded. However, it is worth noting that information that does not meet this standard is behaviorally relevant. This highlights the complexities and pressures that communicating large or complex messages can have on public reception.

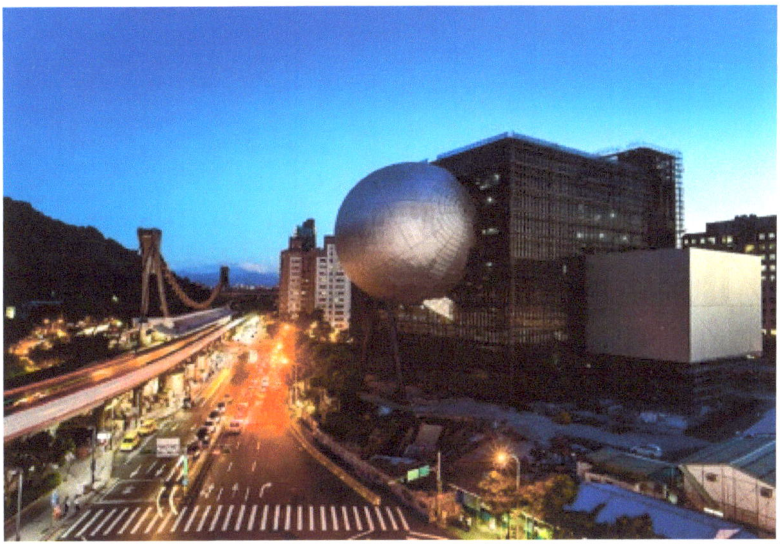

Figure 1. Taipei Performing Arts Center building's exterior with a variety of materials.

The term 'visual complexity' in architecture refers to the level of detail or intricacy that influences people's perception [19,20]. This means that excessive details enhance visual complexity but they also overwhelm the viewer with too much information. Berlyne [21,22] has suggested that a high degree of visual complexity holds people's attention for longer periods. However, it is crucial to balance visual complexity and the amount of information presented. Therefore, it is essential to present information clearly and concisely, avoiding sprawling descriptions and complex terminology. Nasar [23] defined visual complexity as 'diversity' and evaluated the visual quality of residential scenes through surveys based on objective assessment. It is important to use precise terminology when discussing visual complexity and avoid decorative language. In other words, the more complex the appearance of a building, the longer citizens pay attention to it, and the greater the psychological pressure to be caused. This is because the brain requires more time to process complex information.

3. Methodology

3.1. Survey Method

Various studies confirmed that exposure to a natural urban environment led to positive changes in mood and stress reduction as well as a lower heart rate compared to the built environment. Thus, it is needed to make the building relieve the pressure on the citizens. Due to the purpose of the present research and the basis of existing theory, we adopted experimental methods to investigate the stress-relieving building facade.

In past research, we used experimental methods to obtain the subject's views on the decompression structure to obtain the participants' feelings. Therefore, in this study, we used the same research method to examine the impact of the quantity of building materials on high-stress people. For each of the 70 participants, we analyzed their perceptions of stress relief and pressure and investigated how each perception was related to previous and subsequent thoughts and external stimuli. The decompression index of 30 buildings was evaluated through the Decompression Building Scale.

3.2. Participants

To examine the influence of building exterior materials on individuals experiencing high levels of stress, we analyzed the impact of building materials on psychological stress. We recruited 70 Taiwanese office workers, aged 35 on average, with at least 5 years of work experience (Table 1). Semi-structured interviews were conducted individually in the same room. During the interviews, each participant was shown ten architectural images aimed at relieving stress and was interviewed for forty minutes. The selected sample buildings were shown, and participants chose buildings they had seen in person, online, or in their daily lives. These public buildings are located in Taiwan, a culture familiar to the participants.

Table 1. Participants in this study.

Demographic Item		Number	Proportion (%)	Demographic Item		Number	Proportion (%)
Gender	Male	30	42.9	Age	20 or below	2	2.9
	Female	40	57.1		21–30	26	37.1
Profession	Government Official	19	27.1		31–40	30	42.9
	Administrative	18	25.7		41–50	8	11.4
	Project assistant	11	15.7		50 or above	4	5.7
	Business	3	4.3	Highest Education Level	Junior High School or below	3	4.3
	Self-employment	3	4.3		General and vocational High School	12	17.1
	Stewardship	1	1.4		Post-secondary School	7	10
	Others	15	21.4		University/College	39	55.7
					Master or above	9	12.9

We asked 10 experts in architectural design to select representative and relatively stress-relieving buildings from these two types of buildings (Table 2). We used a stress index scale (Health Promotion Agency, Taiwan Ministry of Health and Welfare) to select 10 office workers who showed a stressful lifestyle from the previous 70 participants (Table 3). These 10 participants selected 523 stress relief-related adjectives during a KJ method screening process.

Table 2. List of experts.

Code	Personal Profile	Code	Personal Profile
A1	Mr. Du; Age: 55–60 Occupation: Distinguished Professor	A6	Mr. Ho; Age: 65–70 Occupation: Emeritus Professor
A2	Miss Yang; Age: 50–55 Occupation: Associate Professor	A7	Mr. Liu; Age: 45–50 Occupation: Executive Officer
A3	Mr. Zhang; Age: 40–45 Occupation: Associate Researcher	A8	Mr. Pan; Age: 40–45 Occupation: Associate Professor
A4	Miss Lin; Age: 40–45 Occupation: Architect	A9	Miss Kong; Age: 40–45 Occupation: Environmental Designer
A5	Miss Chen; Age: 45–50 Occupation: Director of Design Company	A10	Miss Zhang; Age: 35–40 Occupation: Executive Officer

Table 3. High-stress assessors.

Code	Personal Profile	Code	Personal Profile
B1	Miss Shen (Tainan); Age: 30–35 Occupation: Project Assistant	B6	Mr. Lee (Fengshan); Age: 40–45 Occupation: Government Administrator
B2	Mr. Xiao (Kaohsiung); Age: 35–40 Occupation: Professional Soldier	B7	Miss Zheng (Yunlin); Age: 35–40 Occupation: Administrative Specialist
B3	Miss Chang (Pingtung); Age: 45–50 Occupation: Public Servant	B8	Miss Young (Hsinchu); Age: 45–50 Occupation: Scholar
B4	Miss Chen (Taipei); Age: 45–50 Occupation: Subject Teacher	B9	Mr. Shen (Pingtung); Age: 45–50 Occupation: Firefighter
B5	Mr. Zhong (Keelung); Age: 40–45 Occupation: Education Staff	B10	Miss Wang (Taichung); Age: 45–50 Occupation: Company Senior Personnel

3.3. Procedure

We obtained the subject's views and feelings on the decompression structure by collecting data on buildings with Taiwanese cultural characteristics for investigation (Figure 2). Each participant was assigned to observe two types of buildings (buildings with more than three materials and less than three materials). Participants chose one of three constructive conditions including (1) no stimuli available (after observation, participants were given only a brief overview of the building's design, e.g., location, building name, and designer's name), (2) restricted access to stimuli (participants have access to the stimulus search tool, but only once per session, i.e., using web pages to retrieve material), and (3) unlimited access to stimuli (we used the search tool multiple times within the access time limit). Then, we studied the stress-relieving architectural choices for the participants. We asked for the judgment of the participants in a short period to obtain the true feelings of the participants.

3.4. Data Analysis

If individuals are exposed to a high-stress environment, either in their personal or professional lives, they may experience cognitive overload and fatigue due to the abundance of visual information. This information can be overwhelming, particularly during the initial stages of reception. Similarly, excessive information, such as overly complex building designs, can cause stress for residents, especially when these elements interact. Simpler buildings are easier to handle and provide a stress-relief effect for residents. In this study, 70 participants assessed stress by using the Stress Index Scale provided by the Department of Health Promotion, Ministry of Health and Welfare, Taiwan. Ten participants showed high scores for stress in the Jiro Kawakita (KJ) method. The top five words expressed by the participants were 'comfortable', 'kind', 'friendly', 'simple', and 'fun' (Table 4).

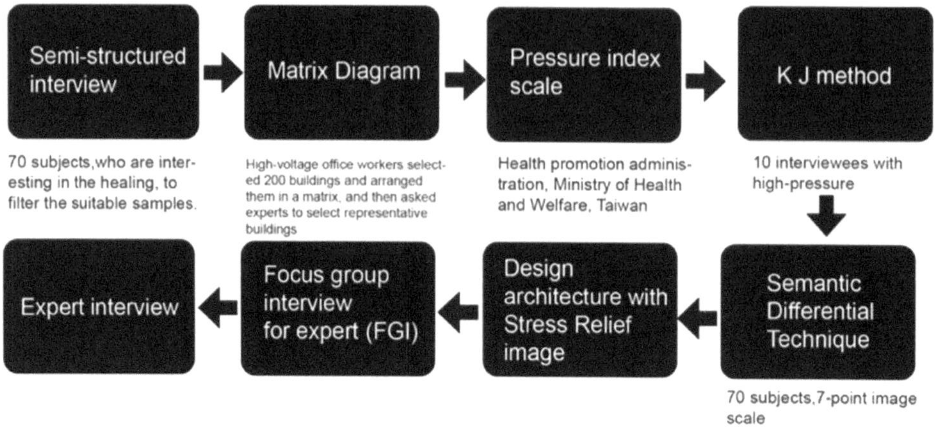

Figure 2. Study procedure.

Table 4. Top five attractive feelings.

Adjective	Votes	Related
Comfortable	101	Satisfied, Easy, Cozy, Cheerful, Quiet
Kindly	80	Safety, Peaceful, Amiable, Gentle, Benevolent, Beneficent
Friendly	73	Nice, Kind, Heavenly, Steady
Simple	68	Bright, Plain, Still, Pure
Fun	39	Happy, Colorful

These two types of buildings have a massive amount of exterior materials. After discussions with experts, more types of different materials were defined to assess the degree of viewers' stress.

In testing, we first selected people who visited test sites (Figure 3). In total, 70 participants (40 women) were office workers. We briefed the evaluation process and asked the participants to choose an adjective or preference to express their feelings about the images to reduce the chances for them to assess the scale of the buildings. After the participants saw the slides for 60 s, they rated the degree of stress reduction (Figure 4). The test results showed that most participants believed that the fewer materials used in the building's exterior, the more stable and relaxing they felt. The more natural the material was, the more comfortable they felt too.

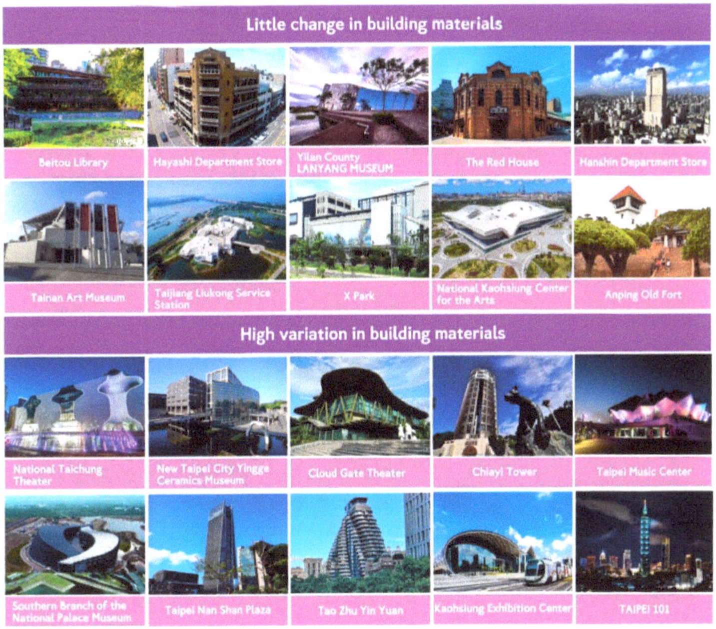

Figure 3. Twenty test buildings.

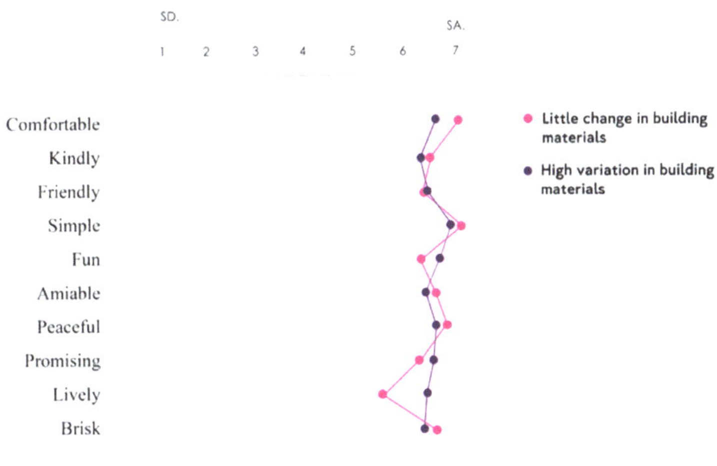

Figure 4. Measurement results of two types of buildings.

4. Discussions

The buildings in cities are shaped by perception-based characteristics such as material, color, shape, form, light, and size [24]. Materials show details [24,25], encapsulating contours and compositions [24,26,27]. Colors reflect the structure of different tones in the scene [24,28]. Material, shape, and color are considered to be the most basic visual elements that represent the built environment [28]. According to Lynch [29], the shape, color, and arrangement of urban environments contribute to the formation of clear and useful mental images, including details such as materials and shapes.

During the COVID-19 pandemic, architectural types were especially associated with stress relief. People's emotions are affected by what they see. Excessive material on the exterior of buildings increases the amount of information, which affects the emotional response of the people. During COVID-19, people were forced not to move around the city. If they saw buildings with many materials from the windows, it affected emotions and reactions. When they walked around, they were more affected. Therefore, people consider the current development and urban form for the judgment standard that is affected by the spiritual interests of citizens. Architecture relieves stress and improves mental health if it is designed with consideration for the spatial environment [30]. It is required for buildings to create a positive atmosphere especially for patients as visual surroundings can significantly impact their mood.

5. Conclusions

Currently, over 50% of the world's population resides in urban areas globally, and the number will increase to 70% by 2050. Despite the increase in urban building and population density, living in cities is linked to higher risks of mental health issues compared to rural areas. For instance, individuals living in cities have an almost 40% higher risk of depression, which is double that of schizophrenia. Anxiety, stress, and isolation are more often observed [31]. This indicates that cities need to exert the most significant psychological pressure on individuals from a social, cultural, or economic perspective. The most immediate form of pressure is visual. Therefore, when creating environments, designers must consider design elements that reduce the impact of external factors on the reception of information.

This study was conducted based on the experience of the participants and their perceptions of building materials. The findings in this study suggested that buildings with excessive decoration and detail are fascinating but cause stress. Too many decorations on buildings overwhelm people with excessive information. Thus, multi-feature visual complexity is required for urban renewal. For instance, when renewing historical streetscapes, the principle of preserving urban memory is required. Instead of reproducing each element in an imitative manner, multi-feature visual complexity is used for buildings, facilities, or furniture to maintain a similar level of complexity by using surface materials with similar textural complexity. It is important to consider the residents' well-being. In the past, urban architecture was often developed solely according to the designer's aesthetics but emphasis was put on functionality and livability recently. It is necessary to include more designs and materials. The building must be isolated from its environment to conduct more organized experiments. We used software to remove things other than buildings in images. The participants were influenced by environmental impressions when judging materials were changed. Therefore, they had different opinions based on their imaginations. However, it was still possible to examine the stress-relieving building's materials. That is, individuals' judgments of material changes depended in part on their mood. There are various emotions involved in these judgments being affected by changes in the environment.

Author Contributions: Conceptualization, M.-C.H. and Y.-C.C.; investigation, Y.-C.C. and Y.-J.J.; methodology, Y.-C.C. and J.-C.T.; writing—original draft, Y.-C.C.; writing—review and editing, Y.-C.C. All authors have read and agreed to the published version of the manuscript.

Funding: This research received no external funding.

Institutional Review Board Statement: Not applicable.

Informed Consent Statement: Not applicable.

Data Availability Statement: Data sharing is not applicable due to privacy.

Conflicts of Interest: The authors declare no conflict of interest.

References

1. Daniel, T.C.; Muhar, A.; Arnberger, A.; Aznar, O.; Boyd, J.W.; Chan, K.M.A.; Costanza, R.; Elmqvist, T.; Flint, C.G.; Gobster, P.H.; et al. Contributions of cultural services to the ecosystem services agenda. *Proc. Natl. Acad. Sci. USA* **2012**, *109*, 8812–8819. [CrossRef] [PubMed]

2. Hegetschweiler, K.T.; de Vries, S.; Arnberger, A.; Bell, S.; Brennan, M.; Siter, N.; Olafsson, A.S.; Voigt, A.; Hunziker, M. Linking demand and supply factors in identifying cultural ecosystem services of urban green infrastructures: A review of European studies. *Urban For. Urban Green.* **2017**, *21*, 48–59. [CrossRef]
3. ESPON. *ESPON QOL—Quality of Life Measurements and Methodology*; Final Report; ESPON: Luxembourg, 2020.
4. Luo, Y. Gender and job satisfaction in urban China: The role of individual, family, and job characteristics. *Soc. Indic. Res.* **2016**, *125*, 289–309. [CrossRef]
5. Costanza, R.; Fisher, B.; Ali, S.; Beer, C.; Bond, L.; Boumans, R.; Snapp, R. Quality of life: An approach integrating opportunities, human needs, and subjective well-being. *Ecol. Econ.* **2007**, *61*, 267–276. [CrossRef]
6. Santos, L.D.; Martins, I.; Brito, P. Measuring subjective quality of life: A survey to Porto's residents. *Appl. Res. Qual. Life* **2007**, *2*, 51–64. [CrossRef]
7. Mouratidis, K. Urban planning and quality of life: A review of pathways linking the built environment to subjective well-being. *Cities* **2021**, *115*, 103229. [CrossRef]
8. Mouratidis, K. Commute satisfaction, neighbourhood satisfaction, and housing satisfaction as predictors of subjective well-being and indicators of urban livability. *Travel Behav. Soc.* **2020**, *21*, 265–278. [CrossRef]
9. Mouratidis, K. Compact city, urban sprawl, and subjective well-being. *Cities* **2019**, *92*, 261–272. [CrossRef]
10. Ulrich, R.S. Effects of interior design on wellness: Theory and recent scientific research. *J. Health Care Inter. Des.* **1991**, *3*, 97–109.
11. Asgarzadeh, M.; Koga, T.; Yoshizawa, N.; Munakata, J.; Hirate, K. A transdisciplinary approach to oppressive cityscapes and the role of greenery as key factors in sustainable urban development. In Proceedings of the 2009 IEEE Toronto International Conference Science and Technology for Humanity (TIC-STH), Toronto, ON, Canada, 26–27 September 2009.
12. Asgarzadeh, M.; Koga, T.; Hirate, K.; Farvid, M.; Lusk, A. Investigating oppressiveness and spaciousness in relation to building, trees, sky and ground surface: A study in Tokyo. *Landsc. Urban Plan.* **2014**, *131*, 36–41. [CrossRef]
13. Asgarzadeh, M.; Lusk, A.; Koga, T.; Hirate, K. Measuring oppressiveness of streetscapes. *Landsc. Urban Plan.* **2012**, *107*, 1–11. [CrossRef]
14. Cohen, S. Aftereffects of stress on human performance and social behavior: A review of research and theory. *Psychol. Bull.* **1980**, *88*, 82–108. [CrossRef] [PubMed]
15. Fleming, I.; Baum, A.; Weiss, L. Social density and perceived control as mediators of crowding stress in high-density residential neighborhoods. *J. Personal. Soc. Psychol.* **1987**, *52*, 899–906. [CrossRef]
16. Tan, Z.; Shi, F.; Zhang, H.; Li, N.; Xu, Y.; Liang, Y. Household income, income inequality, and health-related quality of life measured by the EQ-5D in Shaanxi, China: A cross-sectional study. *Int. J. Equity Health* **2018**, *17*, 1–10. [CrossRef]
17. Glaeser, E. Cities, productivity, and quality of life. *Science* **2011**, *333*, 592–594. [CrossRef]
18. Adriaans, P. Information. In *Standford Encyclopedia of Philosophy*; Zalta, E.N., Ed.; Stanford University: Stanford, CA, USA, 2012.
19. Posner, M.I.; Snyder, C.R.R. Attention and cognitive control. In *Information Processing and Cognition: The Loyola Symposium*; Solso, R.L., Ed.; L. Erlbaum Association: Hillsdale, NJ, USA, 1975; pp. 55–82.
20. Snodgrass, J.G.; Vanderwart, M. A standardized set of 260 pictures: Norms for name agreement, image agreement, familiarity, and visual complexity. *J. Exp. Psychol. Hum. Learn. Mem.* **1980**, *6*, 174–215. [CrossRef]
21. Berlyne, D.E. *Conflict, Arousal, and Curiosity*; McGraw-Hill Book Company: New York, NY, USA, 1960.
22. Berlyne, D.E. Novelty, complexity, and hedonic value. *Percept. Psychophys.* **1970**, *8*, 279–286. [CrossRef]
23. Nasar, J.L. Perception and evaluation of residential street scenes. In *Directions in Person-Environment Research and Practice*; Nasar, J.L., Preiser, W.F.E., Eds.; Ashgate Publishing Ltd.: Surrey, UK, 1999; pp. 229–247.
24. Stamps, A.E. *Psychology and the Aesthetics of the Built Environment*; Springer Science & Business Media: Berlin/Heidelberg, Germany, 2013.
25. Cooper, J.; Oskrochi, R. Fractal analysis of street vistas: A potential tool for assessing levels of visual variety in everyday street scenes. *Environ. Plann. Plann. Des.* **2008**, *35*, 349–363. [CrossRef]
26. Guan, F.; Fang, Z.; Wang, L.; Zhang, X.; Zhong, H.; Huang, H. Modelling people's perceived scene complexity of real-world environments using street-view panoramas and open geodata. *ISPRS J. Photogrammetry Remote Sens.* **2022**, *186*, 315–331. [CrossRef]
27. Liu, Z.; Ma, X.; Hu, L.; Lu, S.; Ye, X.; You, S.; Tan, Z.; Li, X. Information in streetscapes—Research on visual perception information quantity of street space based on information entropy and machine learning. *ISPRS Int. J. Geo-Inf.* **2022**, *11*, 628. [CrossRef]
28. Rossetti, T.; Lobel, H.; Rocco, V.; Hurtubia, R. Explaining subjective perceptions of public spaces as a function of the built environment: A massive data approach. *Landsc. Urban Plann.* **2019**, *181*, 169–178. [CrossRef]
29. Lynch, K. *The Image of the City*; MIT Press: Cambridge, UK, 1964.
30. DuBose, J.; MacAllister, L.; Hadi, K.; Sakallaris, B. Exploring the Concept of Healing Spaces. *HERD Health Environ. Res. Amp Des. J.* **2018**, *11*, 43–56. [CrossRef] [PubMed]
31. Gruebner, O.; Rapp, M.A.; Adli, M.; Kluge, U.; Galea, S.; Heinz, A. Cities and mental health. *Dtsch. Arztebl. Int.* **2017**, *14*, 121. [CrossRef] [PubMed]

engineering proceedings

Proceeding Paper

Color Images in Architecture for Stress-Relief †

Yung-Chia Chiu [1,2,*], Ming-Chyuan Ho [3], Jui-Che Tu [4] and Zhi-Xuan Yang [2]

1 School of Design, National Yunlin University of Science and Technology, Douliu 643, Taiwan
2 Department of MICE Marketing & Event Management, Shu-Te University, Kaohsiung 824, Taiwan; a0987931599@gmail.com
3 Department of Industrial Design, National Yunlin University of Science and Technology, Douliu 643, Taiwan; homc@yuntech.edu.tw
4 Department of Creative Design, National Yunlin University of Science and Technology, Douliu 643, Taiwan; tujc@yuntech.edu.tw
* Correspondence: mk04271@gmail.com
† Presented at the 2024 IEEE 4th International Conference on Electronic Communications, Internet of Things and Big Data, Taipei, Taiwan, 19–21 April 2024.

Abstract: The emotional responses and perceptual preferences of individuals for urban public spaces are shaped by their interactions with the physical environment. Emotions and perceptions are inextricably linked, forming the basis of people's spatial experience. For instance, the presence of dense city buildings can result in feelings of crowding and friction. By improving the urban landscape, it is possible to reduce the stress experienced by citizens. In this study, architectural styles and building facade colors were examined to explore design approaches and features of stress-relieving building facades and identify metrics that measure participants' stress-relief when viewing buildings. The color of 600 buildings in Japan and Taiwan was analyzed to understand stress-relief from architecture. Semi-structured interviews were conducted with 70 participants who viewed images of 30 buildings. The semantic differential method with a seven-point image scale was employed to assess the stress-relieving potential of different architectural styles and colors. The findings of this study indicated that participants perceived that architectural colors influenced feelings of relief. Additionally, they anticipated variations in architectural colors contingent on architectural usage patterns. To substantiate this observation, three principles—city image, identity, and spiritual atmosphere—were identified as fundamental elements in designing cities for livability. The three principles are illustrated by several case studies for a detailed understanding of their applicability in biodesign practices.

Keywords: stress-relief; architecture; color image; environmental sustainability

Citation: Chiu, Y.-C.; Ho, M.-C.; Tu, J.-C.; Yang, Z.-X. Color Images in Architecture for Stress-Relief. *Eng. Proc.* **2024**, *74*, 18. https://doi.org/10.3390/engproc2024074018

Academic Editors: Shu-Han Liao, Teen-Hang Meen and Cheng-Fu Yang

Published: 28 August 2024

1. Introduction

City planners and society at large are increasingly aware of the value of urban stress-relief. Consequently, a variety of services have been transformed in the environmental space, including parks, entertainment, aesthetic, and spiritual experiences [1]. Consequently, it is necessary to determine the impact of the built environment on the physiology and behavior of those exposed to it. Those residing in urban areas frequently contact the built environment. The United Nations Sustainable Development Goals, established in 2015, include Goal 11 to "make cities and human settlements inclusive, safe, resilient, and sustainable," and Goal 8 to "promote sustained, inclusive, and sustainable economic growth, full and productive employment, and decent work for all". Consequently, the construction of a sustainable city necessitates the provision of a perpetually evolving visual landscape. The architectural and landscape design of urban areas plays a pivotal role in the achievement of these objectives. A city whose urban architecture features stress-relieving design elements is likely to have a unique, stress-relieving image.

This article presents the results of a research project investigating the potential of building color to relieve stress. The findings can allow for the planning and design of urban environments to become stress-relieving cities. The concept of quality of life encompasses a multitude of factors, including an individual's physical health, mental state, degree of independence, social relationships, personal beliefs, and relationship to salient features in the environment. Previous studies [2] have mainly focused on the impact of building shape and the addition of green plants on human psychology and physiology. However, we defined the factors of urban stress as the psychophysiological stress of urban people, which exists in a complex matrix of environmental factors (including landscape, architecture, etc.), and socioeconomic and political conditions (such as urban building density). Numerous employment, housing, and workplace issues require attention. The appearance of buildings has always been a prominent feature in people's lives. Nevertheless, there has been a paucity of research investigating the emotional impact of these structures.

According to Michael [3], the performance of buildings and landscapes in cities affects the mood of people and the city atmosphere, which is also the issue of happy cities being discussed in countries. Cells in the human brain's hippocampus interact with the geometry, arrangement, and color of the urban architectural spaces. Therefore, urban architecture must conform to the designer's style and characteristics and affect the visual and emotional state of residents to increase the sustainability of the city. The spirituality of a city includes the observable objects and the spiritual feelings. The spirituality of the city is divided into external performance and internal feeling (Figure 1). Previous research found [4] that shapes can be stored in memory through their emotional and cognitive impact on the viewer, and that buildings can facilitate the formation of memories and emotions of people. The study found that complex shapes are more attractive and influential than simple shapes or straight lines, but also require more mental processing and higher mental effort. This is because complex shapes contain visual information that needs to be processed and retained in memory. Compared with the color of the building, their effect is consistent.

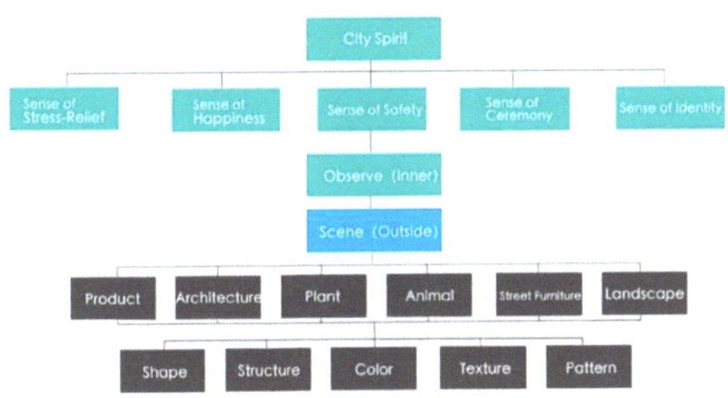

Figure 1. Spirituality of a city.

2. Affective Atmosphere and Material Imagination of Stress-Relieving Architecture

2.1. Stress-Relieving

In addition to shape, urban color is a significant element when planning urban space [5]. The color of urban buildings is a component of the urban landscape, offering residents a distinctive visual experience and perception of the spatial environment. These factors influence residents' emotions and behaviors [6,7]. Consequently, color can evoke and promote emotions, which is a concept that can be employed in urban architecture. The impact of vision is the most direct sensorily [8]. The perceptions and emotions of urban residents, including comfort, safety, vitality, and depression, are influenced by their visual exposure to the built environment [9–13]. When individuals are traversing a city street or pausing in a public square, they may not be aware of a specific color but experience an emotional response to the prevailing ambiance. We observed that expressions such as "this place makes me feel good" or "the surroundings are quite disturbing" can often substitute for the evaluations of the color combinations. Mahnke posited that patterns and color combinations in urban environments elicit both conscious and unconscious emotional responses. The combination of shaped lines and incongruous color schemes results in visual disturbances, disorientation, and stress or depression [14].

According to the "City Pulse Survey 2021" by Gensler, the largest construction company in the United States, many countries have begun to consider future cities that can resist infectious diseases by avoiding loneliness while maintaining personal space as expressed by "physical, not social, distancing." These concepts are components of urban redesign [15]. The movement restrictions during the COVID-19 pandemic caused a rethinking of environmental space planning and design. Designers need to create open spaces that are comfortable and relaxing; enhance social interaction; and reduce antisociality, loneliness, and stress. Urban planning has transitioned to land planning in many countries.

We used the images of large buildings, which increase the pressure on cities. In such a dense city, if the architectural colors are full of changes, it brings a heavy sense of pressure to the citizens. Among buildings, the color of residential buildings is relatively simple as residents do not want overly vibrant colors that may affect their mood in living. A survey of the appearance of 600 buildings revealed that achromatic colors were used, so the residents of these two places tended to have a restrained and conservative disposition.

2.2. Research Framework

As Day [16] posited, the relationships between urban forms, spaces, and color invigorate the individual or sap them of their life force. Ellard [17] researched the impact of design on psychology, demonstrating that individuals were unaware of the ways in which their physical and psychological well-being were influenced by the environment. Ellard corroborated the physiological response with the collected experimental data and found that, regarding their stress levels, respondents perceived it to be a relatively minor issue. However, when physiological responses were measured, they revealed that stress levels were significantly elevated. The research results demonstrated that the psychological mood of citizens is unconsciously influenced by the shape and color of buildings in urban areas. The intricacy of alterations to the external facade of a building necessitates research on cognitive resources and emotional responses. Figure 2 illustrates the framework employed in this research, which shows that the appearance of buildings and the associated mood can interfere with message transmission and affect user perceptions.

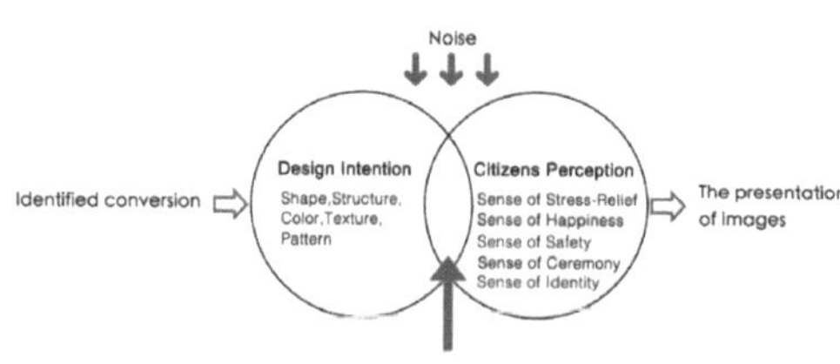

Figure 2. Framework of this research.

3. Materials and Methods

3.1. Research Method

Exposure to a natural urban environment can lead to positive changes in mood and stress reduction, as well as a lower heart rate compared to the built environment. Thus, it is needed to ensure the building is able to relieve the pressure of the citizens. Based on the existing theory, we adopted experimental methods to investigate the stress-relieving building facade. We explored the theoretical background [18] to develop a model to test the hypotheses [19]. We collected a large number of photos of buildings in Japan and Taiwan, compared the use of color of the buildings, and then experimented to understand the subjective feelings of the buildings. We predicted the color of city buildings that affected the stress index of residents.

In our research, the method in Figure 3 was used to obtain the subjects' views and feelings on the decompression structure. We used the same research method to examine the impact of building color on high-stress people. We added a building matrix to explore the impact of architectural styles in different regions. We analyzed the perceptions of stress-relief and pressure of 70 subjects to analyze the difference between previous and present thoughts and external stimuli. The subjects were asked for the decompression index of 30 buildings using the Decompression Building Scale (Figure 3).

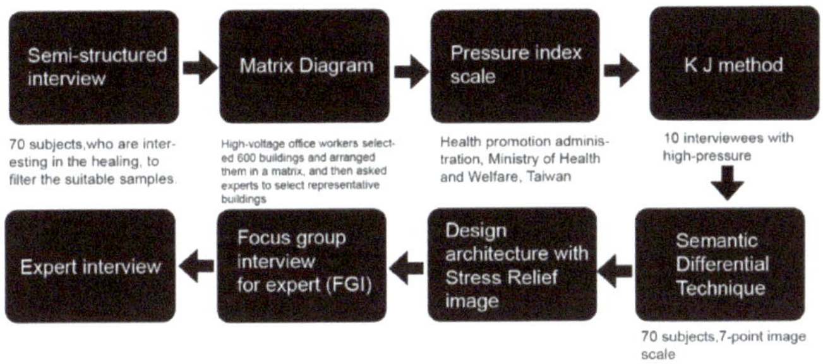

Figure 3. Study procedure.

3.2. Sample and Data

Seventy office workers in Taiwan with over five years of experience participated in the study. Each individual was employed on a full-time basis and worked more than 48 h per week, and their average was 35 years old. Seventy participants (thirty females and forty males) provided informed consent to participate in this research. The experts in the design or creation of spiritual environments with over 10 years of experience were invited to participate in the study.

The participants were interviewed separately in the same room using a semi-structured interview technique. Each participant was presented with ten images of stress-relieving buildings and interviewed for 40 min. The sample buildings were selected through a preliminary screening. The participants were likely to select buildings that they had previously visited or seen on the Internet or in their daily lives. The buildings were selected from Taiwan and Japan as the two countries have similar cultures.

We collected photos of 600 different buildings, removed their backgrounds, and divided them into three groups: public buildings, residential buildings, and religious buildings. We arranged these buildings using a matrix diagram and compared the color characteristics of Taiwanese versus Japanese buildings (Figures 4–6). In Japan, 52% of the buildings used white, gray, and black colors, whereas only 24% of the buildings in Taiwan used these colors. The chromaticity of residential buildings in the two places was low in saturation, whereas the exterior chromaticity of religious buildings was high in saturation. The saturation of religious architecture in Taiwan was higher than that of Japan.

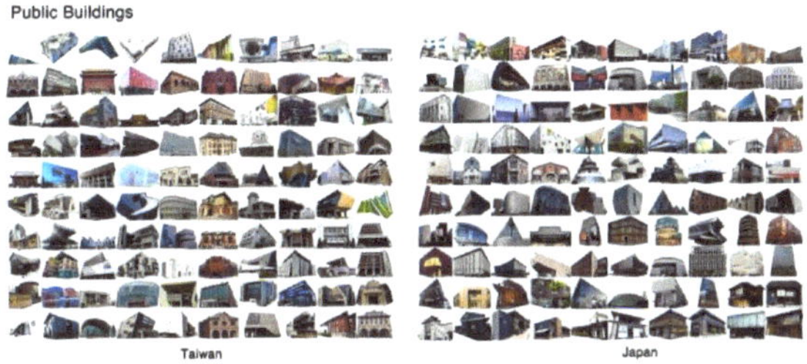

Figure 4. Color comparison of public buildings in Japan and Taiwan.

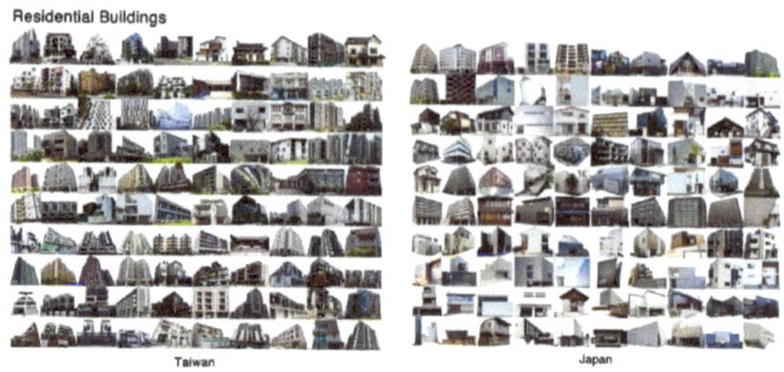

Figure 5. Color comparison of residential buildings in Japan and Taiwan.

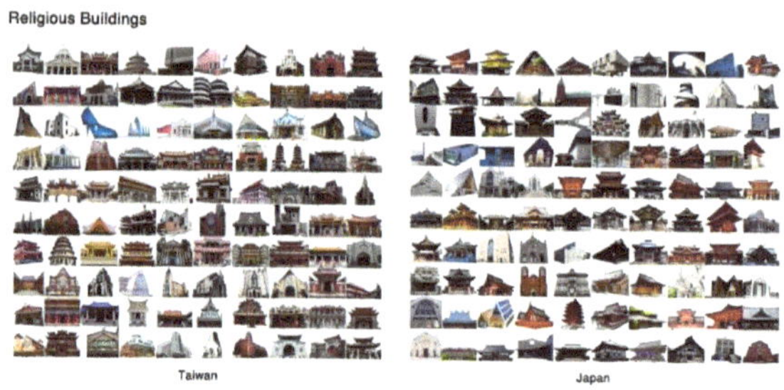

Figure 6. Color comparison of religious buildings in Japan and Taiwan.

We asked experts in architectural design to select representative and relatively stress-relieving buildings. The three types of buildings were subdivided into buildings of high color saturation/high lightness or low color saturation/low lightness. In selecting architectural colors, we excluded buildings that were entirely white, black, or gray. At least 50% of the selected buildings had those colors as displayed in Figures 7–9. We used a stress index scale (Health Promotion Agency, Taiwan Ministry of Health and Welfare) to select 10 office workers who had a stressful lifestyle (Table 1). These 10 participants selected a total of 420 stress relief-related adjectives using the Jiro Kawakita (KJ) method.

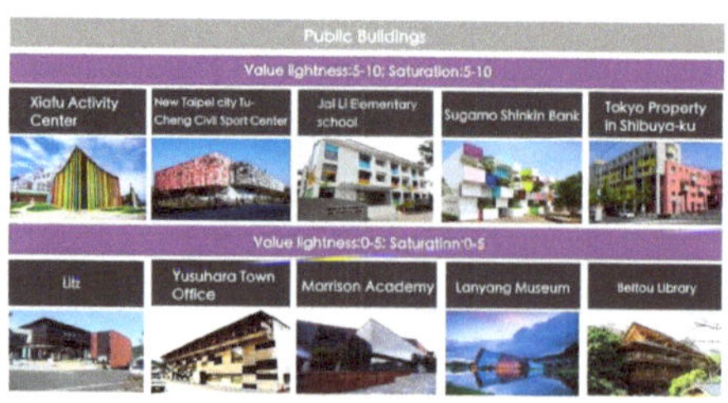

Figure 7. Public buildings.

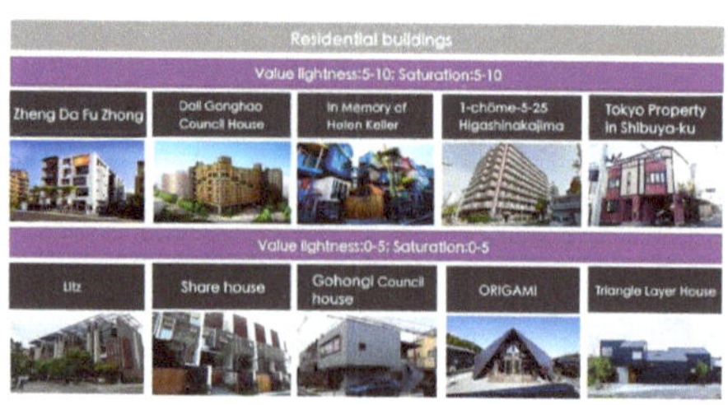

Figure 8. Residential buildings.

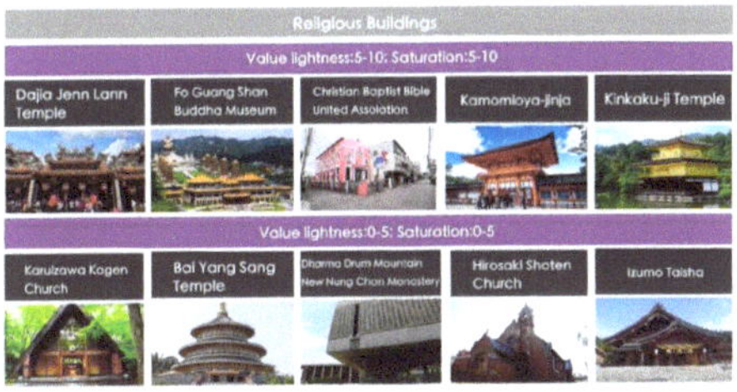

Figure 9. Religious buildings.

Table 1. Ten participants with stressful lifestyles.

Code	Personal Profile	Code	Personal Profile
A1	Mr. Wu (Kaohsiung); Age: 40–45 Occupation: Firefighter	A6	Mr. Wu (Kaohsiung); Age: 40–45 Occupation: Marketing Specialist
A2	Mr. Lin (Tainan); Age: 30–35 Occupation: Career Soldier	A7	Miss Lin (Chiayi); Age: 25–30 Occupation: Executive Assistant
A3	Miss Chen (Tainan); Age: 30–35 Occupation: Freelancer	A8	Miss Pan (Taichung); Age: 35–40 Occupation: Soldier
A4	Miss Lin (Tainan); Age: 25–30 Occupation: Executive Assistant	A9	Miss Chen (Hualien); Age: 40–45 Occupation: Project Planner
A5	Miss Wang (Taichung); Age: 45–50 Occupation: Director	A10	Miss Chang (Pingtung); Age: 35–40 Occupation: Executive Officer

4. Discussion

4.1. Sample Analysis

With high levels of stress in learning, living, or work, the influx of new information can result in cognitive overload. Similarly, an excess of information, such as a building with overly complex colors, may cause stress, particularly if the building elements are interactive. Consequently, simpler buildings are favored by residents for stress-relieving effects. The participants evaluated the buildings using the stress index scale. Ten participants were identified with high-pressure lifestyles using the Jiro Kawakita (KJ) method and were tested to identify the major factors. A total of 420 words were collected and grouped into 15 adjectives. Table 2 presents the five most frequently words identified by the 10 participants, i.e., "comfortable", "kindly", "friendly", "simple", and "fun".

Table 2. Top five words.

Adjective	Votes	Related
Comfortable	102	satisfied, easy, cozy, cheerful, quiet
Kindly	80	safety, peaceful, amiable, gentle, benevolent, beneficent
Friendly	73	nice, kind, heavenly, Steady
Simple	66	bright, plain, still
Fun	45	happy, colorful

Ten pairs of adjectives were chosen from the words collected, and the participant's perceptions of the building images were measured (Table 3). The instructor introduced the evaluation process and clarified that the participants could express their feelings regarding the imagery in each photograph and select adjectives or preferences. This process was adopted to minimize the likelihood of the participant's responses. As the adjective pairs were meaningful, a video was played while the participant performed the tests.

Each video was displayed for 60 s. Following this, the participants selected their rating criteria. The results of the test indicated that the majority of participants perceived religious buildings as providing stress-relief, stability, and joy (Figure 10). A total of 73% of the participants indicated that buildings with lower color saturation provided larger stress-relief. Additionally, the participants indicated that residential buildings with simpler colors were perceived as more comfortable.

Table 3. Sample statistics.

Project		Number of Times	%	Project		Number of Times	%
Gender	Male	30	42.9	Age	20 or below	2	2.9
	Female	40	57.1		21–30	26	37.1
Profession	Government Official	18	25.7		31–40	28	40
					41–50	10	14.3
	Administrative	17	24.3		50 or above	4	5.7
	Project assistant	12	17.2	Highest Education Level	Junior High School or below	3	4.3
	Business	3	4.3		General and vocational High School	12	17.1
	Self-employment	3	4.3		Post-secondary School	7	10
	Stewardship	1	1.4		University/College	37	52.9
	Others	16	22.9		Master or above	11	15.7

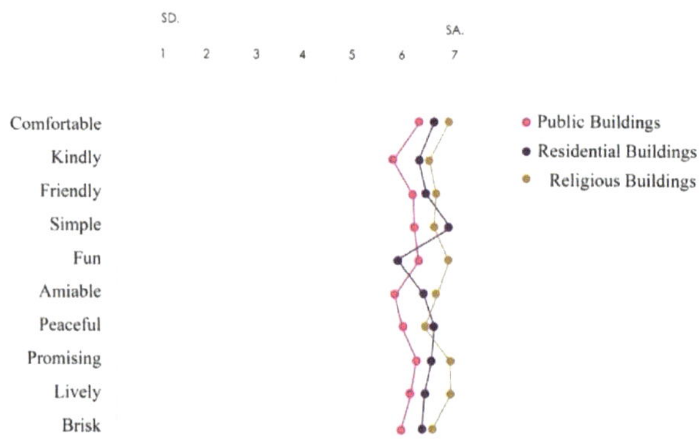

Figure 10. Seven-point scale of building ratings.

4.2. Attractive Factors

The three most prevalent feelings and their corresponding building forms are presented in Table 4. Thirteen images were selected by the design experts as the most stress-relieving (Table 5).

Table 4. Top 5 attractive feelings and their related initial reasons and concrete reasons.

Adjective	Color Image
Comfortable	Warm color; Value lightness: 0–3, 8–10; Saturation: 2–6
Kindly	Warm color; Value lightness: 6–10; Saturation: 7–9
Friendly	Warm color; Value lightness: 6–10; Saturation: 7–9
Simple	Warm color; Cool color; Value lightness: 0–3, 8–10; Saturation: 2–6
Fun	Warm color; Value lightness: 7–10; Saturation: 7–10

Remark: Black/0; White/10.

Table 5. Invited experts in this research.

Code	Personal Profile	Code	Personal Profile
B1	Miss Wu, Age: 45–50 Occupation: Professor	B6	Mr. Ho, Age: 60–65 Occupation: Professor
B2	Mr. Liu, Age: 40–45 Occupation: Professor	B7	Mr. Wu, Age: 45–50 Occupation: Professor
B3	Miss Li, Age: 40–45 Occupation: Designer	B8	Miss Pai, Age: 35–40 Occupation: Professor
B4	Mr. Lin, Age: 35–40 Occupation: Architect	B9	Miss Liu, Age: 40–45 Occupation: Designer
B5	Miss Chen, Age: 40–45 Occupation: Director	B10	Miss Chang, Age: 35–40 Occupation: Assistant Researcher

4.3. Buildings and Environmental Concerns

Architecture and built environments are conducive to stress-relief and mental health if they are designed with a consideration of the environment [20]. This is important for patients as some colors encourage activity, and others encourage rest. We used retouching software to remove things other than buildings. When the participants judged the color images, they were influenced by the impression of the environment and opinions affected by the imagination in their memory. Judgments about color images depended on their mood and involved various emotions affected by the color of the environment.

Architectural experiences are complex. Mental health is closely related to social ties and social capital. In other words, the emotions people experience may be influenced by emotional residue. Designers need to innovate and create functions to promote positive, safe, and natural interactions between people and foster a sense of community. It is difficult for an individual to describe the experience without an understanding of the architecture. The participants in this research experienced or visited the buildings before being tested. Thus, they had a basic judgment of the buildings. Building colors remained in the memory. The ambient color became a stressful color. The participants were also influenced by instructions. The purer the color of the building, the more it slows down the emotional fluctuation of the participants.

5. Conclusions

Today, more than 50% of the global population lives in cities, and this figure is predicted to rise to over 70% by 2050. Urban building and population density will keep increasing. Nonetheless, numerous studies revealed that cities are associated with an increase in risk to mental health, relative to rural areas; depression shows a 40% increase in risk, the risk for schizophrenia is doubled, and the risks for anxiety, stress, and isolation are increased considerably [21]. Therefore, designers must consider the design elements to reduce the influence of the reception of information.

The comparison of the exterior colors of buildings in Japan and Taiwan revealed that 93% of the participants were affected by changes in the color of buildings and the area. They did not prefer buildings with high brightness and chroma. In the second stage of the test, the color area of the buildings was reduced to 40% and the color types were reduced to fewer than four in number; the participants chose buildings with high brightness and high chroma. The test results revealed that excessive exterior color caused the participants to feel emotionally disturbed. That is, the amount of information increased the stress of the participants. Six hundred buildings revealed how a building's appearance is influenced by culture. In other words, each country has its own colors for buildings. The chroma of buildings in Taiwan was between 7° and 8°, and the brightness was 8°–9°, whereas the chroma of buildings in Japan was between 6° and 7° and the brightness was 7°–8°.

An individual's living space is shaped by their work and education. When designing urban buildings, it is also necessary to consider what practical tasks and activities the inhabitants engage in, in addition to creating a positive atmosphere. Beautiful shapes, colors, and feelings are design elements. Designers need to pursue self-realization and consider the changes and feelings of the environment. For example, Tadao Ando's Chapel of Light and I.M. Pei's Miho Art Museum present a sense of tranquility through the use of shapes and colors, all of which embody this concept. The present research results showed that the simplicity of architectural color use made the participants feel happier. The more complex the color used in the building, the more the information in the subjects' brains increases. The simplicity of color depends on the variety and saturation of colors.

In this research, we created a preliminary design based on the experimental results. The quantity of color information influences psychological feelings, while the chroma of the color affects judgment. While buildings with color variations were perceived as enjoyable, they did not relieve stress, as people received more information. An overstimulating environment is characterized by the use of highly saturated colors and complex color combinations. It is important to achieve color harmony to minimize stress. The concept of color harmony is not based on personal preference but on the position of each color within a scientific color system. Color harmony is achieved when the eye is no longer seeking to balance colors. An understanding of color and color systems is important in architecture. The architectural design of a city represents a display of regional culture and life. However, it must not be a burden on people and increase their stress.

Author Contributions: Conceptualization, M.-C.H. and Y.-C.C.; investigation, Y.-C.C. and Z.-X.Y.; methodology, Y.-C.C. and J.-C.T.; writing—original draft, Y.-C.C.; writing—review and editing, Y.-C.C. All authors have read and agreed to the published version of the manuscript.

Funding: This research received no external funding.

Institutional Review Board Statement: Not applicable.

Informed Consent Statement: Not applicable.

Data Availability Statement: Data are contained within the article.

Conflicts of Interest: The authors declare no conflict of interest.

References

1. Daniel, T.C.; Muhar, A.; Arnberger, A.; Aznar, O.; Boyd, J.W.; Chan, K.M.; Costanza, R.; Elmqvist, T.; Flint, C.G.; Gobster, P.H.; et al. Contributions of cultural services to the ecosystem services agenda. *Proc. Natl. Acad. Sci. USA* **2012**, *109*, 8812–8819. [CrossRef] [PubMed]
2. Salingaros, N.A.; Masden, K.G. *Neuroscience, the Natural Environment, and Building Design, Biophilic Design: The Theory, Science, and Practice of Bringing Buildings to Life*; Wiley: Hoboken, NJ, USA, 2008; pp. 59–83.
3. Bond, M. As More of Us Flock to Urban Living, City Designers Are Re-Thinking Buildings' Influence on Our Moods in an Era of "Neuro-architecture", United Kingdom. 2017. Available online: https://www.bbc.com/future/article/20170605-the-psychology-behind-your-citys-design (accessed on 10 March 2021).
4. Ho, M.-C.; Chiu, Y.-C. Evaluating Stress Relief from Architecture: A Case Study Based on Buildings in Taiwan, China and Japan. *Sustainability* **2021**, *13*, 7899. [CrossRef]
5. Markevych, I.; Schoierer, J.; Hartig, T.; Chudnovsky, A.; Hystad, P.; Dzhambov, A.M.; De Vries, S.; Triguero-Mas, M.; Brauer, M.; Nieuwenhuijsen, M.J. Exploring preathways linking greenspace to health: Theoretical and methodological guidance. *Environ. Res.* **2017**, *158*, 301–317. [CrossRef] [PubMed]
6. Gou, A.P.; Wang, J.B. Research on the location characters of urban color plan in China. *Color Res. Appl.* **2008**, *33*, 68–76. [CrossRef]
7. Tosca, T.F. Environmental color design for the third millennium: An evolutionary standpoint. *Color Res. Appl.* **2002**, *27*, 441–454. [CrossRef]
8. Kuo, F.E.; Faber Taylor, A. A potential natural treatment for attention-deficit/hyperactivity disorder: Evidence from a national study. *Am. J. Public Health* **2004**, *94*, 1580–1586. [CrossRef] [PubMed]
9. Jiang, B.; Chang, C.Y.; Sullivan, W.C. A dose of nature: Tree cover, stress reduction, and gender differences. *Landsc. Urban Plan.* **2014**, *132*, 26–36. [CrossRef]
10. Beil, K.; Hanes, D. The Influence of Urban Natural and Built Environments on Physiological and Psychological Measures of Stress—A Pilot Study. *Int. J. Environ. Res. Public Health* **2013**, *10*, 1250–1267. [CrossRef] [PubMed]
11. Berto, R. Exposure to restorative environments helps restore attentional capacity. *J. Environ. Psychol.* **2005**, *25*, 249–259. [CrossRef]
12. Lindal, P.J.; Hartig, T. Effects of urban street vegetation on judgments of restoration likelihood. *Urban For. Urban Green.* **2015**, *14*, 200–209. [CrossRef]

13. Ewing, R.; Hajrasouliha, A.; Neckerman, K.M.; Purciel-Hill, M.; Greene, W. Streetscape Features Related to Pedestrian Activity. *J. Plan. Educ. Res.* **2016**, *36*, 5–15. [CrossRef]
14. Porter, T.; Mikellides, B. (Eds.) *Color for Architecture Today*; Taylor & Francis: London, UK, 2009.
15. Gensler Research Institute. *City Pulse Survey 2021*. 2021. Available online: https://www.gensler.com/blog/insights-from-genslers-2021-city-pulse-survey-and-the-impact (accessed on 15 March 2022).
16. Day, C. *Place of the Soul. Architecture and Environmental Design as a Healing Art*; Elsevier, Architectural Press: Oxford, UK, 2004.
17. Ellard, C.G. A New Agenda for Urban Psychology: Out of the Laboratory and onto the Streets. *J. Urban Des. Ment. Health* **2017**, *2*, 3.
18. Handfield, R.; Melnyk, S.A. The scientific theory-building process: A primer using the case of TQM. *J. Oper. Manag.* **1998**, *16*, 321–339. [CrossRef]
19. Wacker, J.G. A definition of theory: Research guidelines for different theory-building research methods in operations management. *J. Oper. Manag.* **1998**, *16*, 361–385. [CrossRef]
20. DuBose, J.; MacAllister, L.; Hadi, K.; Sakallaris, B. Exploring the Concept of Healing Spaces. *HERD Health Environ. Res. Des. J.* **2018**, *11*, 43–56. [CrossRef] [PubMed]
21. Gruebner, O.; Rapp, M.A.; Adli, M.; Kluge, U.; Galea, S.; Heinz, A. Cities and mental health. *Dtsch. Arztebl. Int.* **2017**, *114*, 121. [CrossRef] [PubMed]

engineering proceedings

MDPI

Proceeding Paper

Gait Analysis and Fall Risk Assessment in Different Age Groups: A Comparative Study †

Thanaporn Sukpramote and Wongwit Senavongse *

Department of Biomedical Engineering, Faculty of Engineering, Srinakharinwirot University, Nakhon Nayok 26120, Thailand; thanaporn.suk@g.swu.ac.th
* Correspondence: wongwit@g.swu.ac.th

† Presented at the 2024 IEEE 4th International Conference on Electronic Communications, Internet of Things and Big Data, Taipei, Taiwan, 19–21 April 2024.

Abstract: Daily walking reflects the quality of life concerning physical status and its association with the risk of falls. Abnormal walking can lead to injuries and increase the likelihood of future falls. It has been found that older adults are more prone to falls than younger persons. However, there is limited research on gait analysis in older adults. Thus, we analyzed gait parameters, involving 10 participants aged between 20 and 30 years old, and 10 participants aged 50 years and older, using the Gait Analysis System (LONGGOOD Meditech Ltd., Taipei, Taiwan), which automatically positions the human body and GaitBEST. GaitBEST is used for analyzing and calculating key timing points and displacement values from the Kinect detector as it captures the location of joint points and adjusts them to the program. After the gait testing, the result is displayed immediately. Each volunteer did not have any surgery that impacted their walking and signed a written informed consent statement before the study. The volunteers walked on a straight flat surface for 4.2 m, repeating the walking test five times at a self-determined comfortable speed. Subsequently, a comparative analysis of the gait parameter outcomes was performed using a parametric test by a *t*-test. The results showed the balance parameters of both groups significantly differed in the head sway range ($p = 0.008$), head tilt range ($p = 0.018$), and pelvis tilt range ($p = 0.003$). The younger group exhibited better postural control than the other group. The spatiotemporal parameters, stride length, and step length during walking were also significantly different at $p = 0.001$. This indicated that the older group had shorter lengths compared to the other group, leading to a significant difference in the percentage of falls and functional loss at $p = 0.021$ and 0.023, respectively. The result of this study assists in examining and assessing the physical condition, preventing falls, optimizing walking efficiency, preventing injuries, and reducing the falling risk.

Keywords: gait analysis; risk of falling assessment; gait analysis system; fall risk

Citation: Sukpramote, T.; Senavongse, W. Gait Analysis and Fall Risk Assessment in Different Age Groups: A Comparative Study. *Eng. Proc.* **2024**, *74*, 19. https://doi.org/10.3390/engproc2024074019

Academic Editors: Shu-Han Liao, Teen-Hang Meen and Cheng-Fu Yang

Published: 28 August 2024

1. Introduction

Walking is a simple physical movement and contributes to long-term physical health when performed correctly in daily life. Walking correctly enhances overall well-being and fortifies muscles and joints. Conversely, abnormal gait patterns can lead to injuries and increase the risk of falls. As individuals age, joints deteriorate due to use [1] and result in degenerative joints combined with abnormal walking in the long term. For people aged 40 years and older, the falls of females occur 2–3 times higher than that of males [2]. Weerapong [3] found that changes in the musculoskeletal system resulting from osteoarthritis are associated with falls. Understanding the impact of abnormal walking on joint health is crucial, not only contributing to the prevention of injuries and the elevated risk of falling.

The previous studies analyzed gait patterns among patients with knee osteoarthritis compared to those with normal people. Additionally, the risk of falls among patients with conditions characterized by abnormal walking such as Parkinson's disease was assessed in comparison to normal individuals. We studied the gait of elderly individuals with normal health compared to young adults, along with evaluating the risk of falls. To examine and evaluate gait, design walking plans, and prevent fall risks that may occur in the future, we used the Gait Analysis System (GaitBEST, LONGGOOD Meditech Ltd., Taipei, Taiwan). The walking data between the two groups of volunteers were compared to assess fall risk. The findings from this study provide a basis for further research.

2. Materials and Methods

2.1. Participants

For the gait testing, volunteers aged 20–39 years (the younger group) and those aged 50 years (the older group) and older were recruited. Each volunteer had not undergone any surgery that impacted their walking. All participants signed a written informed consent before the study. The participant's details are presented in Tables 1 and 2.

Table 1. Characteristics of younger group.

Characteristics	Mean	Range
Age (year)	23	22–27
Heights (cm)	164	153–181
Weight (kg)	59	42–105
BMI * (kg/m^2)	21.59	17.19–33.14

* BMI is Body Mass Index (kg/m^2).

Table 2. Characteristics of older group.

Characteristics	Mean	Range
Age (year)	56	50–61
Heights (cm)	161	150–175
Weight (kg)	74	56–110
BMI * (kg/m^2)	28.02	23.44–35.92

* BMI is Body Mass Index (kg/m^2).

2.2. Gait Analysis

GaitBEST was used in the gait test as it automatically positions the human body. It contains a Kinect detector (Three-dimension Kinect V2) that automatically tracks skeletal data and rebuilds 25 significant reference joint points without markers attaching to the skin of participants. In the detector, a sample rate of 30 Hz, Window 10 operation, i5 CPU or higher, and specialized algorithm are used [4]. GaitBEST analyzes and calculates key time points and displacement values from the Kinect detector, the location of joint points. and fits them into the program. After the gait testing, the result is displayed immediately.

The volunteers with the required qualifications walked with GaitBEST. Then, walking was analyzed using a camera and capturing the walking of volunteers on a straight flat surface for 4.2 m. The result was analyzed to show the result immediately after walking. The method was as follows.

- Walking on a straight flat surface from the starting point to the endpoint for 4.2 m (Figure 1).
- Walking at a natural pace.
- Walking with a normal and relaxed walking posture as in daily life, avoiding any stiff movements.
- Shoes and a face mask were not worn while walking.
- A plain-colored outfit with minimal patterns was worn.

- Test walking using the GaitBEST program. In the program, the Guest user account was selected to prevent the program from saving the walking data of the volunteers for a test walk.
- Walking was tested one or two times, or as per the volunteer's preference to become familiar with the walking procedure.
- Walking was recorded GaitBEST.
- The test was repeated five times. Volunteers took a break between each test. Once they were ready, the next walking test proceeded.

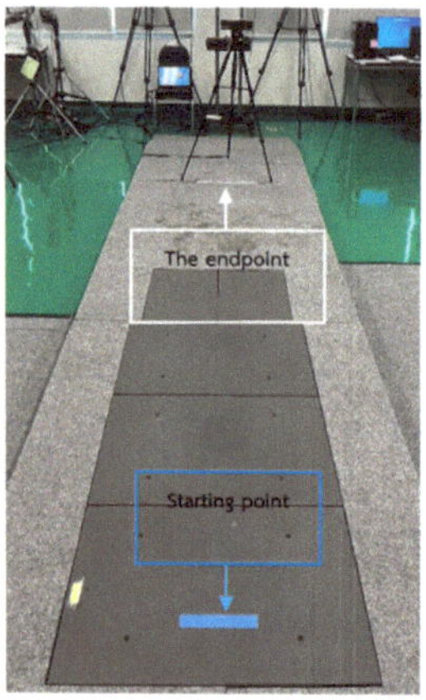

Figure 1. Straight flat floor walkways and starting and ending points for laboratory walking tests.

We analyzed gait parameters and conducted statistical analysis by comparing walking parameters between the two volunteer groups (Figure 2).

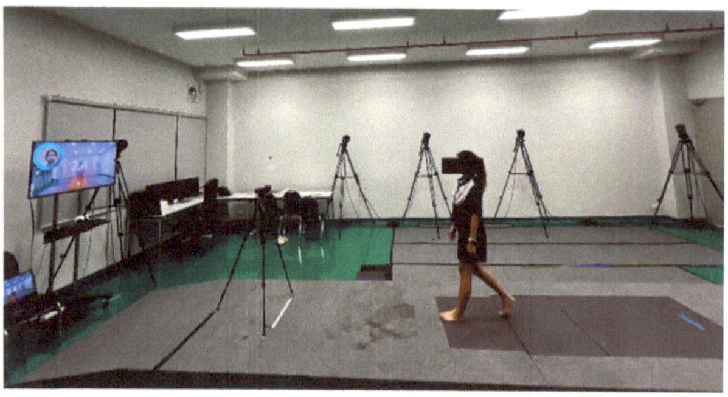

Figure 2. Experiment with walking using the Gait Analysis System.

2.3. Statistical Analysis

Gait parameters were analyzed using a normality test. To test the normal distribution, we used the Kolmogorov–Smirnov test and the Shapiro–Wilk test. The results showed the normal distribution of the collected data. Then, a t-test was conducted to compare the walking data of the two groups. The Statistical Package for the Social Sciences (SPSS) program and Microsoft Excel were used for data analysis.

3. Results and Discussions

When comparing gait between the two groups (Table 3), balance parameters (head sway range, head tilt range, pelvis tilt range, and shoulder obliquity max) in the younger group showed better postural control compared to the older group. In terms of the spatiotemporal parameters (stride length and step length), the older group exhibited shorter lengths than the younger group, while there was no significant difference in cadence and speed, which depended on each person's walking. Therefore, it is not conclusively clear whether the younger walked faster than the older. Both the left and right knee ranges of motion (ROM) for the older group were lower than the other group. As age increases, the ROM of the knee tends to decrease. The older group had a higher risk of falling and functional decline in daily activities.

Table 3. Data of gait parameters obtained from experiment.

Parameters	Range of Average Data	
	Volunteers Aged 20–39 Years	**Volunteers Aged 50 Years and Above**
Balance (The higher the grade, the healthier. (Grade: 1–5))		
Head sway range	1.8–4.6	1.6–4.0
Head tilt range	2.6–4.8	1.6–4.2
Pelvis tilt range	2.4–4.0	1.4–4.0
Shoulder obliquity max	4.4–5	4.2–5
Spatiotemporal		
Cadence (step/s)	1.82–2.05	1.71–2.30
Speed (m/s)	0.95–1.22	0.82–1.32
Stride length (m)	1.03–1.28	0.93–1.18
Step length (m)	0.51–0.64	0.47–0.59
Range of Motion of Knee		
Right knee ROM (deg)	19.04–65.82	32.05–57.28
Left knee ROM (deg)	28.79–127.94	42.71–54.53
Health Risk Score		
Risk of falling (%)	1.54–2.57	1.46–4.00
Functional loss (%)	3.08–5.51	2.92–8.28

When comparing gait between the two groups, the balance of both groups during walking significantly differed. The head sway range ($p = 0.008$), head tilt range ($p = 0.018$), and pelvis tilt range ($p = 0.003$) showed statistically significant differences. The younger group exhibited better postural control. In terms of spatiotemporal parameters, stride length and step length during walking significantly differed between the two groups at $p = 0.001$. The older group had shorter lengths compared to the other group, leading to a higher percentage of falls and functional loss at $p = 0.021$ and 0.023 (Table 4). The balance of the younger group was better (Figure 3). Their median and mean values of the head sway range, the head tilt range, and the pelvis tilt range were higher in the range of grade 3–4, while those of the other group were in the range of grade 2–3. The head sway range of the older group was in the interquartile range (IQR), or 50% (grade 1–3), whereas the other group exhibited an IQR of grade 2–4. The head tilt range of the younger group was grade 4, and 50% of the values belonged to grades 3–5. In contrast, the older group showed an IQR of grade 2–5. A right-skewed distribution was within grades 2–3, and data density was in grades 3–5. For the pelvis tilt range, the younger possessed an IQR of grade 2–5, with the highest grade (5) within the 50% data range. For the older group, the IQR spanned grades 2–3, and the highest grade was 4, with few individuals reaching grade 5.

Table 4. Comparison of gait patterns between the two groups.

Parameters	Class [1]	$\overline{X}$	S.D.	df	t Stat	p (T ≤ t) Two-Tail	t Critical Two-Tail
Head sway range	1 2	3.18 2.48	1.62 1.72	98	2.707	0.008 *	1.984
Head tilt range	1 2	3.8 3.12	1.84 2.19	97	2.396	0.018 *	1.985
Pelvis tilt range	1 2	3.24 2.42	2.06 1.43	95	3.101	0.003 *	1.985
Shoulder obliquity max	1 2	4.86 4.84	0.12 0.46	73	0.185	0.854	1.993
Cadence (step/s)	1 2	1.92 1.96	0.03 0.06	88	−1.180	0.241	1.987
Speed (m/s)	1 2	1.07 1.02	0.02 0.04	86	1.434	0.155	1.988
Stride length (m)	1 2	1.12 1.04	0.01 0.02	95	3.297	0.001 *	1.985
Step length (m)	1 2	0.56 0.52	0.003 0.004	95	3.281	0.001 *	1.985
Right knee ROM (deg)	1 2	47.98 49.97	334.12 182.33	90	−0.617	0.539	1.987
Left knee ROM (deg)	1 2	55.80 49.41	2894.28 208.91	56	0.811	0.421	2.003
Risk of falling (%)	1 2	1.90 1.35	0.45 1.38	78	−2.365	0.021 *	1.991
Functional loss (%)	1 2	4.00 4.95	2.36 6.12	82	−2.316	0.023*	1.989

* p-value < 0.05 which means the data is statistically significant. (If the p-value is less than 0.05, it is judged as "significant", and if the p-value is greater than 0.05, it is judged as "not significant [5]".). [1] Classes 1 and 2 are groups of volunteers aged 20–39 years and aged 50 years and above, respectively.

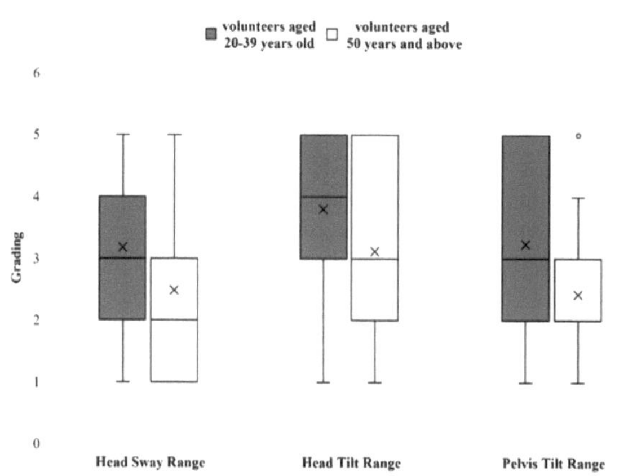

Figure 3. Comparison of significant balance parameters, which includes head sway range, head tilt range, and pelvis tilt range between the volunteers aged 20−39 years group and volunteers aged 50 years and above group.

Figure 4 shows the median and mean values of stride length and step length which were longer for the younger group. Notably, the stride length of the older group exhibited the lowest maximum value, while the minimum value was higher than that of the younger group. The data within the range from Q1 to the median had a higher frequency than that within the range from the median to Q3, which exhibited greater data variability. The younger group had significantly longer lengths compared to the older group.

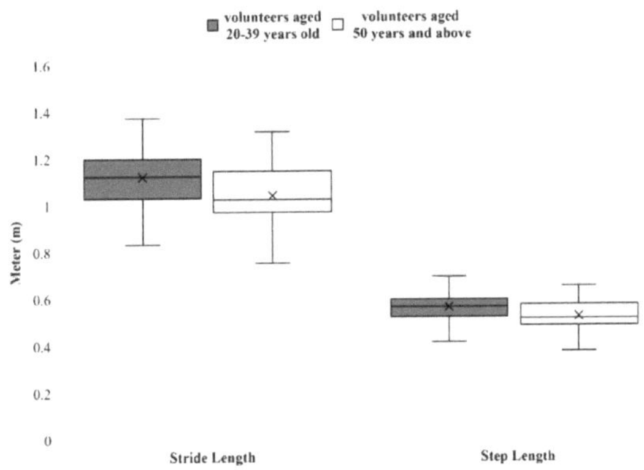

Figure 4. Comparison of the significant spatiotemporal parameters, which includes stride length and step length between the volunteers aged 20–39 years group and volunteers aged 50 years and above group.

The percentage of the risk of falling in the younger group was lower than in the older group. One individual exhibited an abnormal value, which could potentially be an outlier resulting from stiff walking during the experiment (Figure 5). On the other hand, in the older group, there was a higher risk. Several individuals in this group exhibited significantly elevated risks, indicating potential outliers. This suggested increased susceptibility to falls. However, the minimum risk was lower than in the younger group. This implied the presence of individuals with good health or normal walking patterns. The functional loss between the two groups exhibited significant differences, as notably the older group had higher values and abnormal values. However, several participants in this group exhibited good health. Conversely, the younger group had only one abnormal value. For such outliers, careful observation and assessment of participants' walking patterns were essential. If stiff walking was detected, participants were encouraged to walk in a manner to prevent the occurrence of outliers.

The older group showed a slower walking speed, less step length, and less stride length. The stride length of patients with osteoarthritis is reduced compared to healthy people [6,7]. Patients with Parkinson's disease showed decreased stride length, step length, and speed, which are hallmarks of falling and are associated with an increased risk of falling [4]. Falls are associated with aging with stride length being one of the significant parameters associated with falling. Thus, stride length can be used to assess fall risk [8], and step length can used to identify falls between older fallers and non-fallers [9,10]. Older fallers have short steps and less stability in walking [11]. The balance parameters of the younger group had a higher grade (the higher the grade, the healthier) and declined in postural stability resulting in reduced walking stability, which coincided with Ref. [12]. Balance is related to weakness, which is an important predictor of falls [12]. The risk of falling (%) and functional loss (%) of the older group had higher values than those of the younger group. Reference [13] showed that when the function of the body decreased, falls increased.

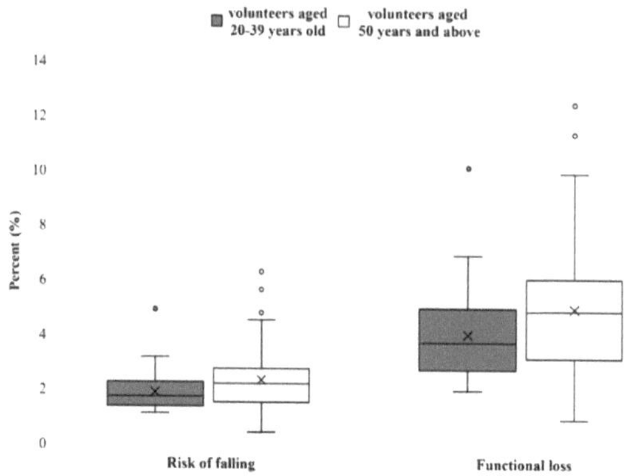

Figure 5. Comparison of the significant health risk score parameters, which includes the risk of falling and functional loss between the volunteers aged 20–39 years group and volunteers aged 50 years and above group.

4. Conclusions

The walking patterns between the two groups were different in walking efficiency, performance, and overall mobility. There was a higher likelihood of falls for the older group, which can result in injuries, disabilities, or loss of functionality. The findings of this study are beneficial for surveillance, fall prevention, and guiding the design of walking interventions. Enhancing walking efficiency is crucial to minimize the risk of future falls and associated injuries, contributing to improved overall well-being. In the future, it is necessary to utilize the parameters obtained from walking analysis to investigate gait patterns in patient groups. This can contribute to a further understanding of walking abnormalities in specific populations for the development of targeted interventions or treatments to improve gait and overall mobility. The Gait Analysis System needs to be studied to increase the reliability of the data and for patients with knee osteoarthritis, which has not been studied yet.

Author Contributions: Conceptualization, W.S. and T.S.; methodology, T.S. and W.S.; software, T.S.; validation, T.S.; formal analysis, T.S.; investigation, T.S.; resources, W.S. and T.S.; data curation, W.S. and T.S.; writing—original draft preparation, T.S.; writing—review and editing, T.S.; visualization, T.S.; supervision, W.S.; project administration, T.S.; funding acquisition, W.S. All authors have read and agreed to the published version of the manuscript.

Funding: This research received no external funding.

Institutional Review Board Statement: Not applicable.

Informed Consent Statement: Informed consent was obtained from all subjects involved in the study.

Data Availability Statement: All data obtained by the gait test of participants in the author's laboratory are presented in the contribution.

Acknowledgments: This work was supported by Pattana Lee from Blue Oak Co., Ltd. for his supporting the Gait Analysis System in this study. The first author was supported by a grant from the Graduate School, Srinakharinwirot University, Thailand.

Conflicts of Interest: The authors declare no conflicts of interest.

References

1. Worawit Louthrenoo. *Osteoarthritis*; Thanabaan Printing: Chiang Mai, Thailand, 2003.
2. Wirot Kawinwongkovit. *Knee Osteoarthritis*; Department of Orthopedics, Faculty of Medicine, Mahidol University: Bangkok, Thailand, 2012.

3. Weerapong, S. Relationship between osteoarthritis and the risk of falls in the elderly: A case study of Kang Aen, Prasat, Surin, Thailand. *Srinagarind Med. J.* **2018**, *33*, 57.
4. Lai, Y.-R.; Lien, C.-Y.; Huang, C.-C.; Lin, W.-C.; Chen, Y.-S.; Yu, C.-C.; Cheng, B.-C.; Kung, C.-T.; Kung, C.-F.; Chiang, Y.-F.; et al. Clinical Disease Severity Mediates the Relationship between Stride Length and Speed and the Risk of Falling in Parkinson's Disease. *J. Pers. Med.* **2022**, *12*, 192. [CrossRef] [PubMed]
5. Kwak, S. Are only *p*-values less than 0.05 significant? A *p*-value greater than 0.05 is also significant! *J. Lipid Atheroscler.* **2023**, *12*, 89. [CrossRef] [PubMed]
6. Esrafilian, A.; Karimi, M.T.; Amiri, P.; Fatoye, F. Performance of subjects with knee osteoarthritis during walking: Differential parameters. *Rheumatol. Int.* **2013**, *33*, 1753–1761. [CrossRef] [PubMed]
7. Weidow, J.; Tranberg, R.; Saari, T.; Kärrholm, J. Hip and knee joint rotations differ between patients with medial and lateral knee osteoarthritis: Gait analysis of 30 patients and 15 controls. *J. Orthop. Res.* **2006**, *24*, 1890–1899. [CrossRef] [PubMed]
8. Ruiz-Ruiz, L.; Jimenez, A.R.; Garcia-Villamil, G.; Seco, F. Detecting Fall Risk and Frailty in Elders with Inertial Motion Sensors: A Survey of Significant Gait Parameters. *Sensors* **2021**, *21*, 6918. [CrossRef] [PubMed]
9. Liebherr, M.; Schubert, P.; Schiebener, J.; Kersten, S.; Haas, C.T. Dual-tasking and aging—About multiple perspectives and possible implementations in interventions for the elderly. *Cogent Psychol.* **2016**, *3*, 1261440. [CrossRef]
10. Sherrington, C.; Fairhall, N.; Wallbank, G.; Tiedemann, A.; Michaleff, Z.A.; Howard, K.; Clemson, L.; Hopewell, S.; Lamb, S. Exercise for preventing falls in older people living in the community. *Cochrane Database Syst. Rev.* **2019**, *54*, 885–891. [CrossRef] [PubMed]
11. Nascimento, M.D.M.; Gouveia, É.R.; Gouveia, B.R.; Marques, A.; Martins, F.; Przednowek, K.; França, C.; Peralta, M.; Ihle, A. Associations of gait speed, cadence, gait stability ratio, and body balance with falls in older adults. *Int. J. Environ. Res. Public Health* **2022**, *19*, 13926. [CrossRef] [PubMed]
12. Delbaere, K.; Close, J.C.; Heim, J.; Sachdev, P.S.; Brodaty, H.; Slavin, M.J.; Kochan, N.A.; Lord, S.R. A Multifactorial Approach to Understanding Fall Risk in Older People. *J. Am. Geriatr. Soc.* **2010**, *58*, 1679–1685. [CrossRef] [PubMed]
13. Rodríguez-Molinero, A.; Herrero-Larrea, A.; Miñarro, A.; Narvaiza, L.; Gálvez-Barrón, C.; León, N.G.; Valldosera, E.; de Mingo, E.; Macho, O.; Aivar, D.; et al. The spatial parameters of gait and their association with falls, functional decline and death in older adults: A prospective study. *Sci. Rep.* **2019**, *9*, 8813. [CrossRef] [PubMed]

engineering proceedings

Proceeding Paper

Preliminary Study on Image Captioning for Construction Hazards †

Wen-Ta Hsiao [1], Wen-Der Yu [1,*], Tao-Ming Cheng [1] and Alexey Bulgakov [2]

1 Department of Civil and Construction Engineering, Chaoyang University of Technology, Taichung 413310, Taiwan; wdshiau@cyut.edu.tw (W.-T.H.); tmcheng@cyut.edu.tw (T.-M.C.)
2 Department of Automation, Robotic and Mechatronic in Construction, South-Russian State Polytechnic University, Novocherkassk 346428, Russia; agi.bulgakov@gmail.com
* Correspondence: wenderyu@cyut.edu.tw
† Presented at the 2024 IEEE 4th International Conference on Electronic Communications, Internet of Things and Big Data, Taipei, Taiwan, 19–21 April 2024.

Abstract: Construction accidents are a major contributor to occupational fatalities. To tackle this issue, improved monitoring for hazard elimination is crucial. By introducing a deep-learning image captioning system, we identified hazards via closed-circuit television in construction sites. By leveraging Inception-v3 for feature extraction and the gated recurrent unit for caption generation, real-time hazard monitoring was enabled. Bilingual evaluation understudy scores were determined for continuous and effective hazard detection, helping construction managers enhance safety.

Keywords: construction safety; image captioning; deep learning; closed-circuit television (CCTV) monitoring

Citation: Hsiao, W.-T.; Yu, W.-D.; Cheng, T.-M.; Bulgakov, A. Preliminary Study on Image Captioning for Construction Hazards. *Eng. Proc.* **2024**, *74*, 20. https://doi.org/10.3390/engproc2024074020

Academic Editors: Shu-Han Liao, Teen-Hang Meen and Cheng-Fu Yang

Published: 28 August 2024

1. Introduction

Construction accidents are a major cause of occupational fatalities worldwide [1–3]. The most effective way to prevent accidents is to eliminate hazards [4]. However, current methods depend on manual inspections by limited safety personnel and are ineffective for real-time monitoring. An alternative to this method is the use of closed-circuit television (CCTV) monitoring [5]. Hazard identification from CCTV images is manually conducted by supervisors, which is impractical for continuous operation [6]. Thus, we explored an AI-based image-captioning approach using a deep learning model with an attention mechanism. It utilizes a pre-trained Inception-v3 network [7] for feature extraction and a gated recurrent unit (GRU) [8] for caption generation. Preliminary tests using bilingual evaluation (BLEU) scores [9] showed promising results regarding the model's effectiveness for captioning hazard images.

2. Literature Review

2.1. Hazard Identification in Construction

A "hazard" is defined as a dangerous condition potentially causing injury, property damage, or environmental impact [10]. According to Heinrich's Domino Theory, accidents can be prevented by removing underlying factors [11]. Traditional identification of hazard images adopts process hazard analysis (PHA) to identify possible hazardous scenarios [12]. However, this method is ineffective in dynamic construction sites where safety measures can be temporarily compromised.

Safety personnel use regular patrols and CCTV to monitor real-time hazards. Additionally, computer vision technologies have been employed to identify hazards [13]. Despite technological advancements, the use of CCTV for real-time hazard detection has been underexplored. Using CCTV effectively, existing safety equipment can be utilized to ensure continuous surveillance to reduce accident risks on construction sites [5].

2.2. Image Caption and Applications

Image captions are generated as descriptive sentences for images using various techniques [14]: (1) template-based methods, which use syntactic parse trees from datasets; (2) image search-based methods, comparing target images against dataset images; (3) deep learning-based methods, utilizing neural networks for multimodal transformations to convert images into text [15]. Recently, deep learning methods have been widely chosen for use over MS COCO image caption generation due to its inherent challenges [16]. The architecture for these models is the encoder–decoder framework, integrating a convolutional neural network (CNN) for image extraction and a recurrent neural network (RNN) for sentence generation [15]. Examples of deep learning-based models include the neural image caption (NIC) model [16], mask RCNN + LSTM with attention mechanisms [17], self-critical sequence training [18], and transformer [19].

Image captioning has shown success in various fields [15–19] but is relatively new in construction engineering. Liu et al. [20] and Wang et al. [17] applied it to describe construction scenes and extract semantic information from images and videos, respectively. Although promising, their results are simple descriptions with limited semantic detail, and thus, are inadequate for complex hazardous construction scenarios. This limitation highlights the importance of the current study.

3. Method

We employed a conventional architecture that combines an Inception v3 deep CNN encoder to extract image features and a GRU recurrent network decoder to generate hazard descriptions. The input images were sourced from CCTV cameras widely used on construction sites.

3.1. Feature Extraction

The proposed model's feature extraction process adopts a pre-trained Inception v3 network, implemented via a MATLAB 2023 program, as detailed in Figure 1. Initially, the model gathers information on the network's input size, constructs a layer graph of the architecture, and removes the classification layers. In the second phase, it introduces a new image input layer matching the original network's dimensions and sets the output size to [8 8 2048], defining the feature maps' dimensions and depth. Finally, the model creates a deep learning network based on Inception v3, specifically adapted for feature extraction by omitting the final classification layers, enhancing its suitability for high-level feature extraction across various computer vision tasks.

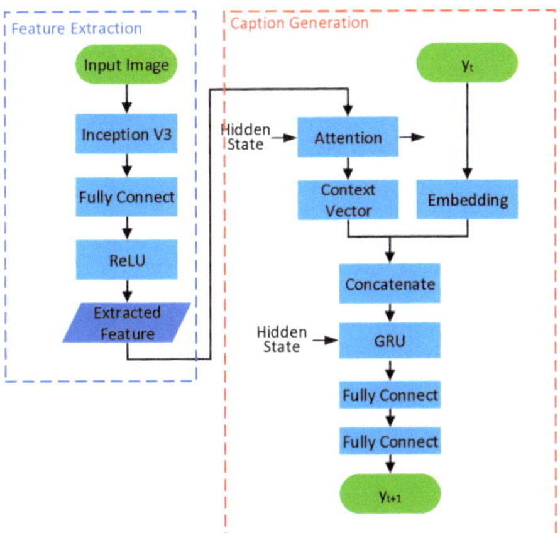

Figure 1. Procedure of proposed method.

3.2. Caption Generation

The process of generating image captions is implemented through a MATLAB program with the following functionalities (Figure 1). The program sets the model's parameters, such as word embedding dimension (256) and the number of hidden units (512), and then initializes encoder and decoder components, including fully connected layers, word embeddings, GRU weights, and attention mechanism weights. Next, it defines two critical functions: one for processing image data through fully connected layers and rectified linear unit (ReLU) activation, and another for generating predictions and attention weights for captioning. The program then sets training parameters and determines the number of epochs, the mini-batch size, and options for visualizing progress, followed by executing a custom training loop that includes data shuffling, preprocessing, loss calculation, gradient computing, and parameter updating via the Adam optimizer. The loop continues through the designated number of epochs, with data shuffling and mini-batch processing occurring during each epoch.

3.3. Performance Evaluation

Four key metrics are commonly used to evaluate natural language processing (NLP) tasks [17]: (1) BLEU, which measures the precision of n-grams in the generated caption and the reference caption; (2) ROUGE, assessing the overlap of n-grams between generated and reference captions; (3) CIDEr, calculating similarity with the reference caption by considering consensus across multiple references; (4) SPICE, evaluating captions by parsing them into semantic propositions and comparing these with reference captions. Each metric has specific strengths and weaknesses.

In this study, we used BLEU to evaluate the accuracy of hazard information extraction and the linguistic quality of the captions in images. We chose BLEU because it effectively evaluates the presence of key terms crucial for describing hazardous scenarios. These descriptions involve key terms including objects (e.g., workers, vehicles, materials), the accident medium (e.g., scaffolding, openness), and location (e.g., top floor, roof). BLEU is outlined in Equation (1), as follows:

$$\mathrm{BLUE} = \mathrm{BP} \cdot \exp\left(\sum_{n=1}^{N} w_n \log p_n\right) \tag{1}$$

where n denotes the n-gram, w_n denotes the weight of the n-gram, BP denotes the short sentence penalty factor (brevity penalty), and p_n denotes the coverage of the n-gram.

4. Preliminary Testing Results

To assess the hazard image caption method, the research team gathered CCTV videos from Chaoyang University of Technology (CYUT) and created a dataset of images and captions using their construction hazard description system (CHDS) [5]. The Matlab® Deep Learning Toolbox's "Image Captioning Using Attention" program was employed to train and test the method on these datasets.

4.1. Image Caption Dataset Generation

Figure 2 illustrates the construction of hazard image caption datasets. The process starts with the caption from an image from a CCTV video, which is then inputted into the construction hazard description system (CHDS) for captioning. Within CHDS, a domain expert marks hazard scenarios with a yellow square frame, identifying and classifying associated objects such as workers and formwork to determine the hazard type. The system generates a caption describing the hazard. In total, we have captioned 1138 hazard images, encompassing 1544 site objects. For each hazard image, we generated four synonymous captions using ChatGPT, resulting in a total of 5690 captions for the 1138 hazard images. These datasets were employed to train the image caption program.

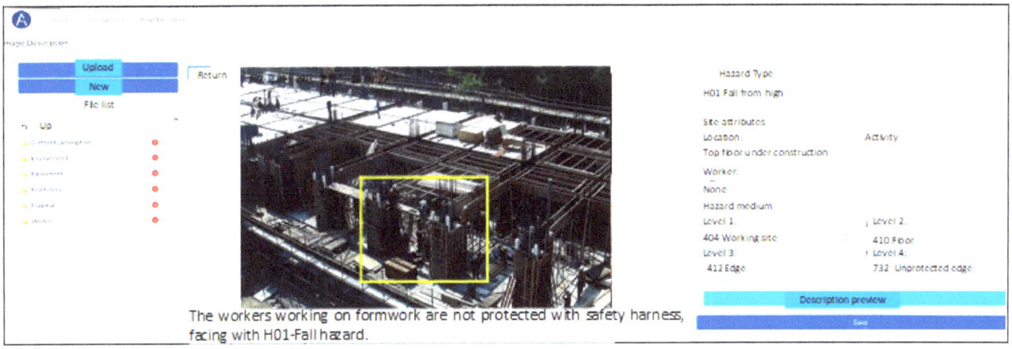

Figure 2. Image caption data generation with CHDS.

4.2. System Training

The "Image Captioning Using Attention" program from the Matlab® Deep Learning Toolbox® was used to test the proposed method. In the testing experiment, model parameters were initialized with 512 hidden units and a word embedding dimension of 256. The fully connected network's weights were initialized using the Glorot initializer. The output size was matched with the decoder's embedding dimension (256), and the input size was aligned with the "mixed10" layer's 2048 output channels from the pre-trained Inception-v3 network. The mini-batch size was set at 128, with a maximum of 30 epochs, and other parameters are detailed in Table 1.

Table 1. Parameters of captions.

Initial Learn Rate	Mini Batch	L2 Regularization	Optimizer
0.0001	30	0.01	rmsprop

The hardware for the training experiment includes (1) CPU: Intel Xeon E5-2620v4 @ 2.10 GHz, (2) RAM: 40 GB at 2400 MHz, (3) Operating System (OS): Microsoft Windows 10, and (4) GPU: NVIDIA Quadro P2000 (5 GB). The training process lasted over 21.5 h, encompassing 30 epochs, and culminated in a final BLEU score of 0.3851. This BLEU score suggests a moderately feasible outcome.

4.3. System Testing

The trained image caption model was evaluated using site hazard images. The caption generation process of the program is illustrated in Figure 3. The initial step involves the identification of site objects, including workers and formwork. Subsequently, the program detects the associated hazard scenario within the image, marked by the yellow-dot square area. Finally, it proceeds to generate a caption, word by word, to describe the hazard scenario.

Figure 4 shows a test result of a site image, where a worker standing beside a mobile crane, without protective barriers, is at risk of being struck.

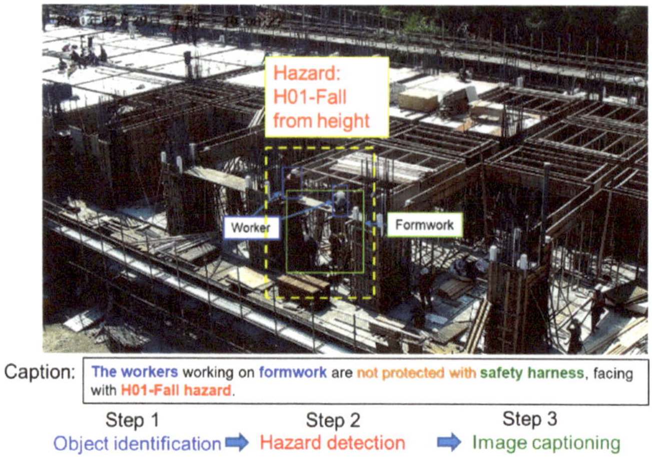

Figure 3. Image caption generation process.

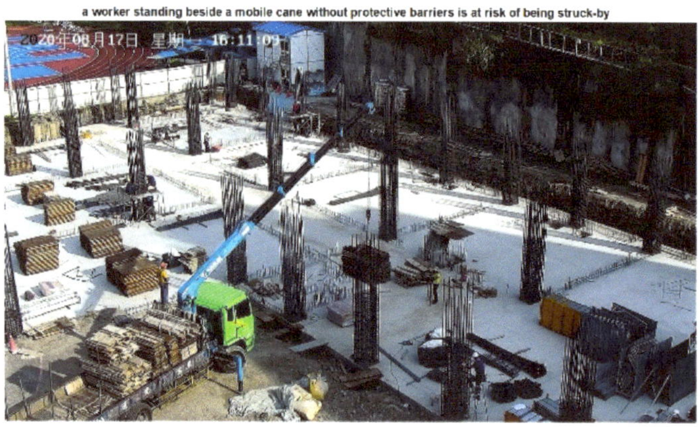

Figure 4. Sample testing hazard image.

5. Conclusions

We explored the generation of image captioning for the construction industry. The approach involved a traditional encoder–decoder architecture, where an Inception-v3 model was utilized for image feature extraction, while a GRU recurrent network was used for caption generation. The method was tested on a dataset comprising 1138 hazard images, 1544 site objects, and 5690 captions, resulting in a moderate BLEU score of 0.3851. While the results are promising, limitations exist. Firstly, the performance of the pre-trained Inception-v3 model for object recognition needs refinement. Despite an improvement from an initial accuracy of 74.4 to 92.53%, enhancement is still demanded. Additionally, it is essential to enhance the caption generation accuracy of the GRU model, which necessitates a more extensive image caption dataset surpassing the current 5690 captions. Furthermore, the feature extraction capability of the encoder requires enhancement to increase its performance.

Author Contributions: Research conceptualization, W.-D.Y.; conceptualization refinement, T.-M.C.; methodology, W.-D.Y. and W.-T.H.; CHDS program preparation and performance, W.-T.H.; validation, W.-D.Y. and W.-T.H.; formal analysis, W.-T.H.; investigation, W.-T.H.; resources, T.-M.C.; data curation, W.-T.H.; writing—original draft preparation, W.-D.Y. and W.-T.H.; writing—review and editing, T.-M.C. and A.B.; visualization, W.-D.Y.; supervision, T.-M.C.; project administration, W.-D.Y.; funding acquisition, W.-D.Y. All authors have read and agreed to the published version of the manuscript.

Funding: This project (MOST 111-2221-E-324-011-MY3) was funded by the National Science and Technology Council of Taiwan. The authors gratefully acknowledge this support.

Institutional Review Board Statement: Not applicable, for this study does not involve humans or animals.

Informed Consent Statement: Not applicable.

Data Availability Statement: The data are available upon request to the corresponding author.

Acknowledgments: The case study construction site was provided by Chaoyang University of Technology. The authors would like to express their sincere gratitude to the provider.

Conflicts of Interest: The funders had no role in the design of the study; in the collection, analyses, or interpretation of data; in the writing of the manuscript; or in the decision to publish the results.

References

1. Kang, K.; Ryu, H. Predicting types of occupational accidents at construction sites in Korea using random forest model. *Saf. Sci.* **2019**, *120*, 226–563. [CrossRef]
2. Chiang, Y.-H.; Wong, F.K.-W.; Liang, S. Fatal Construction Accidents in Hong Kong. *J. Constr. Eng. Manag.* **2018**, *144*. [CrossRef]
3. TOSHA. 2020 Labor Inspection Annual Report. Occupational Safety and Health, Taiwan. 2020. Available online: https://www.osha.gov.tw/1106/1164/1165/1168/34345/ (accessed on 24 October 2022).
4. Yu, W.D.; Wang, K.C.; Wu, H.T. Empirical Comparison of Learning Effectiveness of Immersive Virtual-Reality-Based Safety Training for Novice and Experienced Construction Workers. *J. Constr. Eng. Manag.* **2022**, *148*, 04022078. [CrossRef]
5. Yu, W.D.; Hsiao, T.; Cheng, T.M.; Chiang, H.S.; Chang, C.Y. Describing Construction Hazard Images Identified from Site Safety Surveillance Video. In Proceedings of the 3rd International Civil Engineering and Architecture Conference (CEAC 2023), Kyoto, Japan, 17–21 March 2023.
6. Ding, L.; Fang, W.; Luo, H.; Love, P.E.D.; Ouyang, X. A deep hybrid learning model to detect unsafe behavior: Integrating convolution neural networks and long short-term memory. *Autom. Constr.* **2018**, *86*, 118–124. [CrossRef]
7. Szegedy, C.; Vanhoucke, V.; Ioffe, S.; Shlens, J.; Wojna, Z. Rethinking the Inception Architecture for Computer Vision. *arXiv* **2023**, arXiv:1512.00567v3.
8. Cho, K.; Van Merri, B.; Gulcehre, C.; Bahdanau, D.; Bougares, F.; Schwenk, H.; Bengio, Y. Learning phrase representations using rnn encoder-decoder for statistical machine translation. *arXiv* **2014**, arXiv:1406.1078.
9. Papineni, K.; Roukos, S.; Ward, T.; Zhu, W.-J. BLEU: A Method for Automatic Evaluation of Machine Translation. In Proceedings of the 40th Annual Meeting of the Association for Computational Linguistics (ACL), Philadelphia, PA, USA, 7–12 July 2002; pp. 311–318.
10. Heinrich, H.W. *IFRCRCS Public Awareness and Public Education for Disaster Risk Reduction*; International Federation of Red Cross and Red Crescent Societies: Geneva, Switzerland, 16 June 2021; pp. 7–9. Available online: https://www.ifrc.org/sites/default/files/2021-06/04-HAZARD-DEFINITIONS-HR.pdf (accessed on 11 November 2023).
11. Heinrich, H.W. *Industrial Accident Prevention*; McGraw-Hill: New York, NY, USA, 1931.
12. Cameron, I.; Mannan, S.; Németh, E.; Park, S.; Pasman, H.; Rogers, W.; Seligmann, B. Process hazard analysis, hazard identification and scenario definition: Are the conventional tools sufficient, or should and can we do much better? *Process Saf. Environ. Prot.* **2017**, *110*, 53–70. [CrossRef]
13. Zhang, L.; Wang, J.; Wang, Y.; Sun, H.; Zhao, X. Automatic construction site hazard identification integrating construction scene graphs with BERT based domain knowledge. *Autom. Constr.* **2022**, *142*, 104535. [CrossRef]
14. Hossain, M.Z.; Sohel, F.; Shiratuddin, M.F.; Laga, H. A comprehensive survey of deep learning for image caption. *ACM Comput. Surv.* **2019**, *51*, 1–36. [CrossRef]
15. Li, S.C. Image Caption with Object Detection and Self-Attention Mechanism Integration and Model Analysis. Master's Thesis, Graduate Program in Artificial Intelligence Technology and Applications, National Yang Ming Chiao Tung University, Hsinchu, Taiwan, July 2021. (In Chinese).
16. Vinyals, O.; Toshev, A.; Bengio, S.; Erhan, D. Show and Tell: A Neural Image Caption Generator. *arXiv* **2015**, arXiv:1411.4555.
17. Wang, Y.; Xiao, B.; Bouferguene, A.; Al-Hussein, M.; Li, H. Vision-based method for semantic information extraction in construction by integrating deep learning object detection and image caption. *Adv. Eng. Inform.* **2022**, *53*, 101699. [CrossRef]
18. Rennie, S.J.; Marcheret, E.; Mroueh, Y.; Ross, J.; Goel, V. Self-critical Sequence Training for Image Caption. *arXiv* **2016**, arXiv:1612.00563.

19. Vaswani, A.; Shazeer, N.; Parmar, N.; Uszkoreit, J.; Jones, L.; Gomez, A.N.; Kaiser, L.; Polosukhin, I. Attention Is All You Need. *arXiv* **2017**, arXiv:1706.03762.
20. Liu, H.; Wang, G.; Huang, T.; He, P.; Skitmore, M.; Luo, X. Manifesting construction activity scenes via image caption. *Autom. Constr.* **2020**, *119*, 103334. [CrossRef]

engineering proceedings

Proceeding Paper

Application of Multi-Diamond Processing Model to Hairstyling †

Shih-Wen Hsiao and Yu-Jie Tsai *

Department of Industrial Design, National Cheng-Kung University, Tainan 701, Taiwan; swhsiao@mail.ncku.edu.tw
* Correspondence: p36111141@gs.ncku.edu.tw
† Presented at the 2024 IEEE 4th International Conference on Electronic Communications, Internet of Things and Big Data, Taipei, Taiwan, 19–21 April 2024.

Abstract: In 2003, the British Design Council advocated for strategic design and its management. They researched ways to create a universal framework for describing the design process and came up with the Double Diamond Model, which became a part of the universal design language. The Double Diamond Model applies to innovation and problem-solving involving divergence and convergence at four stages: Discover, Define, Develop, and Deliver. Continuous divergence, convergence, and iteration are necessary at each stage of the design process. Therefore, we reinterpreted design process methods to optimize and apply the entire design process in various fields. A case study applying the Multi-Diamond Model to users' experiences during a hairstyling appointment was conducted to understand user needs and behavioral differences. Users' behaviors and their understanding of hairstyling were analyzed by employing the fuzzy comprehensive evaluation method to choose hairstyles that were suitable for various face shapes at different perceived difficulty levels.

Keywords: design process; multi-diamond modeling; design thinking; user experience

Citation: Hsiao, S.-W.; Tsai, Y.-J. Application of Multi-Diamond Processing Model to Hairstyling. *Eng. Proc.* **2024**, *74*, 21. https://doi.org/10.3390/engproc2024074021

Academic Editors: Shu-Han Liao, Teen-Hang Meen and Cheng-Fu Yang

Published: 28 August 2024

1. Introduction

The Double Diamond Model was proposed by the Design Council of the United Kingdom in 2005 to understand a problem and identify potential challenges. It is a design process model consisting of four phases: Discover, Define, Develop, and Deliver [1]. Various solutions were generated during the development phases through prototyping, testing, and evaluation [2]. These phases belong to a cycle of divergence and convergence. The first diamond model defines the problem, while the second diamond model explores possibilities through iterative computation, testing, and development. Widely applied in designing products and services, the Double Diamond Model provides a structured approach to the design process [3] (Figure 1).

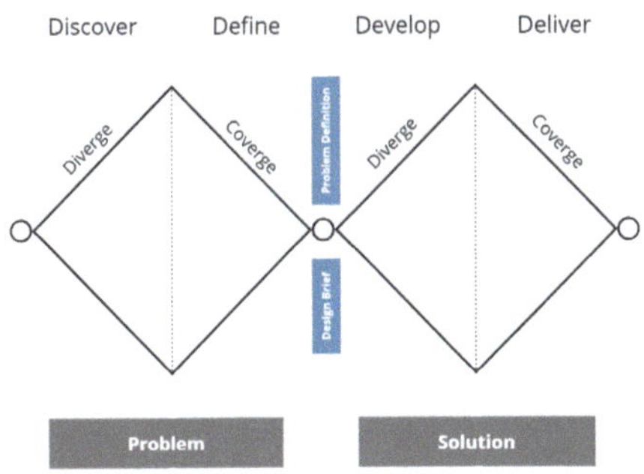

Figure 1. Double Diamond Model design process.

A three-diamond design model was also proposed as the two-diamond model is usually employed for problem discovery and problem-driven solutions in the design process. Data are used for computation, analysis, or planning to represent and quantify the problem. By incorporating data on user needs and data constraints, the third diamond model is introduced to enhance the framework of the two-diamond model in the design process. Design experiences involve diverse processes with divergences and convergences in continuous iterations. A simple two or three-diamond model cannot fully capture the complexities of a design project. Teachers often outline phased objectives in product design courses, breaking each phase down for better comprehension for students. The Double Diamond Model is applied to each design stage with dispersion, convergence, and iteration.

In the beauty industry, a user service process can include choosing a hairstyle and hair color that expresses individual personality and style. Satisfaction hinges on an individual's expectations regarding image, style, and personality. Effective communication ensures that serviced hairstyles and colors align with client expectations.

We delved into how to select design thinking methodologies to support human-centered artificial intelligence and innovation. Using a multi-diamond design framework, we reinterpreted the Double Diamond Model as seven phases: Observation, Requirements, Market Research, Design Goals, Conceptual Solution, Conceptual Evaluation, and Solution Validation. Each phase involves divergence, convergence, and iteration. Black box system analysis, the six-whys questioning method, and a goal tree were applied in each diamond model to illustrate divergence and convergence actions. Using the user's hair experience as a case study, customer behavior was analyzed by gender, age, and profession. Customer understanding of face shape and hair color, difficulty level, and personal evaluation were used to verify the feasibility of the model and understand the customer's experience during the process, their comprehension of hairstyle and color, and the difficulty.

2. Theoretical Background

2.1. Maslow's Theory of Needs

Maslow's Theory of Needs was developed by psychologist Abraham Maslow to outline human motivations based on inherited, instinctive needs. These needs encompass physiological (air, water, food), safety (personal and property safety), social (relationships, love), respect (self-worth, achievement), and self-actualization (personal potential, dreams realization). Physiological and safety needs are basic, social and respect needs are psychological, and self-actualization needs are self-satisfaction. The theory provides a framework for understanding universal human needs and the development of higher-level emotions.

2.2. Black Box System

In the design process, various constraints make reliance on intuition and subjectivity difficult. System theory is used to recognize and analyze problems such as data collection, organization, and goal establishment in design. A system is a conceptual entity with no independent existence, focusing on understanding its characteristics of input, output, and conversion. The purpose of the conversion process is to establish connections with other elements (Figure 2). In the system, substances, energy, and information undergo orderly flow and conversion in the interactive process (Figure 3), representing the essence of black box analysis [4].

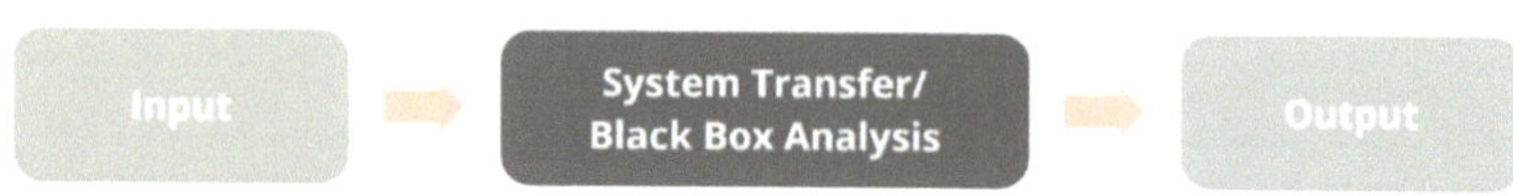

Figure 2. Basic Flowchart of Black Box System Analysis.

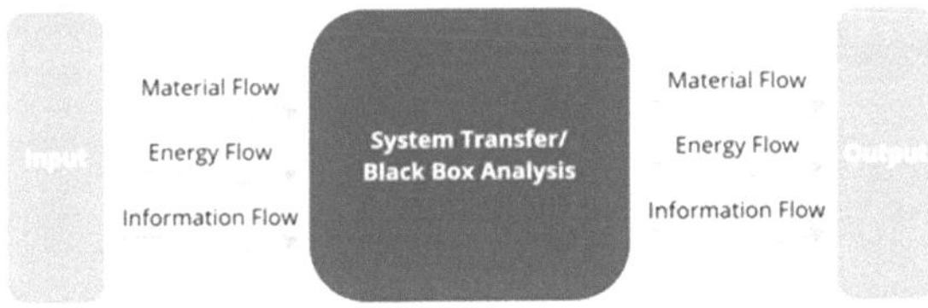

Figure 3. The Transformation Process in Black Box System.

2.3. Objective Tree

An objective tree is used to set goals which are categorized into primary and secondary goals in a hierarchical structure [5]. The goals are interrelated to ensure consistency and validity. When creating an objective tree, the following points are usually included (Figure 4).

(1) Determine the overarching goal to achieve, whether it is an organizational, team, or individual objective aligned with the long-term strategic direction.
(2) Define key objectives by splitting the final goal into several primary objectives, which are the stages or nature of the end goal to be achieved.
(3) Define secondary objectives to segment each primary goal into specific, quantifiable, measurable, and achievable secondary goals.
(4) Establish a hierarchy of objectives according to the logical relationship between the primary and secondary objectives and establish a hierarchical structure of objectives, usually in the form of a tree diagram.
(5) Determine the relevance and constraints within the objective tree and identify associations and constraints among the objectives, including sequential relationships, dependencies, or conditional factors.

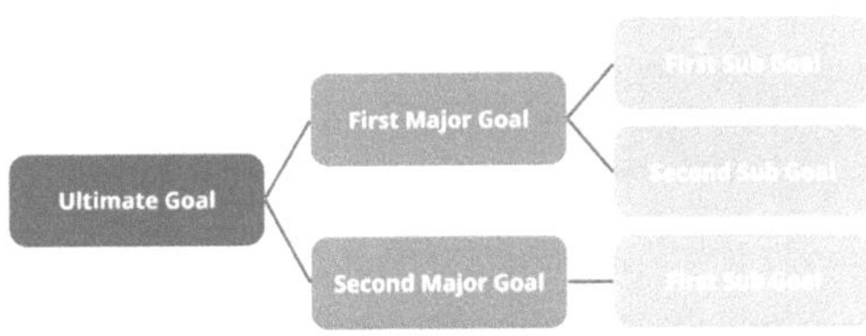

Figure 4. Structure of objective tree.

2.4. Evaluation Using Fuzzy Theory

Zadeh introduced 'fuzzy sets' to explore quantitative processing in human cognitive processes and created a new branch of mathematics. Practical phenomena are categorized as definite, random, and fuzzy in the fuzzy set. Mathematical tools such as geometry and algebra address definite objects, probability theory deals with random phenomena, and fuzzy mathematics is used to explain fuzzy phenomena [6]. In assessing entities with multiple attributes and diverse influences, the Fuzzy Comprehensive Evaluation involves six main steps [7].

(1) Establishment of factor sets

$$U = \{u_1, u_2, \ldots, u_m\} \tag{1}$$

(2) Creating weight sets

$$\underset{\sim}{A} = (a_1, a_2, \ldots, a_m) \tag{2}$$

(3) Creating a rating set

$$V = \{V_1, V_2, \ldots, V_n\} \tag{3}$$

(4) Single Factor Fuzzy Evaluation

$$\underset{\sim}{R}_i = \left(\frac{r_{i1}}{V_1} + \frac{r_{i2}}{V_2} + \ldots + \frac{r_{in}}{V_n}\right) \tag{4}$$

$$\underset{\sim}{R} = \begin{pmatrix} r_{11} & r_{12} & \cdots & r_{1n} \\ r_{21} & r_{22} & \cdots & r_{2n} \\ \cdots & & & \\ r_{m1} & r_{m2} & \cdots & r_{mn} \end{pmatrix} \tag{5}$$

(5) Fuzzy Comprehensive Evaluation

$$\underset{\sim}{B} = \underset{\sim}{A} \circ \underset{\sim}{R} \tag{6}$$

$$\underset{\sim}{B} = (a_1, a_2, \ldots, a_m) \circ \begin{pmatrix} r_{11} & r_{12} & \cdots & r_{1n} \\ r_{21} & r_{22} & \cdots & r_{2n} \\ \cdots & & & \\ r_{m1} & r_{m2} & \cdots & r_{mn} \end{pmatrix} = (b_1, b_2, \ldots, b_n) \tag{7}$$

included among these

$$b_j = \bigvee_{i=1}^{m} (a_i \wedge r_{ij})(j = 1, 2, \ldots, n) \tag{8}$$

3. Methods

For the foundational design flow, we developed the stages of dispersion, iterative computation, convergence, and delivery in design. At each stage, outputs were used as inputs. In this approach, we used a multi-diamond model and employed the methodology in Section 2 for the research, analysis, and evaluation of the model's feasibility.

3.1. Multi-Diamond Model

The design framework of the Multi-Diamond Model comprises seven stages: observation, requirement proposal, market research, design objectives, conceptual proposals, concept evaluation, and proposal validation. In the Double Diamond Model's design process, the discovery phase corresponds to observation, requirements, and market analysis. The definition phase aligns with design objectives derived from market analysis, while the development phase corresponds to conceptual solutions. The delivery phase aligns with evaluating conceptual solutions, involving testing and feasibility assessment. The process starts with an input point, flowing through the diamond, generating an output (Figure 5). This output becomes the input for the next stage, continuing the process within the diamond. Iteration results in a complete result denoted by a bolded hollow circle, symbolizing integrated output and input. In the figure, arrows present the potential for backtracking and iteration when facing challenges.

In the observation phase, everyday experiences or Maslow's hierarchy of needs are presented for inspiration. The emphasis is on identifying and exploring issues and understanding stakeholder perspectives using surveys, interviews, and the 5W1H technique. Simultaneously, market analysis and target trees are used to shape the final design. Utilizing image boards, design scripts, and scenario planning, conceptual design solutions are envisioned within specific contexts. By evaluating these solutions using merits, drawbacks, and feasibility, followed by prototyping for validation, the groundwork is established for subsequent development and assessment.

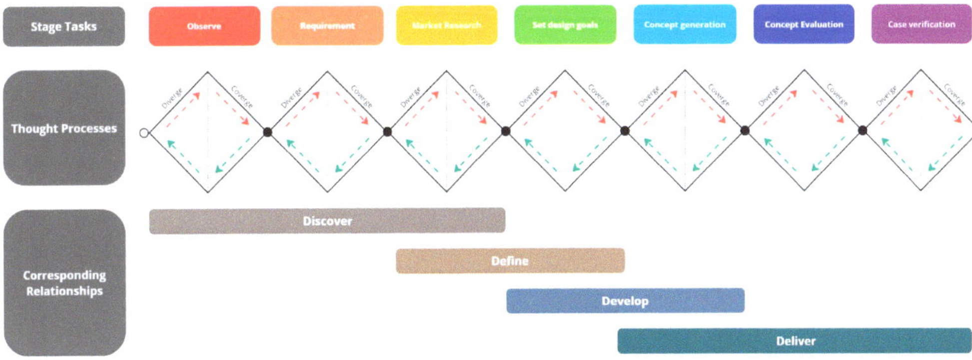

Figure 5. Flowchart of Multi-Diamond Modeling.

3.2. Detailed Process

Using Maslow's hierarchy of needs, life's different facets, personal experiences, behaviors, emotions, inner feelings, and preferences are determined and documented. This process generates meaningful and interesting problem requirements for further exploration. After identifying the requirement, we employed the 5W1H method to analyze each item and presented the results in a target tree to identify design targets and requirements. Utilizing the organized design targets and potential problem requirements, we interviewed and administered a questionnaire survey on the design targets. Data were collected to understand the importance of the requirement items. This process aided in determining the design objectives. The fuzzy theory or grey theory was applied to analyze the data to explore behavioral patterns, design objectives, and demand values. After setting the design objectives, a literature review was conducted to identify relevant technologies and methods. We set design boundaries by defining the research scope for convergence. With these conditions, the conceptual design phase was initiated to generate multiple conceptual solutions. We evaluated the strengths and weaknesses of these concepts. For the evaluation, the PUGH evaluation method was used to analyze data based on weights or degrees, simplifying the process of ranking and selecting the final solution. Following the selection of the final solution, feasibility was validated. A retrospective examination of the preceding stage was performed, followed by iterative corrections for the final product.

4. Case Study

Instagram and TikTok are vital for personalized communication. Maslow's Needs Theory and the first diamond model were used for such social media to investigate appearance anxiety regarding hairstyles and hair color.

Process

The output from the first diamond model was used to summarize problems and demands as the input for the next diamond model through divergence and convergence. The second diamond model was used to explore consumer demands, employing the 5W1H analysis. For each goal, divergence and convergence were conducted in a target tree to illustrate their relationship at each level. Systematically analyzing potential consumer needs, design objectives, and potential demand was obtained as the final output. In the second diamond model, the output comprised design objectives and problem demands. Transitioning to the third diamond model of the market survey, the input was derived from the output of the second stage. Based on the results of divergence and convergence from the second stage, potential problems were analyzed further through a questionnaire survey and interviews such as a market survey. Interviews with hairstylists revealed that customers browsed hairstylists' portfolios on social media, using images for communication. The questionnaire was designed to understand how customers chose hairstyles and colors, identified their problems, and validated the consistency of the requirements in the second stage. The questionnaire consisted of basic demographic information, a survey on face shape and hairstyle/hair color preferences, and customers' feelings regarding their appearance. Integrating the findings, demands, and customer behavior patterns was confirmed as the final output.

According to the survey results (Figure 6), 80% of the respondents conducted research before visiting a hair salon. The primary methods included using social media and referencing hairstylist portfolios. Approximately 20% did not perform pre-research due to a lack of ideas or a preference for direct communication with hairstylists. These findings represent the customer experience process before visiting a hair salon.

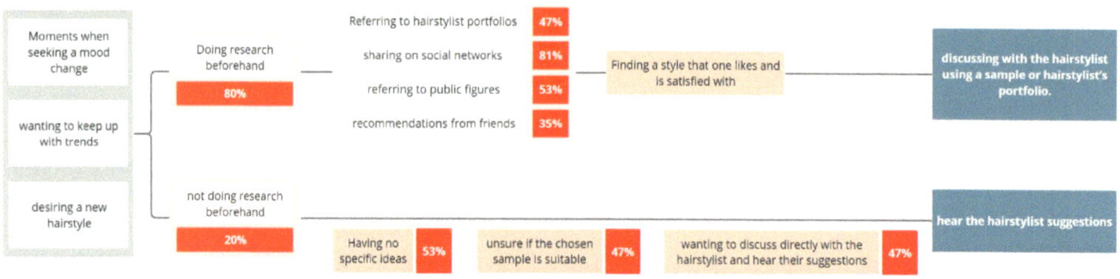

Figure 6. Flowchart of customer experience.

The design objective of the fourth diamond model was to confirm the ultimate purpose of the analysis by analyzing users' understanding of their hairstyles, face shapes, and behaviors to explore their needs and entry points for hairstylists. The fifth to seventh diamond models involved a coherent operation that converted qualitative text into quantitative data. In the approach, the fuzzy logic of the fuzzy evaluation method was used to understand and analyze subjective user feedback involving qualitative concepts.

In the questionnaire, customers were asked about their understanding of their face shape, hairstyle, and hair color, as well as the difficulty in selecting a hairstyle and hair color. Scores of 0, 0.25, 0.5, 0.75, and 1 were used, ranging from "not at all understanding" to "very understanding," and from "not at all difficult" to "very difficult." Tables 1 and 2 present the percentage results of these scores.

Table 1. Understanding face shape, hairstyle, and hair color.

	Not at All Understanding	Not Understanding	Average	Well Understanding	Very Well Understanding
Face Shape	0.15	0.15	0.26	0.43	0.11
Hair Shape	0.16	0.21	0.29	0.29	0.05
Hair Color	0.26	0.3	0.12	0.25	0.07

Table 2. Difficulty in choosing hairstyle and hair color.

	Very Little Difficult	Not Difficult	Average	Difficult	Very Difficult
Hair Style	0.09	0.23	0.18	0.36	0.14
Hair Color	0.1	0.27	0.11	0.33	0.19

5. Results and Discussion

The fuzzy comprehensive evaluation was used as follows.

The customer's knowledge of face shape, hairstyle, and hair color was analyzed.

(1) Factor set $U1 = \{$ Face Shape, Hair Style, Hair Color $\}$

(2) Weight set $\underset{\sim}{A}_1 = (0.3, 0.35, 0.35)$

(3) Ratings V_1 = { Very unaware, unaware, average, aware, very aware }

(4) Single Factor Fuzzy Evaluation: Face Shape ($x1$), Hair Shape ($x2$), Hair Color ($x3$), we get

$$\underset{\sim}{R}(x1) = (0.05\ 0.15\ 0.26\ 0.43\ 0.11)$$
$$\underset{\sim}{R}(x2) = (0.16\ 0.21\ 0.29\ 0.29\ 0.05)$$
$$\underset{\sim}{R}(x3) = (0.26\ 0.3\ 0.12\ 0.25\ 0.07)$$

Therefore, the one-factor evaluation matrix is given by

$$\underset{\sim}{R}_1 = \begin{pmatrix} 0.05 & 0.15 & 0.26\ 0.43 & 0.11 \\ 0.16 & 0.21 & 0.29\ 0.29 & 0.05 \\ 0.26 & 0.3 & 0.12\ 0.25 & 0.07 \end{pmatrix}$$

(5) Fuzzy Comprehensive Evaluation $\underset{\sim}{B} = \underset{\sim}{A} \circ \underset{\sim}{R}$

$$\underset{\sim}{B} = \left(\frac{0.26}{\text{Very unaware}} + \frac{0.21}{\text{unaware}} + \frac{0.29}{\text{average}} + \frac{0.3}{\text{aware}} + \frac{0.11}{\text{very aware}} \right)$$

Since the sum of the values of the factors in the evaluation result exceeded 1, normalization was required.

$$\because\ 0.26 + 0.21 + 0.29 + 0.3 + 0.11 = 1.17$$

The rating result was adjusted to

$$(0.22\ 0.18\ 0.25\ 0.26\ 0.09)$$

The results of this evaluation were as follows.

- In total, 22% of people did not understand their face shape and suitable hair style and color at all.
- In total, 18% did not understand their face shape and hair color.
- In total, 25% understood their face shape and hair color.
- In total, 26% understood their face shape and hair color well.
- In total, 9% understood their face shape and hair color very well.

The customer's difficulty in choosing their own hair style and color was as follows.

(1) Factor set $U2$ = { Hair Style, Hair Color }

(2) Weight set $\underset{\sim}{A}_2 = (0.6,\ 0.4)$

(3) Rating V_2 = { Very little difficult, not difficult, average, difficult, very difficult }

(4) Single Factor Fuzzy Evaluation: Face Shape ($x1$), Hair Shape ($x2$), Hair Color ($x3$), we get

(5) $\underset{\sim}{R}\ (x_4) = (0.09\ 0.23\ 0.18\ 0.36\ 0.14)$

$\underset{\sim}{R}\ (x_5) = (0.1\ 0.27\ 0.11\ 0.33\ 0.19)$

Therefore, the one-factor evaluation matrix is given by

$$\underset{\sim}{R}_2 = \begin{pmatrix} 0.09 & 0.23 & 0.18\ 0.36 & 0.14 \\ 0.1 & 0.27 & 0.11\ 0.33 & 0.19 \end{pmatrix}$$

(6) Fuzzy Comprehensive Evaluation $\underset{\sim}{B} = \underset{\sim}{A} \circ \underset{\sim}{R}$

$$\underset{\sim}{B} = \left(\frac{0.1}{\text{Very undifficult}} + \frac{0.27}{\text{not difficult}} + \frac{0.18}{\text{average}} + \frac{0.36}{\text{difficult}} + \frac{0.19}{\text{very difficult}} \right)$$

Since the sum of the values of the factors in the evaluation result exceeded 1, normalization was required.

$$\because\ 0.1 + 0.27 + 0.18 + 0.36 + 0.19 = 1.1$$

The rating result was adjusted to

$$(0.09\ 0.25\ 0.16\ 0.33\ 0.17)$$

The results of this evaluation were as follows.

- In total, 9% felt 'very little difficulty' choosing their hairstyles and colors.
- In total, 25% felt 'no difficulty' in choosing their hairstyles and colors.
- In total, 16% felt 'average difficulty' in choosing their hairstyles and colors.
- In total, 33% felt 'difficulty' in choosing their hairstyles and colors.
- In total, 17% felt 'very difficult' in choosing their hairstyles and colors.

6. Conclusions

In the multi-diamond design, services, event planning, and corporate operational decision-making need to be determined. This flexible and dynamic model provides a framework for adaptability based on different activities in various domains. Divergence, convergence, and iteration are emphasized at each stage, departing from traditional approaches. This approach adds granularity to the design process, enabling designers to address challenges more precisely and adapt to rapidly changing demands. The multi-diamond design model offers a framework for design thinking and integrates divergence, convergence, and iteration. This approach is a problem-solving method for innovation. This model can guide designers to successfully solve diverse challenges in different domains. Simultaneously, it encourages the exploration of new possibilities while solving problems.

Author Contributions: Conceptualization, S.-W.H. and Y.-J.T.; methodology, S.-W.H. and Y.-J.T.; validation, Y.-J.T.; formal analysis, S.-W.H. and Y.-J.T.; investigation, Y.-J.T.; resources, S.-W.H. and Y.-J.T.; data curation, S.-W.H. and Y.-J.T.; writing—original draft preparation, Y.-J.T.; writing—review and editing, S.-W.H. and Y.-J.T.; visualization, Y.-J.T.; supervision, S.-W.H. and Y.-J.T.; project administration, S.-W.H. and Y.-J.T. All authors have read and agreed to the published version of the manuscript.

Funding: This research received no external funding.

Institutional Review Board Statement: Not applicable.

Informed Consent Statement: Not applicable.

Data Availability Statement: The original contributions presented in the study are included in the article, further inquiries can be directed to the corresponding author.

Conflicts of Interest: The authors declare no conflicts of interest.

References

1. Available online: https://www.designcouncil.org.uk/our-resources/the-double-diamond/ (accessed on 1 June 2023).
2. Suoheimo, M.; Määttä, K. Service Design Thinking Method for Educational Leaders. In *Educational Governance Research*; Springer Science and Business Media B.V.: Berlin/Heidelberg, Germany, 2024; pp. 81–100. [CrossRef]
3. Schleith, J.; Tsar, D. Triple Diamond Design Process. In *HCI International 2022—Late Breaking Papers. Design, User Experience and Interaction*; Kurosu, M., Yamamoto, S., Mori, H., Soares, M.M., Rosenzweig, E., Marcus, A., Rau, P.-L.P., Harris, D., Li, W.-C., Eds.; Springer International Publishing: Cham, Switzerland, 2022; pp. 136–146.
4. Jian, Z. *Methodology of Industrial Design*; Beijing University of Technology Press: Beijing, China, 1995. (In Chinese)

5. Cross, N. *Engineering Design Methods: Strategies for Product Design*; Wiley: Hoboken, NJ, USA, 2008.
6. Zadeh, L.A. Fuzzy sets. *Inf. Control* **1965**, *8*, 338–353. [CrossRef]
7. Wang, M.-F.; Hsiao, S.-W.; Zhong, Y. A study on the evaluation method of fuzzy theory on cultural and creative products in Taiwanese aborigines' cultures. In *AICS 2019: Proceedings of the 2019 International Conference on Artificial Intelligence and Computer Science*; Springer: Berlin/Heidelberg, Germany, 2019; pp. 55–61. [CrossRef]

engineering proceedings

Proceeding Paper

Antibacterial and Thermal Insulated Property of Sputtered Copper/Aluminum-Doped Zinc Oxide Films †

Shang-Chou Chang [1,2,*] and Jian-Syun Wu [1]

[1] Department of Electrical Engineering, Kun Shan University, Tainan 71003, Taiwan; kevin88774917@gmail.com
[2] Green Energy and Research Center, Kun Shan University, Tainan 71003, Taiwan
* Correspondence: jchang@mail.ksu.edu.tw
† Presented at the 2024 IEEE 4th International Conference on Electronic Communications, Internet of Things and Big Data, Taipei, Taiwan, 19–21 April 2024.

Abstract: Recent developments in architectural materials emphasize the importance of antibacterial and thermal insulation functions due to the prevalence of diseases such as COVID-19 and influenza. There is a growing expectation for the implementation of constructed glass that possesses antibacterial properties. Low-emissivity (Low-E) glass, known for its ability to reduce infrared radiation penetration through windows, is a focal point of our ongoing research. In this study, we continued our preliminary investigations into the development of Low-E glass by preparing copper/aluminum-doped zinc oxide (Cu/AZO) films on glass substrates through in-line sputtering. Copper was incorporated to provide antibacterial functionality, while aluminum-doped zinc oxide was chosen for its high visible optical transmission, which is crucial for architectural glass, and its low electrical resistivity indicative of thermal insulation properties. A vacuum annealing process was subsequently applied to the Cu/AZO films on glass. The evaluation of these films involved measuring electrical resistivity that correlates with emissivity, as well as assessing average visible transmission and antibacterial effectiveness according to the JIS Z2801:2000 standard. The results of these tests reveal that the vacuum-annealed Cu/AZO films on glass exhibited commendable antibacterial and thermal insulation properties. Specifically, the antibacterial index (R) was determined to be 8.75; the emissivity, calculated from the measured electrical resistivity, was found to be 0.18; and the average visible transmission was recorded at 52.78%. These findings underscore the potential of Cu/AZO films in advancing the functionality of architectural glass.

Keywords: antibacterial; thermal insulated; Cu/AZO

Citation: Chang, S.-C.; Wu, J.-S. Antibacterial and Thermal Insulated Property of Sputtered Copper/Aluminum-Doped Zinc Oxide Films. *Eng. Proc.* **2024**, *74*, 22. https://doi.org/10.3390/engproc2024074022

Academic Editors: Shu-Han Liao, Teen-Hang Meen and Cheng-Fu Yang

Published: 28 August 2024

1. Introduction

In public spaces, numerous bacteria and viruses are present in facilities and equipment. These pathogens are transmitted through contact and potentially become a source of infection. Recent research has focused on the use of copper metal materials for sterilization purposes [1–5]. The literature demonstrates that copper surfaces exhibit reduced bacterial adhesion, thus confirming the outstanding antibacterial properties of copper and its alloys [2].

Among various building materials, low-emissivity (Low-E) glass is distinguished by its high transmittance in the visible light spectrum and high reflectivity in the infrared band. The utilization of Low-E glass not only facilitates optimal indoor lighting but also ensures effective thermal insulation, therefore making it a staple in the construction of green buildings [6–9]. Presently, the radiation coefficient of Low-E glass available in the market serves as a crucial metric for consumers when selecting these products. The lower the emissivity of the glass, the greater its capability to insulate against heat.

In everyday environments, such as public facilities, including libraries and medical institutions, as well as in vehicles, such as buses and MRT systems, glass building materials are extensively used. Glass surfaces in public buildings are contacted by numerous individuals. If these glass materials offer both sterilization and thermal insulation properties, the safety, illumination, and comfort of the interior spaces can be significantly enhanced. Similarly, in public transportation, the glass surfaces that passengers frequently touch have antibacterial properties to prevent bacterial transmission. This functionality is beneficial and essential for maintaining public health and safety, highlighting yet another critical application of Low-E glass.

Based on the previous research result regarding the application of copper/aluminum-doped zinc oxide (Cu/AZO) films to energy-saving glass, we employed linear sputtering techniques to deposit Cu/AZO films. Additionally, we introduced a vacuum annealing process aimed at enhancing the material properties of the samples. The vacuum annealing step was effective in improving the electrical properties of the materials. The experimental analysis involved comprehensive measurements of the electrical, optical, and antibacterial properties of the Cu/AZO films post-vacuum annealing. These assessments were critical in determining the efficacy of the vacuum annealing process in optimizing the performance of Cu/AZO films for application in energy-saving glass solutions.

2. Experiment

Cu/AZO thin films were fabricated on borosilicate glass substrates using a linear sputtering system. Initially, the substrates were methodically cleaned through sequential ultrasonic baths in acetone, isopropyl alcohol, and purified water, followed by drying under a stream of nitrogen. The resulting Cu and AZO layers had thicknesses of 10 nm and 500 nm, respectively. The deposition process began with the application of an AZO thin film onto the glass substrate through in-line sputtering. The AZO layer was deposited using an AZO target material ($ZnO:Al_2O_3$ = 98.5%:1.5% by weight) at a direct current (DC) power setting of 2500 W, an argon (Ar) flow rate of 250 cm^3/min (sccm), and a working pressure of 3 mTorr. Subsequently, a Cu film was deposited on top of the partially deposited AZO film to form the Cu/AZO film. This copper layer was sputtered from a Cu target (99.9% Cu by weight) using a DC power of 1000 W, an Ar flow rate of 250 sccm, and a working pressure of 3 mTorr. We used a vacuum heating system to perform vacuum annealing treatment on the sample. Treatment conditions: annealing time of 1 h and temperature condition of 300 degrees.

The optical transmittance of the Cu/AZO film across the visible spectrum was analyzed using a UV-visible spectrophotometer (Model U-2800A, Hitachi, Tokyo, Japan), specifically within the wavelength range of 400 to 800 nm. The electrical properties, including resistivity, carrier mobility, and carrier concentration, were determined using a Hall measurement system (Model HMS-3000, Ecopia, Gyeonggi-do, Republic of Korea). Additionally, the antibacterial activity of the Cu/AZO film against Escherichia coli ATCC 8739 (E. coli) was assessed following the JIS Z 2801:2010 standard [10] to evaluate its effectiveness in inhibiting bacterial growth on its surface.

3. Results and Discussion

Figure 1 presents the optical transmission spectra of both vacuum-annealed Cu/AZO films and untreated Cu/AZO films. The spectra reveal differences in the visible light transmittance between the two types of films. The data showed that vacuum annealing positively affected the optical properties, as demonstrated by the higher average transmittance recorded for the annealed films. Specifically, the average transmittance of the Cu/AZO films processed by vacuum annealing at 300 degrees Celsius was 52.78%, compared to 50.11% for the untreated films. This improvement in visible light transmittance post-annealing is demonstrated in Figure 1.

Table 1 details the electrical and optical properties of both the Cu/AZO and untreated Cu/AZO films produced by the vacuum annealing process, providing a comprehensive comparison of their performance characteristics. This information is crucial for understanding the impact of the annealing process on the functionality of the films in various applications.

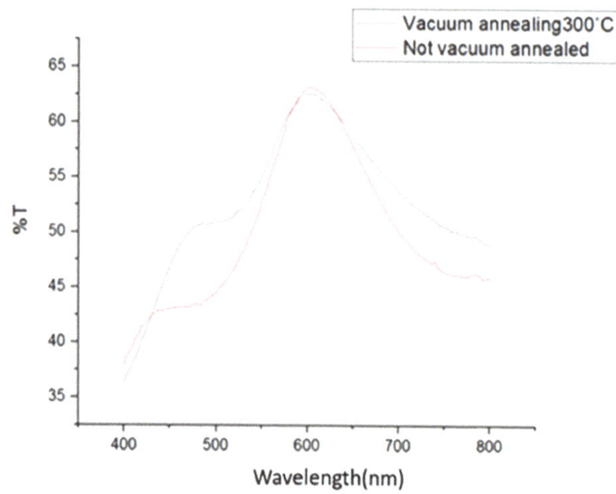

Figure 1. Visible light cross-transmittance of vacuum-annealed 300-degree Cu/AZO samples and unannealed Cu/AZO samples.

Table 1. Structural, electrical, antibacterial, and optical properties of vacuum-annealed Cu/AZO samples at 300 °C and untreated Cu/AZO samples.

Sample	Cu/AZO Films	Cu/AZO Films (Vacuum Annealed 300 °C)
Average optical transmittance (%)	50.11%	52.78%
Carrier concentration (10^{20}/cm^3)	10.65	10.49
Carrier mobility (cm^2/Vs)	4.46	0.6585
Electrical resistivity (10^{-3} Ω-cm)	1.314	9.033
Antibacterial activity (R)	8.66	8.75

Table 1 indicates significant differences in the resistivity and emissivity values between the Cu/AZO films before and after vacuum annealing at 300 degrees Celsius. Specifically, the resistivity of the untreated Cu/AZO films was recorded at 1.314×10^{-3} Ω-cm, whereas the vacuum-annealed Cu/AZO films exhibit a higher resistivity of 9.033×10^{-3} Ω-cm. Additionally, the emissivity of the Cu/AZO films decreases from 0.29 in the untreated state to 0.18 after undergoing vacuum annealing.

The reduction in emissivity observed in the annealed films suggests that vacuum annealing enhances the thermal insulation properties of the Cu/AZO films. This enhancement is likely due to modifications in the film's microstructure and surface characteristics induced by the annealing process, which in turn affect its ability to emit infrared radiation, therefore improving its thermal insulation performance. Such findings underscore the potential benefits of vacuum annealing in optimizing the functional properties of Cu/AZO films for applications requiring efficient thermal management.

Table 1 also displays the antibacterial activity values of Cu/AZO films both before and after undergoing vacuum annealing at 300 °C. The antibacterial activity value of the unannealed Cu/AZO films was 8.66, while the value for the Cu/AZO films vacuum-annealed was 8.75. These values are significantly above the threshold of ≥2.0 as stipulated by the JIS Z 2801:2010 standard, confirming that both sets of films exhibit effective antibacterial properties. The enhanced antibacterial activity in the vacuum-annealed films is attributed to the contact-killing mechanism, a well-documented antimicrobial effect of copper [11,12]. This mechanism involves the release of copper ions that interact with bacterial cells, leading to the disruption of cell membranes, the generation of reactive oxygen species, and, ultimately, the damage to cellular DNA. The slight increase in antibacterial activity following vacuum annealing is caused by changes in the surface structure or the increased availability of copper ions at the surface, which enhances the contact interaction between the copper and microbial cells. These results underscore the dual functionality of Cu/AZO films, offering both improved thermal insulation and effective antimicrobial properties, making them highly suitable for applications in environments where hygiene and temperature control are critical.

4. Conclusions

In this article, for the Cu/AZO samples after the vacuum annealing process, the electrical properties and antibacterial properties were enhanced compared with untreated Cu/AZO. The Cu/AZO sample produced by the vacuum annealing process has low emissivity and high antibacterial properties.

Author Contributions: Conceptualization, investigation, funding acquisition, project administration and methodology, Shang-Chou Chang; validation, formal analysis, writing—review and editing, Shang-Chou Chang and Jian-Syun Wu; resources, Jian-Syun Wu. All authors have read and agreed to the published version of the manuscript.

Funding: This research was funded by the National Science and Technology Commission of Taiwan for financial support under contract no. NSTC 112-2637-E-168-002.

Institutional Review Board Statement: Not applicable.

Informed Consent Statement: Not applicable.

Data Availability Statement: The original contributions presented in the study are included in the article, further inquiries can be directed to the corresponding author.

Acknowledgments: This work was partially supported by the Green Energy Technology Research Center of Kunshan University.

Conflicts of Interest: The authors declare no conflicts of interest.

References

1. Hans, M.; Mathews, S.; Mücklich, F.; Solioz, M. Physicochemical properties of copper important for its antibacterial activity and development of a unified model. *Biointerphases* **2016**, *11*, 018902. [CrossRef] [PubMed]
2. Casey, A.L.; Karpanen, T.J.; Adams, D.; Lambert, P.A.; Nightingale, P.; Miruszenko, L.; Elliott, T.S. A comparative study to evaluate surface microbial contamination associated with copper-containing and stainless steel pens used by nurses in the critical care unit. *Am. J. Infect. Control* **2011**, *39*, e52–e54. [CrossRef] [PubMed]
3. Rtimi, S.; Dionysiou, D.D.; Pillai, S.C.; Kiwi, J. Advances in catalytic/photocatalytic bacterial inactivation by nano Ag and Cu coated surfaces and medical devices. *Appl. Catal. B Environ.* **2019**, *240*, 291–318. [CrossRef]
4. Ondok, V.; Musil, J.; Meissner, M.; Čerstvý, R.; Fajfrlík, K. Two-functional DC sputtered Cu-containing TiO2 thin films. *J. Photochem. Photobiol. A Chem.* **2010**, *209*, 158–162. [CrossRef]
5. Prado, J.V.; Esparza, M.M.; Vidal, A.R. Adherence to copper and stainless steel metal coupons of common nosocomial bacterial strains. *Rev. Med. Chile* **2013**, *141*, 291–297.
6. Horiuchi, T.; Yoshimura, K. Solar heat gain coefficient and heat transmission coefficient of Al-doped ZnO thin-film coated low-emissivity glass. *J. Ceram. Soc. Jpn.* **2020**, *128*, 220–223. [CrossRef]
7. Lee, S.Y. Low Emissivity Property of Amorphous Oxide Multilayer (SIZO/Ag/SIZO) Structure. *Trans. Electr. Electron. Mater.* **2017**, *18*, 13–15. [CrossRef]
8. Baetens, R.; Jelle, B.P.; Gustavsen, A. Properties, requirements and possibilities of smart windows for dynamic daylight and solar energy control in buildings: A state-of-the-art review. *Sol. Energy Mater. Sol. Cells* **2010**, *94*, 87–105. [CrossRef]
9. Hagen, E.; Rubens, H. Über Beziehungen des Reflexions- und Emissionsvermögens der Metalle zu ihrem elektrischen Leitvermögen. *Ann. Phys.* **1903**, *4*, 873–901. [CrossRef]
10. *JIS Z 2801:2010*; Antimicrobial Products—Test for Antimicrobial Activity and Efficacy. Japanese Standards Association: Tokyo, Japan, 2010.

11. Grass, G.; Rensing, C.; Solioz, M. Metallic copper as an antimicrobial surface. *Appl. Environ. Microbiol.* **2011**, *77*, 1541–1547. [CrossRef] [PubMed]
12. Lee, S.Y.; Mettlach, N.; Nguyen, N.; Sun, Y.M.; White, J.M. Copper oxide reduction through vacuum annealing. *Appl. Surf. Sci.* **2003**, *206*, 102–109. [CrossRef]

engineering proceedings

Proceeding Paper

The Relationship between the Risk of Sarcopenia in the Elderly and Autonomic Nervous System Balance †

Chih-Wei Lin [1,2], Chih-Chien Lin [1], Chi-Pei Ou Yang [2], Su-Shiang Lee [1], Tso-Yen Mao [1,*] and Hsuan-Lin Chen [2,*]

1 Department of Leisure Services Management, Chaoyang University of Technology, Taichung 413310, Taiwan; cwlin@cyut.edu.tw (C.-W.L.); gueyu45123@gmail.com (C.-C.L.); sulee@cyut.edu.tw (S.-S.L.)
2 Department of Business Administration, Chaoyang University of Technology, Taichung 413310, Taiwan; sam5008@hotmail.com
* Correspondence: tymao.research@gmail.com (T.-Y.M.); tgtsunny@gmail.com (H.-L.C.); Tel.: +886-4-23323000 (ext. 7468) (T.-Y.M.)
† Presented at the 2024 IEEE 4th International Conference on Electronic Communications, Internet of Things and Big Data, Taipei, Taiwan, 19–21 April 2024.

Abstract: Elderly people with sarcopenia experience symptoms related to dysfunction in the autonomic nervous system (ANS), including rapid or irregular heartbeat, dizziness, and fluctuations in blood pressure. These symptoms may be a result of immune system activation and the impact of the disease, leading to alterations in certain aspects of ANS regulation. There is limited research that discusses the relationship between these factors. Therefore, we investigated the correlation between the risk of sarcopenia and the balance of the autonomic nervous system. The participants included 87 females and 25 males aged between 60 and 79 years old, who were assessed for sarcopenia risk including walking speed, grip strength, muscle mass, and the Appendicular Skeletal Muscle Mass Index (ASM). The collected data were analyzed using descriptive statistics, *t*-tests, one-way ANOVA, and Pearson correlations. The results showed the following: (1) Individuals at a high risk of sarcopenia displayed a slightly greater degree of autonomic nervous system imbalance compared to those at low risk. (2) In the time-domain analysis, sympathetic nervous system activity was higher in males than in females, whereas parasympathetic nervous system activity exhibited the opposite trend. In the frequency-domain analysis, heart rate variability was higher in females than in males, and both genders met the criteria for sarcopenia risk assessment. (3) There were no significant differences in heart rate variability indices among different sarcopenia risk groups. (4) Different levels of sarcopenia risk showed a significant correlation with ANS. Individuals at a higher risk demonstrated an imbalance, while those at a lower risk displayed a more balanced state. Overall, the results of this study confirmed the correlation between sarcopenia risk and heart rate variability among the elderly, further emphasizing the importance of the autonomic nervous system in sarcopenia risk.

Keywords: elderly; sarcopenia risk; heart rate variability; autonomic nervous system

Citation: Lin, C.-W.; Lin, C.-C.; Ou Yang, C.-P.; Lee, S.-S.; Mao, T.-Y.; Chen, H.-L. The Relationship between the Risk of Sarcopenia in the Elderly and Autonomic Nervous System Balance. *Eng. Proc.* **2024**, *74*, 23. https://doi.org/10.3390/engproc2024074023

Academic Editors: Shu-Han Liao, Teen-Hang Meen and Cheng-Fu Yang

Published: 29 August 2024

1. Introduction

Global aging is a significant social issue faced by countries worldwide. By the end of 2021, those of Taiwan's population aged 65 years old and above exceeded 16.59% of the total population, officially indicating an aging society. After 2025, it is projected to become a "Super Aged Society", with the population aged 65 years old and above surpassing 20% of the total population. By 2040, it is estimated to exceed 30%, surpassing the aging rate of countries in Europe and America, and by 2050, it is expected to surpass Japan, becoming the fastest-aging country globally. The challenges associated with aging, particularly issues related to disability in the elderly, have gradually become a concern for most countries around the world.

As people age, their body composition changes, including a gradual reduction in skeletal muscle fibers, a decrease in muscle mass, lower strength, and a decline in muscle endurance and metabolic capacity. These physiological changes contribute to the onset of chronic diseases, cognitive impairments, and diminished physical function. Consequently, this declines in overall mobility and the loss of muscle mass. According to research in the United States and Europe, the prevalence of sarcopenia among the elderly aged 60 to 70 years old is approximately 5 to 13%, while for those aged 80 years old and above, it ranges from about 11 to 50%. Meanwhile, studies in Taiwan indicated that the prevalence of sarcopenia among individuals aged 65 and above is approximately 3.9 to 7.3% (females: 2.5 to 6.5%; males: 5.4 to 8.2%) [1]. According to the European Working Group on Sarcopenia in Older People (EWGSOP), the diagnosis of sarcopenia involves assessing muscle mass, muscle strength, and physical performance, aligning with the understanding of sarcopenia [2]. The Asian Working Group for Sarcopenia (AWGS) adopted a similar approach to diagnosing sarcopenia with differences from EWGSOP. AWGS recommends screening tests that involve the simultaneous measurement of muscle strength (grip strength) and physical performance (gait speed) [3].

We adopted the sarcopenia screening process proposed by AWGS. Individuals with normal grip strength and walking speed are defined to have a low risk for sarcopenia. For those with at least one of either grip strength or walking speed below the normal range, a measurement of skeletal muscle mass is conducted. If muscle mass is normal, it is defined as moderate risk for sarcopenia; otherwise, it is considered high risk. This classification is applied to individuals aged 60 years and above to explore and provide evidence for the early prevention or delay of sarcopenia in the elderly.

Heart Rate Variability (HRV) refers to the variations in the time intervals between each heartbeat. This phenomenon is attributed to the reciprocal interactions of the Sympathetic Nervous System (SNS) and Parasympathetic Nervous System (PNS). It serves as an indicator used to assess the functioning of the Autonomic Nervous System (ANS). The analysis of HRV is conducted through the measurement and observation of continuous electrocardiographic signals. HRV time series are assessed for autonomic nervous system (ANS) activity and quantified using specialized analysis methods. Currently, the most widely used analysis methods are time-domain analysis and frequency-domain analysis. time-domain analysis is conducted using continuous electrocardiogram recordings as the baseline data, offering the advantages of simplicity and speed in calculations. The analysis involves detecting the intervals between each QRS complex wave in the continuous electrocardiogram. The adjacent R waves represent the cycle of heartbeats, and the interval between these cycles is measured in milliseconds (ms), referred to as the R-R interval. Frequency-domain analysis is a common method in HRV that involves decomposing the time series of HRV into composite waveforms containing different frequency components. Currently, the most widely used frequency-domain analysis methods include Fast Fourier Transform and Autoregressive Model Estimation (AR model).

Currently, the frequency-domain analysis of HRV is classified into short-term (3–5 min) and long-term (24–48 h) analyses. The primary indicators for heart rate variability in frequency-domain analysis are as follows:

1. Total Power (TP) refers to the magnitude of normal heartbeat interval amplitudes within the frequency range of $\leq$0.4 Hz for both long-term and short-term HRV time series;
2. High-Frequency Power (HF) refers to the magnitude of normal heartbeat interval amplitudes within the frequency range of 0.15 to 0.4 Hz, representing the PNS activity index;
3. Low-Frequency Power (LF) refers to the magnitude of normal heartbeat interval amplitudes within the frequency range of 0.04 to 0.15 Hz, representing an index jointly regulated by the SNS and PNS;
4. Very Low-Frequency Power (VLF) is typically referenced when analyzing continuous data spanning over 24 h or more;

5. Ultra Very Low-Frequency Power (ULF) is valuable when analyzing continuous data for durations exceeding 24 h;
6. Normalized Low-Frequency Power Ratio (nLF): This refers to LF/(TP − VLF) × 100, representing an indicator of sympathetic nervous system activity;
7. Normalized High-Frequency Power Ratio (nHF): This refers to HF/(TP − VLF) × 100, representing the reciprocal of the parasympathetic nervous system (PNS) activity index;
8. Low/High-Frequency Power Ratio (LF/HF): This represents an indicator of SNS and PNS balance or sympathetic nerve regulation.

The above frequency-domain indicators are widely applied in daily life, clinical assessments, and disease monitoring. For example, during the day, there is a predominance of SNS activity, indicated by a higher LF component. Conversely, during nighttime rest, PNS activity relatively increases, characterized by slower breathing, lower blood pressure, and a slower heart rate, with an enhanced HF component [4]. HRV, as one of the indicators for assessing ANS function, has been widely utilized in clinical applications and research. Its time-domain and frequency-domain indicators show correlations with physiological functions in the human body, providing real-time, reliable, and accurate assessment metrics.

2. Methods

2.1. Procedure

We conducted HRV analysis and sarcopenia risk assessments for the elderly in the community. We compared the correlation and differences between the risk levels of sarcopenia (low risk, moderate risk, and high risk) and obtained HRV indicators using time-domain analysis and frequency-domain analysis (Figure 1).

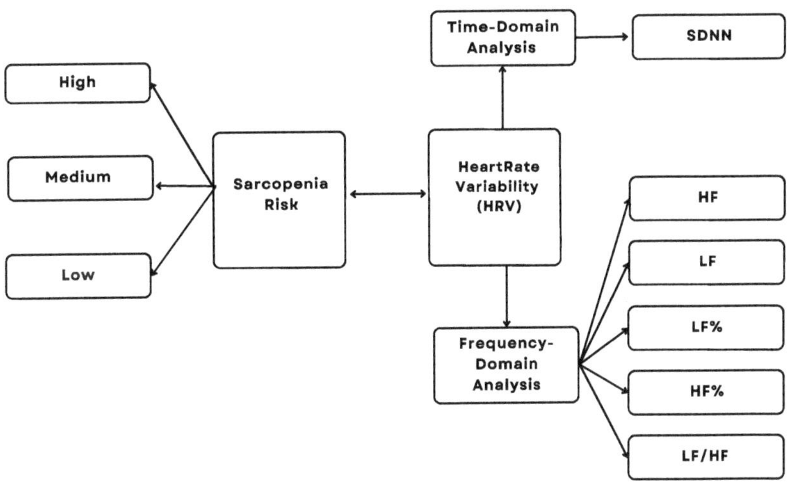

Figure 1. Framework of this research.

2.2. Research Subject

We recruited participants aged 60 years and above in Taiwan. Exclusion criteria included individuals with limited mobility, undergoing dialysis, having chronic conditions (hypertension, hyperlipidemia, hyperglycemia, and chronic kidney disease), cancer, and those unable to cooperate or participate. A total of 112 participants were recruited, and the AWGS screening process [3] was utilized for assessment.

2.3. Sampling Method

We used purposive sampling, and the testing location was the community care center in Taichung City.

2.4. Research Tools

We investigated the association between sarcopenia risk classification, HRV, and the influence on the balance of the ANS for the elderly in Taiwan. The following are the relevant measurement methods and tools.

- Detection of Sarcopenia Risk: (1) A Four-limb Muscle Mass Index was used to measure the four-limb skeletal muscle mass index using a body composition analyzer, (2) Grip Strength was used to measure the grip strength of the dominant hand using a handgrip dynamometer, and (3) a Walking Speed Assessment was used to measure walking speed using a walking activity recorder.
- HRV Instrument Assessment: The VitalScan ANS PWV instrument was used for the measurement of HRV in time-domain and frequency-domain analysis. Time-domain analysis was conducted to assess HRV by examining the intervals between each consecutive QRS complex in the continuous waveform. Frequency-domain analysis was conducted using the Fast Fourier Transform to decompose the composite waveforms of different frequency ranges in the HRV time series. In the time-domain analysis, the standard deviation of normal-to-normal (SDNN) intervals represents the variability of all normal heartbeats. In the frequency-domain analysis, High-Frequency Power refers to the magnitude of normal heartbeat interval and amplitudes within the frequency range of 0.15 to 0.4 Hz as an indicator of PNS activity. Low-Frequency Power presents the magnitude of normal heartbeat interval amplitudes within the frequency range of 0.04 to 0.15 Hz, serving as an indicator of both the SNS and the PNS regulation. nLF represents the ratio of LF divided by the difference between TP and VLF, multiplied by 100. It serves as an indicator of SNS activity.
- nHF represents the ratio of HF divided by the difference between TP and VLF, multiplied by 100. It is the reciprocal indicator of PNS activity. LF/HF represents an index of the balance between the SNS and PNS or an indicator of sympathetic nerve regulation.

2.5. Data Analysis

- Sarcopenia Risk Classification Method

We adopted the sarcopenia screening process proposed by AWGS as the risk classification method [3]. According to this process, grip strength and walking speed were measured for the elderly population. If both measurements were normal, individuals were classified into the low-risk group for sarcopenia. If one of the measurements was below the normal range, a further assessment of muscle mass was conducted. If muscle mass was normal, individuals were classified into the moderate-risk group for sarcopenia. If muscle mass was below the normal range, individuals were classified into the high-risk group for sarcopenia.

- Autonomic Nervous System Balance (ANS)

ANS balance is a crucial mechanism for the body to adapt and regulate in response to environmental changes. We referred to the research conducted by Kou and Yang [4] to assess HRV reference values for healthy adult males and females at various age groups in Taiwan. Based on the assumption of a normal distribution, we asserted with a 95% confidence level so that the values of HF, LF, and LF/HF could be distributed within plus or minus two standard deviations from the mean. Therefore, in this study, values falling within this range were considered indicative of ANS balance, while values outside this range were deemed indicative of ANS imbalance.

2.6. Statistical Methods

SPSS version 23 was used for various statistical analyses. The following are the statistical methods employed in this study.

Descriptive Statistical Analysis: Descriptive statistical analysis, including frequency distribution tables, percentages, means, and standard deviations, was employed to explore the current status of age, height, weight, walking speed, grip strength, and four-limb muscle mass index among individuals classified into sarcopenia low, moderate, and high-risk groups.

Independent Samples t-Test: In an independent samples *t*-test, differences in indicators such as the walking speed, grip strength, and four-limb muscle mass index were examined based on the presence or absence of autonomic nervous system (ANS) balance.

One-Way Analysis of Variance (ANOVA): We employed ANOVA to explore whether there are differences in HRV time-domain analysis and frequency-domain indicators among individuals classified into sarcopenia low, moderate, and high-risk groups.

Pearson Chi-Square Test: We employed the Pearson Chi-Square Test to explore whether there is a correlation between low-, moderate-, and high-risk sarcopenia groups and the presence or absence of autonomic nervous system (ANS) balance.

3. Result and Discussion

3.1. Detection of Sarcopenia Risk

This study included 112 participants with an average age of 72.88 ± 9.27 years, consisting of 25 males and 87 females. The research results indicated differences in sarcopenia risk and HRV indicators among the elderly. Male participants demonstrated better walking speed, grip strength, and four-limb muscle mass index compared to female participants, while female participants exhibited superior HRV indicators compared to male counterparts. These findings provide information for understanding the correlation between sarcopenia risk and autonomic nervous system (ANS) balance in the elderly. Differences were found in sarcopenia risk between elderly males and females, related to gender disparities and physiological decline. In the survey on the distribution of sarcopenia risk that was conducted, 76 participants were classified as low-risk for sarcopenia, 26 as moderate-risk, and 10 as high-risk. In the low-risk sarcopenia group, males constituted 22.4%, and females constituted 77.6%, with an average age of 71.12 years old, an average height of 157.32 cm, and an average weight of 62.41 kg. In the moderate-risk sarcopenia group, males accounted for 26.9%, females accounted for 73.1%, with an average age of 76.58 years, an average height of 153.17 cm, and an average weight of 63.16 kg. In the high-risk sarcopenia group, males comprised 10.0%, females comprised 90.0%, with an average age of 76.60 years, an average height of 148.30 cm, and an average weight of 58.73 kg. We measured grip strength, walking speed, and muscle mass in each group. These results help to understand the sarcopenia situation in different risk groups. The findings of this study provide information on the health status of the elderly and relevant preventive measures.

3.2. Correlation between Sarcopenia Risk and ANS Balance

We investigated the correlation between sarcopenia risk and ANS balance. To mitigate the potential impact of significant variations in measured values, we referred to the values for HRV for classification in different age groups of healthy Taiwanese adults provided by Kuo and Yang [4]. As the reference values were only for the age group of 60–79 years old, we included 81 participants in this study. Assuming that the measured values follow a normal distribution, we considered values within two standard deviations from the mean, accounting for 95% of the distribution, as an indicator of ANS balance. Conversely, values outside this range are classified as indicative of ANS imbalance. However, due to the non-normal distribution of the histogram of measured values, we took the natural logarithm of the values, using ln (ms2) as the unit for more accurate classification.

According to the classification results, we set the standards for the LF values for male participants aged 60 to 64 years old as 2.449 to 6.464, HF values as 1.829 to 5.946, and LF/HF values as 0.853 to 1.991. For male participants aged 65 to 69 years old, the LF values were set between 2.050 and 6.553, the HF values between 1.840 and 5.861, and the LF/HF values between −1.144 and 2.044. For those aged 70 to 74 years old, the LF values were set between 2.335 and 5.680, the HF values between 1.615 and 5.592, and the LF/HF values between −1.159 and 1.967. Finally, for male participants aged 75 to 79 years old, the LF values were set between 1.891 and 6.210, the HF values between 1.146 and 6.129, and the

LF/HF values between −1.066 and 1.892. If the participant's LF, HF, and LF/HF values all fell within the standard range, ANS balance was diagnosed; otherwise, if any of these values were below or above the standard range, it was considered ANS imbalance.

The chi-square test results for the association between ANS balance and sarcopenia risk revealed a significant relationship. The distribution of participants across different risk categories indicated that those with low sarcopenia risk were predominantly in ANS balance (80.0%), while individuals with high sarcopenia risk were primarily in ANS imbalance (83.3%). The participants with low sarcopenia risk showed ANS balance, whereas a higher proportion experienced ANS imbalance in the high sarcopenia risk group. Individuals with low sarcopenia risk were in ANS balance (80.0%), while those with medium and high sarcopenia risk were in ANS imbalance (42.9%). The participants with a low sarcopenia risk showed ANS balance. Conversely, in the high sarcopenia risk group, there was a higher proportion experiencing ANS imbalance.

The independent samples *t*-test results showed no significant difference in walking speed among those in ANS balance. There was no significant difference in walking speed, grip strength, and four-limb muscle mass index among participants, regardless of ANS balance.

Before the measurements, the sample data were not adjusted for participants' gender and external factors. This caused large differences in HRV values. HRV indicators of too high or too low are considered abnormal. The average values are compared to understand the canceling effect of high and low scores and non-significant differences. The observed results are not attributed to participants' abnormal HRV indices or other factors. Previous studies suggested a correlation between sarcopenia and ANS balance [5]. To mitigate potential score cancelation, we used a classification approach to explore the relationship between sarcopenia risk and ANS balance. Previous study results indicated that adults with sarcopenia were older than those without sarcopenia [5–7]. Additionally, a correlation between sarcopenia in older adults and ANS dysregulation was observed [5]. There was an increasing trend in the proportion of ANS imbalance among individuals at a high risk of sarcopenia.

4. Conclusions

We investigated the association between sarcopenia risk and the autonomic nervous system (ANS) balance of the elderly. In total, 23% of the elderly in Taiwan have a moderate-to high-risk of sarcopenia, and about 25.9% exhibit an imbalance in the ANS. Females show higher PNS activity in time-domain analysis compared to men, while their SNS activity showed the opposite trend. In frequency-domain analysis, females exhibited higher HRV than men. Regarding the three indicators of sarcopenia, males and females had normal values for walking speed, grip strength, and four-limb muscle mass index. In the low-risk sarcopenia group, an ANS balance was observed. In contrast, the moderate- and high-risk sarcopenia groups showed an increase in ANS imbalance. Among the overall participants, ANS was balanced in the low-risk sarcopenia group, while the proportion of ANS imbalance increased in the moderate- and high-risk sarcopenia groups. A correlation between sarcopenia risk in the elderly and ANS balance was observed.

Due to limitations in the number of sample and analysis methods, there are constraints in this study. It is necessary to expand the sample size and employ more precise analysis methods to obtain more accurate results. Additionally, it is suggested to apply the research findings in practical healthcare and health management to aid in the prevention and treatment of sarcopenia in the elderly. It is beneficial to understand the physical fitness performance and health education of the elderly. This involves the implementation of community-based exercise programs, with courses tailored to different age groups and health conditions to equip the elderly with accurate knowledge and a heightened awareness of preventive measures. Then, the onset of sarcopenia can be delayed for a healthy and high-quality life.

In community care centers for the elderly, diverse exercise programs are provided, including those focused on physical health, such as reducing blood pressure and improving insomnia, as well as activities such as yoga and meditation. The activities contribute to enhancing overall well-being. These practices help to regulate somatic reflex function, balance the sympathetic and parasympathetic nervous systems, and promote the effectiveness of parasympathetic activity, ultimately addressing situations of autonomic nervous system imbalance.

Author Contributions: Conceptualization, C.-W.L., C.-C.L. and S.-S.L.; methodology, C.-W.L. and T.-Y.M.; writing—original draft preparation, C.-P.O.Y., T.-Y.M. and H.-L.C.; writing—review and editing, T.-Y.M. and H.-L.C. All authors have read and agreed to the published version of the manuscript.

Funding: This research received no external funding.

Institutional Review Board Statement: Not applicable.

Informed Consent Statement: Not applicable.

Data Availability Statement: Data are contained within the article.

Conflicts of Interest: The authors declare no conflicts of interest.

References

1. Benjumea, A.M.; Curcio, C.L.; Duque, G.; Gomez, F. Dynapenia and sarcopenia as a risk factor for disability in a falls and fractures clinic in older persons. *Open Access Maced. J. Med. Sci.* **2018**, *6*, 344. [CrossRef] [PubMed]
2. Cruz-Jentoft, A.J.; Baeyens, J.P.; Bauer, J.M.; Boirie, Y.; Cederholm, T.; Landi, F.; Martin, F.C.; Michel, J.P.; Rolland, Y.; Schneider, S.M.; et al. Sarcopenia: European consensus on definition and diagnosis: Report of the European Working Group on Sarcopenia in Older People. *Age Ageing* **2010**, *39*, 412–423. [CrossRef]
3. Chen, L.K.; Liu, L.K.; Woo, J.; Assantachai, P.; Auyeung, T.W.; Bahyah, K.S.; Chou, M.Y.; Chen, L.Y.; Hsu, P.S.; Krairit, O.; et al. Sarcopenia in Asia: Consensus report of the Asian Working Group for Sarcopenia. *J. Am. Med. Dir. Assoc.* **2014**, *15*, 95–101. [CrossRef] [PubMed]
4. Kuo, B.-J.; Yang, C.-H. *Study on Heart Rate Variability: From Health Maintenance to Disease Treatment*; Ho-Chi Book Publishing Co.: New Taipei City, Taiwan, 2016.
5. de Freitas, V.P.; da Silva Passos, R.; Oliveira, A.A.; Ribeiro, Í.J.; Freire, I.V.; Schettino, L.; Teles, M.F.; Casotti, C.A.; Pereira, R. Sarcopenia is associated to an impaired autonomic heart rate modulation in community-dwelling old adults. *Arch. Gerontol. Geriatr.* **2018**, *76*, 120–124. [CrossRef]
6. Janssen, I. The epidemiology of sarcopenia. *Clin. Geriatr. Med.* **2011**, *27*, 355–363. [CrossRef] [PubMed]
7. Morley, J.E. Sarcopenia: Diagnosis and treatment. *J. Nutr. Health Aging* **2008**, *12*, 452–456. [CrossRef]

engineering proceedings

MDPI

Proceeding Paper

Screening and Isolation of Microbes for Promoting Humification of Agricultural Organic Wastes †

Kai-Siang Chen [1], Sheng-Chin Hu [2,*], Pin-Chen Yeh [2], Jia-Xiang You [2] and Rey-May Liou [2,*]

1 Department of Industrial and Systems Engineering, Chung Yuan Christian University, Taoyuan 320, Taiwan; g10302403@cycu.edu.tw
2 Department of Environmental Engineering and Science, Chia-Nan University of Pharmacyand Science, Tainan 717, Taiwan; olly891020@gmail.com (P.-C.Y.); david90062888@gmail.com (J.-X.Y.)
* Correspondence: jeff891207@gmail.com (S.-C.H.); mrmliou@mail.cnu.edu.tw (R.-M.L.)

† Presented at the 2024 IEEE 4th International Conference on Electronic Communications, Internet of Things and Big Data, Taipei, Taiwan, 19–21 April 2024.

Abstract: Agroecosystems play a crucial role in carbon sequestration and reducing atmospheric CO_2 emissions by storing organic carbon in soil. Soil fertility and productivity are essential for global crop demands and depend on soil organic matter, particularly humic substances (HS). HS is crucial for soil health and carbon sequestration as it involves the carbon cycle, supplies nutrients for plants, and reduces the emission of pollutants through microbial processes for the enhancement of CO_2 sequestration. Humification is a natural process of organic matter stabilization, playing a crucial role in maintaining soil organic content and carbon storage. Laccase is used to polymerize monomeric compounds such as phenols and their derivatives into highly polymerized HS. We screened five cellulose-degrading isolates, among which three strains demonstrate lignin-degrading capabilities. WSC-7 exhibited the highest laccase activity and showed a high similarity [99.51%] to *Arthrobacter defluvii* based on 16S rDNA analysis. Strain LiPK-078-5 in nutrient broth medium and WSC-7 in Difco Sporulation Medium exhibited optimal catalytic activity for catechol, indicating their efficiency for aromatic polymerization of soluble organic carbon. The addition of rice husk biochar with strains LiPK-078-5, WSC-6, and WSC-7 increased organic carbon content effectively. The synthesis of humic substances in soil through microbial processes increases soil carbon sequestration and reduces greenhouse gas emissions in the environment.

Keywords: lignin; cellulose; humification; laccase; catechol

Citation: Chen, K.-S.; Hu, S.-C.; Yeh, P.-C.; You, J.-X.; Liou, R.-M. Screening and Isolation of Microbes for Promoting Humification of Agricultural Organic Wastes. *Eng. Proc.* **2024**, *74*, 24. https://doi.org/10.3390/engproc2024074024

Academic Editors: Shu-Han Liao, Teen-Hang Meen and Cheng-Fu Yang

Published: 29 August 2024

1. Introduction

Human activities have increased carbon dioxide in the atmosphere rapidly from 280 ppm before the Industrial Revolution to 415.48 ppm in June 2021 [1]. Soil stores the most carbon emitted. The carbon storage in the "soil carbon pool" on the earth's surface is as high as 250 billion tons, including about 1550 Gts (gigatons) of soil organic carbon and 950 gigatons of soil inorganic carbon. The soil carbon pool is about 3.3 times larger than that of the atmospheric carbon pool (760 Gts) and 4.5 times larger than that of the biological carbon pool [2]. The increasing rate of humus formation in the soil affects the long-term storage of carbon in the soil. Soil is a huge source of carbon emissions. The rate of soil carbon dioxide (CO_2) emissions is approximately 60 petagram (Pg)/yr, which is 10 times higher than that of fossil fuels [3]. Soil carbon emission fluxes are 6 to 10 times higher than emissions from human activities [4]. Changes in land use and inappropriate agricultural practices, such as improper farming or excessive use of chemical fertilizers, cause large soil carbon emission fluxes. Soil carbon flux management is important to mitigate global warming [2,5–7] and has a significant impact on biodiversity, agricultural productivity, and food security. It is also important for many countries to practice sustainable development.

Soil carbon sequestration is determined based on the total organic carbon (TOC) content in the soil. Carbon with high stability is estimated for soil carbon sequestration [8]. Through the biochemical reactions of microorganisms in the soil, organic matter is converted into a stable form that is difficult for organisms to decompose, as converted organic matter is bonded to soil minerals or is protected by micro aggregates formed by biological debris. The process usually includes the following: (1) microorganisms and their extracellular enzymes, such as laccase, manganese peroxidase, and lignin peroxidase, which decompose cellulose and lignin to form aromatic small molecules; (2) condensation with amino acids, quinones, or reducing sugars to form melanin-type compounds. The substances formed through biochemical reactions are more resistant to biological decomposition and form a stable organic carbon pool in the soil [9]. The contribution of microorganisms to the soil carbon sink depends on the interaction between the number of microorganisms, community structure and their metabolites, and soil properties such as texture, minerals, and pore distribution. The formation of humus matter in the soil is conducive to soil carbon sinks. Humus is formed by the oxidative polymerization of phenolic substances in the soil as a stable organic matter structure in the soil [10]. Microorganisms assist in the humification of biochar, which provides soil carbon sinks and makes the effect of soil carbon sequestration more stable.

In this study, we screened and isolated microorganisms to effectively promote the humification of organic matter and enhance soil carbon sequestration. The results provide a reference for future sustainable agricultural practices.

2. Materials and Methods

2.1. Collection of Soil Samples

Surface soil samples were collected from forest, organic farms, rhizosphere soil, and mature compost. The soil sampling locations included Jiadong Township, Pingtung County, Rende District, Tainan City, and Rende District, Tainan City. These soil samples were used for the isolation and screening of microorganisms which promoted the humification of organic matter.

2.2. Isolation and Purification of Strains

Collected samples were placed in sterile water and shaken at room temperature for 1 h. The supernatant was diluted to a concentration of 10^{-4} to 10^{-5} CFU/mL and spread on sterile mineral salt medium (MSM) plates with 100 mg/L of cellulose, hemicellulose, or lignin as the carbon source. The samples were incubated at 30 °C and shaken at 120 rpm. The culture solution was continuously diluted and spread on modified MSM agar plates for incubation at a constant temperature. Colonies with different morphologies and phenotypes on the agar plates were selected, streaked repeatedly on plates for isolation, and preserved on a slant agar medium.

2.3. Catechol Catalytic Reaction and Dark Reaction

To understand the humification ability of each strain on organic matter, the crude protein from each strain was used to catalyze the reaction of catechol. Then, the humification degree of organic matter was measured over time. The strains were cultured separately in nutrient broth (NB) medium and WSC-7 in Difco Sporulation Medium (DSM) medium or in a catechol catalytic reaction for 20 days. The products of the reaction were obtained on days 3, 7, 10, 14, 17, and 20 for humic substance extraction tests and for the recording of changes in the humification index. A 1 mL sample of the culture was obtained and centrifuged, and 100 μL of the supernatant was diluted to 10 mL with ultrapure water. The changes in chromophores and the formation of brown substances during the aromatization and humification processes of organic matter were measured at the absorbance at 254, 465, and 665 nm.

2.4. Determination of Laccase Activity

Laccase activity was measured by monitoring the oxidation of 1 mM of guaiacol (Hi-Media, Mumbai, India) buffered with 0.2 M sodium phosphate at pH 4.5 and 420 nm for 1 min. The reaction mixture of 900 μL contained 300 μL of 1 mM guaiacol, culture filtrate, and 0.2 M sodium acetate buffer of pH 4.5. One unit of enzyme activity was defined as the amount of enzyme that oxidized 1 μmol of guaiacol per minute. The enzyme activity was expressed in U/mL.

2.5. Bacterial Identification

Identification of the selected strains was carried out using 16S rDNA sequence analysis. The selected strains were grown in nutrient broth, and harvested cells were centrifuged to obtain cell pellets for genomic DNA extraction using the Power Soil DNA kit (MOBIO, Jefferson City, MO, USA) following the manufacturer's instructions. PCR amplification was performed in 25 mL consisting of 10 mM of Universal 16S rRNA bacterial primers 27F (5′-AGAGTSTTGATCCTGGCTCAG-3′) and 1392R (5′-GGTSTACCTTGTSTACGACTT-3′) to amplify the gene using 10 ng of genomic DNA isolated from each strain. Polymerase chain reaction (PCR) products were visualized on a 1% agarose gel stained with ethidium bromide under ultraviolet (UV) light to confirm the presence of up to a 1350 bp band. The PCR products were purified using a kit from Ambion, (Emeryville, CA, USA) before bidirectional sequencing with primers 27F and 1392R. Sanger sequences were generated at the UCSF Genomics Core Facility using an ABI PRISM 3730xl DNA Analyzer (Life Technologies Corporation, (Emeryville, CA, USA). The PCR products were separated in 0.8% agarose gel and observed on a UV transilluminator. The collected DNA bands from the gel were purified by a QIA quick gel extraction kit (Qiagen, Germantown, MD, USA) following the manufacturer's instructions. The purified PCR products were sequenced using an automated DNA sequencer. The partial 16S rDNA sequences were compared with the GenBank database on the NCBI website (http://blast.ncbi.nlm.nih.gov/Blast.cgi, accessed on 27 August 2024) by using the Basic Local Alignment Search Tool (BLAST).

3. Results and Discussion

3.1. Isolation and Selection of Test Strains

We isolated strains from soils and composts from different regions. Seventeen strains were selected based on their activity in lignin peroxidase, laccase, and manganese peroxidase. Strains with higher enzyme activities were identified through 16S rDNA sequencing. The test strains were classified as *Pseudomonas* sp., *Mesorhizobium* sp., *Cupriavidus* sp., and others. The selection of test strains was based on whether the strains decomposed lignin and cellulose and exhibited laccase and/or humification activities. Five selected strains demonstrated a higher increase in the aromaticity of soluble organic carbon in soil. The functions of each test strain are described in Table 1. All five strains decomposed cellulose, with three strains possessing both lignin and cellulose decomposition enzymes. Strain WSC-7 exhibited the highest laccase activity, producing 0.0576 U/L of laccase in the culture medium. Based on 16S rDNA sequence analysis, strain LiPK078-5 was identical to *Pseudomonas* sp. LiPK078-8 was 99.93% similar to *Pseudomonas* sp., RHCS-1 was 99.03% similar to *Cupriavidus* sp., WSC-7 was 93.51% similar to *Arthrobacter* sp., and WSC-6 was 99.86% similar to *Mesorhizobium* sp.

Table 1. 16S rRNA percent identity and functions of the selected strains.

Treatment	Similar Strain	Lignin	Cellulose	Laccase (MAX) (μg/L)
LiPK-078-5	*Pseudomonas* sp.	+	+	0.0504
LiPK-078-8	*Pseudomonas* sp.	−	+	0.0352
RHCS-1	*Cupriavidus* sp.	−	+	0.0573
WSC-7	*Arthrobacter* sp.	+	+	0.0576
WSCCS-6	*Mesorhizobium* sp	+	+	0.0544

3.2. Spectral Characterization of Test Strains

3.2.1. E2/E4

The E2/E4 coefficient is used to characterize the degree of condensation of organic molecules during the humification process, which increases as the E2/E4 value decreases [11]. The test strains were cultured in NB and DSM media at a constant temperature, and the catalytic activity of the crude protein of the strain against catechol was tested periodically. On the 20th day of culture, the E2/E4 coefficient reached a peak value, ranging from 0.49 to 1.60. The E2/E4 coefficient index, acquired by measuring the UV spectrum, is an index describing the degree of humification of organic matter. A higher E2/E4 value means that there are relatively smaller aromatic molecules—such as monomers and low-density polymers—in the organic matter and that the degree of humification is low. A lower E2/E4 value means that there are relatively larger aromatic molecules—such as those of a high polymer value—in the organic matter and that the degree of humification is higher [12]. The catalytic activity of pyrogallol in different strains varied depending on the culture medium. The strain WSC-6 cultured in NB medium and the strain WSC-7 cultured in DSM medium exhibited lower E2/E4 values. This indicates that the WSC-6 and WSC-7 strains have a higher potential for the humification of organic matter (Figure 1).

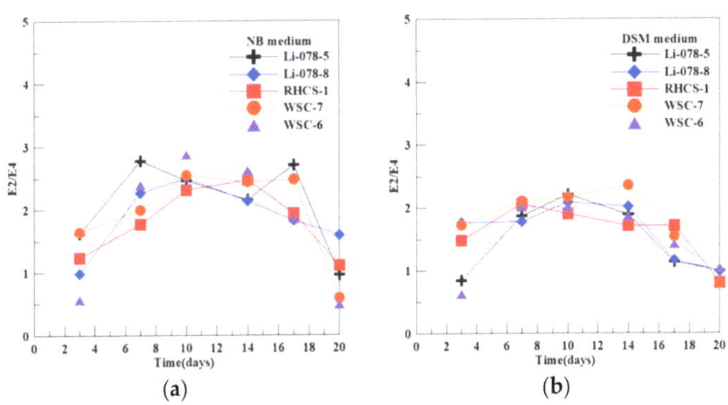

Figure 1. Changes in E2/E4 ratio in the humification index of catechol by crude protein of test strains cultured in (**a**) NB and (**b**) DSM medium.

3.2.2. E2/E6

Humic substances contain conjugated double-bond systems randomly distributed in macromolecules, which are responsible for their brown color. The E2/E6 coefficient is the ratio of initially humified structures to strongly humified ones. Higher E2/E6 values for humic acids (Has) derived from soil suggest more structures of low transformation, typical for lignins [13]. Among the test strains isolated in this study, the catalytic activity of pyrogallol varies in different strains and culture media. The test strains were cultured in NB and DSM media at a constant temperature until the 20th day, and the E2/E6 ratios of each strain ranged from 0.31 to 1.26. The strain WSC-6 cultured in NB medium and the strain LiPK-078-5 cultured in DSM medium exhibited lower E2/E6 values. This indicates that WSC-6, LiPK-078-5, and WSC-7 strains have better potential for the aromatization of organic matter. LiPK-078-5 and WSC-7 strain in NB medium and the WSC-6 strain in DSM medium exhibited the best catalytic activity for catechol, indicating that these strains have the highest capability for aromatization of soluble organic carbon (Figure 2).

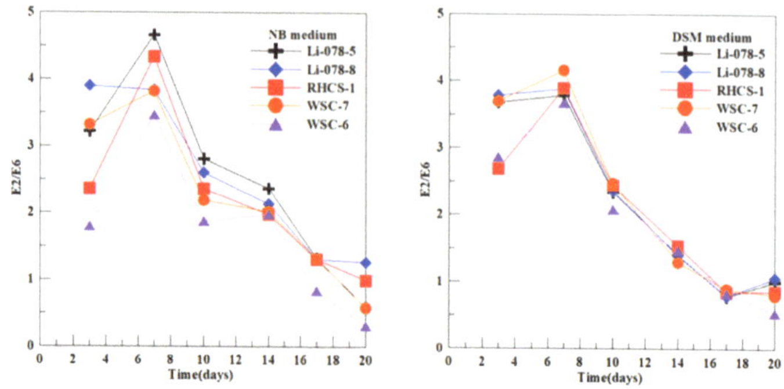

(**a**) (**b**)

Figure 2. Changes in E2/E6 ratio in the humification index of catechol by crude protein of test strains cultured in (**a**) NB and (**b**) DSM medium.

3.2.3. E4/E6

The E4/E6 ratio measured at the absorbances at 465 and 665 nm is used to study the HA fraction. The E4/E6 ratio is inversely related to the degree of condensation and aromaticity of the humic substances and their degree of humification and characterizes the degree of polymerization of the benzene ring C framework [14]. Lower E4/E6 values indicate higher organic matter polymerization levels. The catalytic activity of pyrogallol varied for different strains and culture media in this study. The test strains were cultured in NB and DSM media at a constant temperature for 20 days, and the E4/E6 ratios of each strain ranged from 0.32 to 0.56. The strain WSC-6 cultured in NB and DSM medium showed lower E2/E6 values. This indicates that the WSC-6 strains have better potential for the humification of organic matter (Figure 3).

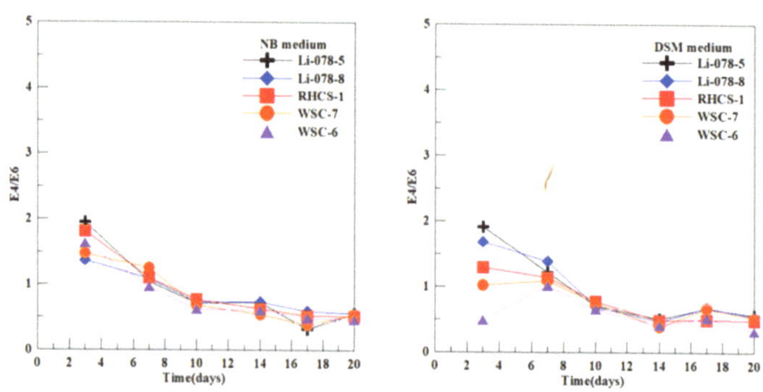

(**a**) (**b**)

Figure 3. Changes in E4/E6 ratio in the humification index of catechol by crude protein of test strains cultured in (**a**) NB and (**b**) DSM medium.

4. Conclusions

The results of this study showed the significant potential of the strain WSC-6 cultured in NB medium and the strain WSC-7 cultured in DSM medium for the humification and aromatization of organic matter. These strains showed lower E2/E4, E2/E6, and E4/E6 values, indicating higher degrees of condensation, polymerization, and aromaticity. Particularly, strain WSC-6 demonstrated the most consistent performance and superior performance across different indices and culture conditions, making it a promising candidate for enhancing the humification process in organic matter treatment.

Author Contributions: Conceptualization, R.-M.L.; methodology, R.-M.L. and K.-S.C.; formal analysis, R.-M.L. and S.-C.H.; investigation, S.-C.H., P.-C.Y. and J.-X.Y.; resources, R.-M.L. and S.-C.H.; data curation, R.-M.L.; writing—original draft preparation, S.-C.H. and K.-S.C.; writing—review and editing, R.-M.L.; visualization, S.-C.H. and K.-S.C.; supervision, R.-M.L.; project administration, R.-M.L.; funding acquisition, R.-M.L. All authors have read and agreed to the published version of the manuscript.

Funding: This research was funded by the National Science and Technology Council and the Ministry of Agriculture of Taiwan.

Institutional Review Board Statement: Not applicable.

Informed Consent Statement: Not applicable.

Data Availability Statement: Data supporting reported results can be made available upon reasonable request from the corresponding author.

Acknowledgments: This research was supported by the National Science and Technology Council and the Ministry of Agriculture of Taiwan.

Conflicts of Interest: The authors declare that they have no known competing financial interests or personal relationships that could have appeared to influence the work reported in this paper.

References

1. Tans, P.; Keeling, R. *Earth System Research Laboratories [ESRL] Global Monitoring Laboratory–Carbon Cycle Greenhouse Gases, National Oceanic and Atmospheric Administration [NOAA]*; US Department of Commerce: Washington, DC, USA, 2021.
2. Lal, R. Soil carbon sequestration impacts on global climate change and food security. *Science* **2004**, *304*, 1623–1627. [CrossRef] [PubMed]
3. Hayes, M.H.; Clapp, C.E. Humic substances: Considerations of compositions, aspects of structure, and environmental influences. *Soil Sci.* **2001**, *166*, 723–737. [CrossRef]
4. Friedlingstein, P.; Jones, M.W.; O'Sullivan, M.; Andrew, R.M.; Hauck, J.; Peters, G.P.; Peters, W.; Pongratz, J.; Sitch, S.; Le Quéré, C.; et al. Global carbon budget 2019. *Earth Syst. Sci. Data* **2019**, *11*, 1783–1838. [CrossRef]
5. Davidson, E.A. Carbon dioxide loss from tropical soils increases on warming. *Nature* **2020**, *584*, 198–199. [CrossRef] [PubMed]
6. Eswaran, H.; Van Den Berg, E.; Reich, P. Organic carbon in soils of the world. *Soil Sci. Soc. Am. J.* **1993**, *57*, 192–194. [CrossRef]
7. Sayer, E.J.; Heard, M.S.; Grant, H.K.; Matthews, T.R.; Tanner, E.V. Soil carbon release enhanced by increased tropical forest litterfall. *Nat. Clim. Chang.* **2011**, *1*, 304–307. [CrossRef]
8. Tang, C.; Yang, F.; Antonietti, M. Carbon materials advancing microorganisms in driving soil. *AAAS Res. Artic.* **2022**, *2022*, 9857374.
9. Li, S.; Sun, K.; Latif, A.; Si, Y.; Gao, Y.; Huang, Q. Insights into the applications of extracellular laccase-aided humification in livestock manure Composting. *Environ. Sci. Technol.* **2022**, *56*, 7412–7425. [CrossRef] [PubMed]
10. Zhao, Y.; Chen, W.; Zhang, P.; Cai, J.; Lou, Y.; Hu, B. Microbial cooperation promotes humification to reduce antibiotic resistance genes abundance in food waste composting. *Bioresour. Technol.* **2022**, *362*, 127824. [CrossRef] [PubMed]
11. Strobel, B.W.; Hansen, H.C.; Borggaard, O.K.; Andersen, M.K.; Raulund-Rasmussen, K. Composition and reactivity of DOC in forest floor soil solutions in relation to tree species and soil type. *Biogeochemistry* **2001**, *56*, 1–26. [CrossRef]
12. Ghabbour, E.A.; Davies, G.; Misiewicz, T.; Alami, R.A.; Askounis, E.M.; Cuozzo, N.P.; Filice, A.J.; Haskell, J.M.; Moy, A.K.; Roach, A.C.; et al. Chapter one—National comparison of the total and sequestered organic matter contents of conventional and organic farm soils. In *Advances in Agronomy*; Sparks, D.L., Ed.; Academic Press: Cambridge, MA, USA, 2017; Volume 146, pp. 1–35.
13. Boguta, P.; Sokołowska, Z. Statistical relationship between selected physicochemical properties of peaty-muck soils and their fraction of humic acids. *Int. Agrophys.* **2014**, *28*, 269–278. [CrossRef]
14. Chin, Y.P.; Ajken, G.; O'Loughin, E. Molecular weight, polydispersity, and spectroscopic properties of aquatic humic substances. *Environ. Sci. Technol.* **1994**, *28*, 1853–1858. [CrossRef] [PubMed]

engineering proceedings

MDPI

Proceeding Paper

Character Building Education through Personalized Programs and E-Learning by Computer Software: A Case Study of Larantuka East Nusa Tenggara in Indonesia †

Isna Fachrur Rozi Iskandar *, Meitty Josephin Balontia, Hari Sriyanto and Jimmy Sapoetra

Character Building Development Center, Bina Nusantara University, Jakarta 11480, Indonesia; meitty.josephine@binus.ac.id (M.J.B.); amroe@binus.ac.id (H.S.); jimmy.sapoetra@binus.ac.id (J.S.)
* Correspondence: isna.fachrur@binus.ac.id
† Presented at the 2024 IEEE 4th International Conference on Electronic Communications, Internet of Things and Big Data, Taipei, Taiwan, 19–21 April 2024.

Abstract: The Indonesian government prioritizes development in the 3T regions: frontier, outermost, and least-developed areas, which are vital for holistic progress. Aligned with the Golden Generation program, it emphasizes education, tech access, and entrepreneurship to empower youth against societal challenges. Larantuka, in East Nusa Tenggara of Indonesia, exemplifies local maritime culture's influence and the need for personalized e-learning which is rooted in tradition. Qualitative research was conducted and identified two key factors: content reflecting collective memory and offline accessibility. Local culture alongside formal education fosters character building and lifelong learning by integrating theoretical teachings with practical applications, based on the cultural value of "gotong royong" (mutual cooperation). This approach ensures that Indonesia's cultural heritage thrives amidst educational progress.

Keywords: online learning; personalized learning; Larantuka; character building

Citation: Iskandar, I.F.R.; Balontia, M.J.; Sriyanto, H.; Sapoetra, J. Character Building Education through Personalized Programs and E-Learning by Computer Software: A Case Study of Larantuka East Nusa Tenggara in Indonesia. *Eng. Proc.* **2024**, *74*, 25. https://doi.org/10.3390/engproc2024074025

Academic Editors: Shu-Han Liao, Teen-Hang Meen and Cheng-Fu Yang

Published: 29 August 2024

1. Introduction

Development brings progress but poses challenges and opportunities to address, especially for remote regions in Indonesia. As a nation with abundant human resources, disparity is a significant issue if every region does not receive equal development and education. Achieving a balance in development requires time and substantial funding. However, it is important to improve education quality through technological advancement with online programs. This argument is supported by the increasing use of internet-connected devices, such as smartphones and tablets, and is further enhanced by government programs that build the telecommunication infrastructure in remote areas of Indonesia.

However, e-learning is not a flawless instructional delivery model and has shortcomings as follows:

1. Accessibility and infrastructure: In several areas, especially in rural or developing regions, access to fast and stable internet remains a problem. Additionally, not all students have the necessary devices (such as computers or tablets) to access e-learning.
2. Limited social interaction: Online learning can reduce social interaction between students and teachers and among students. This lack of social interaction can impact the development of social skills and students' ability to cooperate.
3. Motivation and discipline: Learning independently through e-learning requires a high level of motivation and discipline in students. Several students struggle to maintain motivation for learning without direct supervision from teachers.
4. Quality content: Online learning requires the content to be relevant, interactive, and of high quality. Effective content development demands investments in time and sufficient resources.

5. Evaluation and performance measurement: It is challenging to evaluate students' progress and measure the effectiveness of online learning. Fair and accurate evaluation systems need to be designed to measure students' understanding effectively.
6. Data security concerns: The use of e-learning platforms involves the exchange of personal data and students' academic information. Data security is a major concern, and effective measures need to be in place to protect sensitive information.
7. Educators and technology skills: Teachers and instructors need adequate technology skills to plan, develop, and manage online learning. Proper training and adequate support are necessary to ensure educators have the knowledge and skills required.

These shortcomings need to be studied to create effective personalized e-learning based on specific regions. By studying traditional education systems that are based on local cultures, the idea of character building based on local wisdom and values can be determined and implemented to solve the challenges and obtain the opportunities that arise in their respective regions. Parapat stated that maintaining local wisdom is an effort that can shape the character of the community, especially the local population [1].

Cooperation between existing informal education based on local cultures and the national standard in education helps to build lifelong education. The process of character building through informal education is a strong foundation for the Indonesian people, aligning with human resources and development that encompass skills in hardware and software in the spirit of nationalism. This is inseparable from the fact that maintaining a country must be undertaken by generating human resources who can participate positively in improving people's lives. This also corresponds to lifelong education, forming human beings with useful abilities for the common good. To examine how to shape character building based on personalized e-learning, we used qualitative research methods and extracted data through in-depth interviews, surveys, and literature studies.

2. Background Knowledge

2.1. Lifelong Education

Lifelong education refers to an educational effort that lasts a lifetime to produce individuals to contribute to society. Lifelong education is carried out comprehensively at the formal and informal levels of education. Comprehensiveness means that education is a lifelong learning process for personal, social, and professional development [2]. The process of lifelong education has been improved based on the previous concept of education in two ways. First, the concept of lifelong education contradicts the belief that education is only limited to formal education, namely, schools and universities where both children and young people are prepared for adulthood. Second, the implication of applying this concept is that the formal education system must be regulated flexibly to accommodate individual choices and prepare young people to continue their education as self-directed and competent adult learners [3]. In lifelong education, two types of integration are needed, namely, horizontal integration and vertical integration. Horizontal integration brings all types of education that exist in society together, both in formal education, such as schools, and in informal education so that both can support each other. Furthermore, vertical integration refers to the continuity of each type of education available to each individual throughout their life [2].

2.2. Gotong Royong (Mutual Cooperation): Basis of Character Building and Value

Soekarno, the first president of the Republic of Indonesia, is the one who has sparked "Pancasila" as the nation's ideology. Pancasila is an ideology that contains the following five values extracted from the way of life of the Indonesian people themselves:

- God Almighty group home;
- Just and civilized humanity group;
- Indonesian union group home;
- Democracy led by wisdom of wisdom in representative deliberations group home;
- Social justice for all Indonesian people

In his speech about the idea of Pancasila, Soekarno stated that Pancasila could be squeezed into one virtue, namely mutual cooperation (gotong royong). Gotong royong is one of the local wisdoms of the Indonesian people. Gotong royong can be understood as a way of life for the Indonesian people that encapsulates all the values of Pancasila. The meaning of gotong royong is to help each other in a community. Even though Indonesia has 1340 ethnic groups, gotong royong exists in each of these ethnic groups. Gotong royong has various names depending on the language of the ethnic groups in Indonesia. The Minahasa tribe, one of the Indonesian ethnic groups in North Sulawesi, understands gotong royong with the term "mapalus". Meanwhile, the Minang tribe labels mutual cooperation with the term "manunggal sakato". Every ethnic group in Indonesia has a habit of mutual cooperation in different terms. The practice of gotong royong in every ethnic group of Indonesia shows the values of Pancasila as the way of life of the Indonesian people. This is inseparable from the fact that the five values of Pancasila are rooted in mutual cooperation. Gotong royong is the ideology of the Indonesian nation, namely, Pancasila.

2.3. *Bina Nusantara Character-Building Program*

Since 2014, under Law No. 12 of 2012 regarding higher education and the mandatory teaching of Pancasila education, civic education, religious education, and Indonesian language education to all students, the character-building (CB) curriculum has been adjusted, including its name and content.

Binus University continues to provide character-building education through courses such as Pancasila education, civic education, and religious education as general and compulsory courses. The new courses have new names, such as Character Building: Pancasila, Character Building: Civic Education, and Character Building: Religious Education. The main emphasis in conducting learning activities for the three courses, including social activities conducted outside the classroom, is placed on character formation or improvement. Many fundamental core values are the main topics of discussion in the three courses, which are cultivated within the students through learning activities both inside and outside the classroom.

- Character Building: Pancasila involves a deepening of its noble values, which are articulated in the five principles: the value of the divine, the value of humanity, the value of unity, the value of democracy, and the value of justice. These five values serve as the foundation for character education for all students.
- Character Building: Civic Education focuses on being a good citizen. Through the course, students can possess a strong sense of nationalism and patriotism for the homeland.
- Religious Education: The meaning of faith and religion are emphasized in living. Through the course, students become able to believe and practice their faith in an inclusive, plural, and open manner, while remaining critical and rational. They are also encouraged to understand or interpret religious teachings in situations they are facing.

3. Research Method

Larantuka is located in East Flores district, East Nusa Tenggara, Indonesia, as a sub-district. It is the capital of the district of East Flores. Larantuka comes from the name of the first Catholic kingdom in the archipelago, which was founded in the 13th century, so it is often known as the Vatican foyer. Therefore, this area is a spiritual tourism destination for Catholics. Larantuka is located at the foot of Mount Mandiri and is affected by Portuguese heritage traditions. The area is 75.91 km^2 with a population of 45,515 according to the 2020 census data [4]. Due to its geographical location, before 2020 there was only one mobile telecommunication operator. Their services covered several sub-districts only. The Indonesia Ministry of Communications and Informatics through BAKTI (Accessibility, Telecommunication, and Information Body) provided 753 access points for telecommunication in East Flores in schools, public health centers, municipal buildings, and tourist attractions [5].

Larantuka is a part of East Flores with two original cultures, namely "Lamaholot" and "Malay Nagi Larantuka". Lamaholot is the majority culture of nomadic tribes in the mountains. Meanwhile, Malay Nagi Larantuka is a culture with various cultural adaptations, one of which is Portuguese culture. Judging from its territory, Larantuka has been affected by coastal Malay culture. Over time, both cultures were mixed with due marriages as the most triggering factor. In harmony with Indonesian culture based on gotong royong, the local culture of Larantuka also embraces the value. In Larantuka, gotong royong is called "Gemohing". This word is popularly used to imply a joint activity. Besides that, there is also "Kumpo Kao", which means helping relatives who are experiencing difficulties or solving social agendas altogether, which is manifested in material and physical assistance. The activities are carried out in traditional events, church construction, weddings, and Indonesian proclamation celebrations.

In line with the geographical conditions, the fishing culture in Larantuka is still very strong. Maritime-related matters are popular with all generations in society. The older generation has been traditional or modern fishermen and sailors. Meanwhile, the younger generation, along with globalization and technological developments, continue their studies outside East Nusa Tenggara, and those who stay have maritime professions, including inter-strait sea taxi sailors. This maritime activity has been supported as Larantuka has been a trading center for fish. The "fish market" is classified based on the caught and traded amount.

Social activities in the community at the fish market are closely related to the local culture in Larantuka, where greetings in local languages are still often used among the older generation. Foreign cultures influence the younger generation in Larantuka considerably, but this is not negative for the younger generation for cultural enrichment. This is evidenced by the participation of the younger generation in traditional and customary events, triggered by childhood memories without significant foreign exposure. However, the youth organization in Larantuka, named Simpasio, is maintaining and preserving the indigenous culture of the region. The activities carried out by the organization include the following:

- Exploring local knowledge related to traditional Larantuka medicine;
- Portuguese and Catholic cultural influences;
- Documentation of traditional rituals;
- Audio-visual documentation to meet the needs of the era that contains culture.

The related matters are local content in the region and are used to strengthen and maintain the local culture of the region.

4. Findings and Discussions

Residents, teachers, and government officials in Larantuka were found to communicate about the accessibility and infrastructure of Larantuka. Due to its exposure to foreign cultures and the need to connect with other people in other provinces, it is necessary to communicate through a well-established infrastructure. People in Larantuka, especially younger generations, are aware of data security and how to protect their information. The different views concerning internet security between the older and younger generations are classified into technical and cultural categories. For the older generation, technical issues such as data security, unsecured passwords, and digital footprints are problems since they demand easy access to internet-based technologies. The younger generation has problems such as technological mastery of e-learning, which can be solved using character-building education.

Character-building education in Larantuka is carried out in formal and informal education. These two types of education collaborate as gotong royong is the basis for character building in schools and society. People continue to learn to be social beings and to cooperate. Cooperation is the core of the value of gotong royong and the basic value of the Indonesian nation's ideology, namely Pancasila. For example, gotong royong is informally taught through the practice of cooperation, especially in funerals or wedding ceremonies.

Even though various forms of communication are available through the internet, Larantuka is still a traditional way of communication. This is rooted in cooperation-based education at various levels of formal and informal education. People in Larantuka are used to cooperating with respect to its local culture and familial traits. Learning is effective in the reminiscence of childhood memories, which boosts their motivation. According to our interviews, people in Larantuka find their strength in a group to overcome their weaknesses. Such a way becomes their problem-solving method, in which they discuss their problem and find solutions through "family" discussions. In terms of formal education from pre-school to university, every child is taught the basic values of Indonesian ideology through civic education. The materials are created for the needs of each student at each level of education.

In Indonesia's formal education, local wisdom learning materials are included in the Merdeka curriculum. This implementation allows the regional authority to accommodate local content based on the characteristics and local wisdom in the region. Studies related to local content are based on the nation's culture, which allows the culture to be integrated into the curriculum. The Merderka curriculum provides a learning standard in terms of material development and evaluation. The problem in providing material related to regional culture is the uniformity in schools. In such uniformity, the Medeka Curriculum introduces local excellence and wisdom so that they can be integrated into education. According to the Ministry of Education and Culture of Indonesia, three options exist in the local content integrated into formal education [6]:

- Integration with other subjects;
- Project to strengthen the profile of Pancasila;
- Become a separate subject for two hours.

Local wisdom is associated with Pancasila. Indonesian diversity provides a local and global advantage. In the operational curriculum, institutions integrate local content based on [6] regional characteristics, traditions, and resources. Character education in Indonesia has different characteristics because of its diversity. Gotong royong is a common characteristic. Each region has its characteristics. Such different characteristics cannot be separated from geographical characteristics. Communities in Larantuka are affected by marine cultures. In Larantuka, for example, maritime culture is manifested as a way of making a living. Related to character building in lifelong education, integration between informal education in society is required. Every individual in the area learns maritime culture in everyday life. The integration of informal education in the community is supported by the awareness of the community about maintaining its culture. For example, the Simpasio Institute, an association of young people in Larantuka, maintains culture through various educational activities and explores local knowledge related to traditional Larantuka medicine and traditional rituals. Such efforts cannot be separated from discussions with the local government. The economic benefit from the sea supports informal education at the Simpasio Institute in the community. Character education in Larantuka lasts a lifetime through activities that exist in the community (Figure 1).

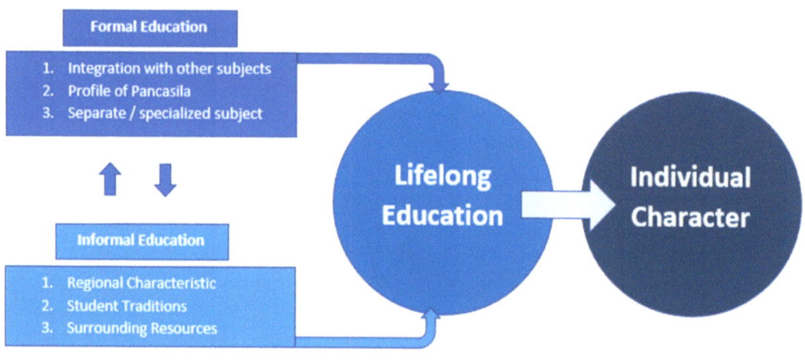

Figure 1. Relationship of individual character in lifelong education at formal and informal educational institutions.

5. Conclusions

Amid globalization and with the influence of foreign cultures, the coastal communities of Larantuka still hold onto their cultural characteristics. People are working at sea for a living. The culture of gotong royong has been implemented in the community. The implementation of mutual cooperation is a form of lifelong education for the residents. The education forms the character of an individual in the region. In terms of character-building education through personalized e-learning, two significant factors are considered: childhood memory, which attracts interest in learning, and methods of learning and materials online, with offline guidance through traditional teaching (Table 1).

Table 1. Teaching-related subjects and means in character-building education.

Items	Means
Accessibility and Infrastructure	Sufficient backup access to local learning centers, schools, or municipal buildings for offline learning
Limited Social Interaction	Required attention through a hybrid approach (offline and online delivery)
Motivation And Discipline	Solution by fostering local culture and familial traits
Quality Content	Content-based local culture and national character-building education to create lifelong and personalized e-learning programs
Evaluation and Performance Measurement	Solution through the Merdeka curriculum
Data Security Concerns	Assistance with existing technology linked to the national database
Educators and Technology Skills	Training with the national standard of the Merdeka curriculum

Author Contributions: Conceptualization, I.F.R.I.; methodology, M.J.B.; software, I.F.R.I. and M.J.B.; validation, I.F.R.I., M.J.B. and J.S.; formal analysis, I.F.R.I.; investigation, I.F.R.I.; resources, M.J.B.; data curation, I.F.R.I.; writing—original draft preparation, I.F.R.I.; writing—review and editing, H.S. and J.S.; visualization, I.F.R.I., M.J.B. and J.S.; supervision, J.S.; project administration, H.S.; funding acquisition, H.S. All authors have read and agreed to the published version of the manuscript.

Funding: This research received no external funding.

Institutional Review Board Statement: This study did not require ethical approval.

Informed Consent Statement: Informed consent was obtained from all subjects involved in the study.

Data Availability Statement: No New Data were created.

Acknowledgments: This research was supported by the Research and Technology Transfer Office, Bina Nusantara University as a part of Bina Nusantara University's Applied Basic Research Grant entitled Pancasila Education and Maritime Culture (Local Culture) as the Foundation for Shaping Society's Character Amidst the Development of Time, with contract no. 060/VR.RTT/IV/2022 and contract date 8 April 2022.

Conflicts of Interest: The authors declare no conflict of interest.

References

1. Parapat, L.H.; Aritonang, D.R. Nilai Kearifan Lokal dan Upaya Pemertahanan Budaya "Marsalap Ari" dalam Menjalin Solidaritas Antar Sesama di Desa Paringgonan sebagai Bahan Ajar Pembentukan Karakter Mahasiswa. *J. Penelit. Pendidik. Bhs. Dan Sastra* **2020**, *5*, 25–28.
2. Iqbal, M.J. Life Long Education: A Conceptual Debate. *Int. J. Media Technol. Lifelong Learn.* **2009**, *5*. [CrossRef]
3. Badan Pusat Statistik Kabupaten Flores Timur. (n.d.). *Kecamatan Larantuka Dalam Angka 2021*; Badan Pusat Statistik: Larantuka, Indonesia, 2021.
4. BPS Nusa Tenggara Barat. (n.d.). *[Sensus Penduduk] Jumlah Penduduk Nusa Tenggara Barat Menurut Kabupaten/Kota dan Jenis Kelamin (Jiwa)*; Badan Pusat Statistik: Kota Mataram, Indonesia, 2020.

5. Andrianto, H. [Esai Foto] Merajut Nusantara Lewat Sinyal Telekomunikasi", Kementerian Komunikasi dan Informasi Republik Indonesia. June 2022. Available online: https://www.kominfo.go.id/content/detail/42651/esai-foto-merajut-nusantara-lewat-sinyal-telekomunikasi/0/artikel (accessed on 2 October 2022).
6. dan Hubungan Masyarakat, B.K.S. Implementasi Kurikulum Merdeka, Muatan Kearifan Lokal Bisa Dimasukan Melalui Tiga Opsi", Kementerian Pendidikan dan Kebudayaan. August 2022. Available online: https://www.kemdikbud.go.id/main/blog/2022/08/implementasi-kurikulum-merdeka-muatan-kearifan-lokal-bisa-dimasukkan-melalui-tiga-opsi (accessed on 2 October 2022).

engineering proceedings

Proceeding Paper

Environmental Movement Regardless of Nationality: International Students' Attitude toward Environmental Protection and Environmental Awareness in Taiwan †

Kai-Fu Yang *, Pei-Rong Liu, Yu-Han Zheng, Yu-Jie Peng, Hai-Yan Wang and Yi-Fang Huang

Department of Applied English, Chaoyang University of Technology, Taichung 413310, Taiwan; s11222605@cyut.edu.tw (P.-R.L.); s10822024@cyut.edu.tw (Y.-H.Z.); s10822030@cyut.edu.tw (Y.-J.P.); s10822008@cyut.edu.tw (H.-Y.W.); s10822020@cyut.edu.tw (Y.-F.H.)

* Correspondence: kaifu0318@gmail.com

† Presented at the 2024 IEEE 4th International Conference on Electronic Communications, Internet of Things and Big Data, Taipei, Taiwan, 19–21 April 2024.

Abstract: In recent years, environmental pollution has become a global concern, but most of the attention has been paid to the impact of garbage pollution on the oceans, and the pollution of mountain areas has rarely been a concern. However, the amount of garbage in the mountains is also considerable. Therefore, in order to make students pay more attention to the issue of environmental protection, we promoted environmental education and increased environmental awareness to encourage green behavior for the goal of environmental sustainability. Foreign students have a better understanding of environmental protection through mountain cleaning, improve their knowledge of garbage sorting, and work together to protect our environment.

Keywords: environmental education; environmental awareness; green behavior; environmental sustainability

Citation: Yang, K.-F.; Liu, P.-R.; Zheng, Y.-H.; Peng, Y.-J.; Wang, H.-Y.; Huang, Y.-F. Environmental Movement Regardless of Nationality: International Students' Attitude toward Environmental Protection and Environmental Awareness in Taiwan. *Eng. Proc.* **2024**, *74*, 26. https://doi.org/10.3390/engproc2024074026

Academic Editors: Shu-Han Liao, Teen-Hang Meen and Cheng-Fu Yang

Published: 29 August 2024

1. Introduction

On the earth, due to over-exploitation and rapid development, many natural ecosystems are destroyed causing many different types of waste on earth, which induces environmental pollution. Thus, resource recycling is used to improve the environment and people's health [1]. Because people are aware of their health and safety, they are actively reducing the use of plastic and starting to buy green products [2]. Only one person will not have any impact on the environmental movement, but if everyone does it together, it can bring unexpected benefits [3]. Environmental protection is an issue of global concern, and we must begin with immediate practical actions for the environment.

Environmental protection has always been a serious issue for Taiwan. Many people do not have the concept of environmental protection awareness, which hurts Taiwan and its environment. It is necessary to advertise the importance of environmental protection through environmental movements. Through these activities, we can protect nature. Coupled with the recent active promotion of the New Southbound Policy by Taiwan, the number of foreign students studying in Taiwan is increasing. Therefore, it is needed to encourage Taiwanese as well as foreign students to collaborate in safeguarding Taiwan.

2. Literature Review

2.1. Environmental Protection

Environmental protection involves the relationship between humans and the natural environment, with a focus on human living habits and behaviors to prevent unnecessary changes to the ecosystem. To enhance environmental awareness and promote appropriate waste disposal, a waste bank has been established, encouraging students to participate in waste sorting in exchange for cash rewards. This initiative benefits the environment and offers opportunities. In the academic year of 2016/2017, Syiah Kuala University (SKU) introduced a mandatory Disaster and Environmental Knowledge (PKL) course for all students to sensitize them to disaster and environmental issues [4]. A policy was enacted in the entire campus community, encouraging the avoidance of plastic bottles and other packaging materials to create a zero-waste campus. In 2018, the university collaborated with the National Electricity Company (PLN) to improve the campus environment following the initiatives proposed on Indonesia's Tree Planting Day on November 18. These institutions planted 1045 trees, contributing to the development of a green campus and environmental protection [5].

2.2. Environmental Education

Environmental education is a transformative process that enables individuals to delve into environmental concerns, actively engage in problem solving, and take proactive measures to enhance the environment [6]. This educational approach fosters an understanding of environmental issues and equips individuals with the capabilities to make informed and responsible choices. As a result, it reshapes people's attitudes and behaviors and establishes a harmonious connection with the natural environment. Environmental education achieves this by imparting knowledge, instilling values, and providing actionable strategies to drive positive environmental changes. Numerous studies support the paramount importance of environmental education in addressing environmental challenges, safeguarding the natural world, and promoting eco-friendly behaviors [7]. Many universities are actively promoting environmental education on campus by adopting various practices such as visiting natural environments or using school settings, planting trees or flowers, opening lectures with an environmental curriculum, forming groups to engage in environmental movements, and establishing Garbage Banks to address concerns for the surrounding environment. We summarized 5 tips for university course material in Table 1.

Table 1. Tips for university course material.

5 Tips for University Course Material	
Plant trees or flowers	Establish a Garbage Bank to concern for the surrounding environment
Form a group to perform some environmental movements	Open lectures with an environment curriculum; class dissemination
Visit natural environments or use places such as school settings	

2.3. Environmental Awareness

In recent years, environmental issues have become a major topic of public opinion. People have begun to develop increasing environmental awareness and a positive attitude towards ecological issues. Many people began to aim for a friendly environment, advocate correct environmental awareness, organize to improve the environment with mountain cleaning, promote the knowledge of correct resource recycling, and work together for the earth. Researchers indicated that environmental awareness refers to a human's understanding of the cognitive level and practical actions of environmental protection [8].

Mountain Riders, an educational organization dedicated to ecological transition, focuses on mountain waste clean-up initiatives that bring together practitioners and mountain enthusiasts to safeguard their natural playgrounds. Their objective is to address mountain litter by reducing its generation at the source. The organization assumes responsibility for education, awareness raising, tool provision, training, and supporting all stakeholders and citizens in the pursuit of a Zero Waste Mountain [9]. The climbers are also called on to take away their garbage and not leave it in the mountains for a comfortable and clean environment [10]. In addition, elementary school students cleaned mountains in an educational activity. Educational meaning was discussed to make students learn effectiveness in environmental education and cherish environmental resources [11]. The International Climbing and Mountaineering Federation (UIAA), which annually convenes nearly a thousand people for these activities, is capable of collecting more than 90 tons of waste each time, with up to 40% of it being recycled. In addition to environmental improvements, its primary mission is to impart relevant knowledge to people [12].

2.4. Green Behavior

The indicators for measuring green behavior include maintaining a positive environmental attitude, taking responsibility for environmental protection, active participation, educational engagement, motivating peers to reduce their carbon footprint, and practicing effective waste sorting and resource recycling [13]. Recycling significantly benefits the environment by reducing landfill waste and conserving limited natural resources, like timber, as well as saving energy. Efforts to recycle waste reflect the commitment to environmental preservation. Major cities have implemented recycling systems to reduce pollution in the atmosphere [14]. We summarized green behavior at university in Table 2.

Table 2. Green behavior at university.

Green Behavior	
The University of George Washington [15]	1. Set up standardized recycling bins 2. Color coding of different waste streams—green for compost, blue for recycling, black for landfill
The University of California Berkeley [16]	Replace the plastic bottles in vending machines with cans and glasses
The University of Waterloo [17]	Hold a garbage marathon for a zero-waste challenge

3. Methodology

The research framework of this study is illustrated in Figure 1. In order to achieve environmental sustainability, we introduced environmental education to university students to raise their environmental awareness and promote green behaviors for the objective of environmental sustainability. Regarding environmental education, we collected foreign university course materials for environmental education, including visiting natural settings, planting trees, opening lectures on the environment to form green behavior groups, and establishing a Garbage Bank. Using these materials, we expanded the curriculum of Chaoyang University of Technology to create awareness among foreign students about the importance of environmental education. To heighten environmental awareness among university students, a series of movements, including activities such as mountain cleaning, have been orchestrated with the explicit objective of not only organizing these environmental movements but also fostering a deeper understanding and commitment to environmental awareness among the student body. In this study, waste sorting knowledge was taught to university students, thereby cultivating and nurturing a more environmentally aware mindset and encouraging the adoption of sustainable practices and green behaviors.

These standards were implemented in three activities: class dissemination for environmental education aimed at students, mountain cleaning to enhance students' environmental awareness, and garbage classification to promote green behavior among students. The standards aim to engage students in practical actions, promoting environmental responsibility on campus. Collaboration between Taiwanese and foreign students emphasized a shared commitment to environmental protection, regardless of nationality. By focusing on these three key points and using practical measures, waste pollution can be reduced to improve the environment not just on the campus but in the surrounding areas.

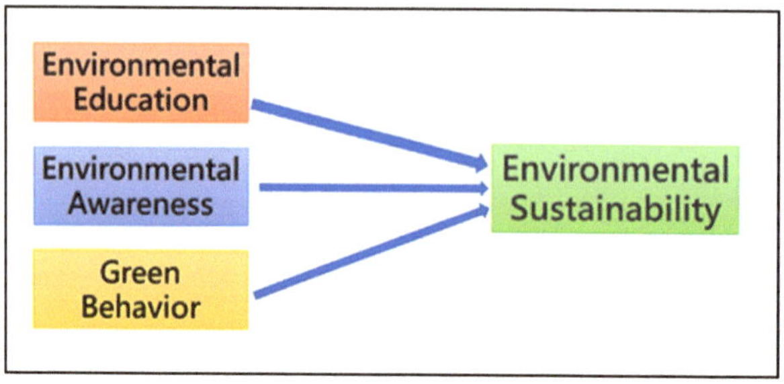

Figure 1. Research framework of this study.

Inspired by Germany's garbage classification, we developed a six-color recycling system: blue, brown, green, yellow, black, and white. Each color represents waste categories and recycling methods for washing and flattening items. We summarized six categories of recycling at CYUT in Table 3.

Table 3. Six categories of recycling at CYUT.

	Recycling at CYUT
Blue	Paper: books, cartons, coated paper, newspapers, photocopying paper, promotional paper, posters, leaflets, etc.
Brown	Aluminum cans: iron cans, bottles and cans of beverages, drinks, cola, cans, beer, etc.
Green	Aluminum foil pack (carton pack with a layer of transparent film): green tea, black tea, milk tea, juice, etc.
Yellow	Plastic bottles and cans that have recycling signs: bottled water, PET bottles, bubble tea, shower, cleaning supplies, straws, etc.
Black	General garbage: toilet paper, garbage bags, plastic bags, leaves, bamboo chopsticks, etc.
White	Glass bottles and cans for beverages: soy sauce, wine bottles, etc.

4. Movements for Environmental Protection

4.1. Class Dissemination

To instill the principles of environmental education among foreign students and foster the habit of garbage classification and recycling, the activity's promotion was conducted through self-created presentation materials and practical demonstrations. In the operational phase, bags were used for five groups: glass, plastic, iron and aluminum, paper, and general waste. These items were presented to foreign students on campus for classification. With such efforts, students comprehended the need to remove straws from aluminum foil beverage packaging, placing them in general waste before flattening them for recycling. However, several students overlooked flattening paper boxes after removing the tape. A Vietnamese student inquired about the correct disposal of paper medicine packaging and was unsure whether it belonged to the paper or general waste category. For those who misclassified garbage or had uncertainties, explanations and practical demonstrations were provided. Through consistent promotion and practice, a clear understanding of garbage classification can be achieved, fostering collective environmental protection, regardless of nationality. Through mountain cleaning activities, garbage classification awareness was enhanced. The promotional videos lasted approximately two minutes, featuring proper garbage classification. These short videos can be played on the campus's TV screens across various locations to familiarize students with these principles, encourage better campus stewardship, and prompt practical implementation of garbage classification in their everyday routines. Initially intending to hold two classes for international students, the class hours were increased to four owing to the outcome, surpassing the expected number of participating students (Table 4, Figure 2).

Table 4. KPI for class dissemination.

	Number of Departments	Number of Students
KPI	2	60
Actual Quantity	4	112

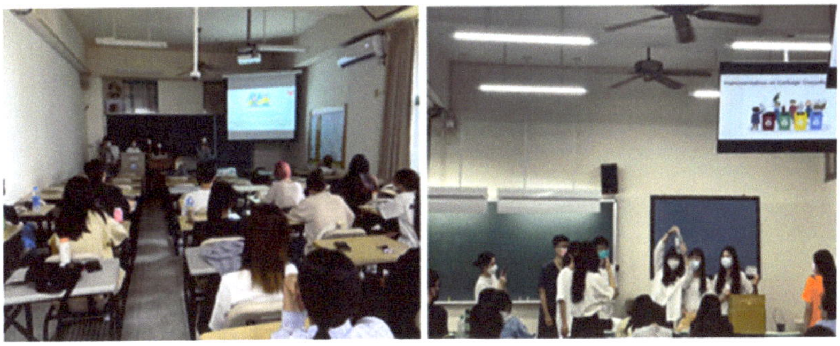

Figure 2. Class dissemination.

4.2. Mountain Cleaning

Foreign students were invited to join the mountain cleaning movement, where, in addition to collecting trash, various games were organized to facilitate cultural exchanges between Taiwanese and foreign students. This collaborative effort not only upheld campus cleanliness but also fostered new friendships. The collected wastes were sorted to reinforce the participants' understanding of garbage classification. This event disseminated knowledge regarding environmental issues and conservation, awakened environmental awareness, and motivated active involvement in environmental preservation.

The mountain cleaning initiative targeted foreign students attending the Chaoyang University of Technology. There were Vietnamese students enrolled in the Department of Marketing and Logistics Management and Mongolian students in the Department of Information Management, encompassing 24 students. The participants in this study are shown in Table 5.

Table 5. Participants in this study.

Department	Grade	Numbers
Department of Marketing and Logistics Management	Freshman	14
Department of Information Management	Freshman Sophomore Junior	10

As depicted in Figure 3, the anticipated participant count was initially 24, yet the actual number of participants was 30. While the projected amount of waste was estimated to reach one ton, the factual accumulation amounted to merely three kilograms. The KPI of mountain cleaning are shown in Table 6.

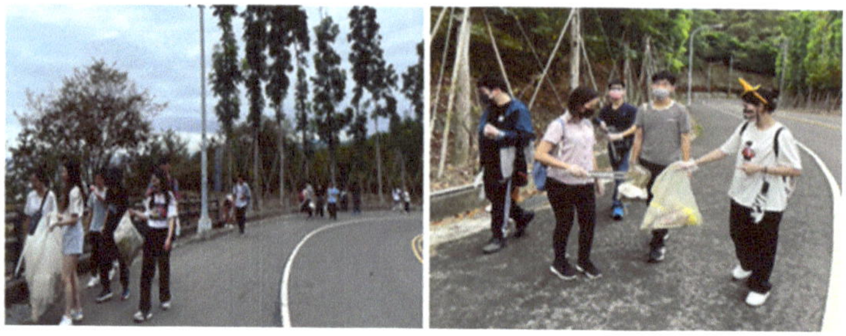

Figure 3. Mountain cleaning.

Table 6. KPI for mountain cleaning.

	Number of Attendances	Amounts of Garbage
KPI	24	5 kg
Actual Quantity	30	6 kg

Foreign students were invited to join in filming promotional videos on purifying the campus. The contents of the three videos are about littering on campus, forgetting to take away the trash in the middle of class, and littering unwashed lunch boxes. These are often overlooked in campus life. The videos allowed them to understand this basic common sense, emphasizing actions within 'green behavior' to take care of the campus and remind others to clean the campus using garbage classification in daily life (Figure 4). The number of cleaned classrooms exceeded that of the initial plan owing to the collaborative involvement of foreign students. This joint effort streamlined the process of cleaning an extra five classrooms. The video showcased substantial garnered attention, with students and teachers frequently pausing to watch as they passed through the area. As a result, the number of viewers exceeded initial expectations (Table 7).

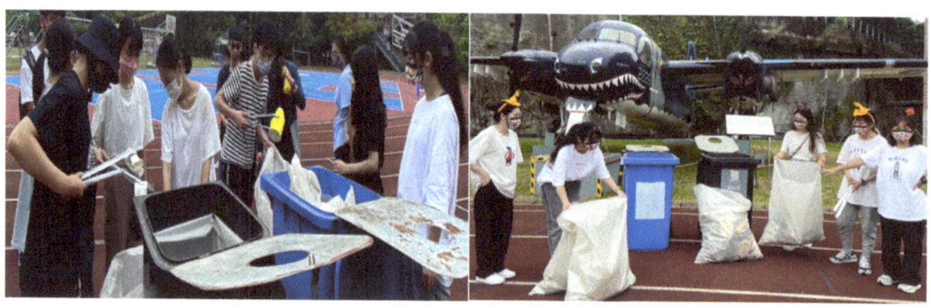

Figure 4. Video recording.

Table 7. KPI for a clean campus.

	Number of Classrooms	Number of Views
KPI	10	500
Actual Quantity	15	800

5. Conclusions and Recommendations

In the program of this study, foreign students came to understand how to classify garbage and the importance of garbage classification. Beyond simply promoting Taiwan's garbage sorting methods, hands-on practice sessions were offered to allow participants from various countries to comprehend classification guidelines. This activity allowed for an understanding of the steps and significance of garbage sorting, aiding foreign students in grasping the intricacies of the future through clean mountains and garbage classification to carry out an environmental movement. In this study, environmental cleanup and cross-cultural communication were executed, heightening participants' awareness of environmental protection. Using the promotional video, waste sorting practices were advertised on campus. International students were invited to participate in this study. The video content highlighted the common neglect of waste sorting during daily garbage disposal. By demonstrating the correct practices in the video, green behaviors were widely adopted.

It is necessary to include more event details to enhance the report's liveliness. Subsequently, to organize a relevant movement, precise time management and the preparation of additional tools for emergencies are demanded. When filming a video, an indoor setting is recommended. Using a more natural approach, authenticity can be added to the content to enhance relatability and avoid an overtly staged appearance. Encouraging student participation and engaging teachers are also recommended. It is necessary to include diverse nationalities. Regarding environmental movements, it is essential to clean mountainous areas and beaches or communities. Additionally, it is recommended to refer to foreign universities' programs, such as a garbage marathon.

Author Contributions: Conceptualization: K.-F.Y.; Methodology: P.-R.L.; Formal analysis: Y.-H.Z.; Data curation: Y.-J.P.; Writing—original draft preparation: H.-Y.W., Y.-F.H., P.-R.L. and Y.-H.Z.; Writing—review and editing: K.-F.Y. All authors have read and agreed to the published version of the manuscript.

Funding: This research received no external funding.

Institutional Review Board Statement: Not applicable.

Informed Consent Statement: Not applicable.

Data Availability Statement: Data available on request from the authors.

Conflicts of Interest: The authors declare no conflict of interest.

References

1. Science Park. The Different Kinds of Waste Produced by Manufacturing Industries. 2019. Available online: https://sciencepark.com.ph/blog/waste-management/ (accessed on 7 January 2020).
2. Olivier, J. For Many Taiwanese, "Buying Green" Has Long Been a Priority. AmCham Taiwan. 19 August 2021. Available online: https://topics.amcham.com.tw/2021/08/taiwanese-buying-green-priority/?fbclid=IwAR25PepbLXUFmdcTr20-CeBx-STfN2FyKaY0_0Uu1AyG0iuXeiy21lSOoV8 (accessed on 19 August 2021).
3. Green Peace. Greenpeace Global Review 2019: The Climate Battle Will Never Give In. 2019. Available online: https://www.greenpeace.org/taiwan/update/12548/%E7%B6%A0%E8%89%B2%E5%92%8C%E5%B9%B32019%E5%85%A8%E7%90%83%E5%9B%9E%E9%A1%A7%EF%BC%9A%E6%B0%A3%E5%80%99%E6%88%B0%E5%BD%B9%E7%B5%95%E4%B8%8D%E8%AE%93%E6%AD%A5/ (accessed on 15 January 2020).
4. Atmaja RT, P.; Sulastri, S.; Nazli, N. Development of students learning module for disaster and environmental knowledge subject for undergraduate students of Universitas Syiah Kuala. *JIPI (Jurnal IPA Pembelajaran IPA)* **2021**, *5*, 48–56. [CrossRef]
5. Syiah Kuala University. USK Waste Management Becomes a Central Reference. Syiah Kuala University. 22 July 2022. Available online: https://usk.ac.id/tata-kelola-sampah-usk-jadi-rujukan-pusat/ (accessed on 22 July 2022).
6. EPA. *What Is Environmental Education?* U.S. Environmental Protection Agency: Washington, DC, USA, 2023. Available online: https://www.epa.gov/education/what-environmental-education (accessed on 2 July 2024).
7. Sharma, N.; Paço, A.; Upadhyay, D. Option or necessity: Role of environmental education as transformative change agent. *Eval. Program Plan.* **2023**, *97*, 102244. [CrossRef] [PubMed]
8. Calculli, C.; D'Uggento, A.M.; Labarile, A.; Ribecco, N. Evaluating people's awareness about climate changes and environmental issues: A case study. *J. Clean. Prod.* **2021**, *324*, 129244. [CrossRef]
9. Mountain Riders. Ensemble Pour Nos Montagnes. 2020. Available online: https://www.mountain-riders.org/ (accessed on 8 April 2020).
10. Geneva Environment Network. Plastic Waste in Mountains | Geneva Beat Plastic Pollution Dialogues & International Mountain Day 2021 Plastic Waste in Mountains. 2021. Available online: https://www.genevaenvironmentnetwork.org/events/plastic-waste-in-mountains-geneva-beat-plastic-pollution-dialogues-international-mountain-day-2021/ (accessed on 10 December 2021).
11. Tsai, P. The Innovation Strategies of Environmental Education and Consciousness of Ecological Protection: A Case Study of the Clean Mountain. Unpublished Master's Thesis, University of Minghsin, Hsinchu, Taiwan, 2020.

12. UIAA. *Mountain Days Campaign for Waste Collection and Sustainable Practices in Europe*; UIAA: Bern, Switzerland, 2021. Available online: https://theuiaa.org/uiaa/mountain-days-campaign-for-waste-collection-and-sustainable-practices-in-europe/ (accessed on 1 August 2016).
13. Shiu, W. A Study of Green Human Resource Management, Green Organizational Climate, and Employees' Green Behavior. Unpublished Master's Thesis, University of Ling Tung, Airiti Library, Taichung, Taiwan, 2022.
14. Ecobin. What Are Green Behaviour? 7 October 2019. Available online: https://www.ecobin.com.au/blogs/blog/what-is-green-behaviour/ (accessed on 7 October 2019).
15. George Washington University. *Trash, Recycling, and Compost at GW*; George Washington University: Washington, DC, USA, 2021. Available online: https://sustainability.gwu.edu/waste (accessed on 1 July 2021).
16. Sumner Byrne. *Chou Hall: Achieving Zero Waste on the UC Berkeley Campus*; U.S. Green Building Council, Inc.: Atlanta, GA, USA, 2022. Available online: https://www.usgbc.org/articles/chou-hall-achieving-zero-waste-uc-berkeley-campus (accessed on 16 June 2022).
17. University of Waterloo. *Zero Waste Week 2019*; University of Waterloo: Waterloo, ON, Canada, 2019. Available online: https://uwaterloo.ca/sustainability/events/zero-waste-week-2019 (accessed on 21 October 2019).

engineering proceedings

MDPI

Proceeding Paper

Using Magnetic Board Media as Complementary Media for Preschoolers' Online Mandarin Learning †

Jureynolds Jureynolds [1,*] and Danielle Crescentia [2]

1 Chinese Department, Bina Nusantara University, Jakarta 11480, Indonesia
2 PT Shan Hai Map, Jakarta 11470, Indonesia; daniellecrescentia@gmail.com
* Correspondence: jureynolds@binus.edu

† Presented at the 2024 IEEE 4th International Conference on Electronic Communications, Internet of Things and Big Data, Taipei, Taiwan, 19–21 April 2024.

Abstract: This research aimed to determine the effect of a magnetic board as an accompaniment to online Mandarin learning and for learning motivation. A one-equivalent control group research model was used. The control and experimental groups of five preschoolers and five accompanying parents participated in this research. Data were collected using observation and interviews conducted for one month. The magnetic board media increased student motivation with an increase of 81.42%. The role of companions was essential in implementing online learning with physical learning media.

Keywords: preschooler; online learning; magnetic board

1. Introduction

In second language acquisition and language development, early childhood is a crucial phase [1]. Frequent exposure is necessary for acquiring language ability [2]. Most parents show a positive attitude towards learning Chinese for children and believe that Chinese is good for their children. China's economic strength is one reason that influences parents' motivation to ask their children to learn Chinese [3]. This also leads to an increase in the number of Chinese language educational institutions opening in Indonesia.

Changes in early childhood education require integrating cutting-edge pedagogical methods and technologies to create a compelling and engaging learning environment. The use of digital media in early childhood education is one of the current research topics. As the online learning environment becomes increasingly common in language learning, researchers and educators are looking for creative methods to improve the efficiency of online learning for young children. Learning for this age group is particularly challenging, which calls for effective teaching strategies and parental involvement [4,5].

One of the Chinese language education centers has a unique way of conducting Chinese teaching and learning activities with magnetic board media. By using this medium, the children's concentration becomes more focused on the learning material, so it slowly fosters children's interest and motivation towards Mandarin learning with activities. Learning activities also involve parents. Physical tools, such as magnetic boards, are multi-sensory elements to enhance learning. Magnetic boards can be used to improve vocabulary acquisition, long-term memory, and children's motivation [6].

This study aims to determine the effect of magnetic board media in increasing motivation to learn Chinese in children aged 4–5 years. Magnetic board media is an additional tool to enhance preschool children's online Mandarin learning experience.

2. Literature Review

2.1. Preschooler Online Learning

Preschooler online learning has been important during the COVID-19 pandemic. Conventional online learning systems are not appropriate for preschoolers, and visualization

Citation: Jureynolds, J.; Crescentia, D. Using Magnetic Board Media as Complementary Media for Preschoolers' Online Mandarin Learning. *Eng. Proc.* **2024**, *74*, 27. https://doi.org/10.3390/engproc2024074027

Academic Editors: Shu-Han Liao, Teen-Hang Meen and Cheng-Fu Yang

Published: 29 August 2024

of teaching materials is critical [7]. Teachers must have digital skills and an open-minded approach to adapt to the needs of children and parents for online learning [8]. Research was carried out to test the effectiveness of online learning media, and digital media was proven to improve language skills [9]. Digital learning media positively impacted learning outcomes [10]. The research development created a new designation for preschooler online learning learners: "digital native" [11]. However, early childhood learning requires sensory motion training because preschoolers have difficulty focusing when learning online [12]. A study showed that movement training is needed in online learning; it can significantly improve focus [13].

2.2. Magnetic Board Media

The use of game boards in learning increased interaction between students and participation in classroom activities [14]. The use of magnetic boards on various subjects and surveys including geology provided visual images to students in a more interactive way [15]. Applying magnetic boards to early childhood learning can increase their creativity [16]. At the same time, using magnetic boards can also improve the teaching and learning process in study groups [17]. Studies on the use of magnetic boards highlighted their effectiveness and potential for early childhood and elementary school groups.

3. Material and Methods

The participants were ten children aged 4–5 years (preschoolers) participating in online Chinese language learning. A parent accompanied each child. Classroom action research was conducted in four steps: planning, action, observation, and reflection. In the planning stage, magnetic boards were used in online Chinese language learning. In the action stage, learning based on planning was implemented. In the observation stage, the children and parents were observed and interviewed. A descriptive qualitative approach was used to process data from observations and interviews with the children and parents. The observation sheet was used for data collection. In the reflection stage, the implementation and observation were discussed focusing on students' enthusiasm and activeness, students' perseverance in doing tasks, the usefulness and benefits of the media used, and students' interest in the media used.

4. Results

4.1. Planning

Learning activities were conducted using the ZOOM platform. The 10 children were divided into the control and the experimental classes. In the control class, they learned without magnetic board media (using animation media), while the experimental class learned with magnetic boards. The magnetic board in the experimental class was used by each child. Teachers and children used the same learning medium, the magnetic board, during learning activities. The control class carried out learning activities using animated media on PowerPoint, a visual medium that the teacher moved through the "share screen" on the ZOOM platform. In the control class, children paid attention to the animated media through their respective screens.

4.2. Action

Learning in the experimental and control classes was conducted online using ZOOM. The differences were interaction and practice. In the experimental class, interaction was conducted with instructions using the physical magnetic board. The exercise was conducted by attaching the pictures to the magnetic board according to the teacher's instructions in Chinese. In addition, question and answer and conclusion sessions were conducted using the magnetic board as a medium. In the control class, the interaction was performed with questions and answers about the PowerPoint presentation slide show. The exercise was conducted with a question-and-answer session according to the material in that session. The observation was carried out directly during class and guided by the observation sheet.

The interview was conducted at the end of the session with each child of the experimental and control classes and their parent parents.

4.3. Observation

The results of the observation were divided into two parts based on the instruments: (1) observation results of the control class and experimental class and (2) interview results of the control class and experimental class. The results of the observation of student activities in the control class and experimental class are presented in Table 1. The average score of the experimental class (81.42%) was higher than that of the control class (65.7%). The learning activities in both classes were carried out satisfactorily. We interviewed five children from each class to explore the children's responses to the learning medium used and its effect on learning motivation. As they were 4–5 years old, we did not use a questionnaire. The interview questions were simple with only two options, "Yes" or "No". In addition, the interview session was conducted with all children. Children could easily understand and answer the questions (Table 1).

Table 1. Student activity observation results.

Observation Indicators	Control Group Scoring	Experimental Group Scoring
Children actively pay attention to the teacher's explanation during learning activities.	3	5
Children actively ask the teacher or friends about material that has yet to be understood.	3	3
Children show interest in various kinds of problems.	3	4
Children enjoy finding and solving problems (questions) from the teacher.	5	5
Children are diligent in doing the tasks given by the teacher.	4	4
Children are encouraged to do something while learning.	2	4
Children strive to get the best grades.	5	5
Children prefer to work on their own.	3	5
Children' desire to do diverse tasks.	4	2
Children are curious about the material being taught.	3	4
Children dare to express their opinions in class.	4	4
Children can defend their opinions in class.	3	3
During teaching and learning activities, some activities attract children' attention.	2	5
Teaching and learning activities are carried out conductively.	2	4
Total Scoring	46	57
Average Score	3.28	4.07
Percentage	65.7%	81.42%

Indicators are determined from the class sit-in observation sheet from the course venue.

Figure 1 shows a summary of the interviews with children and parents of the control group who used magnetic boards. Three factors influenced the children's motivation: rewards and appreciation, hands-on experience, and physical learning tools. "Reward and Appreciation" was the external motivation from the teacher (through ZOOM) and adult assistants through gifts, praise, and help. "Reward and Appreciation" contributed to increasing learning motivation. "Hands-On Experience" is a learning experience of children through physical touch in a project-based oriented activity. "Hands-On Experience" influenced the increase in learning motivation. "Hands-On Experience" was lacking in the control group. It did not increase the children's learning motivation because they observed the computer screen operated by the teacher. Figure 2 shows the interview results for the experimental group showed that three factors, namely, "Reward and Appreciation", "Hands-On Experience", and "Physical Learning Tools", increased learning motivation.

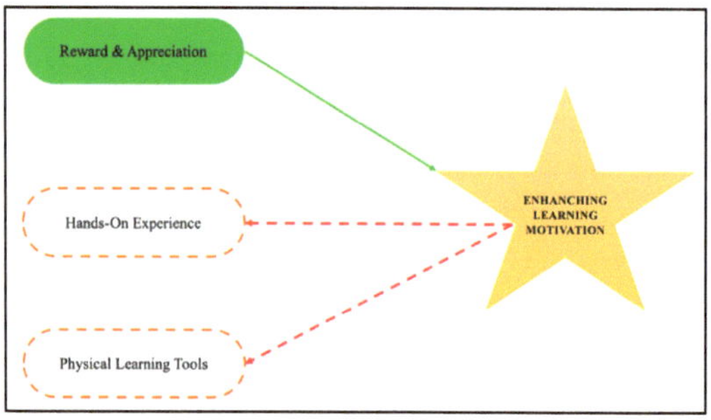

Figure 1. Control group interview summary.

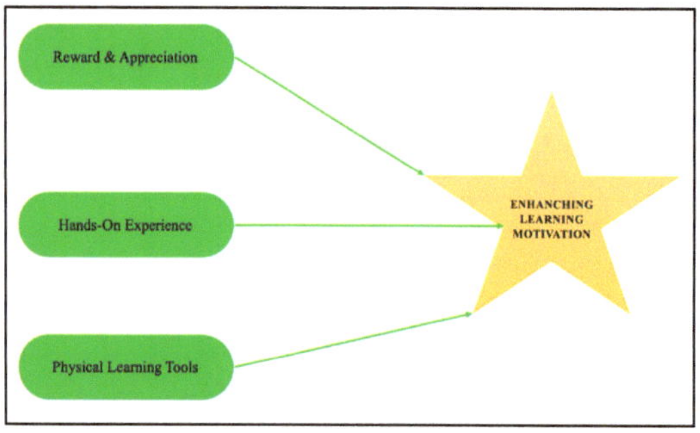

Figure 2. Experimental group interview summary.

5. Discussion

5.1. Enthusiasm and Activeness

Children in the control class were less focused on learning because their focus was distracted by other things. After all, the media could not attract their attention. In the experimental class, children seemed more active in paying attention and following the instructions given by the teacher, answering questions, and working on the problems. With the physical magnetic board, children participated in activities involving handwork and brainwork simultaneously. In learning, there are other things that children can do themselves, and they are actively involved in an object besides listening to the teacher's explanation [18]. In the control class, however, children only listened and paid attention to the material displayed by the teacher through the screen, so this made children quickly bored in the learning process.

5.2. Children's Perseverance

Most children in the experimental class were enthusiastic and preferred to study independently. They were influenced by their curiosity about the media and the material presented. The children preferred to stick to the objects on the magnetic board. In the control class, the level of the children's desire to solve the problems was lower because the children needed help from parents who guided them and from teachers who directed them. However, the level of desire of children in the control class on problems was higher because they felt bored with learning using the same media. When the teacher gave questions to answer, the enthusiasm of children in the control and experimental classes was similar. The children were influenced by the reward. The rewards affected the student's learning motivation [19]. The children were enthusiastic about answering the teacher's questions and greatly desired to answer correctly.

5.3. Usability and Benefits of Media

The media used in the control and experimental classes functioned appropriately. Learning media clarifies learning materials in the classroom [20]. According to the children, learning media, animation media, and physical magnetic boards facilitated their understanding of the material and made it easier for them to answer questions from the teacher. In the experimental class, the media made teaching and learning activities conducive. Meanwhile, in the control class, it was not conducive; children often had to be redirected by teachers or parents who guided them to refocus and pay attention to learning.

5.4. Children's Interest in Media

The children preferred the magnetic board media to the animation media. In addition, children in the experimental class stated that using physical magnetic board media made them happier and more enthusiastic about learning. The children in the experimental class achieved more in several aspects using magnetic board media. Children became more enthusiastic, active, and diligent in doing tasks. A significant aspect was children's pleasure in solving problems and studying alone.

6. Conclusions

The magnetic board was used for learning Chinese online in children aged 4–5 years and affected student learning motivation. Highly motivated students successfully achieved this in several aspects. Classroom action research provides a sustainable improvement in learning planning and implementation. Education institutions need to develop magnetic board media to attract children's attention more creatively and innovatively. Teachers need to explore further teaching techniques using magnetic board media to master materials or combine various learning media. The advice for young parents can be used for successful online learning using physical learning media.

Author Contributions: Conceptualization, J.J. and D.C.; Methodology, D.C.; software, D.C.; validation, J.J.; formal analysis, J.J.; investigation, D.C.; resources, D.C.; data curation, J.J.; writing—original draft preparation, J.J.; writing—review and editing, J.J.; visualization, D.C.; supervision, J.J.; project administration, J.J. All authors have read and agreed to the published version of the manuscript.

Funding: This research received no external funding.

Institutional Review Board Statement: Ethical review and approval were waived for this study because the participants were voluntarily involved. It is because it is a journey for their learning-supported tools.

Informed Consent Statement: Patient consent was waived for this study because the participants were voluntarily involved.

Data Availability Statement: The original contributions presented in the study are included in the article, further inquiries can be directed to the corresponding author.

Conflicts of Interest: The authors declare no conflicts of interest.

References

1. Clark, B.A. First- and Second-Language Acquisition in Early Childhood. In *Early Childhood Education: Curriculum, Teacher Education, & Dissemination of Information*; University of Illinois at Urbana-Champaign: Champaign, IL, USA, 2000; pp. 181–188.
2. Al-Harbi, S.S. Language Development and Acquisition in Early Childhood. *EduLearn* **2019**, *14*, 69–73. [CrossRef]

3. Lin, Y. *A Sociocultural Approach to the Study of Motivation and Attitudes towards the Learning of Mandarin Chinese in the U.S.: Secondary School Children' Perceptions*; Columbia University: New York, NY, USA, 2013.
4. Tatminingsih, S.; Oktarianingsih, T.; Jovanka, D.R. Online Learning for Early Childhood (Case Study in Indonesia). *J. Southwest Jiaotong Univ.* **2021**, *56*, 11. [CrossRef]
5. Lestari, R.; Astuti, B.; Bhakti, C.P. A Comprehensive Teacher Strategy for Successful Online Learning Process. *Int. J. Educ. Insight* **2020**, *1*, 1. [CrossRef]
6. Firdaus, F. Improving Children' Vocabulary Achievement Through Magnetic Board Media. *J. MELT* **2018**, *3*, 173. [CrossRef]
7. Georgiev, V.; Nikolova, A. Tools for Creating and Presenting Online Learning Resources for Preschool Kids. *TEM J.* **2020**, *9*, 1692–1696. [CrossRef]
8. Barabási, T. The Situation of Online Preschool "Learning" from Early Childhood Teachers' Perspective. *ADN* **2021**, *14*, 216–230. [CrossRef]
9. Lieberman, D.A.; Bates, C.H.; So, J. Young Children's Learning with Digital Media. *Comput. Sch.* **2009**, *26*, 271–283. [CrossRef]
10. Bari, S. Using An Effective Online Learning Media on Student's Outcome. *J. Engl. Ibrahimy* **2022**, *1*, 54–60. [CrossRef]
11. Guran, A.-M.; Cojocar, G.S.; Dioşan, L.S. Developing Smart Edutainment for Preschoolers: A Multidisciplinary Approach. In Proceedings of the 2nd ACM SIGSOFT International Workshop on Education through Advanced Software Engineering and Artificial Intelligence, Virtual, 9 November 2020; ACM: New York, NY, USA, 2020; pp. 20–26. [CrossRef]
12. Akbar, Z.; Tohar, K. Fundamental Movement Skills and Sensory Movement Strategies to Support Online Learning in Early Childhood. *JPES* **2021**, *21*, 2364–2371.
13. Hasanah, U.; Umam, A.K.; Muslimah, K.; Rahmatika, A.; Marga, A.A. The Impact of Online Learning on Early Childhood Social Behavior in Tk Pertiwi 2 Sidodadi Pekalongan Lampung Timur. *J. Child. Dev.* **2021**, *1*, 46–52. [CrossRef]
14. Chung, C.M.; Mak, S.Y.; Suen, Y.M.; Sze, P. Game-Display Board Activities for Science Teaching. *J. Sci. Educ. Technol.* **1996**, *5*, 141–154. [CrossRef]
15. Carozzi, A.V. A Magnetic Board as Teaching Aid for Historical Geology. *J. Geol. Educ.* **1964**, *12*, 28–30. [CrossRef]
16. Munawar, M.; Roshayanti, F.; Sugiyanti. STEAM-Based Learning Through Magnetic Book: Efforts to Introduce Science Inquiry for Early Children. In Proceedings of the 2nd International Conference on Education and Social Science Research (ICESRE 2019), Semarang, Indonesia, 19 October 2019; Atlantis Press: Kota Semarang, Indonesia, 2020. [CrossRef]
17. Ismail, M.E.; Yunus, F.A.N.; Sulaiman, J.; Nordin, N.; Sa'adan, N. The Implication of Employing Magnetic Test Kit on Children' Interest, Teachers' Teaching Method and Children' Visualization Ability. *Ujer* **2020**, *8*, 3858–3863. [CrossRef]
18. Susanto, A. *Teori Belajar Dan Pembelajaran Di Sekolah Dasar*; Kencana Prenadamedia Group: Jakarta, Indonesia, 2013.
19. Uno, H.B. *Teori Motivasi Dan Pengukurannya*; Bumi Aksara: Jakarta, Indonesia, 2013.
20. Rusman, M.P. *Belajar Dan Pembelajaran Berorientasi Standar Proses Pendidikan*; Rusman: Jakarta, Indonesia, 2017.

engineering proceedings

Proceeding Paper

Regression Analysis to Identify Relationship between Service Failure, Service Recovery, Customer Satisfaction and Loyalty in Food Delivery Platform †

You-Jie Huang [1,*], Shu-Chia Chang [1], Yi-Shin Lin [2], Ho-Yi Chan [1] and Wei-Ting Chang [1]

1 Department of Leisure Services Management, Chaoyang University of Technology, Taichung 413310, Taiwan; b0237@g.tmhs.tc.edu.tw (S.-C.C.); s11126601@gm.cyut.edu.tw (H.-Y.C.); s11126606@gm.cyut.edu.tw (W.-T.C.)
2 Department of Living Sciences, National Open University, Nantou 540003, Taiwan; yishin10106@gmail.com
* Correspondence: a2470712@cyut.edu.tw

† Presented at the 2024 IEEE 4th International Conference on Electronic Communications, Internet of Things and Big Data, Taipei, Taiwan, 19–21 April 2024.

Abstract: We explored the relationship and impact of service failures, acceptance of service recovery strategy, post-recovery satisfaction, and loyalty in the food delivery service industry. We used the convenience sampling method and adopted an online questionnaire survey on food delivery services for consumers aged 19 to above 30. Service failure, service recovery strategy acceptance, post-recovery satisfaction, and loyalty scales were explored. A total of 128 valid responses were analyzed for descriptive statistics, *t*-test and one-way analysis of variance, Pearson correlation analysis, and regression analysis. Missing food items was the most common and most serious service failure. Providing a refund was the most efficient service recovery strategy. If the service recovery strategy was handled properly, it effectively improved satisfaction and loyalty after service recovery was applied. If the service charge of delivery platforms increased, consumers mostly reduced the usage of the service. Therefore, delivery staff need to check whether the meal was correctly delivered. If service failures occur, active care or apologies must be made with the refund. Delivery platform must avoid increased service change and consumers would use the platform stably.

Keywords: service failures; service recovery strategy; food delivery service

Citation: Huang, Y.-J.; Chang, S.-C.; Lin, Y.-S.; Chan, H.-Y.; Chang, W.-T. Regression Analysis to Identify Relationship between Service Failure, Service Recovery, Customer Satisfaction and Loyalty in Food Delivery Platform. *Eng. Proc.* **2024**, *74*, 28. https://doi.org/10.3390/engproc2024074028

Academic Editors: Shu-Han Liao, Teen-Hang Meen and Cheng-Fu Yang

Published: 29 August 2024

1. Introduction

The world's first online ordering system was launched by Pizza Hut in 1994, and today, online ordering has become a billion-dollar industry. In 2021, the revenue of the global online ordering industry reached USD 302.826 billion, and the growth rate is expected to be 9.89% from 2021 to 2025, of which USD 172.243 billion will come from food delivery services [1]. Nowadays, online ordering through delivery services has become common, and the use of delivery services is even more likely to exceed online ordering transactions directly with stores. Driven by the pandemic, international food delivery service companies such as FoodPanda and UberEats have expanded their business to deliver goods based on online food delivery services [2]. The domestic food delivery service industry is booming with the opportunity given by the epidemic, and the main user group in China is 20–30 years old. The advantage of delivery platforms lies in preferential promotional activities, brand image, and service quality of delivery people in the service process [3,4]. Scholars have proposed that the profit of food delivery service platforms depends on the number of orders, and this type of delivery service is not appropriate for other markets, and a minimum city size is required to maintain operating profits [5]. It is difficult for companies to maintain the penetration rate of food delivery services in the market.

According to the statistics of the Consumer Protection Division of the Executive Yuan (2021), there were 1977 consumer complaints on online food delivery platform services in 2020, while there were 566 consumer complaints from January to April 2021, which was not significantly improved compared with 564 in the same period of the previous year. The service failure of food delivery platforms continues to occur, and the situation of post-recovery satisfaction in service recovery has not been researched. Effective service recovery is important for online traders to maintain customer satisfaction and loyalty [6]. Therefore, in this study, under the shrinkage of food delivery platform services, the current situation of service failures of food delivery services was explored for the post-recovery satisfaction of different service recovery strategies by analyzing the relationship between post-recovery satisfaction and loyalty using food delivery service. We also examined the effectiveness of post-recovery satisfaction after the occurrence of food delivery services failing to provide a reference for operators in their management policies.

2. Literature Review

2.1. Food Delivery Service

The F&B industry is moving from traditional brick-and-mortar operations to online transactions, with alternative systems emerging from supplier procurement to customer-facing ordering, home delivery, and delivery services [7]. In the past, F&B providers provided online ordering services on their official websites, but food delivery service platforms have opened up a new era of online ordering, where customers can choose from different F&B providers on the platform. In the early days, most online ordering platforms were serviced for restaurant reservations, where customers replaced telephone ordering online, and the platform was responsible for collecting customers' orders. After the ordering information was forwarded to the restaurant, customers chose the store or the restaurant to arrange delivery. In contrast, new online delivery platform companies have built their logistics networks to provide delivery services to restaurants that do not have self-delivery [8]. The development of online ordering services is divided into three stages: (1) enterprises operating their online ordering systems, (2) collecting customers' orders through platforms, and (3) collecting customers' orders and arranging delivery services through platforms. Food delivery service platforms enhance the efficiency of market matchmaking and allow consumers to share information through a consumer evaluation mechanism to increase restaurant choices through the platform and obtain a better consumer experience [9].

2.2. Service Failures

Food delivery services have four characteristics, namely Intangibility, Heterogeneity, Inseparability, and Perishability, collectively known as IHIP [10]. From the perspective of the service process, service failures refer to unexpected negative situations during service delivery [11]. If service failures are defined from the perspective of customers, it refers to companies failing to meet customer expectations and requirements [12]. Service failures are inevitable in the service industry [13]. Service failures must be discussed in terms of frequency, time, and severity. From the perspective of social exchange theory, service failure is divided into outcome failure and process failure, outcome failure is related to the economic benefits obtained by customers from services, and process failure is the fault of customers in the process of obtaining services [14,15]. Any service failure in the service process may leave customers with a negative feeling [16], bring negative service evaluation to the enterprise, and reduce customers' willingness to repurchase. Thus, the enterprise needs to manage the different types of service failures through different service recovery strategies to reduce the impact on the enterprise.

2.3. Service Recovery Strategy

Mistakes are inevitable in the service process, and customers are often left dissatisfied and disappointed, and the service provider then needs to take compensatory actions and measures to eliminate negative evaluations by the customer and remedy the relationship between the two parties [17]. This process is called the service recovery strategy [18]. The service recovery strategy is classified into psychological remedies and substantive [15]. Psychological remedies are intangible; i.e., the delivery person shows concern in a respectful and empathetic manner, explains the reason for the mistake, admits negligence, and apologizes. Substantive remedies are physical and tangible compensation measures, including giveaways, discount compensation, proposed discount coupons, refunds, and free or additional monetary compensation.

2.4. Post-Recovery Satisfaction

The degree of customer satisfaction in the service process is called the first satisfaction. In the event of a service failure, the enterprise provides corresponding service recovery actions for the service failure situation, and the customer will be satisfied with the suitability of the service recovery strategy, also known as post-recovery satisfaction [19,20]. If the service recovery is not satisfactory, the post-recovery satisfaction may be lower than the first satisfaction, and conversely, the post-recovery satisfaction will be higher than the first satisfaction if the service recovery strategy is appropriate [21,22]. The effectiveness of a service recovery strategy can be measured by post-recovery satisfaction, which can not only reduce the impact of service failures but also lead to a higher level of recognition. Previous studies confirmed that post-recovery satisfaction affects customers' loyalty to the company, as well as the subsequent trust and commitment relationship with the company [23,24].

2.5. Loyalty

The customer's continuous preference is defined by the product or service and the willingness to repurchase, that is, customer loyalty [25], via four facets: cross-buying intention, price tolerance, willingness to recommend a brand or company to others, and willingness to repurchase [26]. We researched service failures in the context of online shopping, the types of service failures in online transactions, and the impact of service recovery strategy on remediation satisfaction and loyalty. The customers of process failure are biased towards psychological remedies, and substantive remediation can improve remediation satisfaction and loyalty, and remediation satisfaction and loyalty have a significant positive impact. Online merchants need to focus more on the benefits of the service recovery strategy and post-remediation satisfaction [27]. Loyalty must be considered as the concept of whether the food delivery service is regarded as trustworthy and recommended to others, and whether the food delivery service is used if the service fee is increased. Previous studies confirmed that there is a significant positive relationship between post-recovery satisfaction and customer loyalty [26,28,29].

3. Research Methodology

3.1. Subjects

According to the results of an online survey conducted by Kantar Insight and LifePoints in July 2019, young people aged 20–30 used food delivery services mostly (Wang, 2021). The questionnaire in this study was designed for the consumer groups of 19–30-year-olds. It was distributed from 20 October to 20 November 2021, using online questionnaire sampling, and after the formal questionnaire was established and modified by an information and validity analysis, 300 questionnaires were issued and tested (Figure 1).

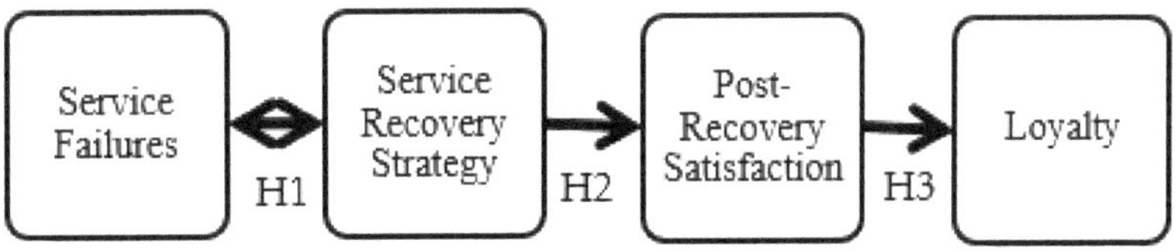

Figure 1. Research framework.

3.2. Research Method

Based on the literature review, the following hypotheses were proposed.

H1: *There is a significant relationship between different service failures and the acceptance of different service recovery strategies.*

H2: *Service recovery has a significant positive impact on post-recovery satisfaction.*

H3: *Post-recovery satisfaction has a significant positive impact on loyalty.*

4. Results and Discussion

This study was conducted from 20 October to 20 November 2021, using a snowballing online questionnaire to explore the relationship between food delivery service failures, service recovery, post-recovery satisfaction, and loyalty. Food delivery service consumers who had experienced service failures were used as the research subjects. A total of 246 questionnaires were collected in this survey, and 221 were validated with a rate of 89.8%. Among them, 128 encountered service failures of the delivery platform.

4.1. Demographics of Subjects

Gender, marital status, age, occupation, average monthly income, weekly food delivery service costs, and service failure experience were analyzed. Overall, 73.4% of the respondents were females and 26.5% were males; 83.6% were unmarried, while 16.4% were married; 31.5% were students, and 1.6% were employed; and 43.8% had an average monthly income of CNY 20,001–40,000, while 2.3% earned CNY 60,001–80,000. For the weekly food delivery service, 35.9% spent CNY 201–500, and 2.3% spent CNY 1101–1400. FoodPanda (76.6%) was the most favored platform.

4.1.1. Service Failure

Service failures included four process failures and seven outcome failures. The largest number of "outcome failures" was three. Missing food and beverage products garnered 86 responses, followed by "process failure" with 2 "improper delivery speeds". A total of 69 respondents experienced "10. No refunds will be given for cancellations" for "process failure". The largest number of the respondents experienced "3. Missing food and beverage products" as the outcome failure of the merchant not preparing the product and the delivery staff not confirming the item, and "2. Improper delivery speed" refers to the process failure of the delivery personnel on the platform who did not deliver on time.

4.1.2. Severity Analysis of Service Failures

The severity of service failures was scored from 1 to 5. The more serious the failure, the higher the score. The more serious ones were "3. Missing food and beverage products", and "10. No refunds will be given for cancellations". The average score was 3.36 for "6. Lack of food hygiene". The item "4. Cutlery problem" under "process failure" scored 3.4. The most serious failure item was "3. Missing food and beverage products", indicating that the respondents could not accept it. The least serious failure item was "4. Cutlery problem", indicating that the respondents did not particularly care about the cutlery problem.

4.2. Number and Severity of Service Errors

Service recovery strategy acceptance refers to which service recovery strategy satisfies customers after encountering service failures. It includes four items for substantive remedies and four items for psychological remedies. The average score was 3.69. From the perspective of "psychological remedies", the average score was 3.79. The failure item "3. The platform gives this consumption free of charge" scored 4.01, and "The platform provides a coupon for the next consumption" scored the lowest. The respondent's favorite service recovery strategy was to be provided free consumption in such an event.

4.3. Acceptance of Service Remediation Strategies

Post-recovery satisfaction included three items. The average score was 3.49. The item "3. Overall, I am satisfied with the remediation of the error" scored 3.51, "1. Overall, I gave a positive rating to the response to the food delivery service's handling error" scored 3.49, and "2. Overall, I am satisfied with the way the service handled the error" scored 3.47 on average. The respondents supported post-recovery satisfaction.

4.4. Loyalty

Loyalty refers to the respondent's use and trust of food delivery service. The average score for loyalty was 3.06. The item "1. I still consider the food delivery service to be trusted" scored 3.33. "3. Assuming the food delivery service charges go up, I will still use the food delivery service" scored 2.55, indicating that if the platform raised charges, the respondents reduced the number of the uses of the platform.

4.5. Service Failures and Service Recovery Strategy Acceptance

Service failures included seven items and outcome failure included three items. The items were multiple-choice questions. The number of choices was the score for the service failures and outcome failure. Pearson correlation analysis was conducted for the service recovery of substantive remedies and psychological remedies. Process failure had a negative correlation with psychological remedies, which means that the respondents wanted to obtain psychological remedies for service failures (Table 1).

Table 1. Correlation between service failures and service recovery strategy acceptance.

		Substantive	Psychological Remedies
Process failure	Pearson correlation	−0.008	−0.257 **
	significance (two-tail)	0.925	0.003
	amount	128	128
Outcome Failure	Pearson correlation	0.026	−0.115
	significance (two-tail)	0.775	0.194
	amount	128	128

** $p < 0.01$.

The item "10. No refunds will be given for cancellations" under "process failure" was significantly different from psychological remedies. The number of the respondents who experienced "10. No refunds will be given for cancellations" was larger than that of those experiencing "10. No refunds will be given for cancellations". When consumers encountered "10. No refunds will be given for cancellations", they were not willing to obtain substantive remedies. Thus, H1 was supported (Table 2).

Table 2. Service failures and service compensation.

Classification	Question	Remedies	T
Process failure	1. The service attitude of the delivery staff is not good	Substantive Psychological	0.300 1.701
Process failure	2. Improper delivery speed	Substantive Psychological	−0.811 0.595
Outcome failure	3. Missing food and beverage products	Substantive Psychological	−0.898 −0.367
Process failure	4. Cutlery problem	Substantive Psychological	0.068 0.724
Outcome failure	5. Lack of food and beverage quality	Substantive Psychological	0.456 1.115
Outcome failure	6. Lack of food hygiene	Substantive Psychological	0.237 0.331
Outcome failure	7. Meals are sold out	Substantive Psychological	−0.337 1.709
Process failure	8. Billing errors	Substantive Psychological	−0.502 0.515
Process failure	9. Orders cannot be canceled	Substantive Psychological	0.010 1.785
Process failure	10. No refunds will be given for cancellations	Substantive Psychological	0.110 2.091 *
Process failure	11. The preferential policies of the platform are not clear	Substantive Psychological	1.176 1.117

* $p < 0.05$.

4.6. Impact of Service Recovery Strategy Acceptance on Post-Recovery Satisfaction

Service recovery (Beta: 0.571) positively impacted post-recovery satisfaction, and the amount of inspection variation was 32.0%, indicating that if the platform improves service recovery, it improves post-recovery satisfaction. This supported H2 (Table 3).

Table 3. Analysis of the impact of service recovery strategy acceptance on post-recovery satisfaction.

Model	Standardized Coefficient Beta Allocation	t	Significance
(Constant)		3.786	0.000
Service recovery	0.571	7.799	0.000
F	60.817		
Significance	0.000		
R^2	0.320		
Dependent variable: Post-recovery satisfaction			

Substantive remedies and psychological remedies positively impacted post-recovery satisfaction. Substantive remedies (Beta: 0.398) had a greater impact than psychological remedies (Beta: 0.271) on post-recovery satisfaction. The inspection variation was 32.4%. The service recovery strategy provided by the platform for substantive remedies improved post-recovery satisfaction (Table 4).

Table 4. Impact of substantive remedies and psychological remedies on post-recovery satisfaction.

Model	Standardized Coefficient Beta Allocation	t	Significance
(Constant)		3.584	0.000
substantive remedies	0.398	4.804	0.000
psychological remedies	0.271	3.274	0.001
F	31.377		
significance	0.000		
R^2	0.324		
Dependent variable: Post-recovery satisfaction			

4.7. Impact of Post-Recovery Satisfaction on Loyalty

Post-recovery satisfaction (Beta: 0.6392) significantly impacted loyalty, and the variation was 47.4%, indicating that the improvement of post-recovery satisfaction improved platform loyalty. Thus, H3 was supported (Table 5).

Table 5. Post-recovery satisfaction on loyalty.

Model	Standardized Coefficient Beta Allocation	t	Significance
(Constant)		1.837	0.069
Post-Recovery Satisfaction	0.692	10.748	0.000
F	115.516		
significance	0.000		
R^2	0.474		
Dependent variable: loyalty			

5. Conclusions

Service failures in online delivery and food and beverage services were explored in this study. The most serious failures include "3. Missing food and beverage products" and "10. No refunds will be given for cancellations". When food and beverage products were missed from orders, the service provider lost customers. In terms of service recovery strategy acceptance, psychological remedies were more important than substantive remedies. "3. The platform gives this consumption for free" was the item with the greatest level of acceptance, and consumers were less likely to obtain psychological remedies when they encountered a process failure, especially for "10. No refunds will be given for cancellations". Post-recovery satisfaction was low, and consumers were negative about the service recovery when they encountered service failures. Consumers thought it was inappropriate and were not satisfied with the way they were handled. Loyalty scores were not high, especially if the delivery service increased its fee. Consumers were found to use food delivery services less often. Service recovery strategies must be considered in food delivery services to improve the post-recovery satisfaction of customers and loyalty.

The most frequent and most severe service failure was "missing food and beverage products". Thus, it is recommended that food delivery service staff need to confirm that the store delivers precisely. If the store is busy and cannot confirm delivery, they need to confirm that the food delivery address is correct. Service recovery highly impacted customer satisfaction, and customers scored highly for "3. The platform gives this consumption for free". Thus, in food delivery services, service failures must be avoided and service recovery must be offered. Consumers were not satisfied with the service recovery of the current food delivery service platforms in general. Therefore, food delivery service platforms must provide service recovery after each service failure to improve customers' evaluations of the platform. Consumers are less likely to have their loyalty affected by fees. Therefore, it is recommended that the adjustment of service fees be minimized so that consumers can use the platform consistently.

Author Contributions: Conceptualization, Y.-J.H. and S.-C.C.; methodology, Y.-J.H. and S.-C.C.; validation, S.-C.C., Y.-S.L., H.-Y.C. and W.-T.C.; formal analysis, Y.-J.H.; investigation, S.-C.C., Y.-S.L., H.-Y.C. and W.-T.C.; resources, Y.-J.H.; data curation, S.-C.C., Y.-S.L., H.-Y.C. and W.-T.C.; writing—original draft preparation, Y.-S.L., H.-Y.C. and W.-T.C.; writing—review and editing, W.-T.C.; supervision, Y.-J.H.; project administration, Y.-J.H.; funding acquisition, Y.-J.H. All authors have read and agreed to the published version of the manuscript.

Funding: This research received no external funding.

Institutional Review Board Statement: Not applicable.

Informed Consent Statement: Not applicable.

Data Availability Statement: Data are contained within the article.

Conflicts of Interest: The authors declare no conflict of interest.

References

1. Statista Market Forecast. Report 2021-Online Food Delivery. Available online: https://www.statista.com/outlook/dmo/eservices/online-food-delivery/worldwide (accessed on 17 October 2021).
2. Branding Now. Branding Now. Epidemic Impact. The Catering Industry Must Recognize: The 4 Major Dietary Trends of Consumers under the Epidemic Have Changed! Available online: https://branding-now.com/case-study/marketing-strategy/4-dining-habits-trend-after-covid-19/ (accessed on 5 October 2021).
3. Chai, K.W.; Ou, W.M.; Li, H.W. The mediator effects of technology readiness on the relationship between use attitude and behavior intention: A study on delivery platform foodpanda. *J. Tour. Leis. Manag.* **2021**, *9*, 11–12.
4. Tsai, Y.J. A Study on Satisfaction and loyalty of Online Delivery Platforms. unpublished.
5. Alvarez-Palau, E.J.; Calvet-Liñán, L.; Viu-Roig, M.; Gandouz, M.; Juan, A.A. Economic profitability of last-mile food delivery services: Lessons from Barcelona. *Res. Transp. Bus. Manag.* **2022**, *45*, 100659. [CrossRef]
6. Chen, Y.F.; Tsai, C.W.; Lin, H.J. An Integrated Model of service recovery Influence on Customer Satisfaction and Reuse Intentions in E-Trading. *J. Perform. Strategy Res.* **2013**, *10*, 73–101.
7. Hossain, F.; Adelaja, A.O. Consumers' Interest In Alternative Food Delivery Systems: Results From A Consumer Survey In New Jersey. *J. Food Distrib. Res.* **2000**, *31*, 1–19.
8. Hirschberg, C.; Rajko, A.; Schumacher, T.; Wrulich, M.; McKinsey & Company. The Changing Market for Food Delivery. Available online: https://www.mckinsey.com/industries/technology-media-and-telecommunications/our-insights/the-changing-market-for-food-delivery (accessed on 27 September 2021).
9. Van Alstyne, M.W.; Parker, G.G.; Choudary, S.P. Pipelines, platforms, and the new rules of strategy. *Harv. Bus. Rev.* **2016**, *94*, 54–62.
10. Parasuraman, A.; Zeithaml, V.A.; Berry, L.L. A conceptual model of service quality and its implications for future research. *J. Mark.* **1985**, *49*, 41–50. [CrossRef]
11. Maxham, J.G., III. Service recovery's influence on consumer satisfaction, positive word-of-mouth, and purchase intentions. *J. Bus. Res.* **2001**, *54*, 11–24. [CrossRef]
12. Bitner, M.J.; Brown, S.W.; Meuter, M.L. Technology infusion in service encounters. *J. Acad. Mark. Sci.* **2000**, *28*, 138–149. [CrossRef]
13. Kelley, S.W.; Davis, M.A. Antecedents to customer expectations for service recovery. *J. Acad. Mark. Sci.* **1994**, *22*, 52–61. [CrossRef]
14. Keaveney, S.M. Customer switching behavior in service industries: An exploratory study. *J. Mark.* **1995**, *59*, 71–82. [CrossRef]
15. Smith, A.K.; Bolton, R.N.; Wagner, J. A model of customer satisfaction with service encounters involving failure and recovery. *J. Mark. Res.* **1999**, *36*, 356–372. [CrossRef]
16. Lin, Y.H.; Huang, D.; Huang, Y.L. An Analysis of the Typology of service failures and Recoveries-A Study of Sit-Down Restaurants in Taiwan. *J. Tour. Stud.* **2003**, *9*, 39–58.
17. Firnstahl, T.W. My employees are my service guarantee. *Harv. Bus. Rev.* **1989**, *67*, 28.
18. Hart, C.W.L.; Heskett, J.L.; Sasser, W.E., Jr. The Profitable Art of service recovery. *Harv. Bus. Rev.* **1990**, *68*, 148–156. [PubMed]
19. Spreng, R.A.; Harrell, G.D.; Mackoy, R.D. Service recovery: Impact on satisfaction & intentions. *J. Serv. Mark.* **1995**, *9*, 15–23.
20. Harris, K.E.; Grewal, D.; Mohr, L.A.; Bernhardt, K.L. Consumer responses to service recovery strategies: The moderating role of online versus offline environment. *J. Bus. Res.* **2006**, *59*, 425–431. [CrossRef]
21. Folkes, V.S.; Kotsos, B. Buyers' and sellers' explanations for product failure: Who done it? *J. Mark.* **1986**, *50*, 74–80. [CrossRef]
22. Smith, A.K.; Bolton, R.N. An experimental investigation of customer reactions to service failure and recovery encounters: Paradox or peril? *J. Serv. Res.* **1998**, *1*, 65–81. [CrossRef]
23. Weun, S.; Beatty, S.E.; Jones, M.A. The impact of service failure severity on service recovery evaluations and post-recovery relationships. *J. Serv. Mark.* **2004**, *18*, 133–146. [CrossRef]

24. Wang, Y.S.; Wu, S.C.; Lin, H.H.; Wang, Y.Y. The relationship of service failure severity, service recovery justice and perceived switching costs with customer loyalty in the context of e-tailing. *Int. J. Inf. Manag.* **2011**, *31*, 350–359. [CrossRef]
25. Gronholdt, L.; Martensen, A.; Kristensen, K. The relationship between customer satisfaction and loyalty: Cross-industry differences. *Total Qual. Manag.* **2000**, *11*, 509–514. [CrossRef]
26. Hsu, S.L.; Doong, H.S.; Lo, Y.P. Customer Satisfaction after Service Failure and Recovery in Online Retailing: Expectancy Disconfirmation and Perceived Justice Perspectives. *J. Perform. Manag Rev.* **2008**, *27*, 1–24.
27. Oliver, R.L. Whence consumer loyalty? *J. Mark.* **1999**, *63*, 33–44. [CrossRef]
28. Boshoff, C. An experimental study of service recovery options. *Int. J. Serv. Ind. Manag.* **1997**, *8*, 110–130. [CrossRef]
29. Kuo, Y.F.; Wu, C.M.; Yang, S.C.; Yen, S.T. Relationships among Online Shopping service failure Types, service recovery Strategies, Perceived Justice, and Satisfaction with service recovery. *J. E-Bus.* **2014**, *16*, 53–84.

engineering proceedings

Proceeding Paper

The Key Factors of Watching Live Streaming in Taiwanese Manufacturing Sectors Identified by the Analytic Hierarchy Process †

Thi-Them Hoang [1], Yung-Fu Huang [2] and Manh-Hoang Do [2,*]

1 Department of Business Administration, Chaoyang University of Technology, Taichung 413310, Taiwan; s11037911@gm.cyut.edu.tw
2 Department of Marketing and Logistics Management, Chaoyang University of Technology, Taichung 413310, Taiwan; huf@cyut.edu.tw
* Correspondence: dohoangtnu@gmail.com; Tel.: +886-4-23323000
† Presented at the 2024 IEEE 4th International Conference on Electronic Communications, Internet of Things and Big Data, Taipei, Taiwan, 19–21 April 2024.

Abstract: Live streaming has become an emerging business with a firm performance. We investigated the key factors that attract audiences to watch live streaming in the Taiwanese manufacturing industry. Nine experts in manufacturing and social media marketing participated in this study. The analytic hierarchy process (AHP) was employed to evaluate the key factors. Three main determinants were determined as a result, including audience motivation, pricing, and branding, each of which was further divided into three sub-factors. Consequently, the results revealed that the most essential factors of these three clusters were social aspects, brand design, and business trend analysis. The results also allow for an understanding of how traditional manufacturers have utilized live streaming to promote products and engage with their audience. These findings serve as a reference for Taiwanese manufacturers to incorporate live streaming into their business promotion strategies.

Keywords: live streaming; manufacturing sector; digital marketing; AHP

Citation: Hoang, T.-T.; Huang, Y.-F.; Do, M.-H. The Key Factors of Watching Live Streaming in Taiwanese Manufacturing Sectors Identified by the Analytic Hierarchy Process. *Eng. Proc.* **2024**, *74*, 29. https://doi.org/10.3390/engproc2024074029

Academic Editors: Shu-Han Liao, Teen-Hang Meen and Cheng-Fu Yang

Published: 29 August 2024

1. Introduction

People receive information through a variety of means as the Internet ecosystem continues to evolve. As a burgeoning industry, live streaming is experiencing the most rapid growth. Live streaming for online shopping has emerged as a popular marketing approach in various businesses, drawing most of its traffic from influencers producing products by live streaming. Live broadcasters use their platform to promote and encourage buyers to try the products they recommend [1]. Initially, the live broadcast presenter focused on product advertising, which led to customers having a negative experience with the product or being emotionally influenced, causing ambiguity in their decision-making. When making a purchase, consumers weigh between assurance and risk [2]. Recognizing these drawbacks, manufacturers have turned to live streaming to enhance authenticity, build customer trust, reduce uncertainty, improve brand reputation, and boost sales [3]. The growing interest of modern consumers in eco-friendly materials has led upstream manufacturers to educate consumers about the use of green products, giving rise to the concept of the green supply chain [4,5].

When the COVID-19 outbreak surged in late 2019 and early 2020, numerous places had to implement epidemic prevention measures [6]. All industries were affected, causing a significant disruption to the globalized infrastructure supporting the expansion of industrial chains [4]. Subsequent epidemic prevention measures and quarantine, alongside supply chain disruptions and other factors, led to drastic changes on both the demand and supply sides [7].

Audiences are drawn to live streaming due to social trends, information acquisition, and attractive product visual design. This form of communication is a novel approach that organizations employ for effective interactions with customers and consumers. Such direct communication yields valuable audience input essential for the business [8–10]. Moreover, analyzing the market, consumer objectives, and business products is pivotal for manufacturers aiming to compete more effectively [5]. Through consumer and live streaming viewer interactions, manufacturers can understand competition. Meanwhile, manufacturers gain by pioneering or initiating trends. Manufacturers effectively delineate their strengths, limitations, opportunities, and challenges, introducing the most competitive products to the market [10–13]. The source of the product and brand promotion hold immense importance, constituting a pivotal component of the brand's marketing strategy. Product promotion plays a significant role in enhancing brand recognition among potential consumers and in nurturing customer relationships through promotional activities or live streaming mini-games [11,14,15].

In this study, we identified and evaluated the important factors influencing live streaming deployment in the manufacturing industry. For this, we investigated what factors arise from the existing literature on live streaming uptake in manufacturing and the important factors to consider to establish live streaming in the manufacturing industry. The characteristics of key factors in the live streaming of the manufacturing industry were identified by the literature analysis and expert interviews. Criteria were determined to design surveys. We employed an analytic hierarchy process (AHP) to comprehend numerous factors and provide a precise direction for the manufacturing industry to perform live streaming in the future.

2. Literature Review

Live streaming is one of the most popular e-commerce sales strategies, significantly shaping both consumers' purchasing behavior and corporate management. It involves the real-time transmission of audio and video content over the Internet [16]. The interactive nature of live streaming allows hosts to engage directly with the audience [17,18]. This form of communication has recently become a fundamental component of e-commerce. With the escalating prevalence of live streaming for shopping, a growing number of manufacturers are establishing channels to directly engage with customers or seek out new agents [16]. Many manufacturers are broadening their reach, integrating live streaming to enhance sales and to bolster consumer understanding of products and brands [19,20].

The impact of live streaming shopping on consumers' purchase intent is significant. Factors such as authenticity, visual appeal, product pricing, design, and authentic engagement have been demonstrated to significantly influence consumers' purchasing decisions [21]. The credibility, impact, and professionalism of the host positively shape customers' buying intent [22]. Hence, live streaming merges the perspectives of hosts and consumers on product quality, enabling manufacturers to refine their optimal strategies [20,23].

In terms of the production industry, live streaming channels exhibit characteristics such as commission rates, fixed fees, and specific fan quotas, alongside unique sales channels or contracts. The potential profitability and advantages of live streaming prompt numerous manufacturers to eagerly initiate their live streaming channels [24]. The competitive intensity concerning pricing, channel market share, and commission rates predominantly shape the sales strategy. Manufacturers establishing direct sales channels yield higher profits for the company [25].

Current research focuses on live streaming by consumer influencers or celebrities. However, we explored aspects of live streaming in the traditional production industry. While previous research was conducted to explore the efficiency of live streaming and the commissions paid by producers to marketing manufacturers, our study delves into the factors that influence live streaming methods in product promotion for production businesses (see Figure 1 and Table 1).

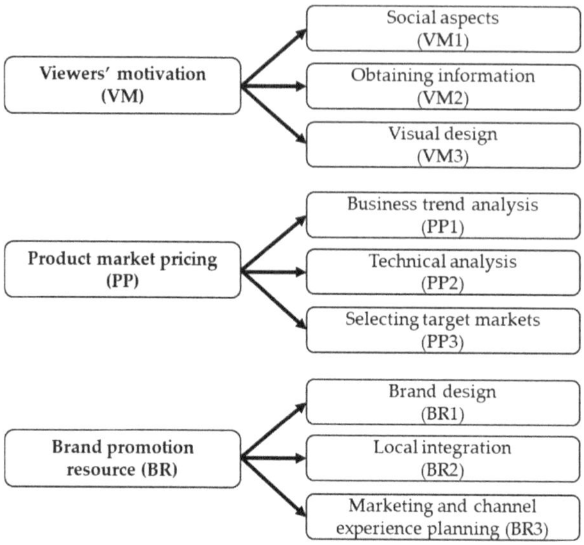

Figure 1. Proposed research model.

Table 1. Identification of critical factors and sub-factors.

No.	Code	Barriers	Description	Reference
		Viewers' motivation to watch live streaming (VM)		
1	VM1	Social aspects	Satisfy and gain social support through live streaming platforms	[8]
2	VM2	Obtaining information	Get new knowledge through live streaming platforms	[9]
3	VM3	Visual design	Viewers and live streaming manufacturers can interact, exchange information, and conduct online teaching	[10]
		Product market pricing (PP)		
1	PP1	Business trend analysis	Enterprises have a grasp of the latest business innovation directions and context. What these refer to are trends like benchmark cases and overall industry trends	[13,23]
2	PP2	Technical analysis	Collect the cross-field technologies required by enterprises when conducting design innovation to understand the implementation methods and feasibility of innovation	[12,26]
3	PP3	Selecting target markets	Strengthen the interactivity of the market, and sociality contributes to the concept of one-to-one marketing	[11]
		Brand promotion resource (BR)		
1	BR1	Brand design	Brand design in a broad sense includes strategic design, product design, and image design. Corporate image design is an aspect of brand design, and its connotation is relatively broad	[15,27]
2	BR2	Local integration	Integrate locally related resources, materials, workforce, expertise, etc. to assist in product manufacturing, sales, promotion, etc.	[14]
3	BR3	Marketing and channel experience planning	Mainly through understanding the positioning of current competitors and overall channel analysis, we develop channel-specific brand strategies, so that the marketing strategy can be fully realized in stores. Channel strategy includes distribution, price, and promotion	[28,29]

3. Research Method

3.1. AHP

The AHP is a multi-criteria decision-making tool developed by Saaty (1990), widely used in domains such as economics and politics [30]. It is a measurement method that uses pairwise comparisons and relies on expert judgment to provide priorities. The AHP method stipulates that a given problem is hierarchically decomposed and partially solved, and then the partial solutions are combined to obtain the solution to the original problem [30,31]. The subjective decision-making process can be formalized through a hierarchical structure, leading to more accurate decision-making [30]. Thus, ensuring consistent decision-making judgments is vital. Breaking down the problem into sub-problems provides a better understanding [32,33]. Comparisons are made by the team or through an iterative procedure until all team members reach an agreement (presented in Table 2). Before finalizing a decision, a sensitivity analysis is conducted to evaluate the data [30,33].

Table 2. Saaty's basic scale.

Intensity of Importance	Definition
1	Equal importance
3	Moderate importance
5	Strong importance
7	Very strong importance
9	Extreme importance

3.2. Questionnaire Design and Survey

The analytic hierarchy process was conducted to assess each component based on the relative importance of paired factors, comparing and judging them based on different facets. The descriptions below cover the purpose of the questionnaire design; its content, revising status, and survey objects; and the methodology for the questionnaire analysis. Each element at every level is an evaluation standard for pairwise comparisons in the content design. The questionnaire on a scale of 1 to 9, designed for professionals and scholars, was distributed via email for assessment. Invited experts completed the questionnaire, and the data were analyzed for multiple pairwise comparisons. The Expert Choice 2000 software was used to calculate the eigenvalues, eigenvectors, and the essential matrix with each ratio. The respondents for this questionnaire comprised executives from manufacturing and digital marketing manufacturers, showcasing their extensive expertise in manufacturing and their ability to effectively evaluate critical aspects in manufacturing live streaming.

4. Result and Discussion

4.1. Ranking

The weight of the "Manufacturing Live-streaming Evaluation Scale" was calculated based on the overall structural weight. Table 3 shows the weights and rankings of the scale components in this study.

Table 3. Ranking of factors.

Factor	Weight	Relative Ranking
Viewers' motivation to watch live streaming (VM)	0.649	1
Product market pricing (PP)	0.247	2
Brand promotion resource (BR)	0.104	3

The relative importance of the factors was determined through the previously established hierarchical evaluation framework using the AHP questionnaire. The Expert Choice 2000 was used to calculate the weight and consistency of each level of the questionnaire and obtain the index weights of each evaluation aspect, as shown in Table 4.

Table 4. Weights and evaluation index of factors.

Code	C.R	Decision
VM	0.030	Accept
VM1	0.001	Accept
VM2	0.003	Accept
VM3	0.004	Accept
PP	0.009	Accept
PP1	0.005	Accept
PP2	0.006	Accept
PP3	0.007	Accept
BR	0.010	Accept
BR1	0.009	Accept
BR2	0.008	Accept
BR3	0.001	Accept

4.2. Discussions

To recognize the need, the manufacturing industry must adapt its business practices for the next generation. Apart from improving performance, industry leaders must prioritize the integration of new technologies to set the pace as a model for future manufacturers. The most essential critical criteria for manufacturing live streaming were "Viewers' motivation to watch live streaming," "product market pricing," and "brand promotion resources." The most essential characteristics of "Viewers' motivation to watch live streaming" were "social aspects", "brand promotion resources", "brand design", product market pricing", and "business trend analysis" (presented in Table 5). The convenience that consumers obtain from retailers' live marketing efforts benefits merchants in a variety of ways (Figure 2). The ability to live stream shopping activities on e-commerce platforms is widely valued [8–10]. Product strategies and business trends used by corporations to deliver benefits and economic benefits to manufacturers are significant, and manufacturers must develop their plans precisely [14,15].

Table 5. Factor weighting and ranking.

Sub-Factor	Weight	Overall Weight	Ranking
VM1	0.663	0.428	1
VM2	0.238	0.154	3
VM3	0.099	0.064	6
PP1	0.652	0.163	2
PP2	0.271	0.068	4
PP3	0.077	0.019	8
BR1	0.647	0.068	4
BR2	0.271	0.029	7
BR3	0.081	0.009	9

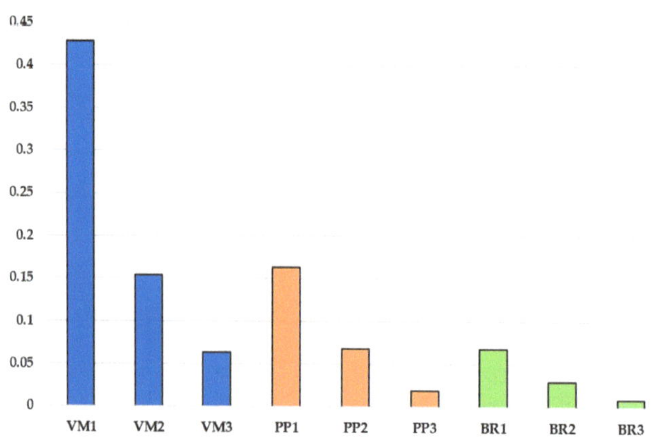

Figure 2. Overall weight ranking of all sub-factors.

COVID-19 has significantly disrupted the operations of numerous industries, leading to the cancellation or postponement of large-scale marketing initiatives and exhibitions. Global supply networks and essential industries have been significantly affected, posing new operational challenges for many small- and medium-sized businesses [7]. This crisis has changed people's purchasing habits from physical to online shopping. To address the challenges posed by the pandemic, many companies have embraced live streaming as an emergent business activity [4,34]. Traditional manufacturing industries have transitioned into providers of manufacturing services. Leveraging live streaming platforms, these industries are exploring new business formats and models to facilitate transformation and upgrading [21]. By investigating the factors of manufacturing live streaming, the result of this study provides a reference for the future development of the manufacturing industry in the direction of live streaming.

5. Conclusions

Online live streaming has emerged as a new and pivotal business activity. In this study, the most effective approach for the manufacturing industry was identified to offer a framework for manufacturing live streaming. The results assist enterprises in mitigating operational blind spots and maximizing commercial rewards. We prioritized the variables of utmost importance, such as "selecting target markets", "marketing and channel experience planning," "business trend analysis", "information acquisition", "local integration", "visual design", "technical analysis", "brand design", and "social aspects". The global epidemic has significantly impacted industries and hindered economic development and the mid- and long-term business goals of manufacturers. Smart manufacturing mitigates losses during this struggle. Manufacturers face significant challenges when the global economy becomes unstable. By adapting and investigating the factors in this study, future research and exploration can be directed. Future research is necessary to include big data, artificial intelligence, cloud computing, and Taiwan's industrial transformation. Then, updated theoretical foundations and practical guidelines can be acquired. The factors of new business activities for traditional manufacturing industries are used for reference. Based on the research findings, the following practical applications are proposed for traditional manufacturing manufacturers.

The professionalization of enterprise's live streaming and the enhancement of the ecosystem are demanded. Live streaming needs to be refined for professional operations, accompanied by a comprehensive industrial chain. To prevent content homogeneity, platforms must differentiate themselves using product and format innovations. Strengthening the anchor ecosystem's construction bolsters platform advantages to gain a competitive edge and win users in a fiercely competitive environment. Various live streaming application scenarios are evolving as the live broadcast market is increasingly segmented and vertically developed, spanning multiple industries such as finance, education, training, and medical care. These scenarios for larger companies are categorized into internal and external services. Internally, companies can utilize live streaming for corporate training, expert lectures, and internal meetings, prioritizing privacy and interaction in the live streaming environment. Externally, the company needs to leverage live streaming technology for marketing in seminars, meetings, events, and exhibitions. In addition to using reliable technical services, a significant focus needs to be put on content promotion and traffic direction to aid businesses in retaining existing clients and attracting new customers. For small- and medium-sized organizations, live video services are emphasized in marketing activities, leveraging public and private traffic sources to promote their activities, empower enterprise development, and achieve traffic conversion.

Author Contributions: Conceptualization, T.-T.H. and Y.-F.H.; methodology, T.-T.H. and M.-H.D.; validation, Y.-F.H. and T.-T.H.; formal analysis, T.-T.H.; investigation, T.-T.H.; resources, T.-T.H.; data curation, T.-T.H.; writing—original draft preparation, M.-H.D. and T.-T.H.; writing—review and editing, T.-T.H. and M.-H.D.; visualization, T.-T.H.; supervision, Y.-F.H.; and project administration, Y.-F.H. and M.-H.D. All authors have read and agreed to the published version of the manuscript.

Funding: This research received no external funding.

Institutional Review Board Statement: Not applicable.

Informed Consent Statement: Not applicable.

Data Availability Statement: Data sharing is not applicable to this article.

Acknowledgments: The authors thank the chief editor and the reviewers for their valuable comments to improve the manuscript.

Conflicts of Interest: All authors declare no conflicts of interest in this paper.

References

1. Zhang, S.; Huang, C.; Li, X.; Ren, A. Characteristics and Roles of Streamers in E-Commerce Live Streaming. *Serv. Ind. J.* **2022**, *42*, 1001–1029. [CrossRef]
2. Hu, M.; Chaudhry, S.S. Enhancing Consumer Engagement in E-Commerce Live Streaming via Relational Bonds. *Internet Res.* **2020**, *30*, 1019–1041. [CrossRef]
3. Ming, J.; Jianqiu, Z.; Bilal, M.; Akram, U.; Fan, M. How Social Presence Influences Impulse Buying Behavior in Live Streaming Commerce? The Role of S-O-R Theory. *Int. J. Web Inf. Syst.* **2021**, *17*, 300–320. [CrossRef]
4. Huang, Y.; Phan, V.; Do, M. The Impacts of Supply Chain Capabilities, Visibility, Resilience on Supply Chain Performance and Firm Performance. *Adm. Sci.* **2023**, *13*, 225. [CrossRef]
5. Van Phan, V.D.; Huang, Y.F.; Do, M.H. Exploring the Effect of Cognitive Factors and E-Social Interactions on the Green Purchase Intention: Evidence from a Transitional Economy. *Young Consum.* **2023**, *24*, 767–785. [CrossRef]
6. Phan, V.-D.-V.; Huang, Y.-F.; Hoang, T.-T.; Do, M.-H. Evaluating Barriers to Supply Chain Resilience in Vietnamese SMEs: The Fuzzy VIKOR Approach. *Systems* **2023**, *11*, 121. [CrossRef]
7. Do, M.-H.; Huang, Y.-F.; Phan, V.-D.-V. Analyzing the Barriers to Green Supply Chain Management Implementation: A Case Study of the Vietnamese Agriculture Sector. *J. Enterp. Inf. Manag.* **2023**, *37*, 125–147. [CrossRef]
8. Vanclay, F. International Principles for Social Impact Assessment. *Impact Assess. Proj. Apprais.* **2003**, *21*, 5–12. [CrossRef]
9. Lv, J.; Yao, W.; Wang, Y.; Wang, Z.; Yu, J. A Game Model for Information Dissemination in Live Streaming E-Commerce Environment. *Int. J. Commun. Syst.* **2022**, *35*, e5010. [CrossRef]
10. Chung, J.J.Y.; Shin, H.V.; Xia, H.; Wei, L.Y. Beyond Show of Hands: Engaging Viewers via Expressive and Scalable Visual Communication in Live Streaming. In Proceedings of the Conference on Human Factors in Computing Systems, Yokohama, Japan, 8–13 May 2021; pp. 1–14.
11. Wongkitrungrueng, A.; Dehouche, N.; Assarut, N. Live Streaming Commerce from the Sellers' Perspective: Implications for Online Relationship Marketing. *J. Mark. Manag.* **2020**, *36*, 488–518. [CrossRef]
12. Rehan, M.M.; Morsi, R.A.; ElNaggar, A. Technical Analysis on Future Challenges and Opportunities in Live P2P Streaming. In Proceedings of the 2014 International Conference on Engineering and Technology (ICET), Cairo, Egypt, 19–20 April 2014; IEEE: Piscataway, NJ, USA, 2014; pp. 1–5. [CrossRef]
13. Schonenberg, H.; Jian, J.; Sidorova, N.; Van Der Aalst, W. Business Trend Analysis by Simulation. In *Advanced Information Systems Engineering*; Lecture Notes in Computer Science (Including Subseries Lecture Notes in Artificial Intelligence and Lecture Notes in Bioinformatics); Springer: Berlin/Heidelberg, Germany, 2010; Volume 6051, pp. 515–529.
14. Selimi, M.; Apólonia, N.; Olid, F.; Freitag, F.; Navarro, L.; Moll, A.; Pueyo, R.; Veiga, L. Integration of an Assisted P2P Live Streaming Service in Community Network Clouds. In Proceedings of the IEEE 7th International Conference on Cloud Computing Technology and Science, CloudCom, Vancouver, BC, Canada, 30 November–3 December 2015; Institute of Electrical and Electronics Engineers Inc.: Piscataway, NJ, USA, 2015; pp. 202–209.
15. Montaña, J.; Guzmán, F.; Moll, I. Branding and Design Management: A Brand Design Management Model. *J. Mark. Manag.* **2007**, *23*, 829–840. [CrossRef]
16. Chou, S.W.; Hsieh, M.C.; Pan, H.C. Understanding Viewers' Information-Sharing in Live-Streaming Based on a Motivation Perspective. *Online Inf. Rev.* **2023**, *47*, 177–196. [CrossRef]
17. Sripanidkulchai, K.; Maggs, B.; Zhang, H. An Analysis of Live Streaming Workloads on the Internet. In Proceedings of the 4th ACM SIGCOMM Conference on Internet Measurement, Taormina, Italy, 25–27 October 2004; pp. 41–54.
18. Smith, T.P.B.; Obrist, M.; Wright, P. Live-Streaming Changes the (Video) Game. In Proceedings of the 11th European Conference on Interactive TV and Video, EuroITV 2013, Como, Italy, 24–26 June 2013; pp. 131–138.
19. Netland, T.; Stegmaier, M.; Primultini, C.; Maghazei, O. Interactive Mixed Reality Live Streaming Technology in Manufacturing. *Manuf. Lett.* **2023**, *38*, 6–10. [CrossRef]
20. Du, Z.; Fan, Z.P.; Sun, F. Live Streaming Sales: Streamer Type Choice and Limited Sales Strategy for a Manufacturer. *Electron. Commer. Res. Appl.* **2023**, *61*, 101300. [CrossRef]
21. Ho, C.I.; Liu, Y.; Chen, M.C. Factors Influencing Watching and Purchase Intentions on Live Streaming Platforms: From a 7Ps Marketing Mix Perspective. *Information* **2022**, *13*, 239. [CrossRef]
22. Hou, J.; Shen, H.; Xu, F. A Model of Livestream Selling with Online Influencers. *SSRN Electron. J.* **2021**. [CrossRef]

23. Wang, S.; Guo, X. Strategic Introduction of Live-Stream Selling in a Supply Chain. *Electron. Commer. Res. Appl.* **2023**, *62*, 101315. [CrossRef]
24. Zhang, T.; Tang, Z. Should Manufacturers Open Live Streaming Shopping Channels? *J. Retail. Consum. Serv.* **2023**, *71*, 103229. [CrossRef]
25. Lin, G.; Xiong, X.; Li, Y.; Zhu, X. Sales Mode Selection Strategic Analysis for Manufacturers on E-Commerce Platforms under Multi-Channel Competition. *Systems* **2022**, *10*, 234. [CrossRef]
26. Vargas, L.G. An Overview of the Analytic Hierarchy Process and Its Applications. *Eur. J. Oper. Res.* **1990**, *48*, 2–8. [CrossRef]
27. Hamilton, W.A.; Garretson, O.; Kerne, A. Streaming on Twitch: Fostering Participatory Communities of Play within Live Mixed Media. In Proceedings of the Conference on Human Factors in Computing Systems, Toronto, ON, Canada, 26 April–1 May 2014; Association for Computing Machinery: New York, NY, USA, 2014; pp. 1315–1324.
28. Hilvert-Bruce, Z.; Neill, J.T.; Sjöblom, M.; Hamari, J. Social Motivations of Live-Streaming Viewer Engagement on Twitch. *Comput. Hum. Behav.* **2018**, *84*, 58–67. [CrossRef]
29. Sjöblom, M.; Törhönen, M.; Hamari, J.; Macey, J. The Ingredients of Twitch Streaming: Affordances of Game Streams. *Comput. Hum. Behav.* **2019**, *92*, 20–28. [CrossRef]
30. Saaty, T.L. How to Make a Decision: The Analytic Hierarchy Process. *Eur. J. Oper. Res.* **1990**, *48*, 9–26. [CrossRef]
31. Baffoe, G. Exploring the Utility of Analytic Hierarchy Process (AHP) in Ranking Livelihood Activities for Effective and Sustainable Rural Development Interventions in Developing Countries. *Eval. Program Plann.* **2019**, *72*, 197–204. [CrossRef] [PubMed]
32. Lahane, S.; Kant, R. Evaluating the Circular Supply Chain Implementation Barriers Using Pythagorean Fuzzy AHP-DEMATEL Approach. *Clean. Logist. Supply Chain* **2021**, *2*, 100014. [CrossRef]
33. Mani, V.; Agrawal, R.; Sharma, V. Supplier Selection Using Social Sustainability: AHP Based Approach in India. *Int. Strateg. Manag. Rev.* **2014**, *2*, 98–112. [CrossRef]
34. He, Y.; Chen, L.; Mu, J.; Ullah, A. Optimal Contract Design for Live Streaming Shopping in a Manufacturer–Retailer–Streamer Supply Chain. *Electron. Commer. Res.* **2024**, *24*, 1071–1093. [CrossRef]

engineering proceedings

MDPI

Proceeding Paper

Utilization of Phototrophic Bacteria to Enhance Carbon Sequestration in Rice Paddy †

Alyssa Katsuyama Wang [1], Kun-Yi Kao [2,*], Yang-Cheng Kuo [3] and Rey-May Liou [2,*]

[1] Taipei American School, Taipei 111, Taiwan; cka200812@gmail.com
[2] Department of Environmental Engineering and Science, Chia-Nan University of Pharmacy and Science, Tainan 717, Taiwan
[3] Bioresource Collection and Research Center, Food Industry Research and Development Institute, Hsinchu 300, Taiwan; yck24@firdi.org.tw
* Correspondence: kristen900525@gmail.com (K.-Y.K.); mrmliou@mail.cnu.edu.tw (R.-M.L.)
† Presented at the 2024 IEEE 4th International Conference on Electronic Communications, Internet of Things and Big Data, Taipei, Taiwan, 19–21 April 2024.

Abstract: Rice paddies are a major source of agricultural greenhouse gas emissions, primarily caused by the proliferation of anaerobic, methanogenic bacteria during prolonged inundation. Phototrophic bacteria utilize light energy for metabolism and are potential candidates for carbon and nitrogen fixation, and reduction of methane gas emissions. We investigated the effect of applying the phototrophic bacterium *Rhodopseudomonas palustris* (PNSB) during the cropping period on soil organic carbon (SOC) and methane emissions for second-crop rice in the Tainan Guantian region. In the experimental group, PNSB was applied five times during the rice cultivation period. Compared to the control group, the experimental group demonstrated a significant reduction in methane emissions, especially in the tillering stage, where emissions averaged 37.26 ± 12.97 g-CH_4/m^2/season compared to 49.48 ± 25.06 g-CH_4/m^2/season of the control group. Over the entire growing season, the experimental group reduced the emission of 3.05 Mg·CO_2e/ha. Additionally, administering PNSB improved soil carbon sequestration, from 4.89 tons-C/ha in the control group to 17.45 tons-C/ha. The phototrophic bacterium PNSB was beneficial for soil carbon sequestration and reducing greenhouse gas emissions. However, further research is required to optimize the methodology of applying phototrophic bacteria for agricultural purposes.

Keywords: phototrophic bacteria; carbon sequestration; paddy fields

Citation: Wang, A.K.; Kao, K.-Y.; Kuo, Y.-C.; Liou, R.-M. Utilization of Phototrophic Bacteria to Enhance Carbon Sequestration in Rice Paddy. *Eng. Proc.* **2024**, *74*, 30. https://doi.org/10.3390/engproc2024074030

Academic Editors: Shu-Han Liao, Teen-Hang Meen and Cheng-Fu Yang

Published: 30 August 2024

1. Introduction

Global warming is mainly caused by the emission of carbon dioxide (CO_2), methane (CH_4), and nitrous oxide (N_2O). It has a large impact on human societal, agricultural, and economic activities, as well as on the global ecosystem. To curtail the greenhouse effect, the Paris Agreement proposed limiting the rise of global temperatures to 1.5 °C above pre-industrial levels. Subsequently, a 2018 report from the Intergovernmental Panel on Climate Change (IPCC) proposed net zero emissions as a goal for climate action.

Methane is a serious greenhouse gas that absorbs and retains heat considerably on the Earth's surface and in the atmosphere [1]. Its global warming potential is 25 times larger than that of carbon dioxide (CO_2) [2]. Agriculture is one of the major contributors to methane emissions, accounting for approximately 20% of global emissions. In particular, the cultivation of rice (*Oryza sativa*), which spans 153 million ha worldwide, is the main source of agricultural methane emissions [3]. In rice cultivation, the soil is constantly flooded, which promotes an anaerobic environment. This anaerobic milieu reduces the oxidative breakdown of organic matter accumulating organic carbon and provides an ideal niche for methanogenic bacteria, which break down the organic material to produce methane. The methane is subsequently released into the atmosphere through bubbling, diffusion, and plant transpiration, resulting in significant greenhouse gas emissions [4]. Therefore, proper management of rice farming must include methods that simultaneously ameliorate methane emissions and sequester organic carbon in the soil [5].

The purple non-sulfur bacteria (PNSB) are a diverse group of microbes that exist as photoautotrophs, photoheterotrophs, chemoautotrophs, and chemoheterotrophs; spanning a variety of habitats in lakes, oceans, and rice paddies. PNSB is capable of promoting plant growth through multiple mechanisms, including fixing atmospheric nitrogen into ammonium or nitrate salts, [6]; solubilizing phosphorous to promote its bioavailability [7]; synthesizing carriers that improve plant iron uptake; as well as synthesizing plant growth hormones such as 5-Aminolevulinic acid (5-ALA) [8] and Indole-3-acetic acid (IAA) [9]. Through these effects, PNSB reduces the reliance on chemical fertilizers by promoting the growth of root systems. Additionally, PNSB is tolerant to hypersaline and poor soil conditions, and aids plant growth in these situations. Considering that the anaerobic milieu of rice paddies provides a suitable niche for PNSB growth, PNSB can be used to outcompete methanogenic bacteria and reduce the breakdown of organic soil material, thus retaining organic carbon in the soil. To prove this, we evaluated the beneficial effects of adding PNSB to rice paddies on reducing methane emissions and increasing soil organic carbon content, compared to a control group of rice paddies without PNSB. The results contribute to the development of agricultural practices to reduce greenhouse gas emissions, improve yields from rice paddies, remedy soil quality, better farmers' incomes, and enhance climate change preparedness.

2. Materials and Methods

2.1. Field Trial

A field trial was conducted on second-crop rice in an experimental field in Guantian District, Tainan City, Taiwan (23°10′00.0″ N and 120°20′43.7″ E), in collaboration with the Taiwan Food Industry Research and Development Institute (FIRDI) and with local farmers. The experimental field was divided into a control group (0.2 ha) and an experimental group (0.3 ha). The fields were separated by ridges, and each possessed a separate water supply. The fertilizer management protocol for the control group was based on recommendations from the Agricultural Research and Extension Station and local farming practices. No pre-planting fertilizer was used, topdressing was applied during the seedling development and tillering phases, and earing fertilizer was used during the young panicle formation stage. Fertilizers dosed 400 kg per hectare of ammonium sulfate and Biotec Organic Compound Fertilizers #39 (Taiwan Fertilizer Co., Taipei, Taiwan). The experimental group was treated with 10–20 L of PNSB (*Rhodopseudomonas palustris*), provided by FIRDI and administered via flood irrigation.

The strain planted was Taiwan Sen glutinous 2 (TCSW2), which was cultivated for 103 days. The fertilizer management protocol for the experimental and control groups was based on recommendations from the Agricultural Research and Extension Station and local farming practices. No pre-planting fertilizer was used. In the seedling development phase, ammonium sulfate and #1 Instant Water Soluble Fertilizer (Taiwan Fertilizer Co., Taipei, Taiwan) were applied. The doses for the experimental and control group were 400 and 640 kg/ha, respectively. During the young panicle formation stage, 300 kg/ha of Biotec Organic Compound Fertilizers #39 (Taiwan Fertilizer Co., Taipei, Taiwan) was used as earing fertilizer. Agricultural pests were managed with pesticides according to best practices. Additionally, the experimental group was treated five times with a compound PNSB formulation provided by FIRDI, administered via flood irrigation. Each dose of PNSB was 200 kg/ha.

2.2. Collection and Analysis of Soil Samples

The sample analysis protocol was adapted from Ref. [10], where five sampling points were selected in each field, with four in the periphery and one in the center (Figure 1). Five samples were collected from each sampling point. To analyze organic carbon content in different soil layers, stainless steel soil core samplers were used to extract soil from three different depths (0–10, 10–20, and 20–30 cm). The samples were stored in individual low-density polyethylene (LDPE) plastic bags and transported to the laboratory.

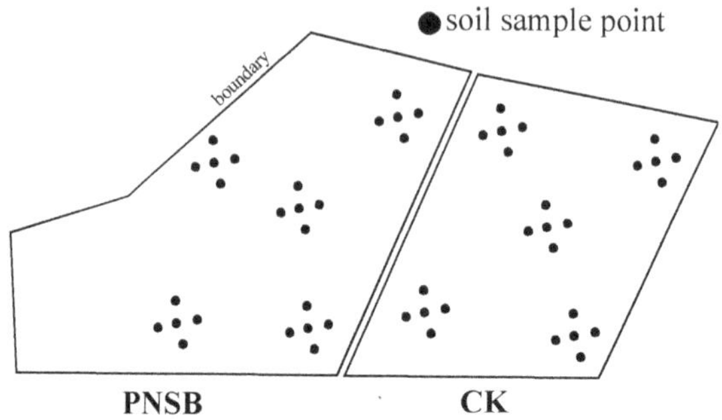

Figure 1. Sample collection points in the experimental field.

For each soil sample, the density, gravel content, organic carbon content, and organic matter content were determined. Samples were weighed and dried, then powdered and sieved through a 2 mm sieve. The amount of gravel and large soil particles larger than 2 mm were weighed and used to adjust the soil density calculation and determine the soil gravel content. The sieved fine sample was ground and homogenized, then analyzed using a Total Organic Carbon (TOC) analyzer. The soil organic carbon content in each soil layer was affected by the soil density and gravel content, which were taken into account using the following equation described by the IPCC in 2006.

$$SOC_{stock} = SOC_{con\ fine\ soil} * FSS \tag{1}$$

(FSS is the fine soil stock.)

$$SOC_i\ stock(Mg\ C\ ha^{-1}) = OC_i * BD_{fine\ 1i} * (1 - C_i) * t_i * 0.1 \tag{2}$$

(SOC_i: soil organic carbon at depth i (mg C ha^{-1})
OC_i: fine-earth organic carbon at depth i (mg C g^{-1} fine earth)
BD_{fine1i}: the overall fine-earth density at depth i (g fine earth, cm^{-3} fine earth)
$1 - vC_i$: the proportion of fine earth by volume (cm^3 fine earth cm^{-3} soil)
vC_i: the proportion of coarse fragments by volume (cm^3 coarse fragment cm^{-3} soil)
t_i: the thickness of soil at depth i (depth, cm)
0.1: the constant used for converting mg C cm^{-1} into Mg C ha^{-1})

2.3. Collection and Analysis of Gas Samples

Gases from the experimental paddies were collected using a close chamber method during the period of rice cultivation. Samples were collected every two weeks, 5 times in total. Methane emissions were collected between 9:30 and 10:30 AM at four locations every 4 m (Figure 2) to obtain results that best correlated with overall emission levels [11]. We collected gas samples from the collection hoods placed horizontally on the field, and methane concentrations were measured at 0, 20, and 40 min after placement.

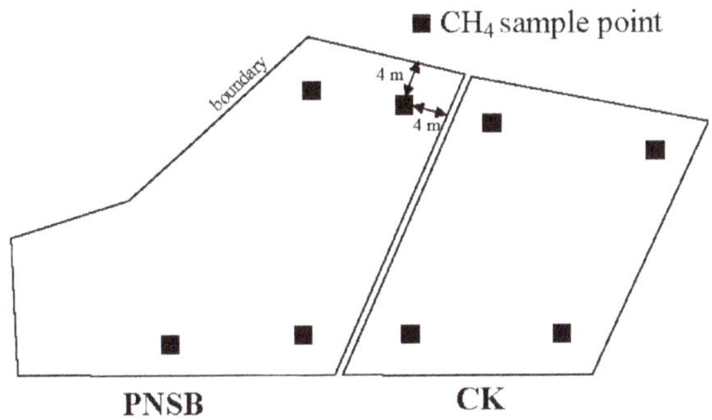

Figure 2. Sampling points for the collection of gas samples.

The sample collection hood was composed of a bottomless acrylic hood and a stainless-steel box that surrounds the rice plant (Figure 3) The acrylic hood contained a thermometer to measure the atmospheric temperature inside the hood, pipes, an airbag for gas collection, a barometer, and a small fan to ensure even mixing of gases in the hood. The size of the stainless-steel box was adjusted to accommodate different rice plant sizes. During sample collection, the sample collection hood was placed horizontally over one rice plant in a stable fashion. The fan in the hood was then powered on to cycle the air inside the hood. A greenhouse gas analyzer (LGR-ICOSTM GLA131-GGA Greenhouse Gas Analyzer) was connected to the hood to obtain instant readings of methane concentrations inside the hood.

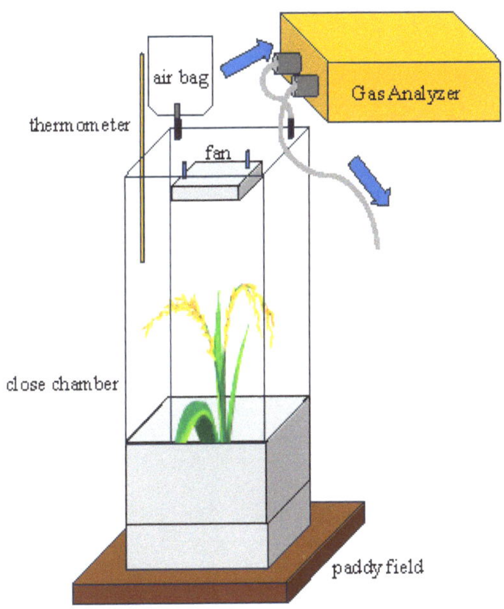

Figure 3. Design of the sample collection hood.

2.4. Calculation of Carbon Dioxide Equivalents

The effect of our intervention on reducing emissions from each hectare of second-crop rice cultivation was calculated from the differential amount of methane between the experimental and control groups, using the following equation:

$$\text{Kg CO}_2\text{e/ha/season} = \text{CH}_4(\text{CK}) - \text{CH}_4(\text{PNSB}) * 25 \tag{3}$$

2.5. Quantification of Soil Carbon Content (SOC)

By comparing the change in SOC and methane emissions between the experimental and control groups, the beneficial effects of PNSB were quantified. SOC was monitored over time in both fields, and the rate of SOC was increased. The annual rate of SOC stock increase was calculated according to an equation published by the IPCC in 2006, by converting SOC (g C kg^{-1}) to SOC per unit area (ton C ha^{-1}) and then dividing by the timespan between measurements.

2.6. Evaluation of Oryza Sativa Growth

On the 90th day of the field trial, a Soil Plant Analysis Development (SPAD) chlorophyll meter was used to measure the chlorophyll content of 20 randomly selected plants in each cohort. The height of the plants, as well as their eventual crop yield, were also collected.

2.7. Analysis of PSNB Content in Soil and Water

After planting, soil samples were collected from five locations in each field, four near the perimeter and one in the center. Three soil cores were collected from each location. After each sample was evenly mixed, 100 g of soil was aliquoted and placed in a sample bottle. The bottles were placed in a low-temperature storage box and then transported to the lab for immediate processing. At the same time, water samples were collected from five locations in each field, four near the perimeter and one in the center. The temperature, pH, and dissolved oxygen (DO) in each sample were quantified on site, and 600 mL of each sample was transported to the lab for immediate processing.

2.8. Analysis of PSNB Content by Most Probable Number (MPN) Method

At the lab, soil and water samples were evenly mixed, serially diluted in NS medium (BCRC 522), and cultured. The most probable number (MPN) method was used to estimate the concentration of photosynthetic bacteria in the samples.

3. Results and Discussion

3.1. SOC

Five samples were collected from each of the five locations in each cohort. The SOC levels are reported in Table 1. The experimental cohort, to which PNSB was added, displayed a slight decrease in the SOC of 0–10 cm deep soil after rice cultivation. The decrease was caused by an increase in water oxygen content caused by PNSB, which promoted aerobic bacterial activity and facilitated the breakdown of soil organic matter. In 10–30 cm, there was a marked increase in SOC in the experimental group after cultivation. The control group did not exhibit significant changes in SOC between the depths of 0–10 cm. Between 10–30 cm, small amounts of SOC increase were observed, the extent of which was less than that of the experimental group. These results suggested that PNSB addition promoted SOC accumulation in 10–30 cm deep soil by reducing methane production and thus curtailing the associated loss of organic matter.

Table 1. SOC (%) in various soil layers.

PNSB	Before cultivation	After cultivation	Difference (%)	Total (%)
0–10 cm	1.433 ± 0.186	1.484 ± 0.14	−0.088	
10–20 cm	1.623 ± 0.227	1.756 ± 0.161	0.209	0.737
20–30 cm	1.763 ± 0.248	2.159 ± 0.141	0.615	
Control group	**Before cultivation**	**After cultivation**	**Difference (%)**	**Total (%)**
0–10 cm	1.448 ± 0.128	1.488 ± 0.051	0.003	
10–20 cm	1.705 ± 0.207	1.779 ± 0.09	0.172	0.209
20–30 cm	2.006 ± 0.154	1.779 ± 0.09	0.034	

The soil density and gravel content (defined as the percentage of particles greater than 2 mm) are shown in Tables 2 and 3. According to TOC calculations, the control group had OC levels of 30.812 and 35.704 tons-C/ha before and after cultivation, respectively, corresponding to a 4.89 tons-C/ha increase. The experimental cohort with PNSB had organic carbon levels of 27.05 and 44.503 tons-C/ha before and after cultivation, corresponding to a 17.45 tons-C/ha increase (Table 4).

Table 2. Overall densities of various soil layers.

PNSB	Before cultivation	After cultivation
0–10 cm	1.433 ± 0.186	1.484 ± 0.14
10–20 cm	1.623 ± 0.227	1.756 ± 0.161
20–30 cm	1.763 ± 0.248	2.159 ± 0.141
Control group	Before cultivation	After cultivation
0–10 cm	1.448 ± 0.128	1.488 ± 0.051
10–20 cm	1.705 ± 0.207	1.779 ± 0.09
20–30 cm	2.006 ± 0.154	1.779 ± 0.09

Table 3. Gravel content (%) of various soil layers.

Depth	**PNSB**	**Control Group**
0–10 cm	0.1959	0.1897
10–20 cm	0.229	0.2012
20–30 cm	0.305	0.4786

Table 4. Soil Organic Carbon Content of various soil layers.

		Soil Organic Carbon Content (tons-C/ha)				**Amount Sequestered (tons-C/ha)**
		(A) [a]	**(B) [b]**	**(C) [c]**	**Total [d]**	
Control group	Before cultivation	15.564	9.530	5.717	30.812	4.89
	After cultivation	15.996	12.832	6.877	35.704	
PNSB	Before cultivation	14.301	9.825	2.929	27.055	17.45
	After cultivation	13.544	14.484	16.475	44.503	

[a.] 0~10 cm, [b.] 10~20 cm, [c.] 20~30 cm, [d.] A + B + C.

3.2. Analysis of Methane Emissions

The amount of emitted methane was measured on five days—17, 29, 34, 48, and 82 days after planting, respectively (Figure 4). During the initial phase of rice cultivation (0–17 days), the control and experimental groups did not exhibit significant differences in methane release. During the tillering phase (17–48 days), the amount of methane released gradually increased. We tallied the methane emissions during the period as a proxy of methane emissions across the entire second crop growth season. The control cohort released 49.48 ± 25.06 g-CH_4/m^2/season, while the PNSB cohort released 37.26 ± 12.97 g-CH_4/m^2/season. PNSB led to a 12.22 g-CH_4/m^2/season (122.2 Kg-CH_4/ha/season) reduction in methane emissions, which is equivalent to 3.05 tons·CO_2e/ha/season in terms of carbon dioxide equivalents.

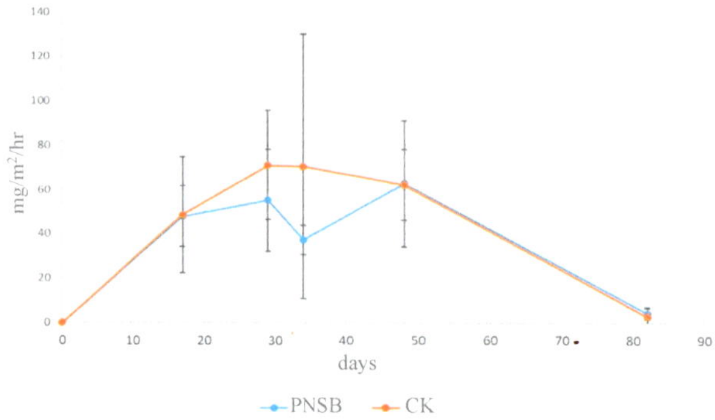

Figure 4. Monitoring of methane emissions in field trials.

3.3. PNSB in Field Trials

PNSB content in water samples was measured using serial dilution followed by MPN. PNSB concentrations in water in the experimental group were higher than those in the control group (Figure 5). The addition of PNSB in this experiment increased the PNSB population size in water. On the contrary, soil PNSB concentrations were not correlated with the presence or absence of PNSB supplementation (Figure 6). Soil PNSB levels were higher during the first 45 days than later. Additionally, the concentrations of PNSB in water were positively correlated with the amount of dissolved oxygen (Figure 7). This indicated that a high PNSB concentration in water increased the amount of DO.

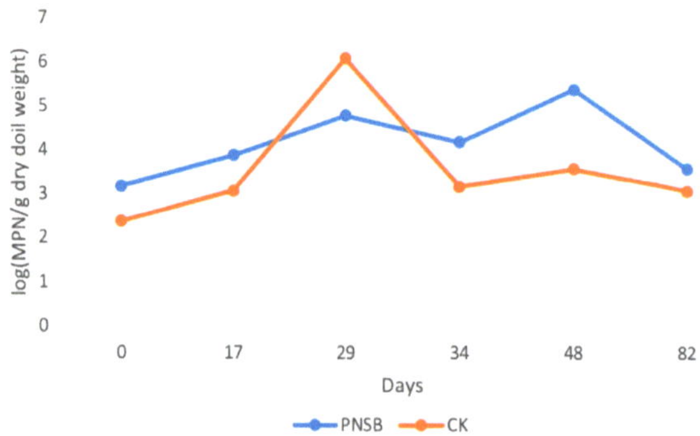

Figure 5. PNSB content in water.

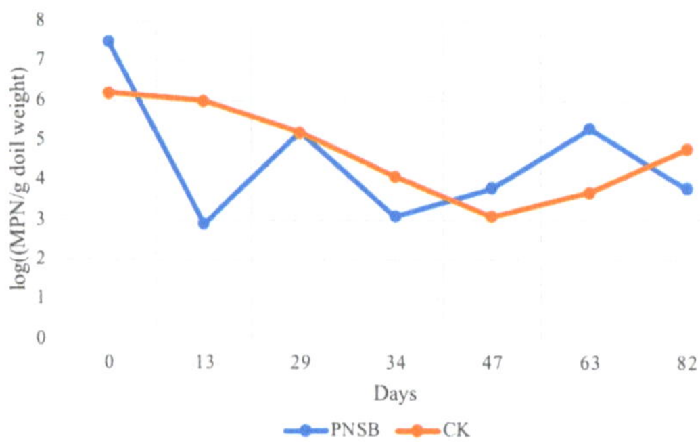

Figure 6. PNSB content in soil.

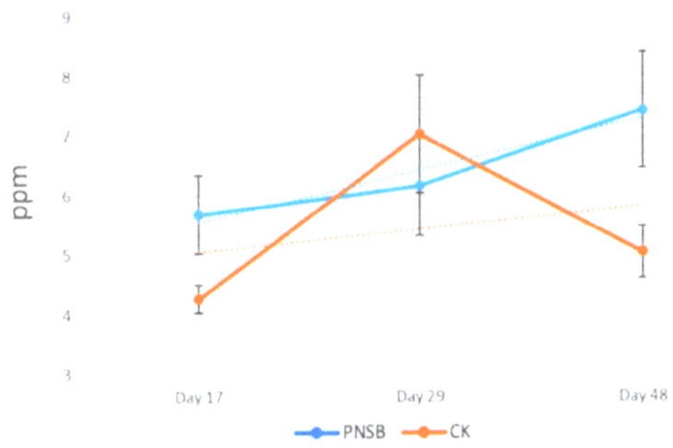

Figure 7. DO in water.

3.4. Evaluation of *Oryza Sativa* Growth

Chlorophyll content and plant height on the 90th day of *Oryza sativa* cultivation are shown in Figures 8 and 9. Measurements from the SPAD chlorophyll meter revealed that plants in the PNSB cohort contained more chlorophyll compared to those in the control cohort (43.7 ± 4.05 and 40.91 ± 3.41, respectively). The average heights of PNSB-treated and control plants were similar (104.64 ± 4.40 and 105.44 ± 6.80 cm, respectively). We harvested the rice on the 103rd day. In the growing season, a hurricane and pests affected the growth, resulting in a reduced yield compared to prior years. The PNSB and control cohorts had yields of 5786.7 and 5645.0 Kg/hectare, respectively, with the PNSB cohort producing a 2.51% higher yield.

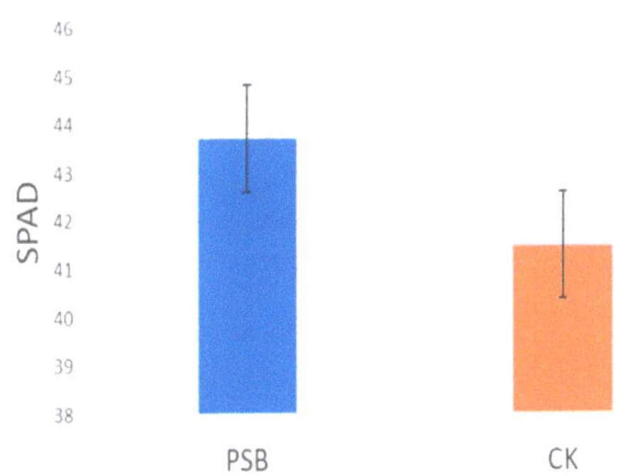

Figure 8. Chlorophyll content on the 90th day of rice cultivation.

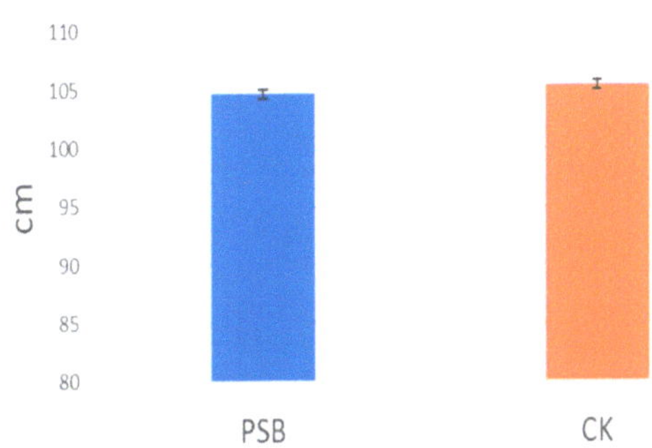

Figure 9. Plant height on the 90th day of rice cultivation.

4. Conclusions

PNSB promoted plant growth, increased nitrogen fixation, and reduced greenhouse gas emissions, which proved that PNSB is a promising candidate for agricultural application. PNSB administration on second-crop rice (*Oryza sativa*) in the Guantian region proved to be effective in its growth. PNSB increased SOC and reduced greenhouse gas emissions. According to the national greenhouse gas inventory reports by the Ministry of Environment in Taiwan, the amount of methane emission coming from rice fields is affected by multiple factors, including climate, organic matter, soil properties, rice strains, and flood management. While the results of this research have demonstrated emission mitigation in the Tainan Guantian region, more field trials are needed in the future to assess the impact of PNSB administration on rice cultivation in other regions. Additionally, SOC contents must be monitored for longer durations to develop PNSB administration methodology for agricultural carbon sequestration.

Author Contributions: Conceptualization, Y.-C.K. and R.-M.L.; methodology, Y.-C.K. and R.-M.L.; validation, Y.-C.K.; formal analysis, Y.-C.K.; investigation, K.-Y.K. and A.K.W.; resources, Y.-C.K., R.-M.L., and K.-Y.K.; data curation, Y.-C.K.; writing—original draft preparation, K.-Y.K. and A.K.W.; writing—review and editing, Y.-C.K. and R.-M.L.; visualization, K.-Y.K. and A.K.W.; supervision, Y.-C.K.; project administration, Y.-C.K. and R.-M.L.; funding acquisition, Y.-C.K. and R.-M.L. All authors have read and agreed to the published version of the manuscript.

Funding: This research was funded by the National Science and Technology Council and Ministry of Agriculture.

Institutional Review Board Statement: Not applicable.

Informed Consent Statement: Not applicable.

Data Availability Statement: Data supporting reported results can be made available upon reasonable request from the corresponding author.

Acknowledgments: This research acknowledges BCRC, the Food Industry Research and Development Institute.

Conflicts of Interest: The authors declare that they have no known competing financial interests or personal relationships that could have appeared to influence the work reported in this paper.

References

1. Shindell, D.T.; Faluvegi, G.; Koch, D.M.; Schmidt, G.A.; Unger, N.; Bauer, S.E. Improved attribution of climate forcing to emissions. *Science* **2009**, *326*, 716–718. [CrossRef] [PubMed]
2. Stocker, T.F.; Qin, D.; Plattner, G.K.; Alexander, L.V.; Allen, S.K.; Bindoff, N.L.; Bréon, F.M.; Church, J.A.; Cubasch, U.; Emori, S.; et al. Technical summary. In *Climate Change 2013: The physical science basis. Contribution of Working Group I to the Fifth Assessment Report of the Intergovernmental Panel on Climate Change*; Cambridge University Press: Cambridge, UK, 2013; pp. 33–115.
3. Carlson, K.M.; Gerber, J.S.; Mueller, N.D.; Herrero, M.; MacDonald, G.K.; Brauman, K.A.; Havlik, P.; O'Connell, C.S.; Johnson, J.A.; Saatchi, S.; et al. Greenhouse gas emissions intensity of global croplands. *Nat. Clim. Chang.* **2017**, *7*, 63–68. [CrossRef]
4. Wassmann, R.; Aulakh, M.S. The role of rice plants in regulating mechanisms of methane missions. *Biol. Fertil. Soils* **2000**, *31*, 20–29. [CrossRef]
5. Liu, Y.; Ge, T.; van Groenigen, K.J.; Yang, Y.; Wang, P.; Cheng, K.; Zhu, Z.; Wang, J.; Li, Y.; Guggenberger, G.; et al. Rice paddy soils are a quantitatively important carbon store according to a global synthesis. *Commun. Earth Environ.* **2021**, *2*, 154. [CrossRef]
6. Huang, Y.; Yan, C.F.; Guo, C.Q.; Lu, Z.X.; Shi, Y.; Wang, Z.D. Synthesis of GO-modified Cu2O nanosphere and the photocatalytic mechanism of water splitting for hydrogen production. *Int. J. Hydrogen Energy* **2017**, *42*, 4007–4016. [CrossRef]
7. Li, Y.; Liu, X.; Hao, T.; Chen, S. Colonization and Maize Growth Promotion Induced by Phosphate Solubilizing Bacterial Isolates. *Int. J. Mol. Sci.* **2017**, *18*, 1253. [CrossRef] [PubMed]
8. Lee, D.H.; Jun, W.J.; Shin, D.H.; Cho, H.Y.; Hong, B.S. Effect of Culture Conditions on Production of 5-Aminolevulinic Acid by Recombinant Escherichia coli. *Biosci. Biotechnol. Biochem.* **2005**, *69*, 470–476. [CrossRef] [PubMed]
9. Bric, J.M.; Bostock, R.M.; Silverstone, S.E. Rapid in situ assay for indoleacetic Acid production by bacteria immobilized on a nitrocellulose membrane. *Appl. Environ. Microbiol.* **1991**, *57*, 535–538. [CrossRef] [PubMed]

10. Blake, G.R.; Hartge, K.H. Bulk Density. In *Methods of Soil Analysis: Part 1 Physical and Mineralogical Methods*; American Society of Agronomy: Madison, WI, USA, 1986; pp. 363–375. [CrossRef]
11. Zhang, X.Y.; Qiu, S.Y. Method for on-Site Measurement of Methane in Paddy Fields. Available online: https://www.hdares.gov.tw/upload/hdares/files/web_structure/13721/02%E6%B0%B4%E7%94%B0.pdf (accessed on 29 August 2024).

engineering proceedings

MDPI

Proceeding Paper

Internet Gaming Disorder of Gamers: A Study on Values and Online Gaming Behavior †

Jessica Angelina Ongkowijaya and Esther Widhi Andangsari *

Psychology Department, Faculty of Humanities, Bina Nusantara University, Jakarta 11480, Indonesia
* Correspondence: esther@binus.edu

† Presented at the 2024 IEEE 4th International Conference on Electronic Communications, Internet of Things and Big Data, Taipei, Taiwan, 19–21 April 2024.

Abstract: This research aims to explore the effect of Internet Gaming Disorder (IGD) and online gaming behaviors related to IGD. The explored behaviors were based on games with microtransactions. Using a revised portrait value questionnaire (PVQ-RR), 186 respondents from 18 to 52 years old were asked about gaming behaviors. Online gaming behaviors such as the duration of online gaming and the payment for online games had a reciprocal relationship with IGD. Stimulation, achievement, hedonism, power through dominance, and personal security were correlated with playing paid online games. It is necessary to consider the fact that the values of the games are related to online gaming behaviors. Positive online gaming behaviors need to be developed.

Keywords: gamers; online game; internet gaming disorder; online gaming behavior; values

Citation: Ongkowijaya, J.A.; Andangsari, E.W. Internet Gaming Disorder of Gamers: A Study on Values and Online Gaming Behavior. *Eng. Proc.* **2024**, *74*, 31. https://doi.org/10.3390/engproc2024074031

Academic Editors: Shu-Han Liao, Teen-Hang Meen and Cheng-Fu Yang

Published: 30 August 2024

1. Introduction

An event in a game usually lasts 10 hours. Several players prioritize gaming over other tasks. They can achieve the goal of the game with high engagement but need to consider the consequences of other ignored activities. Many gamers have negative consequences in their lives due to their gaming behaviors. Gaming has become an acceptable activity and has been enjoyed by many people. In 2022, 77.25% of the Indonesian population reported that the Internet was important for accessing entertainment, and 14.23% frequently played online games [1]. There are 40 million frequent gamers in Indonesia, and many of them are addicted to games [2]. Instead of simply restricting their gaming activities to prevent gaming addiction, it is necessary to understand their behaviors for gamers to recover healthier gaming behaviors [3].

Gaming behaviors vary depending on the genres of games. Several games encourage social interaction, while others are played alone. Some gamers play casually, while others spend long hours playing. Sometimes, gamers sacrifice their work or their sleep. Some gamers never spend any amount of real money on games, while others do, and several gamers cannot control their spending and have financial trouble. Recognizing the harm from excessive or uncontrolled participation in online gaming, the American Psychiatric Association included Internet Gaming Disorder (IGD) in a condition of the *Diagnostic and Statistical Manual of Mental Disorders* (DSM-5). One study in Indonesia found that 2.03% of the respondents experienced IGD [4]. When online gaming has negatively impacted their life, IGD is diagnosed. The most relevant criteria in the diagnosis of IGD are to give up other activities, prioritize gaming to result in negative consequences, and continue to play despite knowing the problems [5].

Players playing games excessively often do not have IGD. Gaming is increasingly accepted with the rising number of gamers. Gaming affects the economy [6], both positively and negatively. One possible explanation for human behaviors is the values that individuals hold. Values motivate online gaming behaviors. Among the three clusters of gaming motivation [7], there are no negative motivations that lead gamers to IGD. Researchers have found empirical evidence that prevents gamers from being addicted. Thus, it is important to understand internal psychological factors to predict how gamers keep playing online games without addiction. Therefore, we assumed that the values that gamers hold are used to predict IGD and explored why gamers do not experience IGD even though they often play games.

2. IGD on Values and Online Gaming Behavior

2.1. IGD

IGD has been included as a condition for further study in the DSM-5. IGD is diagnosed when gaming negatively impacts normal life. To be diagnosed, someone must fulfill at least five of the following criteria [5]: (a) preoccupation with online gaming; (b) withdrawal symptoms when unable to play; (c) the need to increase the time spent playing; (d) unsuccessful attempts to control one's gaming; (e) loss of interest in other hobbies as a result of, and except for, gaming; (f) continued gaming despite knowledge of psychosocial problems; (g) deceiving others regarding the amount of gaming; (h) use of online gaming to escape negative moods; and (i) has jeopardized or lost relationship, job, or school/career opportunities because of gaming.

Several factors contributing to IGD have been identified, including impulsivity, dispositional self-control, anxiety, drive to pursue desired goals, amount of money spent on games, duration of weekday gaming, offline game community attendance, and membership in a game community. These are related significantly to IGD [8]. Among motivations for playing [7], achievement is correlated with IGD stronger than other motivations; however, the strongest correlation is escapism, a subcomponent of immersion motivation [9].

A cognitive–behavioral model explains IGD by including the motivating component of gaming (reward and reducing stress), behavioral executive control, and the weighing of rewards and consequences in decision-making [10]. Four groups of cognitions in IGD were determined in Ref. [11] as follows: (a) belief in the value of game rewards, (b) maladaptive and unflexible gaming rules, (c) dependence on gaming for self-esteem, and (d) gaming for obtaining social acceptance. Gamers' metacognitions about gaming may push them to keep playing by making them believe that gaming can reduce negative effects and that it is hard to stop gaming once they start [12,13].

2.2. Values

Value is considered important by an individual. A theory of basic values was developed to describe the basic values that can be recognized by people in all cultures and to find out whether those values are structured to explain the relationship between them [14]. Schwartz identified 10 such basic values and defined values as "desirable, trans-situational goals, varying in importance, that serve as guiding principles in people's lives" [15]. In the refined theory of basic individual values, Schwartz identified 19 different basic values based on the original 10 values [16]. These basic values are structured on a circular motivation continuum [16,17]. Neighboring values have similar motivational content (e.g., both tradition and conformity to the rules are compatible and can be pursued in the same behavior), while values opposing each other usually have conflicting motivations (e.g., interpersonal conformity can conflict with autonomy to choose one's action). This motivational circle can be understood by the four higher-order values [16], which explain the common goal or essence across several adjacent values. These values change and self-enhance with conservation and self-transcendence. Overall, 19 values, except hedonism, face, and humility, fall into one of the four higher-order values. Hedonism falls between openness to change and self-enhancement, while the face is between self-enhancement and conservation, and humility is between conservation and self-transcendence [16]. The 19 values are understood from another set of concepts that characterize the values, namely growth in anxiety-free conditions or self-protection with anxiety avoidance, and a personal or a social focus [16]. All values help to at least correspond to one of the three requirements for human existence, which are individuals' biological needs, coordinated social interaction, a group's survival, and well-being [18]. In other words, none of the values are "bad" since all of them are needed for human survival and well-being. This is also why all the values are recognized across cultures.

For the present research, we chose 11 values relevant to the behaviors of online gamers or the features of online games that motivate gamers to keep playing. These values were self-direction (thought), self-direction (action), stimulation, hedonism, achievement, power–dominance, power (resources), face, security (personal), conformity (rules), and conformity (interpersonal).

2.3. Online Gaming Behaviors

It is important to analyze the online gaming behaviors of gamers, and the result is used to support the assumption that values motivate online gaming behaviors [19]. Online gaming behaviors considered in this research included average online gaming duration in a day, pay-to-play gaming, and using real money in online gaming to buy items for in-game advantage(s) [6,13,20]. These considerations were made based on the observation that online games with microtransactions are popular, and people are motivated by the economic value of games [21].

3. Materials and Method

In total, 190 gamers were invited for the questionnaire survey of this research. The respondents were 18 years and older and had played online games for the last three months at the time of the questionnaires. The games played had at least one of the following features: in-game currency, inventory or collection, and leaderboard. We assumed that those features motivated players to keep playing games. However, one respondent did not give consent to participate, two were under 18 years old, and one did not respond to the instructions. Thus, 186 respondents (33.33% females), aged between 18 and 52 years old (M = 22.93, SD = 5.33) in various areas of Indonesia, participated in the survey. Most respondents were students or undergraduate students (70.43%), which was relevant to the Asosiasi Penyelenggara Jasa Internet Indonesia (APJII) survey in 2022, which showed that the rate of Internet penetration in Indonesia was the highest among students and undergraduate students [1].

3.1. Instruments

IGD was measured using the IGD Test (IGD-20) [22] in the Indonesian version [23]. IGD-20 consists of 20 items on a 5-point scale ranging from 1 (strongly disagree) to 5 (strongly agree). Examples of IGD-20 items in Indonesian are "saya perlu bermain gim daring lebih lama lagi" (I have significantly increased the amount of time I play games over last year), "saya bermain gim untuk melupakan hal yang menganggu saya" (I play games to forget about whatever's bothering me), and "ketika saya sedang tidak bermain gim, saya merasa lebih mudah marah" (when I am not gaming, I feel more irritable). The internal consistency for IGD-20 in this study was $\alpha = 0.85$.

Values were measured using the Indonesian version of the Revised Portrait Value Questionnaire (PVQ-RR) [17]. We measured 11 values from 19 values and used 33 items of PVQ-RR on a 6-point scale (1 = not like me at all, 2 = not like me, 3 = a little like me, 4 = somewhat like me, 5 = like me, 6 = very much like me). The 11 values were relevant to the online behaviors of gamers. Example of PVQ-RR items in Indonesian are "*penting baginya untuk membuat keputusan sendiri tentang hidupnya*" (it is important to him to make his own decisions about his life), "*penting baginya untuk menjadi kaya raya*" (it is important to him to be wealthy), and "*penting baginya untuk tidak pernah direndahkan*" (it is important to him never to be humiliated). The internal consistency of PVQ-RR from this study ranged from $\alpha = 0.429$ to $\alpha = 0.746$.

Data for the online behaviors of gamers were collected by questions such as "Do you play online games every day?", "Have you ever played a pay-to-play online game?", or "Have you ever used real money to buy something in an online game?". The respondents answered those questions with "yes" or "no". Multiple choice questions were given to collect gaming genre preferences, the average duration of playing online games, and motivation for playing.

3.2. Data Collection and Analysis

Data were collected via an online survey using LimeSurvey. We used the snowball sampling method for recruiting the respondents. The hypotheses were tested with multiple regression analysis. Other analysis results and descriptive statistics for demographics and online gaming behaviors were obtained. All analyses were performed using the JASP 0.14.1.0 version.

4. Results and Discussion

The statistics of the scores of IGD-20 and PVQ-RR are shown in Table 1. The three highest average scores were found for personal security, hedonism, and interpersonal conformity. Those values represent safety in one's immediate environment, the pursuit of personal pleasure, and one's conformity with others. The results indicated that gamers seek enjoyment when playing online games and that the enjoyment is to find a sense of safety, both personally and socially, by avoiding negative responses from others.

Table 1. Scores of IGD and values.

Item	Mean	Standard Deviation	Minimum	Maximum
IGD	55.47	11.67	24.00	88.00
Self-direction—thought	4.68	0.81	2.33	6.00
Self-direction—action	4.75	0.80	1.67	6.00
Stimulation	4.19	0.93	1.67	6.00
Hedonism	4.78	0.84	1.67	6.00
Achievement	4.37	0.92	1.67	6.00
Power—dominance	3.14	1.10	1.00	5.67
Power—resources	3.19	1.07	1.00	6.00
Face	4.23	1.06	1.67	6.00
Security—personal	4.84	0.86	2.33	6.00
Conformity—rules	4.59	0.90	1.33	6.00
Conformity—interpersonal	4.76	0.99	1.67	6.00

Multiple regression results are presented in Tables 2 and 3. The regression model was not significant; thus, the hypotheses were not supported.

Table 2. Results of ANOVA.

Model	R	R^2	Adjusted R	Root mean square of errors	p
IGD on Values	0.26	0.07	0.01	11.61	0.32
Model	**Sum of Squares**	**Degree of freedom**	**Mean of Square**	**F**	p
IGD on Values	1725.26	11	156.84	1.16	0.32

With the 11 values, IGD could not be predicted (Table 3). The values present the driving motivation behind human behaviors [17], but do not represent a psychological disorder. Instead, values directly affected IGD. Reasons for playing games were inferred from the values, but the reasons could not explain gamers' pathological online gaming. The relationship between values and behaviors depends on the importance of the values [24] and is weakened by social norms [25]. The online gaming behaviors of the respondents are presented in Table 4. More than half of them played games every day, with an average duration of 6–9 h each day. Most of them played games in a team, with 74 of the respondents playing team games every day. Their preferred game genres varied, but role-playing and action games were the most popular. Overall, 40.32% of the respondents had escapism as their motivation to play games, indicating that the respondents played games to relax or to stop thinking about real-life problems [7]. The escapism explained why most of them were not found to be in the disordered group. From the other aspects of escapism, online gaming was used to escape negative moods, which is one of the IGD criteria [5]. This motivation pushes someone to keep playing games for long hours, leading to IGD. For the respondents, there was a significant positive correlation between IGD and average hours of gaming per day.

Table 3. Results of multiple regression.

Model	B	Standard Error	Standardized	*t*	Significance
H0	59.80	7.31		8.18	<0.001
Self-direction—thought	−1.95	1.45	−0.14	−1.35	0.18
Self-direction—action	−0.95	1.59	−0.07	−0.60	0.55
Stimulation	−0.91	1.11	−0.07	−0.82	0.41
Hedonism	2.02	1.25	0.15	1.62	0.11
Achievement	−0.55	1.34	−0.04	−0.41	0.68
Power—dominance	0.23	0.95	0.02	0.24	0.81
Power—resources	0.32	1.02	0.03	0.32	0.75
Face	0.41	1.01	0.04	0.41	0.69
Security—personal	1.32	1.38	0.10	0.96	0.34
Conformity—rules	−1.62	1.09	−0.13	−1.49	0.14
Conformity—interpersonal	0.72	1.00	0.06	0.72	0.48

Most of the respondents played a paid game (66.13%), bought a game (55.91%), bought items in-game with real money (83.87%), and even played a game to earn money (37.10%). Online gaming behaviors involving real money were familiar to them. In 2019, a report noted that the Indonesian gaming market was the biggest in Southeast Asia, with a total spending of USD 1.1 billion [26]. There was a positive significant correlation (r = 0.149, $p < 0.05$) between IGD and playing a paid online game. The more a gamer played a paid game, the higher the IGD score was. The higher the IGD score was, the more money they paid for the online game. Details of the correlation between IGD and gaming behaviors are presented in Appendix A.

Values were not used to predict IGD. However, there were significant correlations between values and online gaming behaviors. A significant correlation was observed between the stimulation value and playing a pay-to-play online game (r = 0.153, $p < 0.05$, Appendix B). Pay-to-play behavior was correlated significantly with the duration of online gaming (r = 0.344, $p < 0.05$). Similarly, the achievement and hedonism values were correlated significantly with playing a paid game. IGD was correlated significantly with gaming duration (r = 0.300, $p < 0.01$) and with playing a pay-to-play (r = 0.168, $p < 0.05$) or paid game (r = 0.149, $p < 0.05$). Stimulation, achievement, and hedonism were indirectly correlated with IGD, which must gamers must be notified of.

Power (dominance) was correlated with having spent real money in online games (r = 0.151, $p < 0.05$) and buying items in-game (r = 0.152, $p < 0.05$). Power (dominance) means the motivation to control other people to avoid threats to the self. This means that gamers try to exert dominance over other people through their money spending and cosmetics in the games they play. Personal security was correlated significantly with trying a different game genre (r = 0.149, $p < 0.05$) and buying something in-game for advantages over other players (r = 0.182, $p < 0.05$). Personal security motivates gamers to seek personal safety in their immediate environment. This shows that gamers prefer to attain a sense of personal safety, including spending money for an advantage in-game.

Table 4. Online gaming behaviors (N = 186).

Online Gaming Behaviors		Number	Ratio (%)
Online gaming motivation	Advancement	8	4.30
	Mechanics	11	5.91
	Competition	16	8.60
	Socializing	20	10.75
	Relationships	7	3.76
	Teamwork	21	11.29
	Discovery	6	3.23
	Role Playing	11	5.91
	Customization	7	3.76
	Escapism	75	40.32
	Others	4	2.15
Do you play online games every day?	Yes	122	65.59
	No	64	34.41
Preference for playing online games	Play alone	45	24.19
	Play in a team	103	55.38
	Both	38	20.43
Have you ever played a pay-to-play online game?	Yes	123	66.13
	No	63	33.87
Have you ever bought a pay-to-play online game?	Yes	104	55.91
	No	82	44.09
Have you ever played a paid online game (not free-to-play), not necessarily one you bought yourself?	Yes	96	51.61
	No	90	48.39
Have you ever used real money to buy something in an online game?	Yes	156	83.87
	No	30	16.13
Have you ever tried to play a different genre of online game, different from the one you usually play?	Yes	152	81.72
	No	34	18.28
Duration for online gaming (average hours/day)	3–6 h/day	59	31.72
	6–9 h/day	90	48.39
	9–12 h/day	22	11.83
	12–15 h/day	10	5.38
	15–18 h/day	3	1.61
	More than 18 h/day	2	1.08
Have you ever bought cosmetic items in-game (which gives no advantage over other players)?	Yes	105	56.45
	No	81	43.55
Have you ever bought something that gives you advantage/affects the gameplay (such as in pay-to-win games)?	Yes	92	49.46
	No	94	50.54
Have you ever played a play-to-earn game?	Yes	69	37.10
	No	117	62.90
Online game genres	Action	39	20.97
	Role-playing	68	36.56
	Strategy	21	11.29
	Adventure and casual	9	4.84
	Simulation	10	5.38
	Sports and racing	6	3.23
	Others	33	17.74

5. Conclusions

In this research, we assumed that the values of the game players were used to predict IGD. However, the regression result showed that values did not directly influence IGD. Therefore, values neither led gamers towards nor protected them from IGD. Values are the underlying motivation of online gaming behaviors, but these values do not cause IGD. On the other hand, behaviors such as gaming duration and playing a paid online game were correlated with IGD. Gamers must be cautious in their gaming activities, especially in playing a paid online game that makes them lose time. Gamers must pay attention to the values they hold as important, especially the values of power through dominance and personal security. When these values are engaged in playing paid online games, they must be aware of the important values and reduce their gaming duration. Online games are an application of digital technology. Important values of individuals can encourage gamers to have healthier online gaming behaviors.

This research has limitations, such as no strict control over the characteristics of the respondents. The respondents were not grouped according to their online gaming hours or levels of gaming and various online games. Future research is necessary to investigate how gamers develop the symptoms of IGD, such as playing games for excessive hours, or economic benefits.

Author Contributions: Conceptualization, J.A.O. and E.W.A.; methodology, J.A.O. and E.W.A.; software; validation, J.A.O. and E.W.A.; formal analysis, J.A.O. and E.W.A.; investigation, J.A.O.; resources, J.A.O. and E.W.A.; data curation, J.A.O. and E.W.A.; writing—original draft preparation, J.A.O. and E.W.A.; writing—review and editing, J.A.O. and E.W.A.; visualization, J.A.O. and E.W.A.; supervision, E.W.A.; project administration, E.W.A.; funding acquisition, E.W.A. All authors have read and agreed to the published version of the manuscript.

Funding: This research received no external funding.

Institutional Review Board Statement: The study was conducted in accordance with the Declaration of Helsinki and registered and approved from Open Science Framework (OSF) via link https://osf.io/g73w2 (accessed on 26 January 2024) and https://osf.io/9f58v/ (accessed on 22 January 2024) for studies involving humans.

Informed Consent Statement: Informed consent was obtained from all subjects involved in the study.

Data Availability Statement: The data presented in this study are available on request from the corresponding author.

Conflicts of Interest: The authors declare no conflicts of interest.

Appendix A

The Spearman correlation matrix between IGD and online gaming behavior of gamers is show below. The online gaming behavior of gamers consists of daily gaming behavior, preferences in playing, playing with play-to-pay mode, playing with real money, duration of online gaming, genre of game, ever bought pay-to-play, paid for game cosmetics items or something to win, and playing to earn money.

Table A1. Spearman correlation matrix of IGD and online behavior of gamers.

Variable	1	2	3	4	5	6	7	8	9	10	11	12
1. IGD	—											
2. Playing online games every day	0.260 ***	—										
3. Preferences in playing (alone/team/both)	0.070	0.013	—									
4. Ever played a play to pay	0.168 *	0.103	0.082	—								
5. Ever used real money	0.115	0.144	0.131	0.304 ***	—							
6. Duration for online gaming (average hours/day)	0.300 ***	0.370 ***	0.057	0.344 ***	0.131	—						
7. Ever tried a different genre to play	0.101	0.097	0.227 **	0.249 ***	0.209 **	0.204 **	—					
8. Ever bought a pay-to-play	0.116	0.041	0.083	0.554 ***	0.406 ***	0.203 **	0.196 **	—				
9. Ever played a paid game	0.149 *	0.046	−0.004	0.466 ***	0.248 ***	0.204 **	0.154 *	0.549 ***	—			
10. Ever bought cosmetics items	0.114	0.163 *	0.198 **	0.196 **	0.411 ***	0.127	0.146 *	0.334 ***	0.148 *	—		
11. Ever bought something to win	0.086	0.264 ***	−0.070	0.117	0.288 ***	0.102	0.078	0.120	0.183 *	0.023	—	
12. Ever played a play to earn money	0.104	0.064	0.127	0.291 ***	0.125	0.170 *	0.104	0.211 **	0.387 ***	0.248 ***	0.242 ***	—

Note: Significance based on * $p < 0.05$, ** $p < 0.01$, *** $p < 0.001$.

Appendix B

The Spearman correlation between values and online gaming behavior of gamers is shown below.

Table A2. Spearman correlation matrix of values and online behavior of gamers.

Variable	1	2	3	4	5	6	7	8	9	10	11	12	13	14	15	16	17	18	19	20	21
1. Self Direction-Thought	—																				
2. Self Direction-Action	0.595 ***	—																			
3. Stimulation	0.372 ***	0.451 ***	—																		
4. Hedonism	0.330 ***	0.460 ***	0.386 ***	—																	
5. Achievement	0.467 ***	0.487 ***	0.396 ***	0.496 ***	—																
6. Power Dominance	0.015	0.053	0.108	0.195 **	0.215 **	—															
7. Power Resources	0.044	0.122	0.096	0.244 ***	0.340 ***	0.524 ***	—														
8. Face	0.166 *	0.276 ***	0.198 **	0.281 ***	0.413 ***	0.359 ***	0.376 ***	—													
9. Security Personal	0.422 ***	0.507 ***	0.195 **	0.364 ***	0.469 ***	0.098	0.215 **	0.419 ***	—												
10. Conformity Rules	0.337 ***	0.307 ***	0.180 *	0.280 ***	0.386 ***	0.038	0.128	0.275 ***	0.445 ***	—											
11. Conformity Interpersonal	0.273 ***	0.313 ***	0.150 *	0.337 ***	0.236 **	0.013	0.095	0.228 **	0.435 ***	0.314 ***	—										
12. Playing online game everyday	−0.012	0.009	−0.115	0.076	−0.010	−0.136	−0.071	−0.090	−0.015	0.005	0.058	—									
13. Duration for online gaming (average hours/day)	0.072	0.021	0.007	0.108	−0.058	−0.100	0.034	−0.101	−0.020	−0.079	0.118	0.370 ***	—								
14. Ever played a pay-to-play	0.031	0.033	0.153 *	0.066	−0.064	0.049	0.025	−0.121	−0.078	−0.067	0.116	0.103	0.344 ***	—							
15. Ever used real money	−0.118	−0.080	−0.002	−0.113	0.012	−0.151 *	−0.046	−0.075	−0.127	−0.107	−0.148 *	0.144	0.131	0.304 ***	—						
16. Ever tried a different game genre	0.155 *	0.085	0.090	0.128	0.144 *	−0.022	0.069	0.035	0.149 *	0.055	0.103	0.097	0.204 **	0.249 ***	0.209 **	—					
17. Ever bought a pay-to-play	0.028	−0.046	0.024	0.001	−0.030	−0.017	0.048	−0.131	−0.003	−0.011	−0.015	0.041	0.203 **	0.554 ***	0.406 ***	0.196 **	—				
18. Ever played a paid game	−0.019	−0.068	−0.091	−0.175 *	−0.145 *	−0.059	−0.018	−0.139	−0.092	−0.012	−0.025	0.046	0.204 **	0.466 ***	0.248 ***	0.154 *	0.549 ***	—			
19. Ever bought cosmetics in-game	−0.033	−0.033	0.092	0.100	0.032	−0.152 *	−0.028	−0.141	−0.023	0.089	−0.045	0.163 *	0.127	0.196 **	0.411 ***	0.146 *	0.334 ***	0.148 *	—		
20. Ever bought something to win	−0.092	−0.042	−0.019	−0.081	0.021	−0.036	−0.053	−0.054	−0.182 *	−0.105	−0.095	0.264 ***	0.102	0.117	0.288 ***	0.078	0.120	0.183 *	0.023	—	
21. Ever played a play-to-earn game	−0.028	−0.033	2.089×10^{-4}	−0.003	−0.025	−0.033	−0.082	−0.067	−0.099	−0.033	0.028	0.064	0.170 *	0.291 ***	0.125	0.104	0.211 **	0.387 ***	0.248 ***	0.242 ***	—

Note: Significance based on * $p < 0.05$, ** $p < 0.01$, *** $p < 0.001$.

References

1. APJII. Profil. Internet Indonesia. 2022. Available online: https://survei.apjii.or.id/survei/register/16?type=free (accessed on 11 November 2023).
2. Jap, T.; Tiatri, S.; Jaya, E.S.; Suteja, M.S. The Development of Indonesian Online Game Addiction Questionnaire. *PLoS ONE* **2013**, *8*, e61098. [CrossRef]
3. Männikkö, N.; Ruotsalainen, H.; Demetrovics, Z.; Lopez-Fernandez, O.; Myllymäki, L.; Miettunen, J.; Kääriäinen, M. Problematic Gaming Behavior among Finnish Junior High School Students: Relation to Socio-Demographics and Gaming Behavior Characteristics. *Behav. Med.* **2018**, *44*, 324–334. [CrossRef] [PubMed]
4. Siste, K.; Hanafi, E.; Sen, L.T.; Wahjoepramono, P.O.P.; Kurniawan, A.; Yudistiro, R. Potential Correlates of IGD among Indonesian Medical Students: Cross-Sectional Study. *J. Med. Internet Res.* **2021**, *23*, e25468. [CrossRef]
5. Luo, T.; Wei, D.; Guo, J.; Hu, M.; Chao, X.; Sun, Y.; Sun, Q.; Xiao, S.; Liao, Y. Diagnostic Contribution of the DSM-5 Criteria for IGD. *Front. Psychiatry* **2022**, *12*, 777397. [CrossRef]
6. Balakrishnan, J.; Griffiths, M.D. Loyalty towards Online Games, Gaming Addiction, and Purchase Intention towards Online Mobile in-Game Features. *Comput. Hum. Behav.* **2018**, *87*, 238–246. [CrossRef]
7. Yee, N. Motivations for Play in Online Games. *CyberPsychology Behav.* **2006**, *9*, 772–775. [CrossRef] [PubMed]
8. Rho, M.; Lee, H.; Lee, T.-H.; Cho, H.; Jung, D.; Kim, D.-J.; Choi, I. Risk Factors for IGD: Psychological Factors and Internet Gaming Characteristics. *Int. J. Environ. Res. Public Health* **2017**, *15*, 40. [CrossRef] [PubMed]
9. Wang, H.-Y.; Cheng, C. The Associations between Gaming Motivation and IGD: Systematic Review and Meta-Analysis. *JMIR Ment. Health* **2022**, *9*, e23700. [CrossRef]
10. Dong, G.; Potenza, M.N. A Cognitive-Behavioral Model of IGD: Theoretical Underpinnings and Clinical Implications. *J. Psychiatr. Res.* **2014**, *58*, 7–11. [CrossRef]
11. King, D.L.; Delfabbro, P.H. The Cognitive Psychology of IGD. *Clin. Psychol. Rev.* **2014**, *34*, 298–308. [CrossRef]
12. Marino, C.; Spada, M.M. Dysfunctional Cognitions in Online Gaming and IGD: A Narrative Review and New Classification. *Curr. Addict. Rep.* **2017**, *4*, 308–316. [CrossRef]
13. Caselli, G.; Marino, C.; Spada, M.M. Modelling Online Gaming Metacognitions: The Role of Time Spent Gaming in Predicting Problematic Internet Use. *J. Ration. Emotive Cogn. Behav. Ther.* **2020**, *39*, 172–182. [CrossRef]
14. Schwartz, S.H. Universals in the Content and Structure of Values: Theoretical Advances and Empirical Tests in 20 Countries. *Adv. Exp. Soc. Psychol.* **1992**, *25*, 1–65. [CrossRef]
15. Schwartz, S.H. Basic Individual Values: Sources and Consequences. In *Handbook of Value*; Oxford University Press: Oxford, UK, 2015; pp. 63–84.
16. Schwartz, S.H.; Cieciuch, J.; Vecchione, M.; Davidov, E.; Fischer, R.; Beierlein, C.; Ramos, A.; Verkasalo, M.; Lönnqvist, J.-E.; Demirutku, K.; et al. Refining the Theory of Basic Individual Values. *J. Pers. Soc. Psychol.* **2012**, *103*, 663–688. [CrossRef]
17. Schwartz, S.H.; Cieciuch, J. Measuring the Refined Theory of Individual Values in 49 Cultural Groups: Psychometrics of the Revised Portrait Value Questionnaire. *Assessment* **2021**, *29*, 1–15. [CrossRef]
18. Schwartz, S.H. An Overview of the Schwartz Theory of Basic Values. *Online Read. Psychol. Cult.* **2012**, *2*, 11. [CrossRef]
19. Rezaei, S.; Ghodsi, S.S. Does Value Matters in Playing Online Game? An Empirical Study among Massively Multiplayer Online Role-Playing Games (MMORPGs). *Comput. Hum. Behav.* **2014**, *35*, 252–266. [CrossRef]
20. Wohn, D.Y. Spending Real Money: Purchasing Patterns of Virtual Goods in an Online Social Game. In *Proceedings of the SIGCHI Conference on Human Factors in Computing Systems*; New York, NY, USA, 26 April 2014, pp. 3359–3368.
21. Yoon, G.; Duff, B.R.L.; Ryu, S. Gamers Just Want to Have Fun? Toward an Understanding of the Online Game Acceptance. *J. Appl. Soc. Psychol.* **2013**, *43*, 1814–1826. [CrossRef]
22. Pontes, H.M.; Király, O.; Demetrovics, Z.; Griffiths, M.D. The Conceptualisation and Measurement of DSM-5 IGD: The Development of the IGD-20 Test. *PLoS ONE* **2014**, *9*, e110137. [CrossRef]
23. Aryoseno, A. Gambaran IGD Dan Internet Gambling Disorder Pada Pemain Game Gacha. Unpublished undergraduate thesis, Universitas Bina Nusantara, West Jakarta, Indonesia, 2018.
24. Lee, J.A.; Bardi, A.; Gerrans, P.; Sneddon, J.; van Herk, H.; Evers, U.; Schwartz, S. Are Value–Behavior Relations Stronger than Previously Thought? It Depends on Value Importance. *Eur. J. Pers.* **2022**, *36*, 133–148. [CrossRef]
25. Bardi, A.; Schwartz, S.H. Values and Behavior: Strength and Structure of Relations. *Pers. Soc. Psychol. Bull.* **2003**, *29*, 1207–1220. [CrossRef] [PubMed]
26. Zhou, D. Insights into the Indonesian Games Market. Available online: https://newzoo.com/resources/blog/insights-into-the-indonesian-games-market (accessed on 17 July 2023).

engineering proceedings

MDPI

Proceeding Paper

Implementation of Environmental Management System: A Case Study for Construction Companies in the Philippines †

Marlon C. Leyesa

Bulacan State University—Malolos Campus, City of Malolos 3000, Philippines; marlon.leyesa@bulsu.edu.ph

† Presented at the 2024 IEEE 4th International Conference on Electronic Communications, Internet of Things and Big Data, Taipei, Taiwan, 19–21 April 2024.

Abstract: This study aims to design an environmental management information system (EMIS) by integrating all necessary environmental documents for project implementation based on ISO 14001:2015 and using an exploratory sequential mixed method of research. The agile project management methodology was also used to speculate how a project must be managed using environmental information. The problems with the current operation in compliance with ISO 14001:2015 were addressed using EMIS with the participation of IT professionals. The end-users assessed the functionality, efficiency, compatibility, usability, reliability, security, maintainability, and portability of EMIS. A computer system is required for EMIS for accurate and effective document storage and updates. EMIS can be developed based on coding and simulation to make it simpler to save, retrieve, and update documents. EMIS needs to have functionality, efficiency, compatibility, usability, reliability, security, maintainability, and portability.

Keywords: environmental management information system; agile project management methodology; application software

Citation: Leyesa, M.C. Implementation of Environmental Management System: A Case Study for Construction Companies in the Philippines. *Eng. Proc.* **2024**, *74*, 32. https://doi.org/10.3390/engproc2024074032

Academic Editors: Shu-Han Liao, Teen-Hang Meen and Cheng-Fu Yang

Published: 30 August 2024

1. Introduction

Many construction companies are experiencing an industrial revolution. The construction industry adheres to the international standards for regulating measures, whereas other businesses are bound only by their areas of operation [1]. Realizing environmental threats is a top priority in the construction industry, yet others focus on day-to-day operations. Environmental risks are neglected and given low priority in other industries. Construction companies must determine internal and external issues of the business environment which affects a company's ability to achieve the intended results or outcomes of an environmental management system.

A management system is the method an organization uses to coordinate the various aspects of its operations to accomplish its goals. The techniques for carrying out the business are defined by the policies and procedures [2]. It is important to have a reliable, user-friendly, and efficient management information system to improve the accuracy of environmental reports and efficiently monitor projects related to the environment [3,4]. Most businesses require fast and reliable management information systems for processing and monitoring their environmental requirements [5]. Companies continually need to follow the standards for the environment. Thus, there is a demand to establish an environmental management information system (EMIS) for construction companies [6] to offer differentiated services from small- to large-scale infrastructures [7].

Construction companies must refer to documents for the environmental issues provided by the Environmental Management Bureau (EMB) of the Department of Environment and Natural Resources, which are the following: Environmental Compliance Certificate, Certificate of Non-Coverage, Permit to Operate Air, Certificate of Conformity, Hazardous Waste Management Permit, Water Quality Management Permits, and Self-Monitoring

Report [8]. The reports of monitoring, evaluation, health and safety, and project performance of every project must be submitted. Therefore, it is important to use a system to manage these documents effectively [9]. In this regard, it is necessary to build a system to integrate the environmental documents into a single system that incorporates the necessary processes.

2. Methodology

2.1. Framework of Study

Figure 1 shows the agile project management methodology (APMM) used to develop the environmental management information system (EMIS) in this study. The framework is easy to use and organizes the development of EMIS [10].

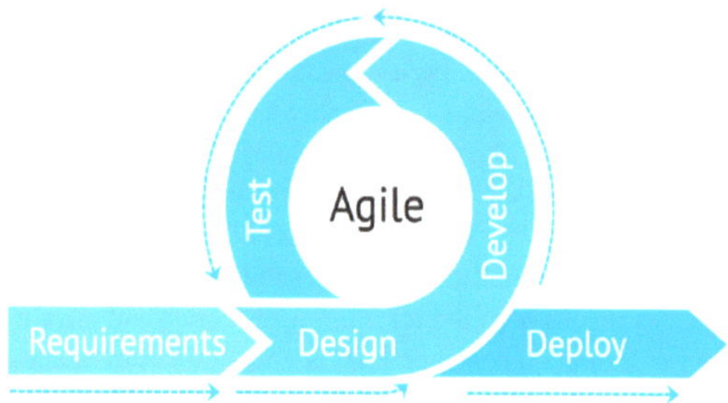

Figure 1. Agile project management methodology (APMM).

APMM is composed of five phases: requirements, design, development, test, and implementation. APMM illustrates the development process in iteration in a productive environment. The iterative phases in APMM are as follows.

1. Requirements and Planning Phase

In this phase, the environmental requirements needed for every project are identified for the company to acquire. This can be completed by conducting a focus group discussion with the engineering and operation departments. Solutions are offered for the identified requirements. The solutions may be in the form of tasks or activities considering the provisions of ISO14001:2015 [11] from the planning phase to the closing phase.

2. Design Phase

Software is used in designing the templates of the expected reports in the proposed system, following the standards in the information technology for software and hardware component requirements for the system. Detailed design of the system is created using flowcharts, diagrams, and other modeling tools.

3. Development and Testing Phase

Software for the coding and simulation of the proposed system is indispensable. Simulation is conducted to ensure the system is error- and bug-free.

4. Deployment Phase

The developed system is installed in the company for utilization. The system's functional suitability, performance efficiency, compatibility, usability, reliability, security, maintainability, and portability are assessed.

The process shows the behavior of the flow from one to the other phases. This process was created in this study to manage the changing requirements of the system without impacting the outcome of the company.

2.2. Software of EMIS

EMIS was constructed for construction companies in the Philippines. The system provides a simple, reliable, user-friendly, and efficient management system for users to access all environmental documents necessary for a project. The procedure to access the EMIS for construction is shown in Figure 2.

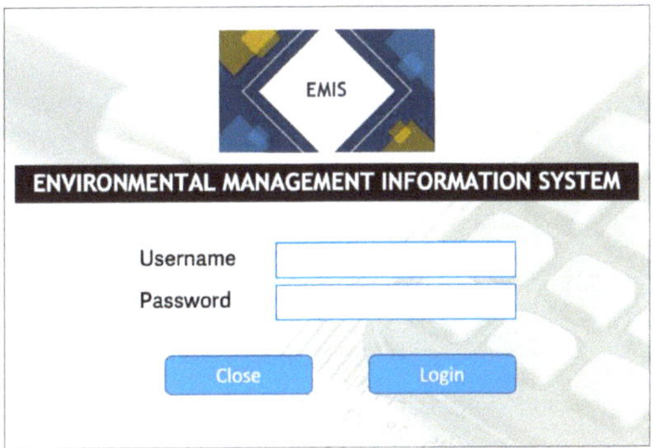

Figure 2. Log-in module of EMIS.

The first step is to collect data from the user, which includes a username and password. The information is sent to the database. If the information matches the data in the system, the user is granted full access to the system, as shown in Figure 3. Figure 3 shows the EMIS project folder with forms and templates. It provides a compilation of reports needed in the initiating stage, delivery stage, and closing stage of every project in compliance with legal and other requirements. Each template records and responds to user actions in the database. All templates needed from the initiating stage to the closing stage of a project are based on the requirements of the client and/or government.

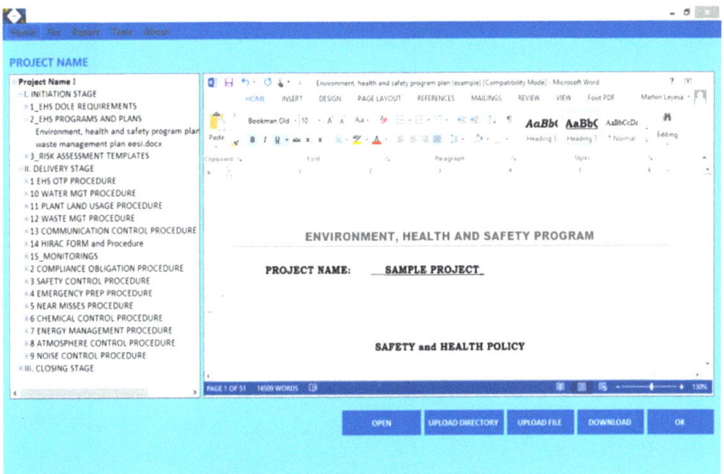

Figure 3. Front graphic user interface of EMIS.

Figure 4 shows the initiation stage subfolders, which compile reports needed in the initiating stage of every project. The initiating stage subfolders consist of the EHS DOLE requirements, EHS programs and plans, and risk assessment templates.

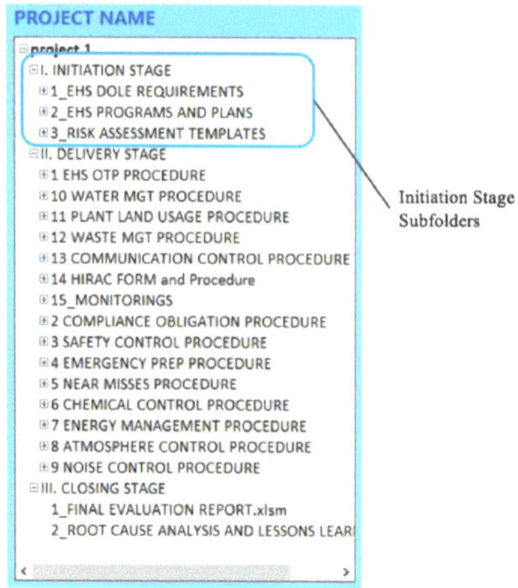

Figure 4. Initiation stage subfolders.

Figure 5 shows the delivery stage subfolders. These subfolders contain the forms and templates that compile reports needed during the delivery stage of every project. Delivery stage subfolders comprise the following: 1. EHS OTP procedure, 2. compliance obligation procedure, 3. safety control procedure, 4. emergency preparation procedure, 5. near misses procedure, 6. chemical control procedure, 7. energy management procedure, 8. atmosphere control procedure, 9. noise control procedure, 10. water management procedure, 11. plant land usage procedure, 12. waste management procedure, 13. communication control procedure, 14. hirac form and procedure, and 15. monitoring report.

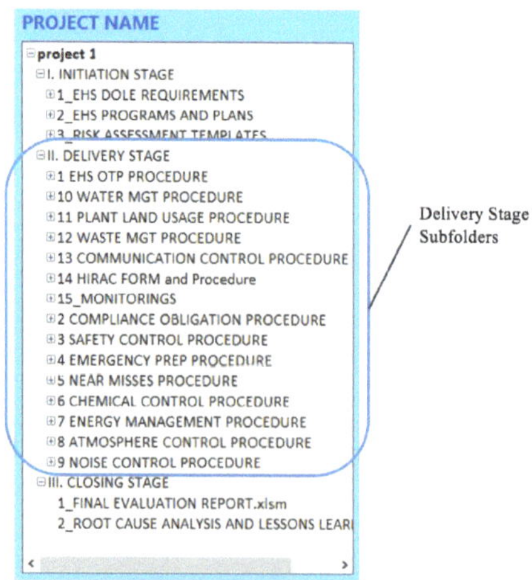

Figure 5. Delivery stage subfolders.

Figure 6 shows the closing stage templates that compile reports needed during the closing stage of the project. The closing stage templates include the final evaluation report, root cause analysis, and lessons learned.

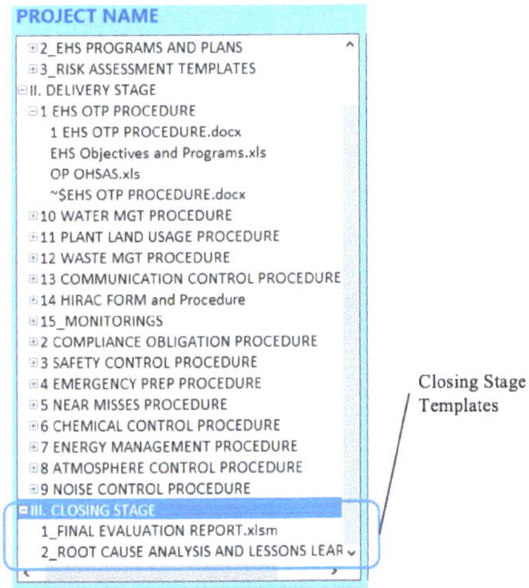

Figure 6. Closing stage subfolders.

2.3. Project Evaluation

The evaluation of EMIS involves assessing the tools and techniques required for project management. EMIS was evaluated by top and middle management as well as the pollution control officer (PCO) of twenty construction companies in the Philippines, as shown in Table 1.

Table 1. Respondents of this study.

Respondents	Percentage of Respondents
Top Management (President/Board of Directors/Project Sponsors/Program Managers/Project Directors)	30%
Middle Management (Project Managers/Supervisors/Project In-Charge)	30%
Pollution Control Officers (PCO)	40%
Total	100%

Table 2 shows the rating scale and criteria for the system evaluation questionnaire. The degree of acceptability of the respondent for each statement was selected in the evaluation to effectively collect sufficient quantitative data for evaluation. The evaluation questionnaire was created to assess the level of satisfaction with the system in terms of functional suitability, performance efficiency, compatibility, usability, reliability, security, maintainability, and portability.

Table 2. Rating scale and description for the system evaluation questionnaire.

Rating Scale	Verbal Interpretation	Description
5	Very Satisfactory	The EMIS is highly functional, efficient, compatible, usable, reliable, secure, portable, and maintainable in providing environmental processes relative to the client and government's requirements.
4	Satisfactory	The EMIS features are enough to provide a functional, efficient, compatible, usable, reliable, secure, portable, and maintainable system. A few limited features need to be upgraded and updated.

Table 2. *Cont.*

Rating Scale	Verbal Interpretation	Description
3	Moderately Satisfactory	EMIS shows fair specifications and physical features. There are still a few important functions that require improvement and enhancement.
2	Poor	The respondents are not satisfied with the demonstration and testing of the EMIS. Some parts malfunctioned.
1	Very Poor	The EMIS is not applicable, not reliable and not useful.

3. Results and Discussion

EMIS provides the methods and results of compilation, computation, and evaluation of every project and allows the user to open, create, update, print, and store the environmental reports of the project. The embedded mixed method was used for qualitative and quantitative assessments for recommendations and the evaluation of the decision support system for the company. The invited IT experts evaluated the design and development of the EMIS. The current environmental practice of construction companies in the Philippines was analyzed based on RA 6969, " An Act to Control Toxic Substances and Hazardous and Nuclear Wastes, Providing Penalties for Violations thereof, and other purposes", RA 9003, "An Act Providing for an Ecological Solid Waste Management Program, Creating the Necessary Institutional Mechanics and Incentives Declaring Certain Acts Prohibited and Providing Penalties, Appropriating Funds thereof, and the other purposes", RA 8749, "Philippine Clean Air Act: An Act Providing Comprehensive Air Quality Management Policy and Program, which Aims to Achieve and Maintain Healthy Air for All Filipinos.", RA 9275, "Environmental Management Bureau: An Act Providing for a Comprehensive Water Quality Management and for other purposes", and PD 1586, "Presidential Decree for Establishing an Environmental Impact Statement System, including other Environmental Management Related Measures and for other purposes". The solution to the existing system is described under ISO14001:2015's Environmental Management System [11].

The design of EMIS was assessed in terms of the hardware, software, and templates. For the hardware, the weighted mean of the score was 4.90, which implied that the existing hardware was highly sufficient with the features of the system. For the software requirements, the weighted mean score was 4.94, which showed that the software design was highly sufficient with the features of the system. The templates were designed according to common templates of the companies and adopted from the Department of Environment and National Resources. The weighted mean score was 4.66, which showed that the proposed template was highly sufficient with the legal and other requirements.

The development of the EMIS was described in terms of coding and simulation. The EMIS was coded based on the limited use of global, standard headers for different modules/forms, naming conventions for local variables, constants and functions, indention, error return values, and exception handling conventions. A simulation was conducted to obtain feedback. The developed EMIS was assessed in terms of functional suitability, performance efficiency, compatibility, usability, reliability, security, maintainability, and portability. Functional suitability and usability shine were the most important criteria, as the respondents rated the system very satisfactory, with a weighted mean score of 4.80. However, for reliability and performance, the score was 4.66. Compatibility was scored 4.64. The portability and security were scored 4.58, and maintainability was ranked eighth with a weighted mean score of 4.52. Overall, the system scored 4.66, which was equivalent to the rate of very satisfactory. The results showed that the EMIS for construction companies in the Philippines is highly recommendable based on the evaluation results.

4. Conclusions and Recommendations

The current environmental management system of the construction companies in the Philippines requires a computer system to aid in the storage, retrieval, and updating of relevant documents. The ISO14001:2015 Environmental Management System standard was adopted to retrieve, create, modify, and update environmental documents and records in the EMIS. The EMIS was designed with high sufficiency in terms of hardware and software for each project and developed using coding and simulation standards. The EMIS facilitates easier storage, retrieval, and the update of pertinent documents in terms of functional suitability, performance efficiency, compatibility, usability, reliability, security, maintainability, and portability. The EMIS can be implemented in companies to improve project processing. A separate unit or team is needed to manage the EMIS to monitor the project in terms of the initiating to closing stages. The EMIS can be used to assess other projects before implementation to avoid unnecessary delays and problems. Further study is needed to provide additional features of the EMIS to enhance the system.

Funding: This research received no external funding.

Institutional Review Board Statement: The study was conducted and approved by the Research Management Office of Bulacan State University.

Informed Consent Statement: Not applicable.

Data Availability Statement: The data presented in this study are available on request from the corresponding author.

Conflicts of Interest: The author declare no conflict of interest.

References

1. Leyesa, M.C.; Florencondia, N.T.; Villar, M.J.M.; Galman, S.M.A. Decision Support System in Environmental, Health and Safety (DSS-EHS) Management Systems. In Proceedings of the 2020 IEEE 12th International Conference on Humanoid, Nanotechnology, Information Technology, Communication and Control, Environment, and Management (HNICEM), Manila, Philippines, 3–7 December 2020.
2. ISO Secretariat. Management System Standards. 2001. Available online: https://www.iso.org/management-system-standards.html (accessed on 14 July 2020).
3. Leyesa, M.C.; Mariano, O.R.; Galvez, R.L. Project Cost Processing System for Electronics Systems Integrator. In Proceedings of the 2022 IEEE 10th Region 10 Humanitarian Technology Conference (R10-HTC), Hyderabad, India, 16–18 September 2022.
4. Abella, & Abella. Permits Issued by the Department of Environment and Natural Resources–Environmental Management Bureau (EMB). 2022. Available online: https://greendevsolutions.com/all-environmental-permits-ph/ (accessed on 15 January 2023).
5. Yin, Y.; Yin, L.; Wang, C. The whole process cost management of construction project based on business process reengineering. In Proceedings of the 2010 International Conference on Logistics Systems and Intelligent Management (ICLSIM), Harbin, China, 9–10 January 2010; pp. 412–415.
6. Isenmann, R. Scholar Archive. July 2008. Available online: https://scholarsarchive.byu.edu/cgi/viewcontent.cgi?article=2886&context=iemssconference#:~:text=Environmental%20Management%20Information%20Systems%20(EMIS)%20are%20socio-technological%20systems,with%20other%20actors%20in%20industry (accessed on 8 February 2023).
7. DPWH. List of Registered Contractors with valid PCAB License as of 2017. Department of Public Works and Highways, Republic of the Philippines. Available online: https://www.dpwh.gov.ph/DPWH/business/procurement/civil_works/contractors (accessed on 16 February 2023).
8. DENR. Environmental Management Bureau. Department of Environment and Natural Resources, Republic of the Philippines. Available online: https://emb.gov.ph/ (accessed on 8 February 2023).
9. Dehao, G. Analysis and improvement of construction project management system based on network information. In Proceedings of the 2020 12th International Conference on Measuring Technology and Mechatronics Automation (ICMTMA), Phuket, Thailand, 28–29 February 2020.
10. Rajdeep, S. Top Agile Software Development Companies for Startups. October 2021. Available online: https://medium.com/@sneharajdeep/top-agile-software-development-companies-for-startups-32cc2285fa8b (accessed on 28 February 2023).
11. *ISO 14001:2015*; Environmental management systems—Requirements with guidance for use. International Organization for Standardization: Geneva, Switzerland, 2015.

engineering proceedings

MDPI

Proceeding Paper

A Preliminary Study on Exploring the Use of Translation Apps and Post-Editing Strategies of University Students †

Ya-Ting Zhan and Hsiao-Tung Hsu *

Department of Applied English, Chaoyang University of Technology, Taichung 413310, Taiwan; s11122603@gm.cyut.edu.tw
* Correspondence: hthsu@cyut.edu.tw

† Presented at the 2024 IEEE 4th International Conference on Electronic Communications, Internet of Things and Big Data, Taipei, Taiwan, 19–21 April 2024.

Abstract: In the digital age, finding technology for English learning experience is imperative. With various language learning technologies emerging, many students are using translation applications (apps) as indispensable tools in their English learning. Previous research has primarily focused on the translation strategies for learners of English as a foreign language (EFL) and post-editing strategies using machine translation and the practices of professional post-editors and translators. We explored students' utilization of translation apps in the context of English language learning and their application of post-editing strategies to understand their perspectives on technology's role. A questionnaire survey was conducted to collect data from university students in Taiwan, which was analyzed utilizing descriptive statistics and one-way ANOVA via SPSS version 23. Students used translation apps to learn vocabulary and comprehend English articles. Post-editing strategies such as punctuation and terminology correction were not used frequently by the students. Most of them agreed that translation apps serve as valuable English learning supplements. By understanding the prevailing learning dynamics of university students, the results of this study lay a foundation for more investigations.

Keywords: translation apps; English learning; post-editing strategies

Citation: Zhan, Y.-T.; Hsu, H.-T. A Preliminary Study on Exploring the Use of Translation Apps and Post-Editing Strategies of University Students. *Eng. Proc.* **2024**, *74*, 33. https://doi.org/10.3390/engproc2024074033

Academic Editors: Shu-Han Liao, Teen-Hang Meen and Cheng-Fu Yang

Published: 2 September 2024

1. Introduction

In the digital era, acquiring language skills has become ubiquitous with the help of various high-end technologies and applications (apps). Software is designed and available on mobile devices such as smartphones and tablets with versatile functions for various purposes [1]. Technology is seamlessly integrated into the language learning experience. With the advancement of translation tools, translation apps (e.g., Google Translate, DeepL Translate, and ChatGPT) assist students in learning English. For instance, teachers apply Google Translate in the classroom and teach students reading, writing, vocabulary skills, and translation. Students are not inclined to use them in translation assignments and writing assignments [2,3]. They can improve their language learning to indulge in their learning and better understand their abilities [3].

Given the inferior translation quality, post-editing is an imperative procedure. Post-editing (also called machine translation post-editing) is defined as the correction of the output produced by machine translation (MT), and based on the requirement of the final product, the target text is amended for translation quality [4,5]. Chang et al. [6] suggested that students must enhance their abilities in machine translation post-editing because they can learn how to recognize the quality of AI-generated texts. MT and translation apps assist students with their translation. Students can accelerate their work and strengthen their competence in transcreation.

Previous research has focused on the translation strategies utilized by learners of English as a foreign language (EFL) [7–10] and the post-editing strategies applied in MT. Researchers have delved into the practices of professional post-editors and translators [11,12]. We explored translation apps in the context of English language learning and investigated their application of post-editing strategies to understand technology's role in their English language learning. Post-editing originally refers to the modification of machine-generated texts. Since MT embodies many translation tools, we used the translated texts generated by translation apps for this study. Based on the purpose of the study, the following research areas for analysis were proposed:

1. Situations where students learn English with translation apps;
2. Post-editing strategies that students adopt after using translation apps;
3. Students' perceptions of using translation apps as an English learning supplement.

2. Literature Review

2.1. Translation in English Learning Strategy

Translation is widely used in English training and facilitates learners' English learning as long as teachers use it for teaching particular English skills [13]. Translation is advantageous for learners to acquire a second language (L2). For instance, they learn new vocabulary, grammatical structures, idiomatic expressions, reading and listening contexts, writing, and the differences and similarities between their first language (L1) and L2 [8,13,14]. Many researchers view translation as a beneficial and supporting method for language learning [7–9,13,15]. It is unavoidable for learners to use their mother tongue to think and comprehend the contexts while learning foreign languages [7,9,15]. On the other hand, several researchers have negative beliefs about using translation as a language-learning strategy because they regard it as a hindrance to their language acquisition [10,15]. Even so, they still think that translation helps them. Highly proficient learners prefer using English directly and translation strategies to find the differences and similarities between the two languages and improve their English skills. This causes them to rarely use translation strategies compared to those with low English proficiency [9,16,17]. Regardless of disparate opinions on strategy use, translation plays a significant role in language learning.

2.2. Post-Editing Strategies

In language learning, students use self-monitoring strategies to ensure that they comprehend correctly and regulate their ways of study [18,19], similar to the machine translation post-editing procedure. Students monitor and control their learning and reflect, improving their language learning outcomes and translation quality [20]. Machine translation post-editing is necessary for correcting a raw output [21,22]. A post-editor needs to ensure the MT-generated text fits the intended meaning of the source language and correct errors appearing in the target language [23,24]. When the post-editors conducted light post-editing, the translation text presented information appropriately and kept it semantically correct, including correcting words, grammar, and punctuation (i.e., linguistic MT errors). As for the full post-editing, the contexts must be grammatically correct and stylistically acceptable with translation quality, so the strategy of adding supplementary explanation (i.e., the correction of pragmatic errors and affective errors) is adopted [21,25–28].

It is essential to educate students to apply MT and post-edit its output. To guarantee the fluency and accuracy of the MT, students use various resources and MT tools to crosscheck [29,30]. In post-editing practices, students can notice different strategies in distinct fields, gain linguistic knowledge and translation skills exploited in both L1 and L2, and enhance the productivity and quality of translation texts [31–34]. Nonetheless, several researchers are concerned about the translation technology in language teaching and learning [33,35]. Although the quality of neural machine translation (NMT) has improved a lot, it cannot translate as well as humans. Students are inclined to rely exclusively on its outcomes but without an excellent language proficiency level and translation competence, contributing to the translation with errors [34–36]. Despite different factors that make the results of post-editing questionable, students have a positive attitude toward post-editing [33,34,37].

2.3. Translation Tools

MT is a digital device to translate texts from one language into another without human intervention [38,39]. Owing to the large amount of MT, we used translation apps to help students translate using mobile devices such as smartphones and tablets. Teachers use translation apps in their teaching, impacting students' language learning [40–42]. Students showed progress in their translation performances and enhanced translation skills, promoting better conversational competence and cultivating linguistic skills [40,41,43,44]. Thus, translation apps need to be utilized in translation classes, and teachers must be open-minded with the use of translation apps in class and teach students how to use them wisely [41,43]. Researchers have a positive attitude toward using Google Translate because they regard it as a significant tool for improving language competence.

3. Methodology

We collected data from university students in Taiwan using a questionnaire survey, which consisted of seven demographic questions and 42 questions related to English learning, post-editing strategies, and students' perspectives. A five-point Likert scale was used in the survey: 5 = Strongly Agree, 4 = Agree, 3 = Neutral, 2 = Disagree, and 1 = Strongly Disagree. The questionnaire was modified for learning strategies [9] and post-editing strategies [12,45]. The survey was administered online, and the data collected were analyzed using descriptive statistics and one-way ANOVA via SPSS version 23.

Thirty-two students were randomly selected for the preliminary questionnaire study. Reliability and consistency were assessed for the quality of research [46]. To test the reliability, Cronbach's α was adopted in this study. Generally, Cronbach's α of 0.7 is deemed acceptable, and a value greater than or equal to 0.9 stands is regarded as excellent. The Cronbach's α of this questionnaire was 0.936, revealing a high level of consistency for 42 items in the questionnaire. Considering the value of Cronbach's α and the types of questions, items 13 (Cronbach's α if Item Deleted = 0.936) and 14 (Cronbach's α if Item Deleted = 0.936) were deleted. Hence, there were seven demographic questions and 40 questions in total. Three professors specializing in English teaching evaluated this questionnaire's validity and provided suggestions for improving its validity, referring to how accurately a measure reflects the reality of the sampled items [47]. The order of questions was reorganized and divided into four sections: (1) background information, (2) the use of translation apps in English learning, (3) post-editing strategies, and (4) students' perspectives.

The research was conducted in the following six steps as depicted in Figure 1. First, we identified the problems. Second, the literature review was conducted. Third, a questionnaire was devised. Fourth, the questionnaire survey was conducted. Fifth, the questionnaire was modified for the survey (Figure 1).

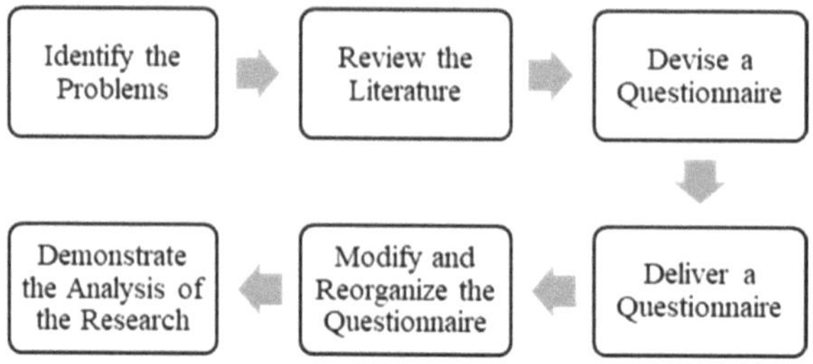

Figure 1. Flow chart of procedure of this study.

4. Results and Discussion

The respondents included 28 females (87.5%) and 4 males (12.5%). To distinguish students' English proficiency, they were assessed for language ability using the Common European Framework of Reference for Languages (CEFR). Students at CEFR B1 (Threshold) level represented the majority (N = 12), followed by CEFR A2 (Waystage) level (N = 8), CEFR A1 (Breakthrough) level (N = 5), CEFR B2 (Vantage) level (N = 5), CEFR C1 (Effective Operational Proficiency) level (N = 2), and CEFR C2 (Mastery) level (N = 0).

The situation of students' English learning with translation apps was revealed in items from 1 to 26 except items 13, 14, 23, and 24. The average score was 3.63, and the score ranged from 2.75 to 4.44. Item 26 (M = 4.44), item 8 (M = 4.28), item 7 (M = 4.03), and item 2 (M = 4.03) showed higher scores. The respondents used translation apps for vocabulary learning and understanding English articles. They did not use it before reading English articles as presented in item 1 (M = 2.75). There was a statistically significant difference in English proficiency (item 19). The threshold was set at 0.05. One-way ANOVA results showed that translation apps helped to recall the content of English lessons (at a significance of 0.014 ($p < 0.05$)). In addition, multiple comparisons of Scheffe's test revealed that students at the CEFR A2 level significantly differed from those at the CEFR C1 level ($p = 0.047 < 0.05$). Students at the CEFR A2 level were more serious and better than those at the CEFR C1 level in using translation apps to recall the content of English lessons.

The average score of students' post-editing strategies for translation apps was 3.75. Most students perceived that post-editing strategies after using translation apps helped them accomplish their translation more quickly (item 36, M = 4.06). The standard deviation (0.95) presented a concentrated distribution. The scores for items 30, 31, 33, and 32 elucidated that students rarely corrected the punctuation (M = 3.31), terminology use (M = 3.44), cultural references and metaphorical expressions (M = 3.47), and added supplementary information or explanations (M = 3.72). There was a significant difference between item 32 and English proficiency ($p = 0.012 < 0.05$). Students' post-editing of supplementary information or explanations in the translation text was significant compared with different English proficiency. According to the results of multiple comparisons of Scheffe's test, learners at the CEFR B1 level and those at the CEFR C1 level showed significant differences ($p = 0.043 < 0.05$). Students at the CEFR B1 level added supplementary information or explanations in the translated text better than those at the CEFR C1 level during strategy use.

Items 23, 24, 27, 40, 41, and 42 were asked to examine students' perceptions. The average score was 3.57, ranging from 3.06 to 4.06. Most participants thought translation apps were helpful English learning supplements (4.06), and the standard deviation (0.91) indicated a relatively concentrated distribution. They had concerns with the translation quality produced by translation apps (item 23, M = 3.06 and item 27, M = 3.09). The correlation between the score of item 24 (I think translation apps are good English learning supplements) and English proficiency was 0.024 ($p < 0.05$), demonstrating that they were significant. The correlation was significant ($p = 0.045 < 0.05$) for students at the CEFR A2 level and CEFR C1 level and was more significant for students at the CEFR A2 level (MD = 2.1250*). The overall descriptive statistics are presented in Table 1.

Table 1. Descriptive statistics of students at three levels in variance.

Item	Mean	Standard Deviation	N
A	3.63	1.12	32
B	3.75	1.16	32
C	3.57	1.04	32

(A: the situation of students' English learning with translation apps, B: post-editing strategies, and C: students' perspectives).

5. Conclusions

Most students learn vocabulary and comprehend reading passages via translation apps. In the question survey, item 19 (I use translation apps to recall the content of English lessons better) was related to English proficiency. Students with low English proficiency preferred to use translation apps to recall the content of English lessons to those with high English proficiency. Most students seldom added supplementary information or explanations, modified cultural references and metaphorical expressions, or corrected the terms and punctuation. Item 32 (I add supplementary information or explanations in the translation done by translation apps to ensure the completeness of the translation work) was significantly different among students at different levels. Students at the CEFR B1 level adopted this strategy more frequently than students at the CEFR C1 level when post-editing the texts. Moreover, they were positive about using translation apps as English learning supplements. Students with low English proficiency were more agreeable to the statement. Students who were not skilled in English had more positive attitudes toward English learning and post-editing strategies with translation apps.

Due to the limitations of this study, the results of this study cannot be generalized for all university students. Accordingly, it is necessary to conduct further research with more samples and questions. Then, the prevailing learning dynamics of university students can be elucidated to understand more about the use of English learning apps.

Author Contributions: Both authors contributed equally to this work. All authors have read and agreed to the published version of the manuscript.

Funding: This research received no external funding.

Institutional Review Board Statement: Not applicable.

Informed Consent Statement: Not applicable.

Data Availability Statement: Data are contained within the article.

Conflicts of Interest: The authors declare no conflicts of interest.

References

1. Lu, Y.; Xiong, T. The attitudes of high school students and teachers toward mobile apps for learning English: A Q methodology study. *Soc. Sci. Humanit. Open* **2023**, *8*, 100555. [CrossRef]
2. Alhaisoni, E.; Alhaysony, M. An investigation of Saudi EFL university students' attitudes towards the use of Google Translate. *Int. J. Engl. Lang. Educ.* **2017**, *5*, 72–82. [CrossRef]
3. Bahri, H.; Mahadi, T.S.T. Google Translate as a supplementary tool for learning Malay: A case study at Universiti Sains Malaysia. *Adv. Lang. Lit. Stud.* **2016**, *7*, 161–167. [CrossRef]
4. O'Brien, S. Methodologies for measuring the correlations between post-editing effort and machine translatability. *Mach. Translat.* **2005**, *19*, 37–58. [CrossRef]
5. Tezcan, A.; Hoste, V.; Macken, L. Estimating post-editing time using a gold-standard set of machine translation errors. *Comput. Speech Lang.* **2019**, *55*, 120–144. [CrossRef]
6. Chang, C.-C.; Chen, B.-J.; Chen, P.-W.; Chin, C.-C.; Liao, P.-S.; Lin, C.-L.; Shih, C.-L. How does translation education face the challenge of AI and use AI. *Compil. Transl. Rev.* **2021**, *14*, 157–181. [CrossRef]
7. Edelia, A.D.; Maharsi, I. A survey on translation as a learning strategy by EFL higher education students in English learning. *Pedagog. J. Engl. Lang. Teach.* **2022**, *10*, 111–122. [CrossRef]
8. Khan, R.M.I.; Kumar, T.; Supriyatno, T.; Nukapangu, V. The phenomenon of Arabic-English translation of foreign language classes during the pandemic. *Ijaz Arab. J. Arab. Learn.* **2021**, *4*, 570–582. [CrossRef]
9. Liao, P. EFL learners' beliefs about and strategy use of translation in English learning. *RELC J.* **2006**, *37*, 191–215. [CrossRef]
10. Thani, A.S.; Ageli, N.R. The use of translation as a learning strategy: A case study of students of the University of Bahrain. *Int. J. Linguist. Lit. Transl.* **2020**, *3*, 87–101. [CrossRef]
11. Girletti, S. Working with pre-translated texts: Preliminary findings from a survey on post-editing and revision practices in Swiss corporate in-house language services. In Proceedings of the 23rd Annual Conference of the European Association for Machine Translation, Ghent, Belgium, 1–3 June 2022; pp. 271–280.
12. Hong, J.; Lee, I.J. A satisfaction survey on the human translation outcomes and machine translation post-editing outcomes. *Int. J. Adv. Smart Converg.* **2021**, *10*, 86–96. [CrossRef]

13. Samardali, M.F.S.; Ismael, A.M.H. Translation as a tool for teaching English as a second language. *J. Lit. Lang. Linguist.* **2017**, *40*, 64–69.
14. Alaboud, A. The positive effect of translation on improving reading comprehension among female Arabic learners of English as foreign language. *Arab. World Engl. J.* **2022**, *13*, 424–436. [CrossRef]
15. Tze Ying, B.; Lay Hoon, A.; Abdul Halim, H.; Majtanova, M. Students' beliefs on translation strategy in learning German language. *GEMA Online J. Lang. Stud.* **2018**, *18*, 69–86. [CrossRef]
16. Qassem, M. Translation strategy and procedure analysis: A cultural perspective. *Asia Pac. Transl. Intercult. Stud.* **2021**, *8*, 300–319. [CrossRef]
17. Yulita, D. The correlation of English proficiency level and translation strategies used by Indonesian EFL learners. *Lang. Lang. Teach. J.* **2021**, *24*, 240–248. [CrossRef]
18. Cárdenas, A.M. Tackling intermediate students' fossilized grammatical errors in speech through self-evaluation and self-monitoring strategies. *Profile Issues Teach. Prof. Dev.* **2018**, *20*, 195–209. [CrossRef]
19. O'Malley, J.M.; Chamot, A.U. *Learning Strategies in Second Language Acquisition*; Cambridge University Press: Cambridge, UK, 1990.
20. Yang, Y.; Wang, X. Predicting student translators' performance in machine translation post-editing: Interplay of self-regulation, critical thinking, and motivation. *Interact. Learn. Envir.* **2020**, *31*, 340–354. [CrossRef]
21. Chang, Y. Differences in Machine Translation Post-Editing (MTPE) Strategies between Technical and Tourism Texts: Analysis from the Perspective of Register Theory. Master's Thesis, National Kaohsiung University of Science and Technology, Kaohsiung, Taiwan, 2020.
22. Ye, N.; Jiang, L.; Ma, D.; Zhang, Y.; Zhao, S.; Cai, D. Predicting post-editing effort for English-Chinese neural machine translation. In Proceedings of the 2021 International Conference on Asian Language Processing, Singapore, 11–13 December 2021; pp. 154–158.
23. Carl, M.; Bangalore, S.; Schaeffer, M. *New Directions in Empirical Translation Process Research: Exploring the CRITT TPR-DB*, 1st ed.; Springer: Cham, Switzerland, 2016; pp. 77–94.
24. do Carmo, F.E.M. Post-editing: A theoretical and practical challenge for translation studies and machine learning. Ph.D. Dissertation, University of Porto, Porto, Portugal, 2017.
25. Koponen, M. Is machine translation post-editing worth the effort? A survey of research into post-editing and effort. *J. Spec. Transl.* **2016**, *25*, 131–148.
26. Krings, H.P. *Repairing Texts: Empirical Investigations of Machine Translation Post-Editing Processes*; The Kent State University Press: Kent, OH, USA, 2001.
27. Massardo, I.; Meer, J.V.D.; O'Brien, S.; Hollowood, F.; Aranberri, N.; Drescher, K. *MT Post-Editing Guidelines*; TAUS Signature Editions: Amsterdam, The Netherlands, 2016.
28. Shih, C. Re-looking into machine translation errors and post-editing strategies in a changing high-tech context. *Compil. Transl. Rev.* **2021**, *14*, 125–166. [CrossRef]
29. Chang, L.-C. Chinese language learners evaluating machine translation accuracy. *JALT CALL J.* **2022**, *18*, 110–136. [CrossRef]
30. Tavares, C.; Tallone, L.; Oliveira, L.; Ribeiro, S. The challenges of teaching and assessing technical translation in an era of neural machine translation. *Educ. Sci.* **2023**, *13*, 541. [CrossRef]
31. Cui, Y.; Liu, X.; Cheng, Y. A comparative study on the effort of human translation and post-editing in relation to text types: An eye-tracking and key-logging experiment. *SAGE Open* **2023**, *13*. [CrossRef]
32. Harto, S.; Hamied, F.A.; Musthafa, B.; Setyarini, S. Exploring undergraduate students' experiences in dealing with post-editing of machine translation. *Indones. J. Appl. Linguist.* **2022**, *11*, 696–707. [CrossRef]
33. Jia, Y.; Lai, S. Post-editing metaphorical expressions: Productivity, quality, and strategies. *J. Foreign Lang. Cult.* **2022**, *6*, 28–43. [CrossRef]
34. Varela Salinas, M.-J.; Burbat, R. Google Translate and DeepL: Breaking taboos in translator training. Observational study and analysis. *Ibérica* **2023**, 243–266. [CrossRef]
35. Liu, K.; Kwok, H.L.; Liu, J.; Cheung, A.K.F. Sustainability and influence of machine translation: Perceptions and attitudes of translation instructors and learners in Hong Kong. *Sustainability* **2022**, *14*, 6399. [CrossRef]
36. Yu, Z.; Lu, Y. Post-editing performance of English-major undergraduates in China: A case study of C-E translation with pedagogical reflections. In Proceedings of the 17th International Conference on Computer Science and Education, Zhejiang, China, 18–21 August 2022; pp. 408–420.
37. Jia, Y.; Carl, M.; Wang, X. How does the post-editing of neural machine translation compare with from-scratch translation? A product and process study. *J. Spec. Transl.* **2019**, *31*, 60–86.
38. Kornacki, M. *Computer-Assisted Translation (CAT) Tools in the Translator Training Process*; Peter Lang: Berlin, Germany, 2018.
39. Potapova, R.; Potapov, V.; Kuzmin, O. Logistics translator. Concept vision on future interlanguage computer assisted translation. In Proceedings of the International Conference on Speech and Computer, Gurugram, India, 14–16 November 2022; pp. 579–589.
40. Chen, Y. Using a game-based translation learning app and Google apps to enhance translation skills: Amplification and omission. *Int. J. Hum.-Comput. Int.* **2023**, *39*, 3894–3908. [CrossRef]
41. Lake, V.E.; Beisly, A.H. Translation apps: Increasing communication with dual language learners. *Early Child. Educ. J.* **2019**, *47*, 489–496. [CrossRef]

42. Ross, R.K.; Lake, V.E.; Beisly, A.H. Preservice teachers' use of a translation app with dual language learners. *J. Digit. Learn. Teach. Educ.* **2020**, *37*, 86–98. [CrossRef]
43. Alotaibi, H.; Salamah, D. The impact of translation apps on translation students' performance. *Educ. Inf. Technol.* **2023**, *28*, 10709–10729. [CrossRef]
44. Bin Dahmash, N. I can't live without Google Translate: A close look at the use of Google Translate app by second language learners in Saudi Arabia. *Arab. World Engl. J.* **2020**, *11*, 226–240. [CrossRef]
45. Yang, Z.; Mustafa, H.R. On postediting of machine translation and workflow for undergraduate translation program in China. *Hum. Behav. Emerg. Technol.* **2022**, *2022*, 5793054. [CrossRef]
46. Cronbach, L.J. Coefficient alpha and the internal structure of tests. *Psychometrika* **1951**, *16*, 297–334. [CrossRef]
47. Almanasreh, E.; Moles, R.; Chen, T.F. Evaluation of methods used for estimating content validity. *Res. Soc. Adm. Pharm.* **2019**, *15*, 214–221. [CrossRef]

engineering proceedings

Proceeding Paper

Constructing a Flexible Framework of Spatial Planning and Design for Theme Parks †

Daniel Sutandio [1,*] and Sheng-Jung Ou [2]

1 Department of Architecture, Chaoyang University of Technology, Taichung 41349, Taiwan
2 Department of Landscape and Urban Design, Chaoyang University of Technology, Taichung 41349, Taiwan; sjou@cyut.edu.tw
* Correspondence: s11112906@gm.cyut.edu.tw
† Presented at the 2024 IEEE 4th International Conference on Electronic Communications, Internet of Things and Big Data, Taipei, Taiwan, 19–21 April 2024.

Abstract: Theme parks have been constantly updated and modified to maintain their attractiveness while managing seasonality and fluctuating visitors. Flexibility must be considered in spatial planning, design, and operations to meet the evolving daily and seasonal requirements and ensure long-term adjustability. Nonetheless, the flexibility remains unclear due to variations in its interpretation among different authors, thus hindering its adoption. Its application in spatial planning and design is still limited, primarily seen in the housing sector. This research aims to establish a framework for integrating and evaluating flexibility in the planning and design of a theme park based on the diverse interpretations of flexibility in residential and urban sectors. These interpretations were distilled into three primary dimensions: function, access, and transformation.

Keywords: theme park; flexibility; spatial planning; spatial design; framework

Citation: Sutandio, D.; Ou, S.-J. Constructing a Flexible Framework of Spatial Planning and Design for Theme Parks. *Eng. Proc.* **2024**, *74*, 34. https://doi.org/10.3390/engproc2024074034

Academic Editors: Shu-Han Liao, Teen-Hang Meen and Cheng-Fu Yang

Published: 2 September 2024

1. Introduction

The development of a theme park requires decades to complete. It demands a substantial investment and a sizable area of land. Ongoing updates are necessary in the long run to sustain and enhance its appeal to visitors. Planners must deal with multiple factors to generate the initial design and devise a future development strategy in a constrained space [1]. Designers are required to forecast future scenarios without the assurance of implementation. Given the constrained space, theme parks have challenges such as fluctuations in the number of visitors. There are predetermined maximum numbers of visitors at any given moment without considering visitor satisfaction; although, the number of visitors fluctuates considerably with the season, day, and even hour [2,3]. A gradual or abrupt surge in tourism demand also poses a challenge. Fully developed theme parks must plan for expansion. While capacity management strategies such as the integration of a virtual queuing system and the provision of a waiting experience mitigate visitors' perceptions of overcrowding and increase the capacity temporarily, expansion and modifications with a spatial arrangement are still necessary [2].

A flexible design strategy is demanded for theme parks as a solution for daily operations and the fluctuation in the number of visitors. Thus, strategic planning is needed to respond to the potential increase in demand. A design with flexibility enhances operational efficiency and prolongs the period of service due to its ability to adapt to changes at a reduced expense for sustainability [4]. Nevertheless, flexibility is ambiguous and devoid of a precise definition, hindering its adoption [5]. The existence of multiple and overlapping definitions for flexibility-related terms (e.g., "adaptability", "flexibility", and "polyvalence") renders a universally accepted vocabulary nearly unattainable [6]. Moreover, flexibility costs are high due to its application redundant to designers who disregard its long-term financial benefits [7].

In light of this, we compiled concepts of flexibility and organized them into a framework to assess the flexibility of theme parks and provide solutions for their problem using the overlapping theory. We proposed suggestions on how to implement flexibility into the design of theme parks.

2. Research Method

2.1. Theme Park

A theme park is a confined space with a controlled entrance for recreation. It possesses a thematic identity and features for attractions or entertainment, consumption facilities, merchandise, and, occasionally, performative labor. According to the scale, a theme park is classified as a niche or indoor park, a regional and urban park, or a destination park. The term "theme park" ranges from theme cities, conventional theme parks, themed amusement parks, and amusement parks in general, all of which are defined by their characteristics [8]. The establishment of a theme park needs considerable capital for land and equipment. To ensure that the parks continue to attract a sufficient number of visitors, especially returning ones, new investment is required to finance ongoing development and improvement [9]. Similar to other tourism businesses, seasonality is a significant challenge. Temporal variations due to climate, season, and vacations affect the operation of theme parks [9].

2.2. Flexibility

The concept of flexibility is often discussed in the context of housing. The broad definition of flexible housing is a house that can adapt to shifting needs (such as user, need, and technological change) and patterns (such as demographic, economic, and environmental change). It pertains to housing that responds to the volatility of habitation [7]. There are three issues in that flexibility: system, environment, and user. Flexibility is defined as the capacity of a system (house) to change according to users' needs, responding to the physical and cultural environment, and user changes [10]. The term "flexibility" encompasses a range of design decisions to ease rigid functionality [6,7]. This concept flourishes with the emergence of modern architecture characterized by limited and narrow space, the industrialization of housing, and the trend toward user participation.

Flexibility can be acquired through either soft or hard methods. Soft methods grant the user control and indeterminacy while necessitating minimal flexibility-led design, whereas hard methods impose flexibility-specific technologies and limitations on how flexibility can be attained. Hard methods are favored by architects because they maintain large control over the architecture and guide the user toward "good" design in their scenarios. This tendency brings the belief that flexibility necessitates a substantial amount of initial investment and that the flexibility provided by flexible design is not substantial. The achievement of a flexible design is significantly predicated on the collaboration of multiple stakeholders throughout the procedure, which explains why rigid approaches often prove ineffective in practice [6,7]. Conversely, the alternative perspective regards flexibility as a mere space or skeleton. The idea of "overprovision first, division later", which is one of the most prevailing soft methods, transforms into irresponsible flexibility-themed planning, providing inadequate building systems and resulting in empty yet inflexible spaces [6,11]. Therefore, a balance between what and how flexibility is provided to a spatial design and planning is crucial.

To understand the essence and different methodologies or approaches of flexibility, its advantages need to be understood, including sustainability. Flexibility, in general, increases the users' long-term appreciation for architecture by meeting users' evolving needs and removing elements that make a building obsolete. In the short term, adaptable housing is efficient. Flexible and adaptable structures optimize space utilization, increase lifespan, and improve performance. Consequently, flexibility reduces the construction's material and energy consumption [4,12,13].

2.3. Concepts

We reviewed the literature containing the terms 'flexibility' and 'adaptability'. We focused on housing and urban spaces with the spatial planning and design of the theme park. Publications containing flexibility strategies for the theme park and its spatial planning were analyzed to determine the key concept. Fifteen appropriate publications were selected: twelve about housing and three about urban space. The key concept and a list of publications are presented in Table 1.

Table 1. Reviewed Paper and Key Concepts.

Year	Source	Title	Realm	Key Concept(s)
2000	[14]	Designing Flexibility into Airport Passenger Buildings: The Benefits of Multifunctional Space and Facilities	Housing	K1. Spare Capacity; K2. Shared multifunction space; K3. Expandable non-fixed capacity; K4. Adaptability; K5. Development expandability
2001	[15]	Design strategies to increase building flexibility	Housing	K6. System interaction and component; K7. Access, layout, flow, and area for a system; K8. Phased installation and demolition
2001	[4]	Assessing the Adaptability of Buildings	Housing	K9. Convertibility; K10. Expandability; K11. Independence; K12. Upgradability; K13. Lifetime compatibility; K14. Record keeping
2005	[7]	Flexible housing: opportunities and limits	Urban Space	K15. Adaptable; K16. Flexible
2006	[16]	Frame and Generic Space	Housing	K17. Polyvalence; K18. Alterability; K19. Extend-ability; K20. Frame and generic space
2008	[6]	Design for flexibility	Housing	K21. Distribution of design control
2012	[17]	A method for evaluating the degree of housing unit flexibility in multi-family housing.	Housing	K22. Orientation of housing unit; K23. Geometry of plan; K24. Structure and size of the flat; K25. Number and disposition of the entrance; K26. Position of technical services; K27. Building structure; K28. Achieved degree of freedom of interior space; K29. Potential for multifunctional use of space; K30. Changes in the number and size of the rooms
2013	[11]	On Flexibility in Architecture focused on the Contradiction in Designing Flexible Space and Its Design Proposition.	Urban Space	K31. Multifunction; K32. Polyvalence; K33. Contextual relations
2014	[10]	Flexible Spatial Configuration in Traditional Houses, The Case of Sabzevar	Housing	K34. Nested space; K35. Multiple entrances for each space; K36. Selective connectability and disconnectability; K37. Multifunctionality
2015	[18]	Flexible House Attributes as Perceived by The End-Users	Housing	K38. Demountable Partitions; K39. Flexible Furniture
2015	[19]	Flexible Housing: The Role of Spatial Organization in Achieving Functional Efficiency	Housing	K40. Multifunction during different times; K41. Interrelated spatial organization
2016	[20]	Explaining the Concept of Flexibility in Urban Spaces	Urban Space	K42. Permeability; K43. Versatility; K44. Legibility; K45. Multifunction; K46. Convertibility; K47. Expansibility; K48. Positive outdoor space; K49. Spaces with multimodal behavior pattern; K50. Multifunctional structures; K51. Active frontage; K52. Fine amenities

Table 1. *Cont.*

Year	Source	Title	Realm	Key Concept(s)
2017	[21]	A Review of Flexibility and Adaptability in Housing Design	Housing	K53. Visitability; K54. Convertibility, Neutral-functionality, and Multifunctionality; K55. Combinability; K56. Connectability and divisibility/partitionability; K57. Upgradability and Refittability; K58. Design for disassembly/demountability/dismantlability; K59. Lifetime compatibility; K60. Durability; K61. Disaggregatability/recyclability; K62. Transferability; K63. Transformability, rearrange-ability, redesign-ability; K64. Expandability, Expansion rejection, scalability
2019	[22]	Ideas or reality? Flexible space—flexible people?	Housing	K65. Open Space; K66. Standardisation; K67. Excess capacity
2022	[23]	What Affects the Use Flexibility of Pocket Parks? Evidence from Nanjing, China	Housing	K68. Paved diverse-functioned Ground; K69. Boundaries and opening balance

3. Discussion

Sixty-nine key concepts were extracted from the publications. These concepts overlapped meanings that differed between authors. They were grouped following the focus group discussions. The focus group consisted of architects and urban designers. They rearranged the key concepts with similar terms and categorized them into groups with similar ideas. These groups were examined using essence concepts [14]: "operational", denoting daily implementation of flexibility strategies, and "strategic", denoting a flexibility strategy for planning and/or future development.

Eight main strategies were derived from the concepts using the "generic flexibility principles" [13] and the "type of change in-built facility" [15]. The eight main strategies are as follows.

- Space: Greater flexibility is achieved by incorporating less specified spaces and greater usability freedom;
- Typical Plan: Flexibility is accomplished through the utilization of typical space, which enables the provision of room options in anticipation of future scenarios;
- Design for Adaptation: Flexibility is achieved by providing a space with the ability to change its function through internal arrangement;
- Function: The same ideas are shared in the three preceding strategies: space, typical plan, and design for adaptation, adhering to the principle that space functions are upgradable, supplementary, and modifiable;
- Service: The intelligent disposition of service facilitates easier upgrades and modifications;
- Construction: Flexibility is provided by creating structures that allow easy access for intervention and maintenance;
- Flows: Changeable environment, people, and things are provided;
- Layers: The segregation between the building component layers—skin, structure, and so forth—enables flexibility, promoting easier modification of components within the spaces;
- Capacity: A space is subject to varying conditions or loads, or its size may be transformed.

The concepts were grouped into three dimensions: function, access, and transformation (Table 2).

Table 2. Concept grouping.

<table>
<tr><th rowspan="2">Key Concepts</th><th rowspan="2">Grouped Essence Concept(s)</th><th rowspan="2">Timing</th><th>Generic Flexibility Principles [13]</th><th>Type of Change in Built Facility [15]</th><th rowspan="2">Dimension</th></tr>
<tr><th colspan="2">Main Strategy</th></tr>
<tr><td>K2, K29, K37, K40, K43, K45, K49, K65, K68</td><td>Multifunction shared open space</td><td>Daily</td><td rowspan="2">Space</td><td rowspan="7">Function</td><td rowspan="7">Function</td></tr>
<tr><td>K4, K15, K17, K31, K32, K34, K50</td><td>Polyvalence</td><td>Strategic</td></tr>
<tr><td>K23, K24</td><td>Geometry of plan</td><td>Strategic</td><td rowspan="3">Typical plan</td></tr>
<tr><td>K54, K66</td><td>Standard convertibility</td><td>Strategic</td></tr>
<tr><td>K55</td><td>Component variety</td><td>Strategic</td></tr>
<tr><td>K9, K28, K30</td><td rowspan="2">Alterability</td><td>Daily</td><td rowspan="2">Design for adaptation</td></tr>
<tr><td>K16, K18, K46, K63</td><td>Strategic</td></tr>
<tr><td>K7, K26</td><td>Position and access of technical services</td><td>Strategic</td><td rowspan="2">Service</td><td rowspan="4">-</td><td rowspan="7">Access</td></tr>
<tr><td>K22</td><td>Orientation of space</td><td>Strategic</td></tr>
<tr><td>K13, K21, K59, K60</td><td>Design control over time</td><td>Strategic</td><td rowspan="2">Construction</td></tr>
<tr><td>K6, K12, K14, K57</td><td>Upgradability and Refittability</td><td>Strategic</td></tr>
<tr><td>K25, K35, K42, K44, K53</td><td>Multiple permeable entrances</td><td>Daily</td><td rowspan="3">-</td><td rowspan="3">Flows</td></tr>
<tr><td>K36, K38, K56, K69</td><td>Selective connectability and disconnectability</td><td>Daily</td></tr>
<tr><td>K33, K41, K48, K51</td><td>Interrelated spatial organization connection</td><td>Daily</td></tr>
<tr><td>K39, K52</td><td>Demountable, movable</td><td>Daily</td><td rowspan="3">Layers</td><td rowspan="3">-</td><td rowspan="6">Transformation</td></tr>
<tr><td>K8, K58, K61, K62</td><td>Layering of frame and generic space</td><td>Strategic</td></tr>
<tr><td>K11, K20, K27</td><td rowspan="2">Spare capacity</td><td>Strategic</td></tr>
<tr><td>K67</td><td>Daily</td><td rowspan="3">-</td><td rowspan="3">Capacity</td></tr>
<tr><td>K1, K3, K5</td><td rowspan="2">Expandability</td><td>Strategic</td></tr>
<tr><td>K10, K19, K47, K64</td><td>Strategic</td></tr>
</table>

4. Conclusions

In addition to ensuring long-term adaptability, theme parks require a high degree of flexibility to accommodate daily and seasonal demands that are varying. Thus, it is necessary to apply flexibility in space planning and the design of theme parks. Nevertheless, flexibility has been applied within the housing industry with ambiguities and a lack of clarity, leading to the misunderstanding of significance and advantages. Of the fifteen selected publications containing flexibility concepts, twelve pertained to residential domains and three to urban domains. Following the review, a framework for flexibility was developed, consisting of 69 key concepts that were then reduced to 18 essential concepts in three dimensions: function, access, and transformation. The framework was used to assess flexibility in theme park design and planning. To use the framework effectively, experts for theme parks rearranged the concepts. Subsequent investigations are needed to improve the framework and expand the application of flexibility in the spatial planning and design of the theme park. Modifications and additions are needed for the framework with more literature reviews. The importance-performance analysis and analytic hierarchy process (AHP) techniques can be used to improve the framework.

Author Contributions: Conceptualization, D.S. and S.-J.O.; methodology, D.S.; software, D.S.; validation, D.S. and S.-J.O.; formal analysis, D.S.; investigation, D.S.; resources, D.S.; data curation, D.S.; writing—original draft preparation, D.S.; writing—review and editing, D.S.; supervision, S.-J.O. All authors have read and agreed to the published version of the manuscript.

Funding: This research received no external funding.

Institutional Review Board Statement: Not applicable.

Informed Consent Statement: Not applicable.

Data Availability Statement: Data are contained within the article.

Conflicts of Interest: The authors declare no conflict of interest.

References

1. Dzeng, R.-J.; Lee, H.-Y. Activity and value-orientated decision support for the development planning of a theme park. *Expert Syst. Appl.* **2007**, *33*, 923–935. [CrossRef]
2. Zhang, Y.; Li, X.R.; Su, Q. Does spatial layout matter to theme park tourism carrying capacity? *Tour. Manag.* **2017**, *61*, 82–95. [CrossRef]
3. Ahmadi, R.H. Managing capacity and flow at theme parks. *Oper. Res.* **1997**, *45*, 1–13. [CrossRef]
4. Moffatt, S.; Russell, P. Assessing the adaptability of buildings. *IEA Annex* **2001**, *31*, 1355–1755.
5. De Paris, S.R.; Lopes, C.N.L. Housing flexibility problem: Review of recent limitations and solutions. *Front. Archit. Res.* **2018**, *7*, 80–91. [CrossRef]
6. John Habraken, N. Design for flexibility. *Build. Res. Inf.* **2008**, *36*, 290–296. [CrossRef]
7. Schneider, T.; Till, J. Flexible housing: Opportunities and limits. *Arq: Archit. Res. Q.* **2005**, *9*, 157–166. [CrossRef]
8. Liang, Z.; Li, X. What is a theme park? A synthesis and research framework. *J. Hosp. Tour. Res.* **2023**, *47*, 1343–1370. [CrossRef]
9. Heo, C.Y.; Lee, S. Application of revenue management practices to the theme park industry. *Int. J. Hosp. Manag.* **2009**, *28*, 446–453. [CrossRef]
10. Estaji, H. Flexible spatial configuration in traditional houses, the case of Sabzevar. *Int. J. Contemp. Archit. New Arch.* **2014**, *1*, 26–35.
11. Kim, Y.-J. On flexibility in architecture focused on the contradiction in designing flexible space and its design proposition. *Archit. Res.* **2013**, *15*, 191–200. [CrossRef]
12. Wong, J.F. Factors affecting open building implementation in high density mass housing design in Hong Kong. *Habitat Int.* **2010**, *34*, 174–182. [CrossRef]
13. Till, J.; Schneider, T. Flexible housing: The means to the end. *ARQ Archit. Res. Q.* **2005**, *9*, 287–296. [CrossRef]
14. Belin, S.C. Designing Flexibility into Airport Passenger Buildings: The Benefits of Multifunctional Space and Facilities. Master's Thesis, Massachusetts Institute of Technology, Cambridge, MA, USA, 2000.
15. Slaughter, E.S. Design strategies to increase building flexibility. *Build. Res. Inf.* **2001**, *29*, 208–217. [CrossRef]
16. Leupen, B. *Frame and Generic Space*; 010 Publishers: Rotterdam, The Netherlands, 2006.
17. Živković, M.; Jovanović, G. A method for evaluating the degree of housing unit flexibility in multi-family housing. *Facta Univ. -Ser. Archit. Civ. Eng.* **2012**, *10*, 17–32. [CrossRef]
18. Alaraji, K.; Jusan, M.B.M. Flexible house attributes as perceived by the end-users. *Int. J. Appl. Eng. Res.* **2015**, *10*, 18313–18324.
19. Raviz, S.R.H.; Eteghad, A.N.; Guardiola, E.U.; Aira, A.A. Flexible housing: The role of spatial organization in achieving functional efficiency. *ArchNet-IJAR Int. J. Archit. Res.* **2015**, *9*, 65. [CrossRef]
20. Ardeshiri, M.; Esteghlal, A.; Etesam, I. Explaining the Concept of Flexibility in urban spaces. *Int. J. Appl. Arts Stud. (IJAPAS)* **2016**, *1*, 79–91.
21. Estaji, H. A review of flexibility and adaptability in housing design. *Int. J. Contemp. Archit.* **2017**, *4*, 37–49.
22. Søiland, E.; Hansen, G.K. Ideas or reality? Flexible space–flexible people? *Intell. Build. Int.* **2019**, *11*, 145–157. [CrossRef]
23. Zhou, C.; Xie, M.; Zhao, J.; An, Y. What affects the use flexibility of pocket parks? Evidence from Nanjing, China. *Land* **2022**, *11*, 1419. [CrossRef]

engineering proceedings

MDPI

Proceeding Paper

Online Learning with Digital Technology and Computer Software: New Experiences for Indonesian Students in Education Institutions †

Agus Masrukhin

Character Building Development Center Information Systems Department, School of Information Systems, Bina Nusantara University, Jakarta 11480, Indonesia; agus@binus.ac.id

† Presented at the 2024 IEEE 4th International Conference on Electronic Communications, Internet of Things and Big Data, Taipei, Taiwan, 19–21 April 2024.

Abstract: The experiences of students in the online lectures of Binus University, Indonesia, were analyzed using a qualitative descriptive approach. Offline and online interviews were conducted for data collection. Interviewed students had different backgrounds and experiences studying online. The perspective of the distance learning program was explored using the Binus Online (BOL) class method. Obstacles were determined for students and lecturers as students did not complete their assignments because they were busy with their work.

Keywords: Indonesian students; higher education institution; Binus online employee class

Citation: Masrukhin, A. Online Learning with Digital Technology and Computer Software: New Experiences for Indonesian Students in Education Institutions. *Eng. Proc.* **2024**, *74*, 35. https://doi.org/10.3390/engproc2024074035

Academic Editors: Shu-Han Liao, Teen-Hang Meen and Cheng-Fu Yang

Published: 2 September 2024

1. Introduction

The development of information and communication technology, such as Android and Zoom, is advanced in the areas of life regarding the economy, society, and culture, which makes education adapt and integrate with technology [1–3]. Employees with limited time are helped by these technological advances as there is no need for them to leave their job to obtain a bachelor's degree. Technology is needed in education, so the government permitted universities to open online lectures after the COVID-19 pandemic in early 2020. The educational process is changing to online learning with the help of communication and information technology [4]. The results of this study showed that the educational process is a new model with conveniences but also with challenges, shortcomings, and obstacles.

The aspects of online learning with new digital technology have not been studied extensively yet. Previous researchers viewed technology linearly, especially the implications of technology in online education. Fundamental issues in the relationship between technology and student status have not been researched yet. Previous research showed three trends in which the difficulty and unpreparedness of using applications [5] and satisfaction with learning experiences were analyzed [6]. Educational technology is analyzed from the perspective of enriching skills and knowledge [6,7]. Technology helps students learn and plays an influential role for teachers to enrich teaching abilities, improve product quality, and make the learning process more effective in an argumentative culture [8–10].

This study aims to complement the shortcomings of previous studies which did not analyze how lecturers control the academic process with new technology. The perceptions of students and lecturers about technology and lectures need to be analyzed because student employees find it more difficult to follow lectures. In line with this, we need to study how to adopt technology for online lecture learning, the challenges for students in their ability to adopt online lecture technology, and lecturers' complaints and difficulties that influence the online class method. The result of this study provides a basis for policy formulation and social engineering in achieving the goals of implementing online class technology. This study was conducted to determine the role of online learning with digital technology for employee students as they have different situations from regular students and the use of technology is a mandatory prerequisite in the online class model.

2. Method

This research was conducted using a qualitative descriptive method to reveal students' experiences in online class learning. Students from Binus University in Jakarta, Indonesia, were invited to participate in the research. This college was chosen because it has good distance-learning programs in various regions. The majority of students were company employees who had limited time to study. They depended on the flexibility of the study time, either in the afternoon after work or on weekends. The students had various backgrounds. Apart from students, lecturers were also invited. Students' experiences were collected using offline interviews via WhatsApp as face-to-face interviews were not possible. The majority of students were working, so lecturers also used WhatsApp for teaching. Data were also collected through observations of the learning process. The role and assistance of lecturers for their students were also observed and recorded.

The data collected was analyzed according to the stages of qualitative descriptive research, including data reduction and presentation [4,11,12]. Data reduction was carried out by selecting and sorting available data and excluding data that were not relevant.

3. Result

3.1. Student's Experiences in Online Lecturing

Students' experiences in online lectures have changed the culture of lectures. Face-to-face classes are no longer mandatory at various institutions in Indonesia, and digital-based learning has been introduced. This shift can be a challenge for universities and students who have a low level of technological literacy. Online lectures are flexible and fun, but seriousness is demanded. The data on students' experiences in online learning are presented in Table 1.

Table 1. Students' experiences in online lecturing.

No	Experience	Code
1	"While taking online lectures, there are many learning resources available on the Internet (articles, electronic books, journals) that I can study, apart from that I am flexible in submitting assignments and taking exams. My sad experience is that I don't socialize enough with my fellow students because they are busy, especially students who are working".	Technological legality
2	"The ups and downs may be greater when doing group assignments. When you get a member who has a large contribution, it's quite good, if you get a member who is easily lost and doesn't have a contribution, it's not good".	Loss of communication
3	"Time is flexible, lecturers understand students' busy schedules, so grades are usually balanced".	Flexibility
4	"The sad thing is that sometimes there is a lot of material that you don't understand and it's difficult to ask questions from lecturers or fellow students. The good thing is that it's very flexible and can be done anywhere the lecture takes place".	Flexibility
5	"Online lectures make us have a lot of time, because the lecture hours are flexible and we are not required to attend lectures in person. The sadness is that socialization is lacking, because there is no direct interaction with lecture friends".	Loss of learning enthusiasm
6	"Actually, online lectures are very difficult, we are required to always be independent, especially when there is a vicon schedule, sometimes I forget".	Loss of discipline
7	"With online lectures, we, students who attend lectures, can work while paying for tuition fees. The sadness is that study hours clash with work".	Not conducive
8	"If you have a zoom meeting while you're still in the office, you will be less focused and you won't be able to optimally understand the lecture topic".	Loss of enthusiasm
9	"The sadness, not being able to meet face to face with classmates, feeling like studying alone even though you have friends".	Loss of enthusiasm
10	"I don't make many friends because they have their own busy lives".	Loss of enthusiasm

3.2. Challenge in Online Lecturing

The change in the learning system demands student independence for their success. This provides obstacles and difficulties. Students are required to be clever in managing their time because they also have obligations as employees. Apart from having to attend online lectures, they have assignments from lecturers on the Binusmaya application for personal and group assignments. They are required to join forums every week. As a result of the online learning system, students encountered many difficulties, as shown in Table 2.

Table 2. Challenges in online lecturing.

No	Challenge Online Lecturing	Code
1	"The challenge of time management is something we always face, where as office workers we also have to complete office work on time and then work on campus assignments so that they are completed on time".	Having limitations
2	"My challenges are in expanding relationships or during group work".	Having limitations
3	"First, from within me, a feeling of laziness and poor management. Second, external factors, such as the material presented is not of high quality, a group of friends who are lazy/not united, network connections that are sometimes slow".	Note professional
4	"The challenge during online lectures is that we are required to be smart in dividing our time between studying and work".	Having limitations
5	"When studying online there were questions that I didn't know, I was confused about what to do, because I'm the type of child who rarely wants to ask my friends".	Having limitations
6	"The challenge faced in online lectures is that we are required to explore more of the subjects we are studying because the number of meetings with lecturers is very limited".	Having limitations
7	"Feeling like you don't need college and sometimes taking it for granted. There needs to be a strong desire and awareness to undertake this online lecture".	Note professional
8	"I study while working. When you have a lot of assignments at college and at work, it is quite a big challenge".	Having limitations
9	"Studying after coming home from work, where you are physically and mentally tired but still have to continue studying at night. The vicon who followed while on the way, was not very concerned about hearing the lecturer, especially if the connection was unstable on the road".	Having limitations
10	"As an office worker, you also have to complete office work on time and then work on campus assignments so that they are completed on time".	having limitations
11	"The biggest challenge in online lectures is taking classes via Zoom while working. Focus will be a big problem in this case and will have an impact on the material presented. Apart from that, group assignments are a challenge because not everyone has the same time to complete the assignments that have been distributed which results in the submission of assignments having to be close to the deadline".	Note professional

At the same time, the students in this program were also required to have an understanding of each subject. JNT said, "I study while working. When you have a lot of assignments at college and work, it's quite a big challenge". AS said, "Studying after work, when you are physically and mentally tired but still have to continue studying at night. The vicon who followed while on the way, was not very attentive to hearing the lecturer, especially if the connection was unstable on the road".

The demand for learning various subjects was a burden for students. They could not follow the lessons, which made them feel depressed and hesitant to do their assignments. When there was a group assignment, they learned together with group friends. For exams, they answered questions that did not match the meaning of the questions. In other words, the role of lecturers was still necessary (Table 3).

Table 3. Obstacles of student.

No	Lecturers' Experiences as Online Learning Companions	Code
1	"The lack of communication between lecturers and students makes lecturers worried that their students will not understand what is being said".	Quality
2	"Usually, when answering questions, many students do not include more references".	Not professional
3	"Students do not turn on cameras during lectures. Several are angry because students do not and the questions before answering. They seem to answer carelessly".	Not conducive
4	"During the video conference session, some students were unable to activate the camera because they were still at work".	Not professional
5	"Many students are not committed to the assignments they have been, so students often miss the assignment deadlines given by the lecturer".	Not professional
6	"Maybe more frequent connection problems".	Not conducive
7	"The lecturer doesn't interact much during class and doesn't even turn on the camera".	Not conducive
8	"Several students submit assignments incorrectly to the LMS and do not submit assignments on time".	Not professional
9	"There are many students who are traveling".	Not professional

3.3. *Lecturers' Experiences as Online Learning Companions*

An obstacle faced by lecturers is their inability to control students so that they can be focused on studying. Online lectures made it easy for employees to continue their studies, which resulted in the obstacles shown in Table 3.

The lecturers hoped to control class conditions during classes and the campus provides mandatory rules for turning on the camera. Even though lecturers often apply discipline, several students actively attend classes. Students sometimes logged in without turning on the camera. Several students were busy playing games without paying attention to the lecturer. These were challenges for lecturers to find effective online learning methods.

These were stated by a lecturer as follows: "Several obstacles when teaching online: Lecturers cannot control the class as a whole as during face to face lectures, Lecturers do not know whether students' attention is focused on the lecture, Lectures are often interrupted by an internet connection that is sometimes not good". Another obstacle is students' seriousness during lectures via video conference. When lecturers send lectures via the Zoom application, many are late for various reasons, either because they are still working or because they are on their way home. This complaint is similar to what US lecturers complained about: "During online learning, students are less focused on following the material. Even though they are asked to be on camera, they will only activate the camera for a maximum of 5 min after it is closed again. Apart from that, because the interaction is not direct, there is less nuance compared to face-to-face meetings".

This makes lecturers unable to control, direct, and condition students [13]. This obstacle is the one faced by lecturers mostly. Many lecturers felt the same without being able to provide optimal action to ensure better online learning conditions.

4. Conclusions

The results of this research showed that online lectures are technically complex for employee class students, which reduces the essence of understanding the learning topics. Lectures are offered through video conference, which requires students to access the information autonomously. As a result, the learning objectives were achieved less than the lecturers had expected. New technologies in education need students to have technological literacy by accessing material and explanations independently, even with obstacles. This research was conducted from the perspective of lecturers and students of Binus University. Thus, a complete and broad picture of learning cannot be provided. Therefore, it is necessary to involve more research objects to collect more data on technology-based education.

Funding: This research received no external funding.

Institutional Review Board Statement: Not applicable.

Informed Consent Statement: Not applicable.

Data Availability Statement: Data can be made available upon request.

Conflicts of Interest: The author declare no conflicts of interest.

References

1. Priyatna, C.C.; Prastowo, F.A.A.; Syuderajat, F.; Sani, A. Optimization of information technology by government agencies in publicommunication activities. *J. Kaji. Komun.* **2020**, *8*, 114–127. [CrossRef]
2. Puspitarini, D. Blended Learning as a 21st Century Learning Model. *Ideguru J. Karya Ilm. Guru* **2022**, *7*, 1–6. [CrossRef]
3. Voutama, A. Website-Based Car Wash Queuing System Using CRM Concepts and Application of UML. *Komputika J. Comput. Syst.* **2022**, *11*, 102–111. [CrossRef]
4. Muassomah, M.; Abdullah, I. Learning with Technology: New Experiences for Indonesian Children During COVID-19. In Proceedings of the International Conference on Engineering, Technology and Social Science, Tangerang, Indonesia, 25 November 2021.
5. Cahyadi, A.; Susanto, D.A.; Wekke, I.S. Obstacles and Challenges of Information Technology Application on the Online Lecturing during COVID-19 Pandemic Outbreaks. *Psychol. Educ.* **2021**, *58*, 1070–1077.
6. Li, N.; Marsh, V.; Rienties, B.; Whitelock, D. Online learning experiences of new versus continuing learners: A large-scale replication study. *Assess. Eval. High. Educ.* **2017**, *42*, 657–672. [CrossRef]
7. Budiman, H. The Role of Information and Communication Technology in Education. *Al-Tadzkiyyah: J. Pendidik. Islam Educ.* **2017**, *8*, 31–43. [CrossRef]
8. Harahap, L. The Role of Information and Communication Technology in Education. In Proceedings of the National Seminar on Postgraduate Educational Technology, 30 November 2019; Available online: https://digilib.unimed.ac.id/id/eprint/38785 (accessed on 6 March 2020). (In Indonesian)
9. Mustofa, M.I.; Chodzirin, M.; Sayekti, L.; Fauzan, R. Formulation of Online Lecture Models as an Effort to Reduce Disparities in Higher Education Quality. *Walisongo J. Inf. Technol.* **2019**, *1*, 151–160. [CrossRef]
10. Archila, P.A.; Restrepo, S.; de Mejía, A.-M.T.; Rueda-Esteban, R.; Bloch, N.I. Fostering instructor-student argumentative interaction in online lecturing to large groups: A study amidst the COVID-19 pandemic. *Rev. Eureka Sobre Ensenanza Y Divulg. De Las Cienc.* **2022**, *19*, 110101–110116. [CrossRef]
11. Trianggoro, I.R.W.; Koeswanti, H.D. Evaluation of the School Literacy Movement (Gelis) Program in Elementary Schools. *J. Ilm. Pendidik. Profesi Guru* **2021**, *4*, 355–362. [CrossRef]
12. Mahardini, M.M.A. Situation Analysis of Using Google Classroom in Online Physics Learning. *J. Pendidik. Fis.* **2020**, *8*, 215–224. [CrossRef]
13. Purnomo, A.; Hartatik, H.; Cahyaningsih, I.J.; Hartono, R.; Bawono, S.A.T. Development of High School E-Learning Applications. *Simetri J. Mech. Electr. Comput. Sci. Eng.* **2017**, *8*, 619–628. [CrossRef]

engineering proceedings

Proceeding Paper

Structural Equation Modeling to Construct Customer Behavioral Intentions in Japanese-Style Yakiniku Restaurants: A Case Study of the Umai Chain Brand †

Chih-Wei Lin [1,2], Wen-Goang Yang [1], Wei-Yeng Sia [2], Yi-Ling Liu [1], Yu-Sheng Lin [3,4,*] and Chen-Hsiang Hsieh [2,*]

1 Department of Leisure Service Management, Chaoyang University of Technology, Taichung 413310, Taiwan; cwlin@cyut.edu.tw (C.-W.L.); wayne@cyut.edu.tw (W.-G.Y.); a25773131@yahoo.com.tw (Y.-L.L.)
2 Department of Business Administration, Chaoyang University of Technology, Taichung 413310, Taiwan; wyc147@gmail.com
3 General Education Center, Chaoyang University of Technology Taichung, Taichung 411030, Taiwan
4 Department of Industrial Education and Technology, National Changhua University of Education, Changhua 500207, Taiwan
* Correspondence: lin3117@cyut.edu.tw (Y.-S.L.); teisho2012@gmail.com (C.-H.H.); Tel.: +886-4-23323000 (ext. 3069) (Y.-S.L.)
† Presented at the 2024 IEEE 4th International Conference on Electronic Communications, Internet of Things and Big Data, Taipei, Taiwan, 19–21 April 2024.

Abstract: By constructing a linear structural equation model, we explored the impact of the customer service, food quality, and physical environment on customer behavioral intentions with experiential value and customer satisfaction as mediators. We focused on customers of the renowned Taiwanese franchised restaurant, Umai Yakiniku, in the Taichung area, Taiwan, and its services. Through customer perception and experience, we unraveled the subsequent behavioral dynamics. A total of 337 valid questionnaires were collected through purposive sampling. The participants encompassed customers who had previously dined at the Umai Yakiniku restaurant, excluding those attending corporate events. The overall behavioral model of customers showed a satisfactory level of fit. The customer service, food quality, and physical environment significantly impacted the experiential value. Customer service directly impacted customer satisfaction, while food quality and the physical environment indirectly affected customer satisfaction. Experiential value positively impacted customer satisfaction, and customer satisfaction positively affected behavioral intentions. Such findings provide information for related companies and their strategic management.

Keywords: perceived value; experiential value; customer satisfaction

Citation: Lin, C.-W.; Yang, W.-G.; Sia, W.-Y.; Liu, Y.-L.; Lin, Y.-S.; Hsieh, C.-H. Structural Equation Modeling to Construct Customer Behavioral Intentions in Japanese-Style Yakiniku Restaurants: A Case Study of the Umai Chain Brand. *Eng. Proc.* **2024**, *74*, 36. https://doi.org/10.3390/engproc2024074036

Academic Editors: Shu-Han Liao, Teen-Hang Meen and Cheng-Fu Yang

Published: 2 September 2024

1. Introduction

The Taiwanese catering market is highly competitive with a strong emphasis on service quality. In the intense competition, restaurant operators need to provide personalized products or services tailored to consumer preferences to increase the chances of success [1]. As consumer awareness rises, the solitary and competitive business approach is gradually losing its appeal in the food and beverage industry as a trend of mainstream culinary culture. According to Xiao [2], the dining experience for today's customers has shifted from satisfying physiological needs to seeking higher levels of gratification. Elements such as the taste of the food, distinctive features, interior design, and ambient atmosphere in restaurants have become increasingly crucial. In order to address the challenges of competition and service, the industry's success needs to be connected to distinctive and culinary offerings, or locational advantages, to secure consumers. However, it is needed to achieve efficiency and service excellence.

According to a report by ET, nine out of the top ten Japanese barbecue restaurants in Taichung are franchised. The characteristic of franchised restaurants lies in their ability to acquire the Know-How of operations. Ninemeier [3] pointed out that franchised restaurants are food service organizations formed by corporate entities, encompassing the adoption of a standardized menu, joint procurement of raw materials and equipment, and the use of consistent operational management. These practices are then transformed into standard operating procedures for each restaurant, contributing to the high operational quality observed.

In this research, Uma Yakiniku, a chain barbecue restaurant, was explored as it operates under a unified company philosophy, comprehensive procurement of raw materials and equipment, and a consistent management operating model as the top chain barbecue restaurant in Taichung. Based on previous research, the personnel service, food quality, and physical environment, and the relationship between value and customer satisfaction, were explored. The essence of experiential marketing lies in the consumer's experience, as consumers are influenced by both rational and emotional factors. Therefore, the shaping of the "consumer context" is deemed crucial in this context. Li [4] found that customer satisfaction significantly influenced customer loyalty and behavioral intention.

This research was conducted to (1) understand the current status of the personnel service, food quality, physical environment, experiential value, customer satisfaction, and behavior intention; (2) explore the impact of the personnel service, food quality, and physical environment on experiential value; (3) explore the impact of the personnel service, food quality, and physical environment on customer satisfaction; (4) explore the impact of experiential value on customer satisfaction; and (5) explore the impact of customer satisfaction on behavioral intent.

2. Literature Review

2.1. Perceived Quality

Liu [5] and Chen [6] posited that perceived quality is a factor directly evaluated by customers through their five senses. The five senses of sensory experience refer to visual, auditory, olfactory, gustatory, and tactile pressure perceptions. For customers, the perceived quality of a restaurant extends beyond the quality of its food, encompassing service quality and the overall physical environment of the establishment. We asserted that restaurant quality must encompass the service quality of personnel, the food quality of the dishes, and the physical environment of the restaurant, elaborated as follows.

2.1.1. Personnel Service Quality

Parasuraman, Zeithaml, and Berry [7] proposed that service quality is assessed by the perceived service performance by customers. Service quality depends on the customer's satisfaction with the service, representing the comparison between customer expectations and the perceived service and indicating that service outcomes meet the established standards [8,9].

2.1.2. Food Quality

Liu [5] suggested that factors judged by consumers including their senses, such as color, flavor, cooking, hygiene, and others, constitute food quality. Wu [6] mentioned that quality aspects are judged through the senses, including hygiene, price, taste, nutrition, calorie content, portion size, packaging, freshness, utensil quality, and dish presentation.

2.1.3. Physical Environment

Belk [10] claimed that the physical environment refers to visible physical characteristics such as the geographical location, decor, sound, atmosphere, and visible appearance of commodities. Bitner, Barnes, and Ward [11] argued that information about the physical environment influences consumers' perceptions of service providers, impacting their consumption behavior. The physical environment combines different elements into a whole [12], and different types of restaurants have corresponding elements. Thus, we defined the physical environment as tangible or intangible entities visible or perceptible to customers.

2.2. Experiential Value

2.2.1. Definition of Experiential Value

In relationship marketing, value is a pivotal factor. According to Ravald and Grönroos [13], the ability of companies to provide exceptional value was considered one of the most successful strategies of the 1990s. Value is a motivator influencing contemporary consumer purchasing behavior and a fundamental basis for consumer purchasing decisions [14,15]. Experiential value encompasses sensory experiences such as emotions, touch, taste, and smell. It allows customers to perceive and form impressions of products or services [16]. Therefore, we defined experiential value as the recognition, preference, and satisfaction generated by customers through sensory experiences.

2.2.2. Measurement of Experiential Value

Holbrook [17] proposed that value is categorized into intrinsic and extrinsic value, along with an activity dimension in a value theory framework. Holbrook suggested that the value theory framework includes (1) Extrinsic versus Intrinsic Value, (2) Self-oriented versus Other-oriented Value, and (3) Active versus Reactive Value. These three combinations intertwine, resulting in a framework comprising eight forms. Due to the complexity of Holbrook's value theory, Mathwick, Malhotra, and Rigdon [18] simplified the framework and introduced the term "experiential value." They defined experiential value as a relative preference developed by individuals during the experiential process with products or services, subsequently enhancing or diminishing the consumption value attributed to products or services. Experiential value is categorized into Consumer Return on Investment, Service Excellence, Aesthetics, and Playfulness.

- Aesthetics: Overall sensory attractiveness of specific visual elements to consumers.
- Playfulness: The intrinsic psychological feelings and enjoyment are generated when consumers participate in activities.
- Consumer Return on Investment (ROI): The rewards obtained by consumers concerning financial and time costs and behavioral input.
- Excellent Service: Consumers' self-directed responses to market service efficiency and marketing capabilities.

2.3. Satisfaction

Spreng, MacKenzie, and Olshavsky [19] stated that the sensation of satisfaction arises from customers comparing the performance of a service or product with their internal expectations for that service or product. If the performance of the product or service exceeds the consumer's expectations, then the customer experiences satisfaction. Satisfaction is the psychological state of an individual after the experience of a product or service and is influenced by various social and psychological factors [20]. Therefore, we defined satisfaction as the overall assessment by customers after receiving the products or services of the restaurant.

2.4. Behavior Intention

Behavioral intention is the degree to which an individual expresses the intention or inclination to engage in a specific behavior before making a decision [21]. In other words, the stronger the willingness to engage in a particular behavior, the more likely the individual is to perform that behavior. Behavioral intention encompasses a willingness to recommend to others, loyalty to the product or company, willingness to speak positively about the product or company, willingness to continue purchasing, and willingness to pay a higher price [22]. Therefore, we defined behavioral intention as the willingness of customers to continue dining at the restaurant.

2.5. Perceived Quality, Experiential Value, Customer Satisfaction, and Behavior Intention

Wu [23] found that in the exploration of customer behavior in restaurants, service personnel impact experiential value, especially the interaction between service personnel and customers, which proves beneficial for experiential value and the emotions of the customers. Thus, we proposed the following hypotheses.

- H1: Perceived quality has a significantly positive impact on experiential value.
- H1-1: Personnel service has a significantly positive impact on experiential value.
- H1-2: Food quality has a significantly positive impact on experiential value.
- H1-3: The physical environment has a significantly positive impact on experiential value.

Liu [24] explored the relationships between the service quality, food quality, environmental atmosphere, consumer satisfaction, and consumer loyalty. He revealed a positive correlation among the service quality, food quality, environmental atmosphere, consumer satisfaction, and consumer loyalty. Thus, we proposed the following hypotheses:

- H2: Perceived quality has a significantly positive impact on customer satisfaction.
- H2-1: Perceived personnel service has a significantly positive impact on customer satisfaction.
- H2-2: Perceived food quality has a significantly positive impact on customer satisfaction.
- H2-3: The perceived physical environment has a significantly positive impact on customer satisfaction.

In the study conducted by Chen, Hu, and Lin [25] on tourists, it was found that experiential quality affects their experiential value. Furthermore, experiential value influences satisfaction, and ultimately, satisfaction affects loyalty. Thus, we proposed the following hypotheses:

- H3: Experiential value has a significantly positive impact on customer satisfaction.
- H4: Customer satisfaction has a significantly positive impact on behavior intention.

3. Research Method

We adopted a purposive sampling method. The participants were customers who patronized the Uma Yakiniku restaurant in the Taichung area and those who visited in the past six months. Those who participated in corporate gatherings were excluded. An online survey was conducted by using Google Forms. All questions were mandatory to answer to avoid any instances of unanswered questions. The official survey was performed online from 1 March to 31 March 2020. A total of 350 responses were collected. After excluding invalid ones, 337 valid responses were obtained with a response rate of 96%.

The questionnaire for this study comprised five sections. The first section covers personal demographic information, and the second section comprises three dimensions of perceived quality: "Personnel Service Quality", "Food Quality", and "Physical Environment". The third section included experiential value, the fourth section included customer satisfaction, and the fifth section included behavior intention. Except for the personal demographic information, the remaining four scales use a Likert five-point scoring system. The content of the questionnaire was created referring to previous study results. After the questionnaire was modified, it was finalized and distributed.

An item analysis was conducted using the correlation with the total score and critical ratio (CR) for item selection. Retaining items showed a CR value greater than 3 and a correlation coefficient above 0.30 at a significant level [26]. The top and bottom 27% in scores were classified in the extreme group. The top 27% were designated in the high-score group, and the bottom 27% in the low-score group. T-tests were then conducted for each factor item between the high- and low-score groups. Statistical analyses were conducted using SPSS 21 and Amos 21 including descriptive statistics, a confirmatory factor analysis, and structural equation modeling.

4. Results and Discussion

4.1. Descriptive Analysis

The males comprised 42.9% of the respondents, while the females accounted for 57.1%. A total of 13.3% were 20–30 years old, and 57.9% were 41 years old and above. In total, 18.4% earned NTD 22,001–32,000 (least), and 28.5% earned NTD 52,001 and more. A total of 69% were military/civil servants and students. In total, 38.4% visited the restaurant for friends/colleagues/family gatherings, and 2.3% visited for marketing events.

4.2. Confirmatory Factor Analysis (CFA)

Amos 21 was used to test the normality of the data, and CFA was used to test whether the measurement tools were appropriate for the research matrix and facets. The reliability and validity were tested for convergent validity, discriminant validity, item reliability, and composite reliability. The standard CR must be above 0.7 [27], and the standard value of the average must be greater than 0.5 [28]. The scale of the customer behavior in this study showed reliability and validity as shown in Table 1.

Table 1. Reliability and convergent validity for customer behavior.

Variables	Item	Factor Loading	CR	Average
Personnel Service	PS 1	0.83	0.895	0.681
	PS 2	0.86		
	PS 3	0.82		
	PS 4	0.79		
Food Quality	FQ 1	0.81	0.899	0.641
	FQ 2	0.75		
	FQ 3	0.81		
	FQ 4	0.83		
	FQ 5	0.80		
Physical Environment	PE 1	0.81	0.877	0.641
	PE 2	0.82		
	PE 3	0.76		
	PE4	0.81		
Experiential Value	Consumer Return on Investment	0.72	0.840	0.568
	Aesthetics	0.83		
	Playfulness	0.73		
	Service Excellence	0.73		
Customer Satisfaction	CS 1	0.69	0.877	0.589
	CS 2	0.77		
	CS 3	0.81		
	CS 4	0.76		
	CS 5	0.80		
Behavior Intention	BI 1	0.91	0.921	0.746
	BI 2	0.95		
	BI 3	0.74		
	BI 4	0.84		

Discriminant Validity Test

Pearson correlation analysis results showed that all variables were significantly correlated, and the coefficient values ranged from 0.462 to 0.865. When using the confidence interval method, the interval that is not 1 indicates a complete correlation between the variables and discriminant validity. In this research, a bootstrapping method was used at a confidence level of below 95%. Estimates were measured using the bias-corrected and percentile methods. The correlation coefficient between variables revealed that the upper bound of the confidence interval was between 0.607 and 0.981, and the lower bound was between 0.437 and 0.949. The result indicated no complete correlation between the dimensions of the behavioral model. Therefore, each variable demonstrated discrimination (Table 2).

Table 2. Pearson Correlation Coefficient.

	Personnel Service	Food Quality	Physical Environment	Consumer Return on Investment	Aesthetics	Playfulness	Service Excellence	Customer Satisfaction
Personnel service								
Food quality	0.641 *							
Physical environment	0.520 *	0.691 *						
Consumer return on investment	0.462 *	0.661 *	0.670 *					
Aesthetics	0.589 *	0.695 *	0.814 *	0.756 *				
Playfulness	0.555 *	0.675 *	0.731 *	0.703 *	0.852 *			
Service excellence	0.621 *	0.692 *	0.716 *	0.709 *	0.836 *	0.818 *		
Customer satisfaction	0.667 *	0.745 *	0.780 *	0.715 *	0.865 *	0.822 *	0.857 *	
Behavior intention	0.487 *	0.669 *	0.665 *	0.723 *	0.725 *	0.730 *	0.733 *	0.734 *

(* $p < 0.05$).

We constructed the behavioral model of Uma Yakiniku customers based on previous research. The analysis was conducted using AMOS 21. In the normality test, although the sample data conformed to the single variance normality, the CR of the multivariate kurtosis was 54.368, which did not conform to the normal distribution. In order to correct the over-inflated chi-square value caused by non-multivariate normality, we used the Bollen and Stine [29] Bootstrap method for modification (Table 3).

Table 3. Model fit of Overall behavior mode.

Indicators	**Criteria**	**Model Fit**	
		Original Fit	**Adjusted by Bootstrap**
REMSEA	<0.08	0.97	0.10
GFI	>0.80	0.789	0.965
AGFI	>0.80	0.746	0.956
NFI	>0.90	0.861	0.965
RFI	>0.90	0.845	0.961
IFI	>0.90	0.891	0.999
TLI/NFI	>0.90	0.878	0.999
CFI	>0.90	0.890	0.999
CN	>200	93	325.449
NC	$1 < x^2/DF < 3$	4.145	1.036

The chi-square value of the original model was 1206.202. The chi-square value revised by the bootstrap was 301.510. The original sample data of this study did not have over-inflated chi-square values; therefore, we used the modified chi-square to test each indicator. The overall behavioral model detection values of the customers met the standard, and the model of this study was acceptable.

The model must meet the following items: (1) all error variations are positive and no negative numbers appear; (2) all error variations are significant; (3) there is standardized regression estimation, and the model is analyzed if the value does not exceed 0.95; (4) there are no excessively large standard errors [30]. The behavioral model in this study met the four conditions recommended in Ref. The model did not differ from the estimation, so the analysis was carried out (Table 4).

Table 4. Hypothesis verification.

Hypothesis	Path		Path Coefficient	S.E.	t	Remarks
H1-1	P.S.	→E.V.	0.243	0.048	4.74 *	Support
H1-2	F.Q.	→E.V.	0.316	0.063	5.21 *	Support
H1-3	P.E.	→E.V.	0.764	0.056	11.89 *	Support
H2-1	P.S.	→C.S.	0.152	0.031	3.46 *	Support
H2-2	F.Q.	→C.S.	0.095	0.040	1.88	Not Support
H2-3	P.E.	→C.S.	0.072	0.050	0.96	Not Support
H3	E.V.	→E.V.	0.830	0.064	9.72 *	Support
H4	C.S.	→B.I.	0.0703	0.080	13.82 *	Support

* $p < 0.05$.

The standardized coefficient of personnel service on experiential value was 0.243, and the t-value was 4.739. The standardized coefficient of food quality on experience value was 0.316, and the t-value was 5.210. The standardized coefficient of the physical environment on experience value was 0.764, and the t-value was 11.892. The standardized coefficient of personnel service on experience value was 0.152, and the t-value was 3.463. The standardized coefficient of experience value on customer satisfaction was 0.830, and the t-value was 9.720. The standardized coefficient of customer satisfaction on behavioral intention was 0.703, and the t-value was 13.822. The result confirmed the significance of the model. Therefore, the first five items were confirmed.

The standardized coefficient of personnel service on experience value was 0.095, and the t-value was 1.882. The standardized coefficient of personnel service on experience value was 0.072, and the t-value was 0.95. Personnel service did not meet the significant standard. The behavior model path analysis is shown in Figure 1.

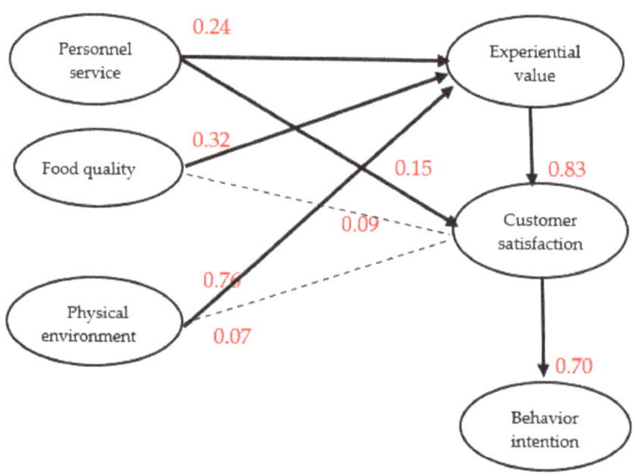

Figure 1. Path analysis of overall behavior model.

In the customer behavior model of the Uma Yakiniku restaurant, the personnel service, food quality, and physical environment positively impacted experiential value. Notably, the impact of the physical environment on experiential value (0.76) was the most substantial, indicating that the restaurant's ambient atmosphere was a primary factor influencing the dining experience. For customer satisfaction, only personnel service was significant (0.16). Although food quality and the physical environment did not impact customer satisfaction, food quality and the physical environment indirectly influenced customer satisfaction through experiential value. Experiential value impacted customer satisfaction (0.83), and customer satisfaction also impacted behavior intention (0.68).

The current food service industry demands experiential marketing. Experiential value is a dynamic experience of satisfaction for lasting memories. These memories encompass the value perceptions before and after visiting [31]. Customer satisfaction is the consumer experience after the consumption of a product or service. Experiential value influences customer satisfaction before and after visiting. Customer behavior is influenced by the "value approach," where satisfaction influences behavioral intent. This aligns with Thompson's [32] results, emphasizing the linkage between customer satisfaction and value to drive purchase behavior and loyalty.

5. Conclusions

We found that the personnel service, food quality, and physical environment impacted experiential value. The impact of the physical environment on experiential value was the most significant. This implied that the restaurant's ambiance influenced the dining experience at Uma Yakiniku. Personnel service significantly impacted customer satisfaction. The performance of the service staff affected customers' satisfaction. While food quality and the physical environment did not directly influence customer satisfaction, they affected experiential value. Experiential value impacted customer satisfaction. This underscored the importance of the dining experience at Uma Yakiniku in customer satisfaction. Customers felt enthusiasm for the service provided by Uma Yakiniku, which was a favored choice. Customer satisfaction influenced behavioral intentions. Despite the higher pricing at Uma Yakiniku, the superior service quality and dishes attracted customers, leading them to express the intention to revisit for dining.

Based on the research results, the following recommendations are proposed for the operations and management of restaurants.

According to the analysis of the overall behavior model, the impact of the physical environment on the experiential value is the most significant. Especially in the competitive landscape of numerous shabu-shabu restaurants in Taichung, the key to attracting customer attention is in the hardware such as the unique design of the restaurant's exterior and thoughtful arrangement of tables and chairs. Personnel services impact customer satisfaction. However, customers scored lower in terms of attention to information related to the restaurant. The main reason was the relatively low interaction between the restaurant and customers, resulting in fewer opportunities for customers to learn about restaurant-related activities. Enhanced on-the-job training can simultaneously be achieved by (1) strengthening future-oriented, sustainable, and relationship-maintaining customer relationships, (2) transitioning from a product–service orientation to an experiential marketing orientation, (3) allowing customers to experience the refined Japanese shabu-shabu dining mode as a genuine source of profit for the restaurant, and (4) continuous innovation in product offerings and dining modes. Then, a high-end consumer base can be secured, thereby increasing market differentiation and positioning the restaurant as a leader beyond price limitations in the market.

Author Contributions: Conceptualization, W.-G.Y., C.-W.L. and Y.-L.L.; methodology, C.-W.L.; writing—original draft preparation, Y.-S.L., C.-W.L. and W.-Y.S.; writing—review and editing, C.-H.H. and Y.-S.L. All authors have read and agreed to the published version of the manuscript.

Funding: This research received no external funding.

Institutional Review Board Statement: Not applicable.

Informed Consent Statement: Not applicable.

Data Availability Statement: Data are contained within the article.

Acknowledgments: All subjects' enthusiastic participation is greatly appreciated.

Conflicts of Interest: The authors declare no conflicts of interest.

References

1. Huang, L.Y. *Theme Restaurant Design and Management*, 1st ed.; Yang Chih Cultural Industry Co., Ltd.: New Taipei City, Taiwan, 2002.
2. Xiao, Y.Q. *Introduction to Catering*, 1st ed.; Yang Chih Cultural Industry Co., Ltd.: New Taipei City, Taiwan, 2000.
3. Ninemeier, J.D. Procurement process in the hospitality industry. In *Planning and Control for Food and Beverage Operation*, 2nd ed.; Educational Institute, American Hotel & Lodging Association: Washington, DC, USA, 2004; p. 4.
4. Li, Y.T. A Study of Service Elements in Sports Themed Restaurant on Customer Satisfaction, Customer Loyalty, Behavioral Intention. Ph.D. Thesis, Fu Jen Catholic University, New Taipei City, Taiwan, 2016.
5. Liu, W.-W. A Study on Consumer Satisfaction of Food Quality of Western Fried Chicken Fast Food Chain Stores. Ph.D. Thesis, Chinese Culture University, Taipei City, Taiwan, 2000.
6. Chen, K.-F. A Study on Consumer Satisfaction of Food Quality of Western Hamburger Fast Food Chain Stores. Ph.D. Thesis, Chinese Culture University, Taipei City, Taiwan, 2002.
7. Parasuraman, A.; Zeithaml, V.A.; Berry, L.L. Servqual: A multiple-item scale for measuring consumer perc. *J. Retail.* **1988**, *64*, 12.
8. Churchill, G.A., Jr.; Surprenant, C. An investigation into the determinants of customer satisfaction. *J. Mark. Res.* **1982**, *19*, 491–504. [CrossRef]
9. Levitt, T. Marketing intangible products and product intangibles. *Cornell Hotel. Restaur. Adm. Q.* **1981**, *22*, 37–44. [CrossRef]
10. Wu, W.-C. The Research with Box Lunch Quality, Customer Satisfaction and Consumer Behavior. Ph.D. Thesis, Chinese Culture University, Taipei City, Taiwan, 1998.
11. Bitner, M.J.; Barnes, J.; Ward, J.C. Measuring the prototypicality and meaning of retail environments. *J. Rretail.* **1992**, *68*, 194–220.
12. Oliveira, V.; Medeiros, V. Morpho: Combining morphological measures. *Environ Plann B Plann Des.* **2016**, *43*, 805–825. [CrossRef]
13. Ravald, A.; Grönroos, C. The value concept and relationship marketing. *Eur. J. Mark.* **1996**, *30*, 19–30. [CrossRef]
14. Berry, L.L.; Yadav, M.S. Capture and communicate value in the pricing of services. *MIT Sloan Manag. Rev.* **1996**, *37*, 41.
15. Parasuraman, A.; Grewal, D. The impact of technology on the quality-value-loyalty chain: A research agenda. *J. Acad. Mark. Sci.* **2000**, *28*, 168–174. [CrossRef]
16. McLuhan, R. Go live with a big brand experience. *J. Mark.* **2000**, *26*, 45–46.
17. Holbrook, M.B. The nature of customer value: An axiology of services in the consumption experience. *Serv. Qual. New Dir. Theory Pract.* **1994**, *21*, 21–71.
18. Mathwick, C.; Malhotra, N.; Rigdon, E. Experiential value: Conceptualization, measurement and application in the catalog and Internet shopping environment. *J. Retail.* **2001**, *77*, 39–56. [CrossRef]
19. Spreng, R.A.; MacKenzie, S.B.; Olshavsky, R.W. A reexamination of the determinants of consumer satisfaction. *J. Mark.* **1996**, *60*, 15–32. [CrossRef]
20. Baker, D.A.; Crompton, J.L. Quality, satisfaction and behavioral intentions. *Ann. Tour. Res.* **2000**, *27*, 785–804. [CrossRef]
21. Fishbein, M.; Ajzen, I. *Belief, Attitude, Intention and Behavior: An Introduction to Theory and Research*, 1st ed.; Issek Ayez; Addison-Wesley Publishing Co, Inc.: New York, NY, USA, 1975; pp. 1–52.
22. Cronin, J.J., Jr.; Brady, M.K.; Hult, G.T.M. Assessing the effects of quality, value, and customer satisfaction on consumer behavioral intentions in service environments. *J. Retail.* **2000**, *76*, 193–218. [CrossRef]
23. Wu, W.Y. Service Encounter in The Luxury Restaurant How to Influence Customer's Experience Value and Positive Emotion. Ph.D. Thesis, Ming Chuan University, Taipei City, Taiwan, 2013.
24. Liu, H.H. The Relationship between Service Quality, Food Quality, Atmosphere, Customer Satisfaction and Customer Loyalty: A Case Study of Mei Mon Restaurant in Chiayi County. Ph.D. Thesis, Taiwan Capital University, Tainan City, Taiwan, 2015.
25. Chen, H.B.; Hu, C.C.; Lin, S.N. Tea Farm Visitors' Travel Experience Quality, Travel Experience Value, Travel Satisfaction and Travel Loyalty. *J. Manag. Pract. Princ.* **2007**, *1*, 107–123.
26. Wu, M.L. *SPSS Statistics Application Learning Practice*; Zhicheng Publishing Co., Ltd.: New Taipei City, Taiwan, 2003.
27. Hair, J.T.; Anderson, R.E.; Tatham, R.L.; Black, W.C. *Multivariate Data Analysis with Readings*, 3rd ed.; Macmillan: New York, NY, USA, 1997.
28. Fornell, C.; Larcker, D.F. Evaluating structural equation models with unobservable variables and measurement error. *J. Mark. Res.* **1981**, *18*, 39–50. [CrossRef]
29. Bollen, K.A.; Stine, R.A. Bootstrapping goodness-of-fit measures in structural equation models. *Sociol. Methods Res.* **1992**, *21*, 205–229. [CrossRef]
30. Hair, J.T.; Anderson, R.E.; Tatham, R.L.; Black, W.C. *Multivariate Data Analysis*, 4th ed.; Prentice Hall: Upper Saddle River, NJ, USA, 1995.
31. Chiang, C.C.; Lee, L.Y.; Chuang, W.T.; Li, K.C. A study on the impact of visitor experience value of Pilgrim Building on satisfaction and revisit intention-Taking the Pilgrim Building of Shunxian Palace in Kaohsiung's inner gate as an example. *J. Sports Health Leis.* **2012**, *20*, 71–84.
32. Thomson, H. What do your customers really want? *J. Bus. Strategy* **1998**, *19*, 17–22.

engineering proceedings

Proceeding Paper

Optimizing Mobile-Assisted Inquiry Learning with Interactive Videos to Boost Scientific Explanation and Understanding of Seventh Graders †

Autchima Thinnongwaeng [1], Niwat Srisawasdi [1,2] and Pawat Chaipidech [1,2,*]

1 Faculty of Education, Khon Kaen University, Khon Kaen 40002, Thailand; autchima_t@kkumail.com (A.T.); niwsri@kku.ac.th (N.S.)
2 Digital Education and Learning Engineering Association, Nonthaburi 11110, Thailand
* Correspondence: pawach@kku.ac.th
† Presented at the 2024 IEEE 4th International Conference on Electronic Communications, Internet of Things and Big Data, Taipei, Taiwan, 19–21 April 2024.

Abstract: Interactive videos and digital technology have been recognized by educators as supportive tools for learning science. To assess their impact, we compared seventh-grade students' abilities to explain scientific phenomena and understand climate change using interactive videos. Eighty-for students from a public secondary school participated in this research. They were divided into two groups, one using KKU iNote (EG1) and the other combining KKU iNote with interactive videos (EG2). Significant differences were observed in the scientific explanation scores between groups, with EG2 outperforming EG1. This suggested that interactive videos boosted students' competency in explaining scientific concepts. Moreover, both groups showed an improved understanding of climate change in post-learning, indicating the positive impact of inquiry-based learning. In particular, EG2 scored higher in their scientific understanding than EG1. This implied that integrating digital technology, particularly interactive videos, effectively enhanced students' scientific explanation and understanding during inquiry-based science learning.

Keywords: explanation; science; digital technology; secondary school

Citation: Thinnongwaeng, A.; Srisawasdi, N.; Chaipidech, P. Optimizing Mobile-Assisted Inquiry Learning with Interactive Videos to Boost Scientific Explanation and Understanding of Seventh Graders. *Eng. Proc.* **2024**, *74*, 37. https://doi.org/10.3390/engproc2024074037

Academic Editors: Shu-Han Liao, Teen-Hang Meen and Cheng-Fu Yang

Published: 2 September 2024

1. Introduction

The rapid development of technology has led to the integration of various technologies into various aspects of daily human life. Simultaneously, education has also incorporated technology to enhance the learning skills of students. Digital technology-integrated teaching methods have been introduced to enhance learners' development. One notable approach is the incorporation of videos in knowledge presentation. Currently, the use of videos in education has increased to improve the efficiency of content delivery, which has proven to be more effective during learning than traditional textbooks [1]. In inquiry-based science learning, students actively participate in activities that involve practicing thinking, observing, analyzing, and presenting. This emphasizes the development of knowledge through the inquiry process. Teachers serve as facilitators, guiding, advising, and assisting students while also fostering collaborative learning. However, since inquiry-based science learning focuses on the process of knowledge acquisition and not on the development of scientific explanation skills, it may not address the development of student's abilities to explain scientific concepts. According to the National Research Council [2], the ability to explain scientifically indicates students' learning skills and fundamental understanding, impacting their engagement in inquiry-based science learning. This, in turn, leads students to understand science content [3,4].

A scientific explanation consists of claims, evidence, and reasoning, which support students in communicating their explanations and arguments. Moreover, the ability to create scientific explanations of phenomena or processes in various scientifically observable forms based on information from research and linking to external experiences is important in developing students' science understanding. Science provides knowledge about phenomena and enhances our understanding of phenomena [5]. In developing students' scientific learning skills through investigation, the mobile application KKU iNote is used, an application designed to facilitate the creation of scientific explanations. In the present day, the utilization of digital technology holds a key position in education. Whether a researcher, an educator, or a science teacher, the emphasis lies in integrating digital technology, as a valuable instrument for fostering inquiry-based science learning, into the science classroom [6].

To reveal the impact of these technologies, we compared seventh-grade students' ability to explain phenomena scientifically and their understanding of climate change. We examined science inquiry-based learning using digital technology, explored the role of interactive videos in the learning process, and evaluated the impact of the mobile application KKU iNote. The findings of this study provide educators and science teachers with a reference to enhance their students' abilities to explain scientifically and understand using digital technology.

2. Literature Review

2.1. Scientific Explanation

The science standards published by the National Research Council [2,7] emphasize that scientific explanations are an essential feature, fundamental ability, and show an understanding of scientific inquiry. Students' explanations that contain flaws, such as citing irrelevant or insufficient data to support their claims, do not necessarily stem from an unscientific way of thinking. Instead, this is attributed to limited opportunities for scientific practices, wherein they can develop, argue, and evaluate explanations through their investigations [8]. Scientific explanations aid in evaluating students' grasp of scientific concepts and reasoning. In addition, the process of constructing such explanations can be used to develop their understanding of science and the scientific practice of explanations. The effectiveness of these scientific expositions can be assessed using targeted indicators to enhance their comprehension and knowledge of scientific principles. When appraising students' scientific commentary, their thinking abilities are stimulated [9]. Additionally, the evidence chosen by students is emphasized to incorporate their explanations into their perceptions of the current phenomenon, determine the relevance of their explanations, and recognize the data chosen [10].

2.2. Interactive Video

Interactive videos incorporate interactive elements and encourage viewers to respond and provide feedback on their responses [11]. Videos represent an enhanced form of digital content and are enriched with various features such as embedded questions, external content links, and additional instructional tools such as instant answers and user statistics for their monitoring. By incorporating extra content and ample guidance, they infuse interactivity into conventional lectures. Viewers engage with the material, participating as passive observers and active participants who answer questions, respond to comments, and access supplementary materials. Notably, video creators can track viewers' progress toward specific objectives by analyzing their data, including answers to questions, responses to comments, and detailed statistics on their viewing behavior. Through the integration of interactive elements, videos empower users to actively engage with the content and the video's creator and fellow viewers, enriching the learning experience. Interactive videos shift individuals from being passive observers to becoming active participants [12]. Additionally, they are utilized to encourage efficient learning. The ability to engage with features in interactive videos while watching them boosts motivation through making this an enjoyable experience [13,14].

3. Materials and Methods

In this quasi-experimental research, we employed a quantitative methodology and evaluated seventh-grade students' ability to articulate scientific explanations of climate change. We investigated the impact of interactive videos on the learning process. The students were divided into two groups: one utilizing KKU iNote (EG1) and the other combining KKU iNote with interactive videos generated by H5P (EG2) (Figure 1). We assessed the students' scientific understanding and their proficiency in grasping scientific concepts related to climate change.

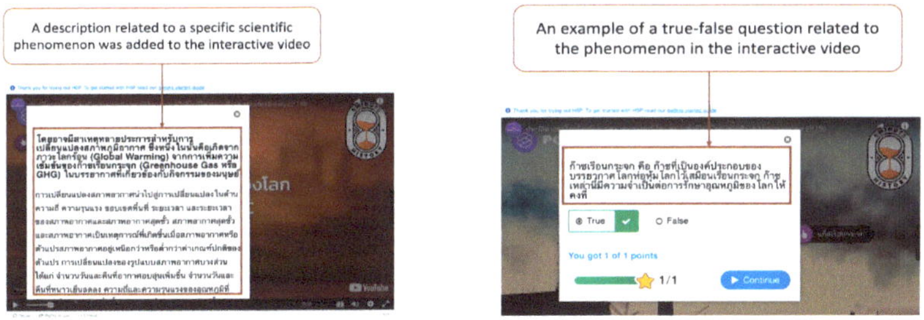

(**a**) (**b**)

Figure 1. Interactive video generated by H5P: (**a**) text added to specific aspects of the video, (**b**) true–false question used for assessment.

3.1. Participants

Eighty-four students from a secondary public school in the northeast of Thailand were selected using a random sampling method. All students were in the seventh grade, with ages ranging from 12 to 13 years. They were divided into EG1 (n = 42) and EG2 (n = 42) and had no prior experience using KKU iNote and interactive videos.

3.2. Materials

Their scientific explanations were collected using the KKU iNote mobile application, which was developed by the Smart Learning Innovation Research Center at Khon Kaen University, Thailand, along with three probing questions. Each question consisted of claims, evidence, and reasoning. These were used to assess their ability to provide scientific explanations. The knowledge of global climate change (KGCC) instrument was designed to evaluate science methods used to enhance students' scientific understanding of climate change and their comprehension of the fundamental science behind understanding weather and climate phenomena and their concepts. The extended-response component was developed using constructive modeling based on four components: (1) the construct map, (2) item design, (3) the outcome space, and (4) the measurement model [15,16]. The KGCC comprises the greenhouse effect, the carbon cycle, the causes of climate change, and the consequences of climate change.

3.3. Methods

Both groups engaged in an inquiry-based learning process using KKU iNote in five stages: (1) engagement, (2) exploration, (3) explanation, (4) elaboration, and (5) evaluation. Each stage was designed to support students in addressing the three key components of scientific explanation. For EG1, the engagement stage was focused on sparking students' interest through targeted questions related to the topic, which were prepared by educators. These included sections for formulating claims in a short-answer format. In the exploration stage, students searched for information from resources to support their claim with evidence. In the explanation stage, students expressed their understanding, which was evaluated using the initial claim. A reasoning-focused short-answer question was posed at this stage. The elaboration stage involved a deeper analysis and discussion of the information gathered, where students, in groups, synthesized their findings on chart paper. The evaluation stage allowed the students to present to the class and assess the knowledge they acquired through inquiry, fostering peer discussion about the learning process.

EG2 followed a similar learning process, which combined KKU iNote with interactive videos. In the engagement stage, interactive videos on global warming were shown, encouraging students to formulate claims relevant to the observed phenomena. Interactive features such as a drag and drop assessment and pop-up questions within the videos were used for evidence collection. The other stages followed the inquiry process adopted by EG1, integrating interactive media into learning (Figure 2). Traditional and multimedia resources were integrated to enhance the educational experience and promote an understanding of scientific concepts.

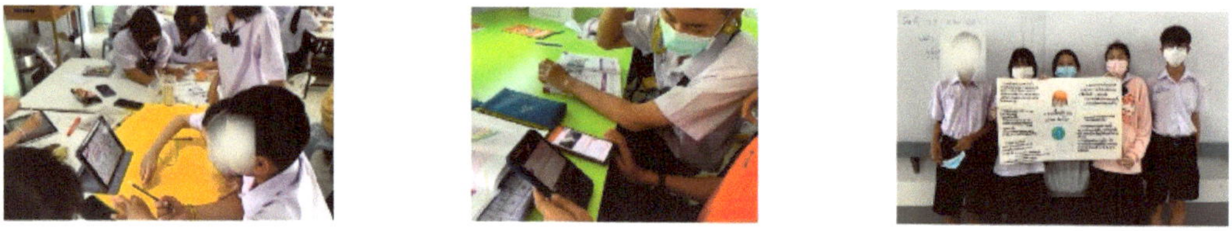

(a) (b) (c)

Figure 2. Student activities in class: (**a**) students exchanging their research knowledge with peers, (**b**) students answering questions in KKU iNote, and (**c**) students summarizing their knowledge and presenting to the class.

3.4. Data Collection and Analysis

We assessed the scientific explanations and understanding of 84 students in EG1 and EG2 who were using the KKU iNote in their science classes. In terms of their scientific explanation, the assessment framework included claims, evidence, and reasoning [9] on a 9-point scale (Table 1). In two sessions of 240 min, students responded to the inquiry questions and stated the three components of the learning process. The scientific understanding assessment was conducted using four extended-response items focusing on climate change, with each item worth 4 points. This scientific understanding test was performed for 40 min as a pre-test. Then, EG1 and EG2 were intervened. After completing the learning process, a 40 min post-test was used to measure the interventions' impact on their scientific understanding. The data were analyzed using the Mann–Whitney U test and the Wilcoxon signed-rank test to assess within-group changes pre- and post-intervention and evaluate between-group differences. SPSS was used to ensure the data's evaluation and interpretation were correct.

Table 1. The criteria for scoring the quality of scientific explanations.

Component	Level of Competency for Scientific Explanation		
	Level 0	Level 1	Level 2
Claim	Does not make a claim or makes an inaccurate claim.	Makes an accurate but incomplete claim, for example, "Caused by solar energy that reaches the atmosphere but cannot be reflected into space".	Makes an accurate and complete claim, for example, "The world's greenhouse effect caused by the Earth's atmosphere being destroyed by CFC and blocking it, making it unable to reflect heat away global warming increases. It also receives radiation from the sun to increase the heat of the earth".

Table 1. *Cont.*

Component	Level of Competency for Scientific Explanation		
	Level 0	Level 1	Level 2
Evidence	Does not provide evidence, or only provides inappropriate evidence (evidence that does not support the claim).	Provides appropriate, but insufficient, evidence to support the claim. May include some inappropriate evidence.	Provides appropriate and sufficient evidence to support the claim.
Reasoning	Does not provide reasoning, or only provides reasoning that does not link evidence to the claim.	Provides reasoning that links the claim and evidence. Repeats the evidence and/or includes some scientific principles, but not a sufficient amount.	Provides reasoning that links the evidence to their claim. Includes appropriate and sufficient principles.

4. Results

4.1. The Comparison of Scientific Explanation

We investigated the scientific explanation abilities of EG1 and EG2 to analyze their claims, evidence, and reasoning. Table 2 presents the results of the Mann–Whitney U-test. EG2 performed significantly better than EG1 in making claims, with a Z-score of −2.526 ($p = 0.012$), and reasoning, with a Z-score of −6.426 ($p < 0.001$), indicating their more effective skills in these areas. However, there was no significant difference in the evidence component. These results highlighted EG2's capabilities in key aspects of scientific explanation, while both groups demonstrated comparable abilities in providing evidence.

Table 2. The result of analyzing students' scientific explanations by Mann–Whitney U-test.

Component	Group (n = 42)	Mean Rank	Mean	Standard Deviation	Z	*p*-Value
Claim	EG1 EG2	36.25 48.75	2.98 3.43	0.91 0.62	−2.526	0.012 *
Evidence	EG1 EG2	41.00 41.00	3.83 3.93	0.69 0.69	−0.615	0.538
Reasoning	EG1 EG2	26.99 58.01	2.02 3.19	0.80 0.45	−6.426	<0.001 *

* $p < 0.05$.

4.2. The Comparison of Scientific Understanding

We assessed the scientific understanding of EG1 and EG2 using pre- and post-tests. The descriptive statistics of both tests are presented in Table 3. For the pre-test, EG1 had a mean score of 3.81 (SD = 1.11) and EG2 had a mean score of 3.02 (SD = 1.30). After the intervention, there was a significant increase in the scores, with EG1 illustrating a mean of 6.14 (SD = 1.69) and EG2 a mean of 7.40 (SD = 1.84) in the post-test.

Table 3. Descriptive statistics of students' scientific understanding.

Component	Group	n	Mean	Standard Deviation
Pre-test	EG1 EG2	42 42	3.81 3.02	1.11 1.30
Post-test	EG1 EG2	42 42	6.14 7.40	1.69 1.84

To analyze the significance of the observed differences, a Wilcoxon signed-rank test was conducted for each group. The results indicated significant increases in scientific understanding for both groups (Table 4). EG1 showed an improvement, with a Z-score of −5.126 ($p < 0.000$), and EG2 demonstrated a more significant increase, with a Z-score of −5.677 ($p < 0.000$). Both groups significantly enhanced their scientific understanding post-intervention. The larger increase in EG2's scores suggested there were differences in the effectiveness of the incorporation of the interactive videos and KKU iNote.

Table 4. Wilcoxon signed-rank test results of the pre–post-test science understanding of the two groups.

Group (n = 42)	Pre-Test		Post-Test		Z	*p*-Values
	Mean	Standard Deviation	Mean	Standard Deviation		
EG1	3.81	1.11	6.14	1.69	−5.126	<0.000 *
EG2	3.02	1.30	7.40	1.84	−5.677	<0.000 *

* $p < 0.05$.

5. Discussion and Conclusions

5.1. Scientific Explanation

This study was carried out to enhance students' abilities to construct scientific explanations specifically related to climate change. The participants constructed scientific explanations of this topic. Several participants struggled with specific concepts such as the greenhouse effect. A notable inconsistency was observed in their understanding of chlorofluorocarbons (CFCs) and their impact on the greenhouse effect. Prior research indicated that misconceptions or alternative conceptions about the greenhouse effect and global warming persisted among secondary school students even after the educational interventions [17]. Moreover, the participants displayed limitations in developing scientific explanations of different components. For instance, their responses often lacked detail in certain areas due to an inaccurate understanding of climate change content. Their ability to effectively link evidence with claims was consequently lacking. The lowest performance was noted in reasoning, where students frequently confused claims with reasons due to unclear distinctions between these elements. The results coincided with those of previous studies. Yu and Lin [18] found that proficiency in creating scientific explanations followed a solid understanding of science, with reasoning consistently scoring the lowest. Lertdechapat [19] discussed how the absence of precise scientific knowledge affected the quality of explanations, leading to incomplete reasoning and inadequate links between claims and evidence. Such results illustrated the need for effective educational strategies that promote scientific explanation skills through scenarios that are combined with students' everyday experiences [20]. EG2 scored higher in both scientific explanation and understanding, emphasizing the impact of constructing scientific explanations on enhancing scientific knowledge [9]. Additionally, EG2's performance in all components was attributed to the integration of interactive video-based learning, which incorporated argumentation and inductive questioning to help students explore hypotheses, build explanations, and expand their understanding [21].

5.2. Scientific Understanding

Inquiry-based learning with digital technology and interactive videos was used to enhance the learning experience in science. This encouraged students to actively inquire about scientific explanations and deepen their scientific understanding [22]. Significant enhancements were observed in both groups in the post-test compared to their pre-tests. This indicated that the incorporation of interactive videos and KKU iNote into inquiry-based learning potentially enhanced its effectiveness. The interactive videos included links. These links were used by the participants to explore related topics from other resources used in their learning. When the video was paused, students contemplated the learning subject extensively and discussed it with classmates. Additionally, they responded to pop-up questions that guided their focus and comprehension [21]. In addition, this interactivity affected the effectiveness of education [23]. Interactivity within educational settings strengthens students' understanding of learning concepts [24]. Daily [25] found that the use of multiple media enriched learning through enhanced visualization and improved learning outcomes. We discovered a significant feature of integrating digital technologies into an inquiry-based learning approach. Students' intrinsic motivation and self-determination increased when using technologies in class [26].

Author Contributions: Conceptualization, N.S. and A.T.; methodology, N.S. and A.T.; software, N.S., A.T. and P.C.; validation, N.S.; formal analysis, P.C. and A.T.; investigation, N.S. and P.C.; resources, A.T.; writing—original draft preparation, P.C. and A.T.; writing—review and editing, P.C.; visualization, P.C. and A.T.; supervision, N.S. and P.C. All authors have read and agreed to the published version of the manuscript.

Funding: This research received no external funding.

Institutional Review Board Statement: Not applicable.

Informed Consent Statement: Not applicable.

Data Availability Statement: The data used in this research are available upon request.

Acknowledgments: This work was supported by the Science and Technology Education Program, Graduate School, Faculty of Education, Khon Kaen University, Khon Kaen, Thailand. The authors would like to thank all participating secondary school students for their cooperation, the research assistants for their analyzing of the scientific conceptual understanding test, and the TELL-STEM Special Interest Group within the Faculty of Education at Khon Kaen University for their assistance with this research.

Conflicts of Interest: The authors declare no conflicts of interest.

References

1. Poquet, O.; Lim, L.; Mirriahi, N.; Dawson, S. Video and Learning: A Systematic Review (2007–2017). In Proceedings of the International Conference on Learning Analytics and Knowledge, Sysney, Australia, 7–9 March 2018; Association for Computing Machinery (ACM): New York, NY, USA, 2018; pp. 151–160.
2. National Research Council. *National Science Education Standards*; National Academies Press: Washington, DC, USA, 1996.
3. Ruiz-Primo, M.A.; Li, M.; Tsai, S.P.; Schneider, J. Testing one premise of scientific inquiry in science classrooms: Examining students' scientific explanations and student learning. *J. Res. Sci. Teach.* **2010**, *47*, 583–608. [CrossRef]
4. McNeill, K.L.; Krajcik, J. *Supporting Grade 5–8 Students in Constructing Explanations in Science: The Claim, Evidence, and Reasoning Framework for Talk and Writing*; Pearson: London, UK, 2011.
5. de Regt, H.W.; Baumberger, C. What is scientific understanding and how can it be achieved? In *What Is Scientific Knowledge?: An Introduction to Contemporary Epistemology of Science*; Routledge: New York, NY, USA, 2019.
6. Srisawasdi, N. Student teachers' perceptions of computerized laboratory practice for science teaching: A comparative analysis. *Procedia-Soc. Behav. Sci.* **2012**, *46*, 4031–4038. [CrossRef]
7. National Research Council. *Inquiry and the National Science Education Standards*; National Academies Press: Washington, DC, USA, 2000.
8. Ruiz-Primo, M.A.; Furtak, E.M. Exploring teachers' informal formative assessment practices and students' understanding in the context of scientific inquiry. *J. Res. Sci. Teach.* **2007**, *44*, 57–84. [CrossRef]
9. McNeill, K.L.; Krajcik, J. Assessing middle school students' content knowledge and reasoning through written scientific explanations. In *Science Assessment, Research and Practical Approaches*; National Science Teacher Association Press: Arlington, VA, USA, 2008.
10. Sandoval, W.A. Students' uses of data as evidence in scientific explanations. In Proceedings of the Annual Meeting of the American Educational Research Association, Seattle, WA, USA, 10–14 April 2001.
11. Stigler, J.; Geller, E.; Givvin, K. Zaption: A platform to support teaching, and learning about teaching, with video. *J. e-Learn. Knowl. Soc.* **2015**, *11*, 13–25.
12. Wachtler, J.; Hubmann, M.; Zöhrer, H.; Ebner, M. An analysis of the use and effect of questions in interactive learning-videos. *Smart Learn. Environ.* **2016**, *3*, 13. [CrossRef]
13. Zhang, D.; Zhou, L.; Robert, O.B.; Jay, F.N. Instructional video in e-learning: Assessing the impact of Interactive Video on learning effectiveness. *Inf. Manag.* **2006**, *43*, 15–27. [CrossRef]
14. Bakla, A. Interactive Videos in foreign language instruction: A new gadget in your toolbox. *Mersin Univ. J. Fac. Educ.* **2017**, *13*, 124–137.

15. Wilson, M.; Bertenthal, M. *Systems for State Science Assessment*; Board on Testing and Assessment, Center for Education, National Research Council of the National Academies; National Academies Press: Washington, DC, USA, 2005.
16. Lambert, V.A.; Lambert, C.E. Qualitative descriptive research: An acceptable design. *Pac. Rim Int. J. Nurs. Res.* **2012**, *16*, 255–256.
17. Mason, L.; Santi, M. Discussing the greenhouse effect: Children's collaborative discourse reasoning and conceptual change. *Environ. Educ. Res.* **1998**, *4*, 67–85. [CrossRef]
18. Yu, K.C.; Fan, S.C.; Lin, K.Y. Enhancing students' problem-solving skills through context-based learning. *Int. J. Sci. Math. Educ.* **2015**, *13*, 1377–1401. [CrossRef]
19. Lertdechapat, K.; Promratana, P.L. Effects of collaborative inquiry on collaborative problem-solving ability of lower secondary school students. *J. Educ. Naresuan Univ.* **2021**, *23*, 1–14.
20. Sirithon, N.; Jantarakantee, E. Implementing argument-driven inquiry approach for developing grade 10th students' ability in making scientific explanation in the topic of force, mass, and law of motion. *Silpakorn Univ. J.* **2019**, *39*, 130–141.
21. Shelton, C.C.; Warren, A.E.; Archambault, L.M. Exploring the use of interactive digital storytelling video: Promoting student engagement and learning in a university hybrid course. *TechTrends* **2016**, *60*, 465–474. [CrossRef]
22. Chaipidech, P.; Srisawasdi, N. A proposal for personalized inquiry-based flipped learning with mobile technology. In Proceedings of the 26th International Conference on Computers in Education, Metro Manila, Philippines, 26–30 November 2018; Wu, Y.T., Srisawasdi, N., Banawan, M., Yang, J.C., Chang, M., Wong, L.-H., Rodrigo, M.M.T., Eds.; Asia-Pacific Society for Computers in Education: Malila, Philippines, 2018; pp. 344–353.
23. Jonassen, D.; Davidson, M.; Collins, M.; Campbell, J.; Haag, B.B. Constructivism and computer-mediated communication in distance education. *Am. J. Distance Educ.* **1995**, *9*, 7–26. [CrossRef]
24. Moore, M.G. Three types of interaction. *Am. J. Distance Educ.* **1989**, *3*, 1–6.
25. Daily, B.; Daily, M. Effectiveness of a multimedia televised distance education program for engineering majors. *J. Eng. Educ.* **1994**, *83*, 383–388. [CrossRef]
26. Srisawasdi, N.; Panjaburee, P. Implementation of game-transformed inquiry-based learning to promote the understanding of and motivation to learn chemistry. *J. Sci. Educ. Technol.* **2019**, *28*, 152–164. [CrossRef]

engineering proceedings

Proceeding Paper

Self-Learning Efficiency in College Virtual Course of Engineering Mathematics on YouTube †

John C.-C. Lu

Department of Civil Engineering, Chung Hua University, Hsinchu 30012, Taiwan; cclu@chu.edu.tw

† Presented at the 2024 IEEE 4th International Conference on Electronic Communications, Internet of Things and Big Data, Taipei, Taiwan, 19–21 April 2024.

Abstract: The author has provided more than 2100 engineering mathematics teaching materials on YouTube since 2014. The viewer information provided by YouTube revealed that (1) 59.16% of viewers were 18 to 24 years old while 23.18% were over 35 years old, (2) the gender ratio was 4:1 (male–female), (3) 9.19% of viewers subscribed to the educational channel, (4) 88.13% of viewers were from Taiwan and 1.97% from Hong Kong, and (5) the proportion of "External Sources" and "Playlist" was 26.91% and 25.30%, respectively. Such viewer demographics help adjust the principles of tutorial videos. For instance, nearly 60% of the viewers were college students, and their expectations aligned with the grading criteria set by instructors. The majority of college instructors arrange written examinations and present engineering mathematics content in a handwritten manner. Around 25% of the students had richer life experiences and no examination pressure. Therefore, proverbs or idioms related to life philosophy in videos better resonated with these viewers. Tutorial videos were created to assist self-learners in mastering engineering mathematics. The data over the past nine years on YouTube serve as a valuable reference in constructing instructional videos for engineering. This virtual tutorial experience provides a basis to adjust the direction of future tutorial video recordings.

Keywords: engineering mathematics; OpenCourseWare; information technology integrated into instruction; self-study tutoring

Citation: Lu, J.C.-C. Self-Learning Efficiency in College Virtual Course of Engineering Mathematics on YouTube. *Eng. Proc.* **2024**, *74*, 38. https://doi.org/10.3390/engproc2024074038

Academic Editors: Shu-Han Liao, Teen-Hang Meen and Cheng-Fu Yang

Published: 2 September 2024

1. Introduction

An open-course teaching model is used in engineering mathematics. Starting from 21 September 2014, a teaching community for engineering mathematics on YouTube was formed. As of 27 January 2024, this community's instructional videos had attracted 3950 subscribers interested in engineering mathematics. Over 2100 instructional videos were posted on YouTube for engineering mathematics.

Many teachers have used YouTube for instruction and have achieved good results. Kadriu et al. [1] explored tutorial trends using available public YouTube data. This study focused on tutorials for 11 programming languages, and its methodology can be used in any other field of interest. Maziriri et al. [2] suggested that perceived usefulness impacted students' perceptions of learning through YouTube compared to considerations of ease of use. Despite the limitations, Kibirige and Odora [3] indicated that incorporating YouTube videos enhanced students' cognitive achievements. Rigdel et al. [4] concluded that YouTube as supplementary material significantly influenced the improvement of students' learning achievements and their attitudes toward learning geography. Nabayra [5] observed a significant improvement in the performance of students before and after the utilization of teacher-created videos on YouTube for online mathematics learning. Jamil et al. [6] disclosed that STEM students frequently utilized YouTube tutorial videos to learn mathematics, and their performance in mathematics was improved. Pattier [7] pointed out the significant impact of YouTube channels on science with a positive trend and substantial growth in users and educational audiovisual content. Based on interviews with mathematics educators and students, Anisa et al. [8] discovered that YouTube served as a viable platform for mathematical education.

Thus, it is crucial to recognize and assess the diverse advantages and disadvantages associated with YouTube's use. Rahmatika et al. [9] concluded that YouTube functioned as a learning medium and encouraged independent learning for students. Nacak et al. [10] determined that teachers considered YouTube to have suitable educational material for various lessons and believed that it enhanced retention and reinforced learning. Dubovi and Tabak [11] demonstrated that YouTube provided an informal space for scientific deliberation and a forum for collaborative interactions to support lifelong learning. Rachmawati and Cahyani [12] concluded that the use of YouTube videos positively impacted students' pronunciation skills, and YouTube was a significant learning medium for English pronunciation, particularly for non-English department students. Shaikh et al. [13] discovered that the number of video views was crucial in predicting citations and enhancing the popularity of research articles, as well as fostering public engagement with science. Sunday et al. [14] demonstrated that the utilization of YouTube as an online educational tool enhanced the academic achievements of undergraduate students in mathematics education. Toleuzhan et al. [15] suggested that students in secondary education held a positive attitude toward utilizing YouTube videos for learning English speaking skills. Nielsen [16] highlighted a strong negative correlation between the length of a video on YouTube and the portion of that video that students watched per viewing session.

In this study, differences in the learning of self-learners by age, gender, subscription ratio, geographical location, and search methods were explored in the YouTube engineering mathematics community. The results can be used to fine-tune the focal points of instructional videos and provide a reference for developers of similar educational channels.

2. Recorded Information on YouTube

In Taiwanese YouTube teaching channels, a channel with over 1800 subscribers is considered important. As of 27 January 2024, the studied engineering mathematics teaching channel had garnered 3950 subscribers (Figure 1). Figure 2 shows that the readers viewed newly published instructional videos every day. In the latest 7 days (20–27 January 2024), 16.12% of the viewers were subscribed. From September 2014 to January 2024, the proportion of subscribed viewers was 9.19%. During 20–27 January 2024, male students were more inclined to view newly published engineering mathematics videos on YouTube. For these 7 days, 91.58% of viewers were male students (Figure 3). From September 2014 to January 2024, the proportion of male students was 80.36%. The gender ratio of male to female viewers was 4:1.

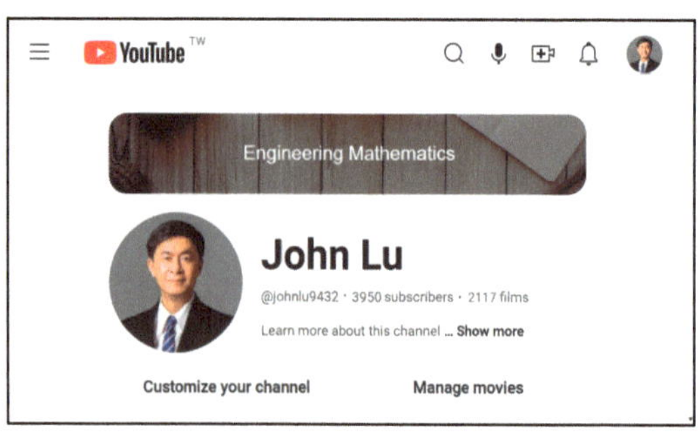

Figure 1. There were 3950 subscribers on a YouTube channel for engineering mathematics (as of 27 January 2024).

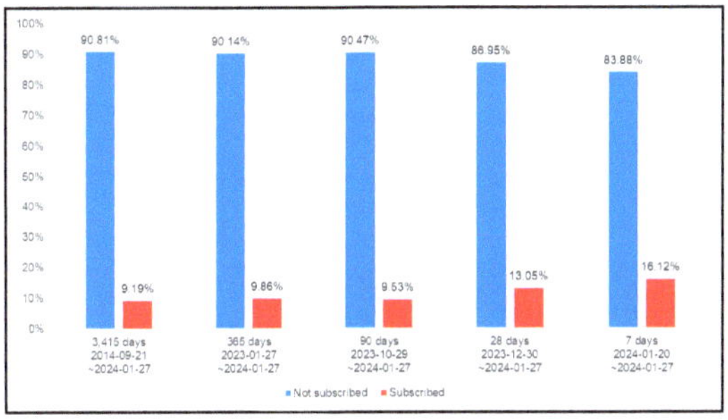

Figure 2. Ratio of subscribers for 7, 28, 90, 365, and 3415 days as of 27 January 2024.

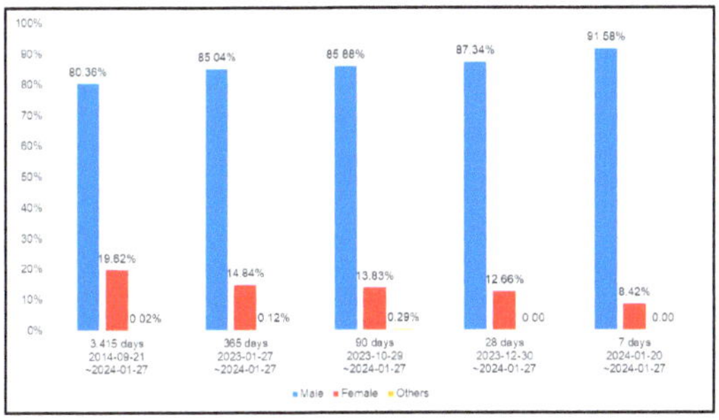

Figure 3. Gender ratio for 7, 28, 90, 365, and 3415 days as of 27 January 2024.

Figure 4 shows that the majority of viewers of the YouTube engineering mathematics channel were 18–24 years old from September 2014 to January 2024, accounting for 59.16%. The viewers were mostly college students studying engineering mathematics in this age group. Viewers over 35 years old accounted for 23.18%. During 20–27 January 2024, the dominant age group was 55–64 years old, constituting 45.70%. These results show the needs of both age groups. As engineering mathematics questions were explained for civil service exams with a proverb (Figure 5) bilingually, this addition attracted more viewers.

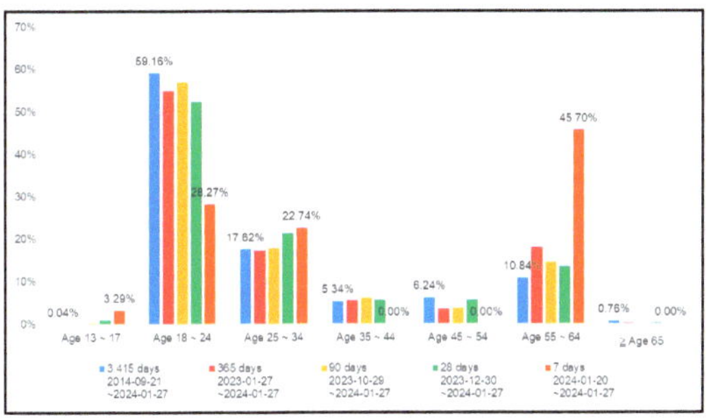

Figure 4. Composition of viewers in various 7, 28, 90, 365, and 3415 days as of 27 January 2024.

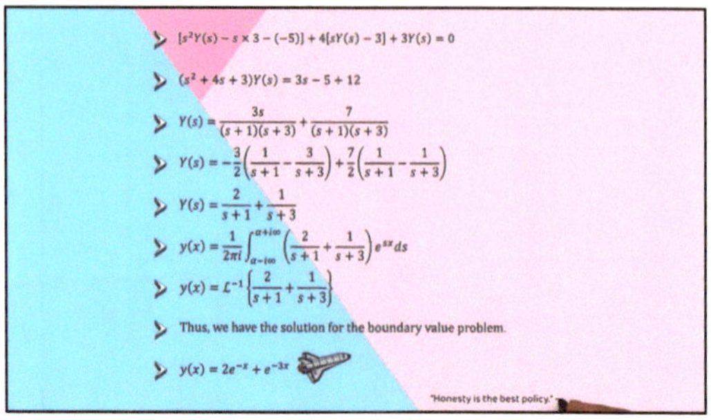

Figure 5. Scene of video with a proverb: "Honesty is the best policy."

From September 2014 to January 2024, most viewers were from Taiwan (88.13%) and Hong Kong (1.97%). Thus, it was necessary to meet the needs of local students. On 20–27 January 2024, there was an increase in the proportion of self-learners from outside Taiwan. Consequently, it was needed to provide the video in a bilingual mode (Figure 6).

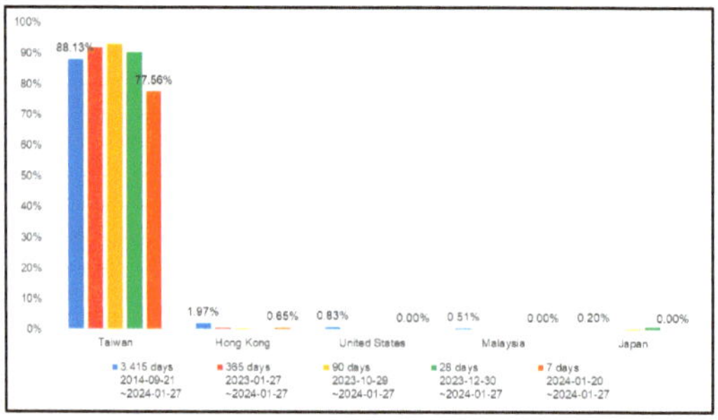

Figure 6. Countries of viewers as of 27 January 2024.

The data in Figure 7 shows that students learning engineering mathematics discover instructional videos on YouTube primarily through "External Sources" and "Playlist", followed by "YouTube Search", "Recommended Videos", and "Browse Features". The proportions of "External Sources" and "Playlist" were 26.91% and 25.30% from September 2014 to January 2024. "External Sources" were used for external websites or apps. During 20–27 January 2024, viewers browsed the videos as "Browse Features". Traffic from "Browse Features" was generated through the homepage, subscription feed, watch later, trending, and explore sections of YouTube.

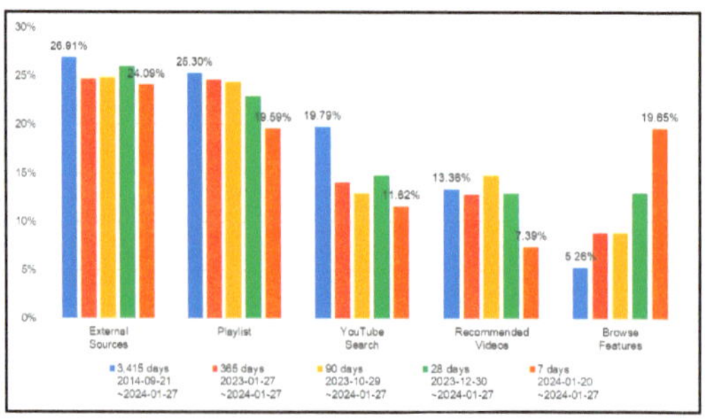

Figure 7. Traffic sources for the created YouTube teaching platform (statistical results on 27 January 2024).

3. Principles of Video

The following factors were considered in creating videos for engineering mathematics.

- **Problem-solving Approach:** In teaching engineering mathematics, examples are often used for explanation. In analyzing each engineering mathematics problem, it is essential to understand the underlying engineering significance. Appropriate mathematical methods are used for this analysis. Theorems also need to be taught for students to grasp the essence of the theorems and handle problem-solving proficiently. When applying formulas to problem-solving, students may find it less engaging. It is recommended to discard formulaic approaches for an enjoyable learning experience.
- **Design-based Teaching Method:** This teaching approach involves the planning of students' learning by themselves. For example, if students want to understand the analytical methods of "first-order ordinary differential equations," they need to review relevant instructional videos and lecture notes. By shortening the learning process, students build confidence and enhance their motivation.
- **Experimental Thinking Teaching Method:** Albert Einstein once proposed the concept of experimental thinking, which implies conducting experiments through thoughtful contemplation. In teaching engineering mathematics, students need experiments. For example, the decay rate of radioactive substances is proportional to the mass of the radioactive substance, and the rate of temperature change in an object is proportional to the temperature difference. These natural laws can be understood through experiments. Students can derive enjoyment from learning through this process.
- **Self-Learning Guidance Method:** In imparting engineering mathematics knowledge, students need to be guided to grasp learning methods and enhance their self-learning capabilities. More than 2100 videos are beneficial for students in previewing, reviewing, and referencing materials.
- **Integration of "Jigsaw" and "Pyramid" Learning:** Based on personal teaching and learning, "Pyramid"- and "Jigsaw"-style teaching are used. Learning engineering mathematics is based on the "Jigsaw" learning method, but each puzzle is a small "Pyramid." When teaching engineering mathematics, teachers need to focus on a single main topic for students to understand fundamental concepts such as calculus or high school mathematics for a specific unit.

The instructional videos on unit topics created by the author were recorded according to such principles.

4. Conclusions

To enhance the strengths and mitigate weaknesses of instructional videos, viewers were analyzed by gender, age, subscription status, and viewing methods. YouTube videos have been used to improve teaching effectiveness. More than 60% of viewers of the created videos were college students, meeting the needs for examinations and further studies. Simultaneously, the videos attracted 25% of viewers who were older than 35 years old with life experience. It is important to include elements to resonate with viewers in instructional videos. For students, detailed solutions for engineering mathematics problems need to be provided for both entrance examinations and civil service examinations. The ratio of male to female self-learners was 4:1, aligning with the common perception of fewer females in learning engineering.

The created videos were perceived as easy to understand, contributing to building learning confidence. This affirms the goal of the videos to assist students in learning engineering mathematics effectively.

Funding: This work is supported by the Ministry of Education of Taiwan, Republic of China, through grants PEE1110397 and PEE1120413.

Institutional Review Board Statement: Not applicable.

Informed Consent Statement: Not applicable.

Data Availability Statement: Data are contained within the article.

Conflicts of Interest: The author declares no conflicts of interest.

References

1. Kadriu, A.; Abazi-Bexheti, L.; Abazi-Alili, H.; Ramadani, V. Investigating trends in learning programming using YouTube tutorials. *Int. J. Learn. Change* **2020**, *12*, 190–208. [CrossRef]
2. Maziriri, E.T.; Gapa, P.; Chuchu, T. Student perceptions towards the use of YouTube as an educational tool for learning and tutorials. *Int. J. Instr.* **2020**, *13*, 119–138. [CrossRef]
3. Kibirige, I.; Odora, R.J. Exploring the effects of YouTube on technology education students' cognitive achievement in a mechanical system module. *Perspect. Educ.* **2021**, *39*, 94–108. [CrossRef]
4. Rigdel, K.S.; Dorji, S.; Rai, D.M. Effectiveness of YouTube as a supplementary material to enhance the students' learning achievement in geography. *Asian J. Educ. Soc. Stud.* **2023**, *47*, 53–72. [CrossRef]
5. Nabayra, J.N. YouTube-based teacher-created videos for online mathematics learning during the pandemic and its effect to students' mathematics performance. *Webology* **2022**, *19*, 1380–1390.
6. Jamil, H.A.H.; Halun, R.A.; Rendiza, A.A. YouTube tutorial videos and mathematics performance. *Asian J. Adv. Multidiscip. Res.* **2022**, *2*, 1–4.
7. Pattier, D. Science on Youtube: Successful edutubers. *TECHNO Rev.* **2021**, *10*, 1–15. [CrossRef]
8. Anisa, Y.; Hafiz, M.; Azmi, F. The potential of YouTube as a source of mathematics learning education. *Asian Res. J. Math.* **2023**, *19*, 1–8. [CrossRef]
9. Rahmatika, R.; Yusuf, M.; Agung, L. The effectiveness of Youtube as an online learning media. *J. Educ. Technol.* **2021**, *5*, 152–158. [CrossRef]
10. Nacak, A.; Bağlama, B.; Demir, B. Teacher candidate views on the use of YouTube for educational purposes. *Online J. Commun. Media Technol.* **2020**, *10*, e202003. [CrossRef]
11. Dubovi, I.; Tabak, I. An empirical analysis of knowledge co-construction in YouTube comments. *Comput. Educ.* **2020**, *156*, 103939. [CrossRef]
12. Rachmawati, R.; Cahyani, F. The use of YouTube videos in improving non-English department students' pronunciation skills. *Alsuna J. Arab. Engl. Lang.* **2020**, *3*, 83–95. [CrossRef]
13. Shaikh, A.R.; Alhoori, H.; Sun, M. YouTube and science: Models for research impact. *Scientometrics* **2023**, *128*, 933–955. [CrossRef] [PubMed]
14. Sunday, Y.; Salami, D.; Olorunishola, O.A.; Arivi, S.S. Influence of YouTube online device on undergraduate students' performance in mathematics education in north-central, Nigeria. *J. Curric. Instr.* **2023**, *14*, 115–124.
15. Toleuzhan, A.; Sarzhanova, G.; Romanenko, S.; Uteubayeva, E.; Karbozova, G. The educational use of YouTube videos in communication fluency development in English: Digital learning and oral skills in secondary education. *Int. J. Educ. Math. Sci. Technol.* **2023**, *11*, 198–221. [CrossRef]
16. Nielsen, K.L. Students' video viewing habits during a flipped classroom course in engineering mathematics. *Res. Learn. Technol.* **2020**, *28*, 1–12. [CrossRef]

engineering proceedings

MDPI

Proceeding Paper

Role of Personalized Learning Program by Learning Management System in Higher Education in Binus Bandung Indonesia †

Agus Masrukhin

Character Building Development Center Information Systems Department, School of Information Systems, Bina Nusantara University, Jakarta 11480, Indonesia; agus@binus.ac.id

† Presented at the 2024 IEEE 4th International Conference on Electronic Communications, Internet of Things and Big Data, Taipei, Taiwan, 19–21 April 2024.

Abstract: This study aims to provide an overview of the effectiveness and responsiveness of the personalized learning model in terms of Industry 4.0. A qualitative and descriptive research method was used as students, staff, and lecturers were interviewed. Campus and journal practices were examined, and peer-reviewed articles in multiple journals, including publications, personal study lectures, and learning analysis, were analyzed. The paradigm shift in curriculum development and personalized learning design, with the help of the learning management system, helped students become more independent and effective in learning.

Keywords: higher education; personalized learning; LMS technology

1. Introduction

Personalized learning (PL) is one of the phenomena of the digital revolution, which is driving important changes in various fields, especially in higher education. In the digital era, college learning does not only happen on campus. Thanks to rapidly developing learning technology, students expect to determine what to learn, when to learn, and how to learn. Students want to determine the learning they want, including the learning resources. PL is the biggest challenge for higher education institutions, which pay attention to student diversity to adapt and utilize technological developments in the learning process.

Binus University captures digital progress in higher education to support student independence by registering for personal study courses for one semester. Students benefit greatly from this personalized learning (PL) model, but creativity, perseverance, and personal responsibility are required for graduation. Students may be bored with ordinary lectures because the graduation requirement is strict attendance. On the other hand, in this PL model, attendance is not a requirement for graduation. Success in assignments or projects is an important part of graduation requirements. The students have the option of one semester in PL for all courses in that semester. Students are not tied to a standard learning process, so they can manage their time during the semester and complete courses in 7–16 weeks, so they can graduate faster.

This study aims to explain how students receive personalized learning innovations, map students' learning expectation models, and analyze how the Binusmaya campus applications and practices support student assignments and projects. It was assumed that the in-depth interview answers given by students reflected the quality of the design of Binusmaya's seven facilities at the school and the quality of other supporting spaces on the campus. In other words, student satisfaction was an indicator of successful academic performance and student growth. However, advances in the application of PL technology also affect student graduation, which is a challenge for future researchers.

According to Ming Chen, on the contrary, most e-learning systems tend to ignore students' abilities and the difficulty level of recommended learning materials that match each other during the learning process. Apart from that, the problem of continuity of

Citation: Masrukhin, A. Role of Personalized Learning Program by Learning Management System in Higher Education in Binus Bandung Indonesia. *Eng. Proc.* **2024**, *74*, 39. https://doi.org/10.3390/engproc2024074039

Academic Editors: Shu-Han Liao, Teen-Hang Meen and Cheng-Fu Yang

Published: 2 September 2024

learning must also be considered, inappropriate lecture material causes cognitive load or disorientation of students in the learning process, thereby weakening learning abilities [1]. Bernacki has noted in various articles on learning adaptation that it is best to focus on an individualized curriculum based on learner characteristics and desired outcomes. Bernacki suggests that a theory-based approach to designing and researching personalized learning can organize efforts to evaluate practice, and creating an explicit theory of change can increase the likelihood of achieving personalized learning goals [2]. Therefore, the curriculum model for each university is different and Binus applies a different PL curriculum for creative entrepreneurship students at the Binus Business School faculty. With the help of personalized learning, students are expected to have the freedom of choice to set their own learning goals, be flexible to take their learning beyond the boundaries of the traditional classroom, and receive feedback to create a process of reflection [3]. With the help of personalized learning, learning needs are tailored to students' interests, talents and abilities, and flexible learning is offered for learning in different conditions. Through personalized learning, specific knowledge or skills are desired by each student. A key component of personalized learning is learner analytics. Learning analytics helps educational institutions analyze students' skill development needs. Learning analysis provides results in the form of learning recommendations tailored to student profiles [4,5]. Student resources are a collection of soft skills and hard skills that students have or the knowledge and skills that a person has. This description is in accordance with the definition of qualifications in Law 14 of 2005 or [6]. Apart from developing skills that match the interests of the major, students are also expected to be able to improve six soft skills: (1) self-management, (2) teamwork, (3) communication skills, (4) initiative and entrepreneurship, (5) problem solving and decision-making skills that must be carried out. the ability to carry out and plan and organize [7–9].

2. Method

Data were collected through observation, interviews, and a literature review. How colleges reacted to new PL policies in the digital era and how students were involved in the learning process were observed. Interviews with students, staff, and teachers revealed various problems related to personalized learning among students and their innovative ideas for implementing personalized learning. The data were obtained from online articles, and several students confirmed the articles as informants. An interview guide was used to formulate questions during data collection. Using open questions, information related to the effectiveness of learning in a private study room was obtained. Second, satisfaction with the Binumaya platform application was investigated. Third, the management of the learning system was adjusted based on the results. The survey was conducted via Google Forms and WhatsApp (WA). At the same time, articles and interview data were categorized and mapped thematically to clarify student responses. Apart from that, adequacy and truth were considered in compiling data. Data were analyzed in three stages: data reproduction, description, and interpretation.

3. Result

The PL design of Binus University in the current digital era has been innovated for e-learning. PL courses have become part of the e-learning model for Binus University students. Students have the opportunity for one semester to take part in PL for all courses. Students are not bound by the regular mode of the learning process. They do not have a class attendance schedule, so they can manage their own time for one full semester and have the opportunity to pass courses between the 7th and 16th weeks (which can be finished sooner). Students can adjust their learning activities to be able to carry out student activities or other self-development activities. Students have the same course qualifications as courses in regular mode.

The different circumstances, social status, and educational background of parents sometimes hinder students' learning processes, including the financial weakness of students' families, the distance between where students live and the campus, students with physical disabilities (disabilities), and students who work part-time. Even parents' educational background can influence parents' attitudes and policies toward their children; some parents are indifferent to their child's achievements in college. These various obstacles make students bored and lazy when it comes studying. The PL lecture program is interesting for students as it saves transportation and accommodation costs for college, and there are no routine lecture activities. Several things make personal study courses interesting: (1) students can learn everything, (2) students can adjust their learning speed, and (3) students can adjust their lecture time to other student activities. Therefore, personal study courses are part of the solution to students' limitations in increasing study resources. There is a problem with the freedom to study lectures individually if students are not disciplined and organized. Therefore, it is necessary to carry out administrative supervision so that student progress can be properly monitored. This is necessary to ensure students follow the lecture process. Without good supervision and monitoring, it is feared that students will get carried away with other activities or socializing with friends.

The application of PL practices by students varies greatly, but in general, students responded well to various narrative responses. Suggestions were proposed by students in interviews as follows:

"I think this personal learning system is very effective for students like me because we can; check the progress of your lecture, there is no minimum number of participants. I think if we decide not to take formal classes, it means we already have other pressing problems. But they feel more productive when they come to study on campus, so I think the PL system is not for all students" (interview, September 2022). NA is a student in Hungary and also a Binus student. According to him, PL is suitable for students like him because he has lecture activities at another campus, so it is not possible to attend regular lectures and attend other classes at the same time. Individual learning is very beneficial for the success of one's studies. Other students acknowledged the effectiveness of OT, although they preferred regular lectures. At Binus Bandung, a student, JS, said:

"PL can be more effective if the student in question knows how to use his time well so that the student can adjust his time and learning abilities, but I like regular classes because I can meet with friends" (interview, September 2022).

There are challenges and difficulties. Students have to be disciplined because there are no regular lectures. Many students attend regular lectures and strictly follow the lecturer's rules, such as submitting assignments on time. Many students rely on assignments from their college friends. Moreover, if students do not ask about lecturers and friends, they have difficulty with subjects. Several students like regular lectures because they can meet friends, socialize, and solve study problems together. However, they acknowledged the effectiveness of PL lectures, especially in terms of time. A student provided a piece of advice based on his interests: "In my opinion, personalized Creative Entrepreneurship learning is effective for students who already have their projects/businesses because PL aims to find out the progress of their business development. Once a week we discuss these developments with the lecturers so that students have a place to consult".

4. Conclusions

The result of this study showed that the current Industry 4.0 era has brought significant changes in higher education. One of the most important impacts of the industrial era is PL at Binus University. Binus University's PL policy illustrates the commitment and challenges of the industrialization era. Students need to focus and be committed to their study goals because of the challenges in PL. The application of PL was interesting for students. Universities need to respond to student expectations and suggestions regarding PL. Constructive and thoughtful policies are needed to ensure that higher education institutions focus on industry market orientation and how PL is used to educate students with hard and soft skills. Therefore, it is necessary to ensure that students, lecturers, and universities utilize education to build personal integrity based on religion. This research is limited to the descriptive analysis of limited data processing. Therefore, further research is needed to explore PL more broadly. Campuses must play a role in overcoming the challenges that students want by increasing self-confidence to raise human resources.

Funding: This research received no external funding.

Institutional Review Board Statement: Not applicable.

Informed Consent Statement: Not applicable.

Data Availability Statement: Data can be made available upon request.

Conflicts of Interest: The author declares no conflicts of interest.

References

1. Chen, C.-M. Intelligent web-based learning system with PL path guidance. *Comput. Educ.* **2008**, *51*, 787–814. [CrossRef]
2. Bernacki, M.L.; Greene, M.J.; Lobczowski, N.G. A Systematic Review of Research on PL: Personalized by Whom, to What, How, and for What Purpose(s)? *Educ. Psychol. Rev.* **2021**, *33*, 1675–1715. [CrossRef]
3. Farisia, H. Membangun Kompetensi Sosial Siswa dalam Pembelajaran IPS melalui PL. *J. Pendidik. Teor. Penelit. Dan Pengemb.* **2021**, *6*, 1588–1592.
4. Gerhana, Y.A.; Kurahman, O.T.; Lukman, N.; Atmadja, A.R. *PL: Tantangan Pengembangan LMS di Era Pendidikan 4.0*; Karya Tulis Ilm. Masa Work from Home COVID-19; UIN Sunan Gunung Djati Bandung: Bandung, Indonesia, 2020; pp. 1–12.
5. Dematrini, C.; Benussi, L. *Do Web 4.0 and Industry 4.0 imply Education 4.0*; IT Professional; IEEE Computer Society: Los Alamitos, CA, USA, 2017.
6. Ismail, I.; Hasan, H.; Musdalifah, M. Pengembangan Kompetensi Mahasiswa Melalui Efektivitas Program Magang Kependidikan. *Edumaspul J. Pendidik.* **2018**, *2*, 124–132. [CrossRef]
7. Arifin, N. *Manajemen Sumberdaya Manusia: Teori Dan Kasus*; Unisnu Press: Kecapi, Indonesia, 2013.
8. Harras, H.; Sugiarti, E.; Wahyudi, W. *Kajian Manajemen Sumber Daya Manusia Untuk Mahasiswa*; Unpam Press: South Tangerang, Indonesia, 2020.
9. Ichsan, R.N.; SEM, M.; Lukman Nasution SE, I.; Sarman Sinaga, S.E. *Bahan Ajar Manajemen Sumber Daya Manusia (MSDM)*; CV. Sentosa Deli Mandiri: Medan, Indonesia, 2020.

engineering proceedings

MDPI

Proceeding Paper

Lighting Design by Computer Software in Teaching and Practice: A Case Study in Vocational Training of Interior Design †

Shaofu Li

Department of Architecture and Urban Planning, Chung Hua University, Hsinchu 30012, Taiwan; shaofu@g.chu.edu.tw

† Presented at the 2024 IEEE 4th International Conference on Electronic Communications, Internet of Things and Big Data, Taipei, Taiwan, 19–21 April 2024.

Abstract: This study aims to compute the display of indoor lighting and compare the performance of different lighting simulations. Students of the two-year vocational training program participated in this study to improve the quality of lighting design and understand lighting simulation programs. The participants learned how to construct 3D models for lighting analysis to acquire the necessary vocational skills. The teaching outcomes of four years were summarized to identify barriers in technical communication. Challenges that teachers face when teaching interior design were determined through discussion to communicate professional skills that were mismatched in teaching and learning. Suggestions were made on how to improve the effectiveness of learning and the quality of teaching in vocational education in online classes.

Keywords: lighting design; lighting simulation; vocational training

Citation: Li, S. Lighting Design by Computer Software in Teaching and Practice: A Case Study in Vocational Training of Interior Design. *Eng. Proc.* **2024**, *74*, 40. https://doi.org/10.3390/engproc2024074040

Academic Editors: Shu-Han Liao, Teen-Hang Meen and Cheng-Fu Yang

Published: 2 September 2024

1. Introduction

A two-year program has been in operation for about 40 years in Taiwan to meet the needs of the young to learn manufacturing and management skills. A few private universities offer such vocational training courses for foreign students according to their abilities. A university in Hsinchu City has developed the Overseas Youth Vocational Training Program (OYVTP) to offer training in various areas. The two-year vocational training courses are adjusted according to the blueprint of the 1st and 2nd years of the Department of Architecture and Urban Planning (DAUP). In terms of cultural literacy, students are familiar with the traditional culture of the East, but their mother tongue is different. Most Chinese students from Malaysia can communicate without barriers. However, for students from other countries, Mandarin is not used, and even English cannot be an alternative. This is challenging for tutors. In this study, indoor lighting was selected as a topic to teach as it demands technical communication to make students understand. Before the advent of computers, the only way to represent the effect of light was to use a model. With the development of digital imaging, various analyses can be presented with hyper-realistic images.

2. Methodology

The DAUP of the school has offered the OYVTP class since 2017 at the College of Architecture and Design. 16 lecturers are responsible for the students each year. The average number of students per year is 20, and the ratio of male to female students is 3 to 1. Table 1 presents the status of students in the OYVTP class in the department.

In addition to exploring the competencies required for the interior design profession and the effectiveness of vocational education, this study was carried out based on pedagogical or structural transformation. In this study, the Focus Group Discussion (FGD)

method was used in interior design. A review was conducted to clarify the study's findings and highlight ideas from experts. In addition to learning the necessary application tools, a satisfaction survey was conducted for students on the applications. It was necessary to optimize the training of graduates of design vocational schools with learning concepts relevant to the needs of the construction industry. Over the past five years, the computer graphics skills of foreign students have been discussed in the department. However, due to the small number of students, the enrollment of foreign students has been allowed since 2021. The university is considering ways to attract more vocational training students to pursue a degree at the university after completing 80 credits.

Table 1. Number of students in OYVTP.

Year of Enrollment (Class)	Total	Continued to Year 3	Transfer Rate (%)
2022 (41st)	16	12	75.0
2021 (40th)	18	12	66.7
2020 (39th)	25	17	68.0
2019 (38th)	0	-	-
2018 (37th)	14	1	7.1
2017 (36th)	16	1	6.3

Source: Office of International and Cross-Strait Affairs and DAUP, 2023.

2.1. Vocational Training and Academic Learning

DAUP is finding a way to absorb OYVTP students into university courses. There is a technical problem to be solved. In Taiwan, school starts in the fall, but OYVTP starts in the spring. The enrollment period for students starts in the second semester of the university. If they successfully study for two years of vocational courses and then enter the university, they need to enter the next semester of their third year. DAUP hopes that these students can change their learning attitude and complete architecture courses in one semester. Figure 1 shows the curriculum planning and progression path, which must be completed in the first semester. This program has been provided to students in the 39th class, after transferring to DAUP.

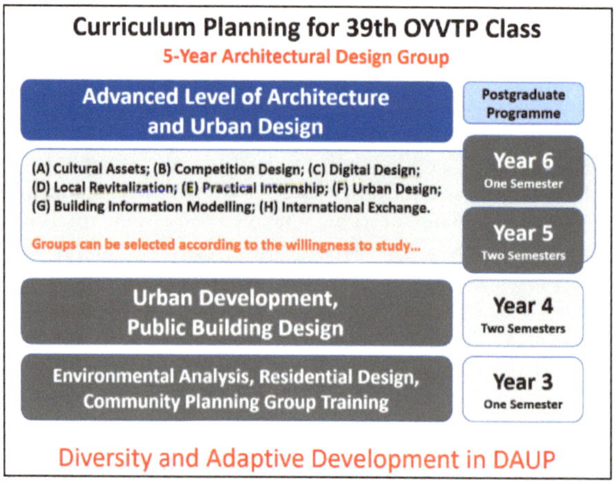

Figure 1. Curriculum planning for the 39th OYVTP students in the 5-Year Architectural Design Group. (Source: DAUP, 2021).

If six semesters are completed, the department encourages students to continue their studies at the Institute of Architecture. Thus, Figure 1 shows the postgraduate program (MArch). It is not difficult to plan the course roadmap, but it is important to adjust the students' mentality. DAUP invited alumni learning architects for intensive training in one semester. The design team of a company can take turns participating in the course and the short-term internship. This enables students to complement their theoretical and practical knowledge of architectural design as well as the concept of large-scale land and site planning. If this experimental arrangement is successful, it will help OYVTP students continue their studies.

2.2. Interior Design Training and Industry Prospects

Art design is an independent discipline, and its research content and service objects are different from traditional art categories. It involves society, culture, economy, market, and technology, and its esthetic standards change with these factors [1]. At the same time, interior design has living space as an object. It requires knowledge of engineering, technology, theory, and art skills. Interior design evolved from the decorative aspects of architectural design and is a recreation of the environment of the building [2]. Interior design is divided into two categories: public building spaces and homes. In interior design, important terms such as movement, space, color, lighting, and function are used. The design depends on creative activities and practices.

2.3. Job Skills

The main job of an interior designer is not easy. In addition to conforming to people's activities and habits, spiritual and esthetic functions need to be satisfied. Designers need to create an artistic conception, which requires talent and cultivation [3]. Therefore, in designing the interior, a designer needs to improve the interior space. The interior is a derivative of architecture [4]. The first thing the designer needs to do is improve the interior space and make the layout reasonable for convenient and comfortable living with complete functions. At the same time, it must be beautiful [2]. The layout must be reasonable, comfortable, convenient, beautiful, generous, and even luxurious. Each designer has new ideas and characteristics. However, for most interior designers, there are a lot of things to do. Interior designers' work includes the following:

- From conception, 3D modeling is necessary to provide complete design solutions, including physical environment planning, interior space separation, decorative image design, interior supplies, and complete configuration.
- Through creativity and design, the sense of space, practicability, superiority, and revolution of home design are demanded for humanization.
- The need to explain and plan creative ideas to coordinate with the decorating personnel.
- The need to coordinate and solve technical problems in the decorating process.
- The need to analyze costs and resources for interior decoration.
- The need to understand the development direction of the industry, from new processes and new technologies to innovative design.

These are also taught in the two-year vocational training courses. Students must obtain 80 credits in two years.

2.4. Industrial Prospects

At present, the rapid development of real estate and construction in mainland China has brought opportunities. The acceleration of urbanization, the prosperity of the housing industry, and the opening of markets make the real estate industry vigorous [5]. Design is the leader of the decoration industry, and the style of interior decoration is determined by design. According to the data of the relevant departments in mainland China, the number of talents that are in demand for interior design reaches 400,000 [6]. The graduates cannot meet the needs of the market in terms of quantity and quality. About a quarter of the graduates of DAUP went to mainland China. There is a demand for spatial design in emerging markets in East Asia, too. Students from Southeast Asia, after the two-year course, can practice at old building renovation sites. For reconstructing old buildings, manpower and financial and material resources are demanded, which allows interior design to have advantages. From a long-term perspective, the construction industry will not shrink as intelligent buildings lead the construction revolution in the 21st century [7] as well as the development of other industries.

3. Lighting Design

Foreign students pursue their goals before coming to Taiwan. On the contrary, teachers at the university are not clear about their role in vocational training. In the sixth year, there are still embarrassing situations. At least half of teachers do not treat OYVTP classes as 4-year students. When it comes to creative design work, a lot of training intimidates students due to communication problems between teachers and students. DAUP has improved this situation, and since the end of 2018, full-time teachers have been assigned. The content of the lectures and the direction of the exercises must meet the requirements of interior design topics. At the same time, the teacher needs to hold regular meetings to track the progress of teaching. Based on the Focus Group Discussions (FGD) in the last three years, the three most frequently discussed topics were teaching, communications, and online teaching methods.

3.1. Learning Content

As all teachers have backgrounds in architectural design, they mainly teach spatial design. Therefore, in the course arrangement, students usually learn architecture. In practice, the master-apprentice teaching method of architecture is used [8]. Students are led by professional designers, and the way of learning is close to the work pattern in a design firm [3]. They behave as employees of the company to complete all the provided work according to the established process. They use presentation boards and scale models to present the interior design process. In addition to drafting, graphic design skills, including typography, color, and text styles, are necessary. In scale models, project display and practice are important. Students must understand details in interior spaces with larger-scale model implementations. Regarding the current requirements of interior design, basic skills are taught. Students are willing to improve their performance by learning the delicacy of the drawings and the meticulousness of the models [9].

3.2. Barriers to Learning

A set of long-term architecture or design training is expected to cultivate innovative or creative design talents [10]. In addition to the exquisite performance, the entire teaching team would like to observe the outstanding design work of the students. Therefore, in teaching or discussion, students are constantly asked to think and verify the best answer. Students think that a general plan can be completed with established progress. A lot of time and energy is spent on the preparation of architectural design drawings and model-making. In terms of the requirements, there is a gap between teachers and students. Normally, academic works of architecture pursue abstract spatial compositions. As long as students have outstanding ideas, even if the drawings and models are difficult, teachers do not mind much. However, if a student makes beautiful models or drawings without any personal design concepts or ideas, it is classified as ordinary work. The two years of vocational training are aimed at teaching skills quickly. Students can study as long as they have high school diplomas. Universities providing vocational training courses accept students in OCAC, so the relevant academic information cannot be obtained until the students submit the related documents.

3.3. Teaching Difficulty

In the Computer-Aided Design (CAD) course, the teaching materials in spatial and lighting are rich, and students' problems can easily be solved. The production of digital models is a demonstration of operating procedures, and the related content can be found on YouTube. Teaching lighting design is easy, but assignments are difficult to complete.

Students need to understand the teacher's opinion. The CAD course coordinates the progress of the interior design class as follows:

- It refers to the substance of the interior design topic and confirms the date of the project review (Crit Day: the work of critique in interior design).
- During the CAD teaching time, about 20 min are provided to share wonderful interior design cases. The selection of cases is designated by the design tutors.
- Before a Crit Day, three cases are introduced, and one simple assessment is reserved. The content of the assessment is based on the cognition of design theory. The questions are created by the teachers of the design class.
- CAD teachers participate in reviews and grading. Generally, at least three teachers participate in the evaluation of the works.

The above practice has been implemented in DAUP's first-year Basic Design class. Given the shortcomings of the design class, equipment is used to conceive the design concept and practice the necessary drawing skills.

4. Application Tools

Interior design training needs a change in curriculum. It is important to have learning objectives so that students can grasp the key learning points and necessary skills in interior design. Lighting design for indoor environments is the most appropriate for professional training. Therefore, from the 39th class, the content and learning progress of the CAD program have been integrated into the design course. In design, the presentation of light is important. Based on the presentation of light in the space, students compare the renderings. Table 2 shows how the lighting tools match the design topics in DAUP. To learn these skills, the following lighting programs related to the visual system were selected as learning tools:

- AutoCAD: a 2D/3D CAD software application for desktop, web, and mobile developed by Autodesk.
- SketchUp: a 3D CAD program for a broad range of drawing and design applications.
- Revit: a BIM software for architects, landscape architects, structural engineers, mechanical, electrical, and plumbing (MEP) engineers, designers, and contractors.
- Kerkythea Rendering System: a standalone rendering system that supports raytracing and Metropolis light transport and uses physically accurate materials and lighting.
- Space Syntax depthmapX: an open-source and multi-platform spatial analysis software for spatial networks of different scales.
- Isovist: one of the two representations of the structure of space, along with the spatial-envelope representation. It is an approach to describing space from the point of view of a person within an environment.
- DIALux evo: to plan, calculate, and visualize lighting for indoor and outdoor areas, from entire buildings and individual rooms to parking spaces or road lighting.
- Radiance (with Ecotect): Using the libraries of materials, glazing, luminaires, and furnishings, realistic lighting models are created. Radiance is a design tool integrated with popular CAD packages to consider energy-efficient lighting and daylighting strategies in building design.

Table 2. Comparison of design topics and lighting design tools.

Semester	Spatial Types for Design Topic	Tools for Modeling and Analysis
1st (Year 1) Basic Design	Simple Booth Ideas (Gallery)	AutoCAD, SketchUp Pro, and Kerkythea Render
2nd (Year 1) Interior Design	Tiny House or Apartment (Residential)	Revit (BIM) with Solar Analysis, Space Syntax, Isovist, and DIALux evo
3rd (Year 2) Interior Design	Commercial Space (Business)	Radiance with Ecotect, Spatial VR, and Microsoft Azure AI
4th (Year 2) Thesis Project	Mixed-Use Property (Shophouses)	Isovist + DIALux evo + Any Renderers

DAUP. 2023.

5. Findings

41 students (39th, 40th, and 41st) responded to the questionnaire surveys at the end of the semester. The questionnaire was generated based on the concept of outcome-based learning and teaching approaches and recent practice. It contained eight closed-ended questions on a five-point Likert scale (where 1 was for 'Strongly Disagree' and 5 was for 'Strongly Agree'). The questionnaire items included the following:

- Q1: Understand how the various applications work and the focus of the course training.
- Q2: The operation of the application is clearly explained.
- Q3: Have detailed feedback that is clearly explained during reviews or critiques.
- Q4: The study of lighting helps to reinforce the knowledge of design.
- Q5: You can use the tools you've learned as you do your homework.
- Q6: Be able to solve problems promptly.
- Q7: This course enhances students' design ability.
- Q8: My abilities meet the basic requirements for employment.

Table 3 shows the average scores of students in the 39th, 40th, and 41st interior design classes. Students agreed with the current learning and training style. The scores ranged from 3.73 to 4.87. The students in the 39th and 40th classes showed an understanding of the course. Students were provided with adequate practical advice during interior design reviews or critiques (Q3, from 3.73 to 4.30). Students sought help with lighting simulations after classes (Q5 and Q6, from 4.22 to 4.82). Well-planned training and appropriate knowledge transfer were confirmed (Q7 and Q8, from 3.89 to 4.87). Students preferred the technical way of lighting design or simulations (Q4, from 3.81 to 4.04). Teachers also agreed that the quality of lighting applications needed to be strengthened.

Table 3. Average scores of students in 39th, 40th, and 41st OYVTP classes.

Class	Q1	Q2	Q3	Q4	Q5	Q6	Q7	Q8
41st	4.01	4.42	3.73	4.04	4.22	4.65	3.89	4.13
40th	3.97	4.11	3.88	3.96	4.39	4.23	4.21	4.02
39th	4.33	4.52	4.30	3.81	4.71	4.82	4.87	4.74

6. Conclusions

The importance of computer graphics skills in interior design was recognized to increase the enrollment of students pursuing a degree. The challenges in transitioning OYVTP students to academic architecture courses were determined, and a curriculum plan to facilitate this transition was outlined in this study. The education of lighting design revealed the evolution of the curriculum to integrate application tools. The results of the student survey indicated overall satisfaction with the learning and training method, with positive responses regarding the clarity of application operation, feedback during reviews, and the enhancement of design knowledge. In vocational training, industry needs, leveraging modern tools, and a smooth transition must be ensured for students in academic courses. The integration of lighting design into the curriculum exemplifies the commitment to providing relevant and practical skills. The findings from student surveys showed the success of the program in achieving its objectives, signaling a positive trajectory for the OYVTP in preparing students for interior design.

Funding: This research received no external funding.

Institutional Review Board Statement: Not applicable.

Informed Consent Statement: Not applicable.

Data Availability Statement: No new data were created or analyzed in this study. Data sharing is not applicable to this article.

Acknowledgments: Special thanks to the 39th, 40th, and 41st OYVTP students for this study, as they stayed and continued their studies, and the related learning experience was recorded. The author is continuing to take over as a mentor to assist this group of students in completing their studies as expected.

Conflicts of Interest: The author declares no conflicts of interest.

References

1. Nicol, D.; Pilling, S. Architectural education and the profession. *Chang. Archit. Educ. Towards A New Prof.* **2000**, *1*, 22.
2. Anthony, K.H. Designing for diversity: Implications for architectural education in the twenty-first century. *J. Archit. Educ.* **2002**, *55*, 257–267. [CrossRef]
3. Bashouri, J.; Duncan, G.W. A model for sharing knowledge in architectural firms. *Constr. Innov.* **2014**, *14*, 168–185. [CrossRef]
4. Lymer, G.; Ivarsson, J.; Lindwall, O. Contrasting the use of tools for presentation and critique: Some cases from architectural education. *Int. J. Comput. Support. Collab. Learn.* **2009**, *4*, 423–444. [CrossRef]
5. Wang, H.; Wang, K. What is unique about Chinese real estate markets? *J. Real Estate Res.* **2012**, *34*, 275–290. [CrossRef]
6. Xu, Z.; Zayed, T.; Niu, Y. Comparative analysis of modular construction practices in mainland China, Hong Kong, and Singapore. *J. Clean. Prod.* **2020**, *245*, 118861. [CrossRef]
7. Elinoff, E.; Sur, M.; Yeoh, B.S. Constructing Asia: An introduction. *City* **2017**, *21*, 580–586. [CrossRef]
8. Schank, R.C.; Berman, T.R.; Macpherson, K.A. Learning by doing. *Instr. Des. Theor. Models A New Paradig. Instr. Theory* **1999**, *2*, 161–181.
9. Steadman, P. *The Evolution of Designs: Biological Analogy in Architecture and the Applied Arts*; Routledge: London, UK, 2008.
10. Biggs, M.; Buchler, D. Architectural practice and academic research. *Nord. J. Archit. Res.* **2008**, *20*, 83–93.

engineering proceedings

MDPI

Proceeding Paper

Impact of Food Delivery Platforms on Consumer Behavioral Intentions During COVID-19 Pandemic †

Chih-Wei Lin [1,2], Yi-An Huang [1], Wei Yeng Sia [2], Kuan-Chuan Tao [1,*] and Yi-Chang Chen [2,*]

1 Department of Leisure Services Management, Chaoyang University of Technology, Taichung 413310, Taiwan; cwlin@cyut.edu.tw (C.-W.L.); s9009281@gmail.com (Y.-A.H.)

2 Department of Business Administration, Chaoyang University of Technology, Taichung 413310, Taiwan; wyc147@gmail.com

* Correspondence: willytao0218@cyut.edu.tw (K.-C.T.); t2003151@cyut.edu.tw (Y.-C.C.)

† Presented at the 2024 IEEE 4th International Conference on Electronic Communications, Internet of Things and Big Data, Taipei, Taiwan, 19–21 April 2024.

Abstract: The COVID-19 pandemic changed people's dining habits and led to the rapid rise of food delivery platforms. Ordering food online and picking it up offline has become an essential dining habit. We applied the stimulus–organism–response model and constructed a model based on factors influencing consumers' continuous use intention from three aspects: store product quality, delivery personnel quality, and delivery platform quality. Through snowball sampling, 321 questionnaires were distributed and collected from consumers who used food delivery platforms in Taiwan. All effective questionnaires were analyzed by structural equation modeling with SPSS 18 and Amos 21. The results showed that (1) the S-O-R theory explained consumer behavior effectively. (2) Store product quality influenced store repurchase intention. (3) Delivery personnel quality and platform quality influenced a platform's continuous usage. (4) Product quality and delivery personnel quality were key factors that influenced store repurchase intention. (5) Platform quality was an important factor that affected platform usage. Finally, recommendations were proposed based on the research findings as a reference for relevant operators in the food delivery platform industry and future researchers.

Keywords: food delivery platform; stimulus–organism–response theory; service quality; repurchase intention

Citation: Lin, C.-W.; Huang, Y.-A.; Sia, W.Y.; Tao, K.-C.; Chen, Y.-C. Impact of Food Delivery Platforms on Consumer Behavioral Intentions During COVID-19 Pandemic. *Eng. Proc.* **2024**, *74*, 41. https://doi.org/10.3390/engproc2024074041

Academic Editors: Shu-Han Liao, Teen-Hang Meen and Cheng-Fu Yang

Published: 2 September 2024

1. Introduction

As of mid-March 2022, data from the World Health Organization (WHO) indicated that there were over 460 million confirmed cases of COVID-19 globally [1]. This led to an increase in the use of food delivery platforms by consumers to avoid direct or indirect social contact. With the rise of the internet generation and the impact of the 2020 pandemic, the food and beverage industry has been prompted to consider digital technologies to adapt to new business models, such as increasing online food delivery services and integrating online-to-offline services to meet consumer demands. Food delivery platforms helped food and beverage enterprises and restaurants survive and grow during the pandemic and fulfill consumer needs [2].

In terms of market value, the global food delivery business reached USD 248 billion in 2022, and it is expected to reach USD 449 billion by 2025 [3]. Taiwan's food delivery industry is also experiencing rapid growth, with a market value that reached USD 707 million in 2022, and it is projected to increase to USD 1.034 billion by 2026 [3]. This makes online ordering and delivery services an integral part of the digital transformation in the food and beverage industry that cannot be ignored.

Service quality is a crucial factor for gaining a competitive advantage in the food and beverage industry [4–6]. With the continuous growth of the delivery industry, service quality has become a significant concern for many consumers. In the past, the service quality of food delivery was often overlooked by food suppliers, decreasing customer satisfaction and consumer willingness. For food delivery, the assessment of various aspects of service quality is necessary [7–9]. Given that service quality in food delivery positively influences customer satisfaction and loyalty [10–12], service quality and satisfaction are factors affecting consumers' subsequent behavioral intentions on food delivery platforms. In this context, using the stimulus–organism–response (S-O-R) model [13], we assessed how environmental stimuli on food delivery platforms influenced consumers' emotional and cognitive states, thereby leading to behavioral responses.

We proposed a structural model to examine the dimensions influencing customer satisfaction and the subsequent construction of behavioral intentions, including intentions for store repurchase and application. Secondly, we identified factors determining consumers' continued intention to use food delivery platforms. Thirdly, we validated the use of promotions on repurchase intention behavior. The results of this study contribute to an understanding and reaffirmation of relationships between the quality of products offered by food delivery stores, the quality of delivery personnel and delivery platforms, satisfaction, and behavioral intentions.

2. Literature Review

2.1. Food Delivery Platforms

Delivery platform applications are an emerging form of online and offline mobile technology that provide a channel between food service businesses and customers. This enables consumers to complete the entire process, from ordering food to having meals delivered to their doorsteps, through the application [2,14]. Moreover, consumers can track their order status, communicate with delivery personnel, and enjoy benefits, such as avoiding waiting in lines, not needing to pick up, and accessing daily promotions or discounts, when ordering meals [15].

2.2. S-O-R Theory

The evolution of the S-O-R theory in psychology has been based on Thorndike's [16] law of effect, or stimulus–response (S–R) theory, which posits that similar stimuli are likely to produce similar responses. Russell and Mehrabian [13] adopted a perspective from environmental psychology. They described a process in which external environmental factors (stimuli) influence the internal states of consumers (organisms), leading to approach or avoidance behaviors (responses). Jacoby [17] reconceptualized the S-O-R model as a Venn diagram rather than a continuous process, illustrating seven domains of psychological dynamics that occur over time. The S-O-R theory is frequently applied in the study of online environments [18], online purchase intentions [19], and consumer behavior [20]. This study invoked the S-O-R framework to describe causal relationships and provide an explanation for how consumers position food delivery platforms. Second, it offers a visualized framework for studying how stimuli influence users' internal psychological responses, subsequently determining their behavioral reactions.

In this context, "stimulus" refers to the social or environmental cues capable of triggering psychological and behavioral responses or changes in individuals [21]. Stimuli can evoke positive or negative emotions in the consumer evaluation process [22], explaining the association between consumer satisfaction and prior expectations of service. Therefore, in this study, stimuli were defined as service quality. "Organism" refers to the intervening internal decision-making processes between stimuli and responses [23], representing the cognition that arises after receiving the service. Organism factors studied in consumer behavior research include attitudes, satisfaction, and perceived value. Thus, in this study, the organism was defined as satisfaction. "Response" refers to the intent, decision, or behavioral change caused by stimuli and organism factors, representing the individual's ultimate reaction to specific stimuli. Therefore, in this study, responses were defined as behavioral intentions, further categorized into intentions to repurchase from a restaurant and intentions to use a platform.

2.3. Service Quality

The current food delivery industry is thriving, and service quality plays a crucial role [24]. Brady and Cronin [25] demonstrated that service quality is a multidimensional, hierarchical concept. Food delivery involves various service factors, including meal quality and hygiene, service convenience, functional attributes of the ordering system, tangible services, professional delivery personnel, and service efficiency [8,9]. The service process in the food delivery industry consists of placing orders through platforms, restaurants preparing meals, and delivery personnel providing delivery services to customers. Therefore, the major distinction in this study was categorizing service quality into three types: restaurant product quality, delivery personnel quality, and delivery platform quality.

Outcome quality is a measure of what consumers receive when a service is provided [25]. For food delivery platforms, customers are most concerned about the quality of the meals (taste, freshness, temperature, etc.), food packaging (hygiene, eco-friendly packaging, etc.), and the consistency of the meal's content [24–28]. Therefore, we defined the quality of the meal, including its taste, freshness, hygiene, and correctness in quantity, as well as the completeness of packaging, as restaurant product quality. This aspect is crucial in assessing the overall quality of food delivery services.

In the food delivery industry, service delivery personnel are essential in providing meal delivery services to customers. Factors such as order consistency, delivery speed, the courtesy and friendliness of delivery personnel, the cleanliness of the meal box, the condition of the delivered food upon receipt, and affordable delivery fees can influence customer behavior [24,29,30]. Hence, in this study, we categorized delivery personnel quality based on the appropriateness of their behavior and communication, delivery speed, meal completeness, and the cleanliness of the delivery environment. Electronic service norms encompass a comprehensive evaluation of services provided by food delivery platforms [31]. When making purchases on a platform, consumers expect high-quality service, and good platform quality enhances consumers' value and satisfaction, subsequently stimulating their behavioral intentions [32].

Platform quality encompasses the accuracy, relevance, and completeness of information provided by a food delivery platform [33]. It also includes the usability of a platform, customer service responsiveness, and the ability to provide diverse information [14,15,34]. For online shopping [35], Kim [36] used SERVQUAL to evaluate platform quality for food delivery, dividing the facets into platform service security, platform vendor professionalism, platform provider user interface, activities and interests, and customer service response time. Therefore, we considered ease of use, diverse meal choices, and prompt responsiveness as indicators of platform quality.

2.4. Satisfaction

Satisfaction has consistently been the central focus of marketing because it has a significant impact on the survival of any business. It is also one of the key constructs used to explain consumer behavior in research models [37]. In the literature on marketing and consumer behavior, customer satisfaction is a crucial predictive indicator for examining behavioral intentions [38,39]. In studies within the restaurant industry, satisfaction positively impacts behavioral intentions, and service quality positively affects both customer satisfaction and behavioral intentions [37,40].

Dash et al. [41] defined the measurement dimensions of customer satisfaction as service quality, professional competence, and frontline staff experience. Liang et al. [42] identified four indicators of satisfaction: dish indicators (taste, quality, hygiene, and freshness), service indicators (speed, attitude, and accuracy), price promotion indicators (price and discounts), and value-added indicators (delivery accessories and packaging). Therefore, in this study, satisfaction was defined as the overall evaluation made by consumers of their entire consumption experience on a food delivery platform after ordering a meal.

Research findings related to satisfaction indicate a positive relationship between store product quality and satisfaction [11,43,44]. When consumers perceive delivery personnel to have quality, satisfaction increases, thereby establishing a positive relationship between delivery personnel quality and satisfaction [26,45]. Additionally, the service quality of delivery platforms positively impacts customer satisfaction [3,34], indicating a positive relationship between delivery platform quality and satisfaction [24]. Based on the aforementioned literature, we proposed Hypotheses 1, 2, and 3.

Hypothesis 1 (H1): *Store product quality has a positive impact on consumer satisfaction.*

Hypothesis 2 (H2): *Delivery personnel quality has a positive impact on consumer satisfaction.*

Hypothesis 3 (H3): *Delivery platform quality has a positive impact on consumer satisfaction.*

2.5. Behavioral Intention

Behavioral intention is an individual's intention to perform specific actions or behaviors towards a product or service [46]. It involves anticipating and planning actions that are likely to occur [47], such as word-of-mouth and repurchase intentions [30]. In this study, behavioral intention was regarded as an outcome between behavior and commitment. Repeat usage, recommendations, and word-of-mouth were employed to explain consumers' behavioral intentions as responses to service quality and satisfaction, distinguishing between store repurchase intention and platform continued usage.

Service quality and satisfaction significantly influence future purchase intentions [48]. When customers are satisfied with products or services they purchase, they tend to make repeat purchases from the same supplier [44]. This satisfaction also enhances their willingness to make online purchases [29,49]. Therefore, we proposed Hypotheses 4 and 5.

Hypothesis 4 (H4): *Satisfaction positively influences consumers' store repurchase intention.*

Hypothesis 5 (H5): *Satisfaction positively influences consumers' platform usage.* Based on the

hypotheses, we developed a research conceptual framework.

3. Research Method

The independent variable in this study was service quality, including three conceptions (store product quality, delivery personnel quality, and delivery platform quality). The mediating variable was satisfaction. The dependent variable was consumer behavior intention, including two conceptions (store repurchase intention and platform usage). These variables were explored using the following methods.

3.1. Data Collection

We distributed a questionnaire via Google Forms using a snowball sampling method. The questionnaire survey was conducted from February to March 2022. Participants were individuals in Taiwan who used food delivery platforms for ordering meals (excluding those who did not use contactless delivery). In total, 350 questionnaires were collected, and, after examination, 321 valid questionnaires were retained.

3.2. Research Tools

Questionnaire items were adapted from existing studies and modified to align with this research's context. References for each construct were as follows: store product quality [24,26], delivery personnel quality [24], platform quality [32], satisfaction [26,29], repurchase intention [16,50], and platform usage [51]. A Likert five-point scale was used, in which 1 represented "strongly disagree" and 5 represented "strongly agree." Descriptive statistics and reliability analyses were conducted using SPSS, and confirmatory factor analysis and structural equation modeling were performed using AMOS.

4. Results and Discussion

4.1. Demographics

A total of 61.4% of participants were female, while 38.6% were male. The majority of participants were 24 years old or younger, accounting for 41.7% of total participants, followed by participants aged 25–34 years (23.7%), 35–44 years (19.0%), 45–55 years (10.9%), and 55 years and above (4.7%). Regarding education levels, there were university graduates (62.3%), holders of master's degrees or above (29.0%), and high school/vocational school graduates (8.7%). The majority of participants were students (39.3%), followed by those in the service industry (20.9%). The majority (69.2%) were not married, and 37.4% had a monthly income below NTD 20,000. Regarding ordering frequency, more than half of participants ordered 2–5 times (55.8%), and the most common spending range was between NTD 201 and 500 (54.5%). The most prevalent dining scenario was regular meals (79.5%), and Foodpanda was the most frequently used delivery platform (70.4%). Overall, the sample was collected to be as evenly distributed across age groups as possible, with a higher representation of young adults in their 20s and 30s, likely attributed to the online data collection method and the context of this study.

4.2. Confirmatory Factor Analysis

Results of the confirmatory factor analysis in this study showed that factor loadings for each factor exceeded 0.5 [52]. Composite reliability (CR) values were above 0.7, and average variance extracted (AVE) values surpassed the threshold of 0.5 [53]. Cronbach's α for each dimension was between 0.904 and 0.943. Thus, the convergent validity of the measurement model was confirmed [54] (Table 1). The multivariate critical ratio (CR) in this study was 2153.47. However, for multivariate normality testing, the CR must be less than 10. To address the issue of non-multivariate normality in sample data, the bootstrap method was employed. The multivariate CR after using the bootstrap method decreased to 487.202, confirming compliance with multivariate normal distribution.

Table 1. Results of confirmatory factor analysis.

Latent Variables	Composite Reliability	Average
Store Product Quality	0.94	0.71
Delivery Personnel Quality	0.93	0.69
Delivery Platform Quality	0.91	0.62
Satisfaction	0.86	0.59
Repurchase Intention	0.86	0.61
Platform Usage	0.89	0.67

4.3. Test Hypothesis

The structural model examination in this study met the standards for various indicators ($\chi2/df = 1.042$, CFI = 0.998, GFI = 0.956, AGFI = 0.948, NFI = 0.956, RMSEA = 0.011, and SRMR = 00.000) [55–59], indicating that the structural model was well fitted for further statistical analysis.

Statistical analysis results revealed that store product quality (H1: $\beta = 0.54$, $t = 8.20$, $p < 0.000$), delivery personnel quality (H2: $\beta = 0.50$, $t = 7.95$, $p < 0.000$), and delivery platform quality (H3: $\beta = 0.42$, $t = 7.17$, $p < 0.000$) positively influenced satisfaction. Additionally, satisfaction positively influenced repurchase intention (H4: $\beta = 0.79$, $t = 9.79$, $p < 0.000$) and continued intention to use a platform (H5: $\beta = 0.71$, $t = 10.48$, $p < 0.000$). Therefore, all hypotheses proposed in this study were supported.

5. Conclusions

Although food delivery platforms have been receiving academic attention, studies on store product quality, delivery personnel quality, and platform quality, along with satisfaction, repurchase intention, and continued use, are scarce. This study employed an S-O-R model to develop a framework explaining the relationships among three stimuli (quality of store products, quality of delivery personnel, and quality of a delivery platform), one emotional state (satisfaction), and two responses (intention to repurchase from a store and intention for continued use of a platform). It was confirmed that assessments of various qualities positively influenced satisfaction, and satisfaction positively influenced subsequent use. These findings align with previous research, indicating store product quality had a direct influence on satisfaction [3,43], delivery personnel quality had an influence on satisfaction [26,45], a positive relationship between delivery platform quality and satisfaction [24], and finally, satisfaction had an influence on both store repurchase intention and platform use intention [29,51]. The S-O-R model was used as a theoretical foundation, and its results can be used to enhance service quality, resource allocation, and marketing strategies for food delivery platforms.

Recently, Taiwan's food delivery industry has been growing rapidly. However, the neglect of service quality in food delivery has decreased customer satisfaction and repurchase intention [24]. Service quality is a crucial factor in customer decision-making. Yet, the service quality of food delivery platforms has unique attributes, encompassing restaurant services, delivery personnel performance, and platform services. This underscores the importance of personnel training and the integration of platform resources. For instance, it is essential to ensure the quality, hygiene, freshness, and completeness of restaurant products. Delivery personnel must be well groomed, courteous, customer-oriented, and empathetic while delivering orders. A platform's customer service must be prompt in response, and platform information needs to be comprehensive and easy to navigate. Failure to meet customer expectations or dissatisfaction may foster a negative attitude toward food delivery platforms, thereby influencing subsequent usage behavior. Customers may choose not to repurchase, or switch to alternative platforms. Therefore, platform managers must ensure that restaurants maintain a certain level of quality, that delivery personnel possess necessary qualities, and that their platform functions smoothly to meet customer expectations and provide excellent service. This ensures that the amount paid by customers corresponds to their expected service quality, potentially surpassing the perceived value of the payment. Ultimately, managers should establish consumer confidence and trust in their platforms.

Data for this study were collected in Taiwan, so its results cannot be generalized. Secondly, data were collected through an online questionnaire, which can be a limitation in using the results of this study. Thirdly, we focused only on users of Foodpanda and Uber Eats. Customer perceptions of each platform may vary. Therefore, it is essential to investigate the predictors influencing user behavior across various food delivery platforms. different food delivery platforms. Finally, as platform interfaces and usage evolve in response to varying temporal and spatial contexts, it will be essential to integrate data from different time periods to enhance the model's validation.

Author Contributions: Conceptualization, C.-W.L., Y.-A.H., and K.-C.T.; methodology, C.-W.L.; writing—original draft preparation, Y.-C.C., Y.-A.H., and W.Y.S.; writing—review and editing, Y.-C.C. and W.Y.S. All authors have read and agreed to the published version of the manuscript.

Funding: This research received no external funding.

Institutional Review Board Statement: Not applicable.

Informed Consent Statement: Not applicable.

Data Availability Statement: The original contributions presented in the study are included in the article.

Acknowledgments: We sincerely acknowledge the enthusiastic participation of all subjects involved in this study. Their willingness to contribute their time and effort was essential to the success of our research. We are grateful for their invaluable support and cooperation.

Conflicts of Interest: The authors declare no conflicts of interest.

References

1. WHO Coronavirus Disease (COVID-19) Dashboard. Available online: https://covid19.who.int/?gclid=CjwKCAjwh7H7BRBBEiwAPXjadiKtb7aw1BDI7iFNjj4pF-b5J-k-VgJVmkC6MmqL8F34DBOxHnX6_BoC2rwQAvD_BwE (accessed on 15 March 2022).
2. Zhao, Y.; Bacao, F. What factors determining customer continuingly using food delivery apps during 2019 novel coronavirus pandemic period? *Int. J. Hosp. Manag.* **2020**, *91*, 102683. [CrossRef]
3. Statistia eServices Report 2020—Online Food Delivery. Available online: https://www.statista.com/study/40457/food-delivery/ (accessed on 17 November 2021).
4. Cheng, C.C.; Chen, C.T.; Hsu, F.S.; Hu, H.Y. Enhancing service quality improvement strategies of fine-dining restaurants: New insights from integrating a two-phase decision-making model of IPGA and DEMATEL analysis. *Int. J. Hosp. Manag.* **2012**, *31*, 1155–1166. [CrossRef]
5. Cheng, C.C.; Chang, Y.Y.; Tsai, M.C.; Chen, C.T.; Tseng, Y.C. An evaluation instrument and strategy implications of service attributes in LOHAS restaurants. *Int. J. Contemp. Hosp. Manag.* **2019**, *31*, 194–216. [CrossRef]
6. Kim, W.G.; Ng, C.Y.N.; Kim, Y.S. Influence of institutional DINESERV on customer satisfaction, return intention, and word-of-mouth. *Int. J. Hosp. Manag.* **2009**, *28*, 10–17. [CrossRef]
7. Cho, M.; Bonn, M.A.; Li, J.J. Differences in perceptions about food delivery apps between single-person and multi-person households. *Int. J. Hosp. Manag.* **2019**, *77*, 108–116. [CrossRef]
8. Fancello, G.; Paddeu, D.; Fadda, P. Investigating last food mile deliveries: A case study approach to identify needs of food delivery demand. *Res. Transp. Econ.* **2017**, *65*, 56–66. [CrossRef]
9. Roh, M.; Park, K. Adoption of O2O food delivery services in South Korea: The moderating role of moral obligation in meal preparation. *Int. J. Inf. Manag.* **2019**, *47*, 262–273. [CrossRef]
10. Annaraud, K.; Berezina, K. Predicting satisfaction and intentions to use online food delivery: What really makes a difference? *J. Foodserv. Bus. Res.* **2020**, *23*, 305–323. [CrossRef]
11. Saad, A.T. Factors affecting online food delivery service in Bangladesh: An empirical study. *Br. Food J.* **2021**, *123*, 535–550. [CrossRef]
12. Yusra, Y.; Eko, C.R.; Agus, A.; Azmi MA, A.; Ugiana, G.P.; Ching, C.R.; Lee, Y. An investigation of online food aggregator (OFA) service: Do online and offline service quality distinct? *Serbian J. Manag.* **2020**, *15*, 277–294. [CrossRef]
13. Russell, J.A.; Mehrabian, A. Distinguishing anger and anxiety in terms of emotional response factors. *J. Consult. Clin. Psychol.* **1974**, *42*, 79. [CrossRef] [PubMed]
14. Ray, A.; Dhir, A.; Bala, P.K.; Kaur, P. Why do people use food delivery apps (FDA)? A uses and gratification theory perspective. *J. Retail. Consum. Serv.* **2019**, *51*, 221–230. [CrossRef]
15. Hong, C.; Choi, H.H.; Choi EK, C.; Joung HW, D. Factors affecting customer intention to use online food delivery services before and during the COVID-19 pandemic. *J. Hosp. Tour. Manag.* **2021**, *48*, 509–518. [CrossRef]
16. Thorndike, E.L. Animal intelligence: An experimental study of the associative processes in animals. *Psychol. Rev. Monogr. Suppl.* **1898**, *2*, 4–160.
17. Jacoby, J. Stimulus-organism-response reconsidered: An evolutionary step in modeling (consumer) behavior. *J. Consum. Psychol.* **2002**, *12*, 51–57. [CrossRef]
18. Wang, Y.J.; Minor, M.S.; Wei, J. Aesthetics and the online shopping environment: Understanding consumer responses. *J. Retail.* **2011**, *87*, 46–58. [CrossRef]
19. Brewer, P.; Sebby, A.G. The effect of online restaurant menus on consumers' purchase intentions during the COVID-19 pandemic. *Int. J. Hosp. Manag.* **2021**, *94*, 102777. [CrossRef]
20. Sultan, P.; Wong, H.Y.; Azam, M.S. How perceived communication source and food value stimulate purchase intention of organic food: An examination of the stimulus-organism-response (SOR) model. *J. Clean. Prod.* **2021**, *312*, 127807. [CrossRef]
21. Eroglu, S.A.; Machleit, K.A.; Davis, L.M. Empirical testing of a model of online store atmospherics and shopper responses. *Psychol. Mark.* **2003**, *20*, 139–150. [CrossRef]
22. Sezgen, E.; Mason, K.J.; Mayer, R. Voice of airline passenger: A text mining approach to understand customer satisfaction. *J. Air Transp. Manag.* **2019**, *77*, 65–74. [CrossRef]
23. Loureiro, S.; Ribeiro, L. The effect of atmosphere on emotions and online shopping intention: Age differentiation. In Proceedings of the Australian and New Zealand Marketing Academy Conference, Perth, Australia, 28–30 November 2011.
24. Cheng, C.C.; Chang, Y.Y.; Chen, C.T. Construction of a service quality scale for the online food delivery industry. *Int. J. Hosp. Manag.* **2021**, *95*, 102938. [CrossRef]
25. Brady, M.K.; Cronin, J.J., Jr. Some new thoughts on conceptualizing perceived service quality: A hierarchical approach. *J. Mark.* **2001**, *65*, 34–49. [CrossRef]
26. Ganapathi, P.; Abu-Shanab, E.A. Customer satisfaction with online food ordering portals in Qatar. *Int. J. E-Serv. Mob. Appl. (IJESMA)* **2020**, *12*, 57–79. [CrossRef]
27. Yang, F.X.; Li, X.; Lau VM, C.; Zhu, V.Z. To survive or to thrive? China's luxury hotel restaurants entering O2O food delivery platforms amid the COVID-19 crisis. *Int. J. Hosp. Manag.* **2021**, *94*, 102855. [CrossRef]
28. Lu, C.Y.; Suhartanto, D.; Gunawan, A.I.; Chen, B.T. Customer satisfaction toward online purchasing services: Evidence from small & medium restaurants. *Int. J. Appl. Bus. Res.* **2020**, 1–14. [CrossRef]
29. Fakfare, P. Influence of service attributes of food delivery application on customers' satisfaction and their behavioural responses: The IPMA approach. *Int. J. Gastron. Food Sci.* **2021**, *25*, 100392. [CrossRef]

30. Chen, A.H.; Peng, N.; Hackley, C. Evaluating service marketing in airline industry and its influence on student passengers' purchasing behavior using Taipei–London route as an example. *J. Travel Tour. Mark.* **2008**, *25*, 149–160. [CrossRef]
31. Ramesh, R.; Prabhu, S.V.; Sasikumar, B.; Devi, B.K.; Prasath, P.; Kamala SP, R. An empirical study of online food delivery services from applications perspective. *Mater. Today Proc.* **2023**, *80*, 1751–1755. [CrossRef]
32. Lin, C.W.; Tan, W.P.; Lin, Y.H.; Tseng, Y.C.; Lee, S.S. Exploring the consumer behavior of online platform by using information system success model. In Proceedings of the 2017 International Conference on E-Business and Internet, Taichung, Taiwan, 25–27 May 2017; pp. 12–16.
33. Patrada, R.; Andajani, E. Effect and Consequence e-Customer Satisfaction for e-Commerce Users. *IPTEK J. Proc. Ser.* **2021**, 219–227. [CrossRef]
34. Dsouza, D.; Sharma, D. Online food delivery portals during COVID-19 times: An analysis of changing consumer behavior and expectations. *Int. J. Innov. Sci.* **2021**, *13*, 218–232. [CrossRef]
35. Parasuraman, A.; Zeithaml, V.A.; Malhotra, A. ES-QUAL: A multiple-item scale for assessing electronic service quality. *J. Serv. Res.* **2005**, *7*, 213–233. [CrossRef]
36. Kim, M. Conceptualization of e-servicescapes in the fitness applications and wearable devices context: Multi-dimensions, consumer satisfaction, and behavioral intention. *J. Retail. Consum. Serv.* **2021**, *61*, 102562. [CrossRef]
37. Konuk, F.A. The influence of perceived food quality, price fairness, perceived value and satisfaction on customers' revisit and word-of-mouth intentions towards organic food restaurants. *J. Retail. Consum. Serv.* **2019**, *50*, 103–110. [CrossRef]
38. Oliver, R.L. A cognitive model of the antecedents and consequences of satisfaction decisions. *J. Mark. Res.* **1980**, *17*, 460–469. [CrossRef]
39. Teeroovengadum, V. Service quality dimensions as predictors of customer satisfaction and loyalty in the banking industry: Moderating effects of gender. *Eur. Bus. Rev.* **2022**, *34*, 1–19. [CrossRef]
40. Han, H.; Hyun, S.S. Impact of hotel-restaurant image and quality of physical-environment, service, and food on satisfaction and intention. *Int. J. Hosp. Manag.* **2017**, *63*, 82–92. [CrossRef]
41. Dash, G.; Kiefer, K.; Paul, J. Marketing-to-Millennials: Marketing 4.0, customer satisfaction and purchase intention. *J. Bus. Res.* **2021**, *122*, 608–620. [CrossRef]
42. Liang, D.; Dai, Z.; Wang, M. Assessing customer satisfaction of O2O takeaway based on online reviews by integrating fuzzy comprehensive evaluation with AHP and probabilistic linguistic term sets. *Appl. Soft Comput.* **2021**, *98*, 106847. [CrossRef]
43. Belarmino, A.; Raab, C.; Tang, J.; Han, W. Exploring the motivations to use online meal delivery platforms: Before and during quarantine. *Int. J. Hosp. Manag.* **2021**, *96*, 102983. [CrossRef]
44. Zibarzani, M.; Abumalloh, R.A.; Nilashi, M.; Samad, S.; Alghamdi, O.A.; Nayer, F.K.; Ismail, M.Y.; Mohd, S.; Akib, N.A.M. Customer satisfaction with Restaurants Service Quality during COVID-19 outbreak: A two-stage methodology. *Technol. Soc.* **2022**, *70*, 101977. [CrossRef]
45. Uzir MU, H.; Al Halbusi, H.; Thurasamy, R.; Hock RL, T.; Aljaberi, M.A.; Hasan, N.; Hamid, M. The effects of service quality, perceived value and trust in home delivery service personnel on customer satisfaction: Evidence from a developing country. *J. Retail. Consum. Serv.* **2021**, *63*, 102721. [CrossRef]
46. Ajzen, I. The theory of planned behavior. *Organ. Behav. Hum. Decis. Process.* **1991**, *50*, 179–211. [CrossRef]
47. Lam, T.; Hsu, C.H. Predicting behavioral intention of choosing a travel destination. *Tour. Manag.* **2006**, *27*, 589–599. [CrossRef]
48. McAlexander, J.H.; Kaldenberg, D.O.; Koenig, H.F. Service quality measurement. *J. Health Care Mark.* **1994**, *14*, 34–41.
49. Abumalloh, R.A.; Ibrahim, O.; Nilashi, M. Loyalty of young female Arabic customers towards recommendation agents: A new model for B2C E-commerce. *Technol. Soc.* **2020**, *61*, 101253. [CrossRef]
50. Allah Pitchay, A.; Ganesan, Y.; Zulkifli, N.S.; Khaliq, A. Determinants of customers' intention to use online food delivery application through smartphone in Malaysia. *Br. Food J.* **2022**, *124*, 732–753. [CrossRef]
51. Rita, P.; Oliveira, T.; Farisa, A. The impact of e-service quality and customer satisfaction on customer behavior in online shopping. *Heliyon* **2019**, *5*, e02690. [CrossRef]
52. Hair, J.F.; Black, W.C.; Babin, B.J.; Anderson, R.E.; Tatham, R.L. *Multivariate Data Analysis*, 6th ed.; Pearson Prentice Hal: Upper Saddle River, NJ, USA, 2006.
53. Fornell, C.; Larcker, D.F. Evaluating structural equation models with unobservable variables and measurement error. *J. Mark. Res.* **1981**, *18*, 39–50. [CrossRef]
54. Hair, J.F. *Multivariate Data Analysis*; Pearson: London, UK, 2009.
55. Carmines, E.; Mclver, J. Analyzing models with unobserved models: Analysis of covariance structures. In *Social Measurement*; Sage Publications, Inc.: Beverly Hills, CA, USA, 1981; Current Issues; pp. 65–115.
56. Bentler, P.M. Comparative fit indexes in structural models. *Psychol. Bull.* **1990**, *107*, 238. [CrossRef]
57. Bagozzi, R.P.; Yi, Y. On the evaluation of structural equation models. *J. Acad. Mark. Sci.* **1988**, *16*, 74–94. [CrossRef]
58. Hu, L.T.; Bentler, P.M. Cutoff criteria for fit indexes in covariance structure analysis: Conventional criteria versus new alternatives. *Struct. Equ. Model. A Multidiscip. J.* **1999**, *6*, 1–55. [CrossRef]
59. Browne, M.W.; Cudeck, R. Alternative ways of assessing model fit. *Sociol. Methods Res.* **1992**, *21*, 230–258. [CrossRef]

engineering proceedings

Proceeding Paper

Loneliness and Psychological Well-Being in Early Adulthood †

Muhamad Nanang Suprayogi * and Luthfi Nisrina Hamidah

Department of Psychology, Faculty of Humanities, Bina Nusantara University, Jakarta 11480, Indonesia; luthfi.hamidah@binus.ac.id
* Correspondence: msuprayogi@binus.edu

† Presented at the 2024 IEEE 4th International Conference on Electronic Communications, Internet of Things and Big Data, Taipei, Taiwan, 19–21 April 2024.

Abstract: We examined the relationship between loneliness and psychological well-being in early adulthood in Jakarta, Indonesia. Using a quantitative method and the UCLA loneliness scale with 212 participants in early adulthood in Jakarta, Indonesia, we measured psychological well-being and loneliness. Ryff's Scale of Psychological Well-Being was also used. A measuring scale was re-formulated in the Indonesian language. Loneliness and psychological well-being were negatively correlated ($r = -0.692$, $p < 0.05$). This result can be used to increase psychological well-being in early adulthood and maximize their productivity.

Keywords: loneliness; psychological well-being; early adulthood; Indonesia

Citation: Suprayogi, M.N.; Hamidah, L.N. Loneliness and Psychological Well-Being in Early Adulthood. *Eng. Proc.* **2024**, *74*, 42. https://doi.org/10.3390/engproc2024074042

Academic Editors: Shu-Han Liao, Teen-Hang Meen and Cheng-Fu Yang

Published: 3 September 2024

1. Introduction

The transition from the adolescent phase to early adulthood affects individuals in terms of relationships with people. Santrock [1] explained that individuals in the early adult phase tend to sort out their social sphere more as they grow older. In this phase, there is the sixth stage of development, namely, intimacy vs. isolation. Meilia [2] confirmed that early adulthood is critical in life as it is characterized by individuals re-adapting themselves to the environment and social desires. In addition, according to Permana & Astuti [3] the early adult phase is the phase when a person is in a period of displacement in deepening identity, lifestyle, and relationships. In the early adult phase, individuals tend to experience difficulties [1]. One of the difficulties that often occurs in early adulthood is loneliness [1].

A survey result conducted to see the phenomena in January 2023 with 19 individuals consisting of 10 women (52.6%) and 9 men (47.4%) in Jakarta showed that individuals at the age of 19−32 years experienced loneliness in the last 6 months. Ten out of the nineteen individuals had difficulty connecting or interacting with other people. Moreover, 42.1% felt that they did not have anyone to ask for help, and 42.1% felt lonely. This showed that loneliness is felt in all developmental periods including early adulthood [4]. Russell [5] defined loneliness as a subjective feeling caused by not achieving intimacy in a relationship. The situation is tentative due to drastic changes that occur in individual social activities. This was evidenced by 42.1% of the participants in the survey who were in a relationship with another individual or group but still felt lonely. Additionally, 10 out of the 19 participants felt incompatible, anxious, and uncomfortable in their social sphere.

Loneliness is felt when individuals feel useless, not accepted by their environment, and confused [6]. Russell [7] reaffirmed that the lack of meaningful social relationships and support is known as social isolation, which is a prime example of the unintentional onset of the experience of loneliness. Psychological well-being is a multidimensional form of interpretation created from decisions related to things experienced regarding daily routines. This refers to a description of the feelings felt based on experiences in life. Individuals who fulfill the six dimensions of psychological well-being tend to be independent and develop self-skills to manage the social environment, establish good relationships with others, and have a sense of self-acceptance [8]. Individuals with high psychological well-being are satisfied to define happiness in life and avoid mental disorders, especially loneliness [9].

In this study, we identified the relationship between loneliness and psychological well-being in early adults to help early adults improve psychological well-being and minimize loneliness. The hypotheses in this study were proposed as follows.

H0. *There is no significant relationship between loneliness and psychological well-being among early adults in Jakarta.*

H1. *There is a significant relationship between loneliness and psychological well-being among early adults in Jakarta.*

2. Method

2.1. Participants

A total of 212 participants were selected according to predetermined criteria. The demography of the participants is presented in Table 1. The participants were selected using a non-probability sampling method. The female participants consisted of 57.1% and the male participants consisted of 42.9% of the total participants. The participants at the age of 20−25 years were 69.3%. The majority of the participants had a bachelor's degree (47.6%). The most common type of employment of the participants was students (47.2%). Employees, entrepreneurs, civil servants, and policemen were also included. In addition, the majority of the participants resided in South Jakarta (54.7%).

Table 1. Demography of participants.

Category	Description	Frequency	Percentage
Gender	Female	121	57.1%
	Male	91	42.9%
Age	<20 years	19	9%
	20–25 years	147	69.3%
	26–30 years	38	17.9%
	31–35 years	5	2.4%
	>35 years	3	1.4%
Education	SMA/SMK/Equivalent	98	46.2%
	D1/D2/D3/D4	11	5.2%
	S1	101	47.6%
	S2	2	0.9%
Occupation	Student	100	47.2%
	Private Employee	77	36.3%
	Entrepreneur	13	6.1%
	Civil Servant/TNI/Police	13	6.1%
	Other	9	4.2%
Domicile	West Jakarta	31	14.6%
	Central Jakarta	17	8%
	South Jakarta	116	54.7%
	East Jakarta	23	10.8%
	North Jakarta	16	7.5%
	Thousand Island	9	4.2
Total		212	100%

2.2. Research Design

We used descriptive statistics and analyzed correlation using the data collected through a questionnaire survey. Non-probability sampling was used in this study as it provides equal opportunities for all participants to be included. The non-probability method is convenient, affordable, easy, and fast [10].

2.3. Measuring Instruments

The instrument used to measure loneliness was the University of California Los Angeles (UCLA) Loneliness Scale version 3 [5]. It consists of 20 items: 9 favorable items and 11 unfavorable items. The scale was modified and translated in this study (Table 2). The scale was used to obtain the data in two dimensions of emotional and social isolation with a validity of >0.40 and reliability at an alpha coefficient value of 0.92. Experts at the Psychology Department of Bina Nusantara University, Indonesia, were invited to validate the scale.

Table 2. Loneliness scale.

Aspect	Indicator	Favorable	Unfavorable	Total
Emotional isolation	The lack of achieving an intimate emotional connection and not having emotional clones with others.	2, 3, 4, 7	15, 16	6
	The individual lacks participation within the group.	12, 17, 18	1, 10	5
Social isolation	The individual does not actively involve themselves within the group.	8	5, 6, 19, 20	5
	The individual feels deliberately excluded from the social sphere.	11, 13, 14	9	4
Total		**11**	**9**	**20**

We tested reliability using Cronbach's alpha. The value was 0.950, which indicated that the survey was reliable. We used a four-point Likert scale: Never = 1, Rarely = 2, Often = 3, Very Often = 4.

Psychological well-being was measured using Ryff's Scale of Psychological Well-Being [11]. This scale encompasses six dimensions: self-acceptance, positive relations with others, autonomy, personal growth, environmental mastery, and purpose in life (Table 3). Reliability was calculated per dimension with values for each dimension as follows: 0.85 for self-acceptance, 0.83 for positive relations with others, 0.88 for autonomy, 0.81 for environmental mastery, and 0.82 for purpose in life. The lowest correlated item scored 0.226, while the highest reached 0.802.

Table 3. Blueprint of psychological well-being scale.

Dimension	Favorable	Unfavorable	Total
Autonomy	1, 7, 25, 37	13, 19, 31	7
Environmental Mastery	2, 20, 38	8, 14, 26, 32	7
Personal Growth	9, 21, 33	3, 15, 27, 39	7
Positive Relations	4, 22, 28, 40	10, 16, 34	7
Purpose in Life	5, 11, 29, 35	17, 23, 41	7
Self-acceptance	6, 12, 24, 42	18, 30, 36	7
Total	22	20	42

3. Result

3.1. Normality Test

We tested normality to test whether the independent and dependent variables were normally distributed [12] using the Kolmogorov–Smirnov method. The asymptotic significance (2-tailed) was 0.060. As it was higher than 0.05, the data were regarded to be normally distributed (Table 4).

Table 4. Result of one-sample Kolmogorov–Smirnov test.

Unstandardized Residual		
N		212
Normal Parameters	Mean	0.0000000
	Standard deviation	1.874278
Most Extreme Differences	Absolute	0.060
	Positive	0.060
	Negative	−0.060
Test Statistic		0.060
Asymptotic significance		0.060

3.2. Correlation

We conducted the correlation analysis as presented in Table 5. Loneliness and psychological well-being were negatively correlated (r = −0.692, p <0.05).

Table 5. Correlation analysis results.

		Loneliness	Psychological Well-Being
Loneliness	Pearson Correlation	1	−0.692 **
	Sig. (2-tailed)		0.000
	N	212	212
Psychological Well-Being	Pearson Correlation	−0.692 **	1
	Sig. (2-tailed)	0.000	
	N	212	212

** Correlation is significant at $p < 0.01$ (2-tailed).

4. Discussion and Conclusions

The results of this study indicated a significant relationship between loneliness and psychological well-being in early adults in Jakarta. The higher the level of loneliness, the lower the level of psychological well-being. This coincides with the results of Hapsari and Ratriana [13] and Halim and Dariyo [14]. This correlation in the males and the females was −0.689 and −0.687, respectively. Such coefficients are regarded to be high [15]. Loneliness can occur to anyone regardless of gender [16]. Thus, gender is not a factor affecting the level of loneliness. The coefficient of the participants younger than 20 years old was −0.420. The results of this study provide a reference in clinical psychology and research on loneliness and psychological well-being. It is important to increase psychological well-being so that young adults can maximize their productivity and achieve goals in life. Individuals can improve psychological well-being by accepting themselves, realizing their goals in life, having independence, developing positive relationships, and controlling the environment. Individuals must have a desire to continue to become a better person. By realizing and applying this, individuals can minimize the level of loneliness.

There are limitations, as psychological well-being in each dimension was not analyzed in detail. The selection of the participants was also limited in Jakarta. For further research, it is necessary to analyze loneliness and psychological well-being in each dimension with more participants in various regions.

Author Contributions: Conceptualization, M.N.S. and L.N.H.; methodology, M.N.S. and L.N.H.; software, M.N.S. and L.N.H.; validation, M.N.S.; formal analysis, M.N.S. and L.N.H.; data collection, L.N.H.; writing, M.N.S. and L.N.H. All authors have read and agreed to the published version of the manuscript.

Funding: This research received no external funding.

Institutional Review Board Statement: This study was conducted in accordance with the Declaration of Helsinki and all subjects gave their informed consent before they participated in this study.

Informed Consent Statement: Informed consent was obtained from all subjects involved in the study.

Data Availability Statement: The data is available at https://bit.ly/4g24gKN.

Conflicts of Interest: The authors declare no conflicts of interest for research and publication for this research article.

References

1. Santrock, J.W. *Life-Span Development*, 17th ed.; McGraw-Hill: New York, NY, USA, 2019.
2. Meilia, A. Pengaruh kesepian sebagai salah satu faktor risiko pengalaman psikotik pada dewasa awal. *Bul. Ris. Psikol. Dan. Kesehat. Ment.* **2021**, *1*, 1207–1217. [CrossRef]
3. Permana, M.F.; dan Astuti, M.Z. Gambaran Kesepian Pada Emerging Adulthood. *Proyeksi* **2021**, *16*, 133. [CrossRef]
4. Anggraeni, N. Hubungan Kesepian Dengan Pengungkapan Diri di Instagram Pada Dewasa yang Belum Menikah. Doctoral Dissertation, University of Muhammadiyah Malang, Malang, Indonesia, 2018.
5. Russell, D.W. UCLA Loneliness scale (version 3): Reliability, validity, and factor structure. *J. Personal. Assess* **1996**, *66*, 20–40. [CrossRef] [PubMed]
6. Domagala-Krecioch, B.; Majerek, A. The issue of loneliness in the period of emerging adulthood. *Eur. Sci. J.* **2013**, *13*, 534–541.
7. Russell, D. Living arrangements, social integration, and loneliness in later life: The case of physical disability. *J. Health Soc. Behav.* **2009**, *50*, 460–475. [CrossRef]
8. Aulia, R.U. Panjaitan Kesejahteraan psikologis dan tingkat stres pada mahasiswa tingkat akhir. *J. Keperawatan Jiwa* **2019**, *7*, 127–134. [CrossRef]
9. Winefield, R.M.; Gill, H.R.; Taylor, T.K.; Pilkington, A.W. Psychological well-being and psychological distress: Is it necessary to measure both? *Psychol. Well-Being: Theory Res. Pract.* **2012**, *2*, 3. [CrossRef]
10. Etikan, R.S.; Musa, S.; Alkassim, A. Comparison of convenience sampling and purposive sampling. *Am. J. Theor. Appl. Stat.* **2016**, *5*, 1–4. [CrossRef]
11. Ryff, C.D. Happiness Is Everything, or Is It? Explorations on the Meaning of Psychological Well-Being. *J. Personal. Soc. Psychol.* **1989**, *57*, 1069. [CrossRef]
12. Ghozali, I. *Aplikasi Analisis Multivariate Dengan Program IBM SPSS 25;* Badan Penerbit Universitas Diponegoro: Semarang, Indonesia, 2018.
13. Hapsari, Y.E.K.; Ratriana, S. Hubungan antara Psychological Well Being dan Kesepian pada Lansia di Desa Ringinawe Kota Salatiga. *J. Ilm. Bimbing. Konseling Undiksha* **2022**, *13*, 2. [CrossRef]
14. Halim, A.; Dariyo, C.F. Hubungan psychological well-being dengan loneliness pada mahasiswa yang merantau. *J. Psikogenesis* **2016**, *4*, 170–181. [CrossRef]
15. Hasan, I. *Analisis Data Penelitian Dengan Statistik;* Bumi Aksara: Jakarta, Indonesia, 2010.
16. Febriani, Z. Perbedaan tingkat kesepian pada remaja ditinjau dari jenis kelamin. *J. Pendidik. Tambusai* **2021**, *5*, 7032–7037.

engineering proceedings

Proceeding Paper

Thematic Analysis of Technology Use by Urban Couples in Stress Management †

Pingkan Cynthia Belinda Rumondor [1,*], Sheilla Lim Omar Lim [2], Ross Azura Zahit [3], Andre Ferdinand Julianto [1], Charoline Xessa [1], Khansa Najla Pramesti [1] and Martinus Fieser Sitinjak [4]

1 Psychology Department, Faculty of Humanities, Bina Nusantara University, Jakarta 11480, Indonesia; andre.julianto001@binus.ac.id (A.F.J.); charoline.xessa@binus.ac.id (C.X.); khansa.pramesti@binus.ac.id (K.N.P.)
2 Human Resource Development Program, Universiti Malaysia Sarawak, Kota Samarahan 94300, Malaysia; olslim@unimas.my
3 Psychology Program, Universiti Malaysia Sarawak, Kota Samarahan 94300, Malaysia; zrazura@unimas.my
4 Global Business Marketing Program, Bina Nusantara University, Jakarta 11480, Indonesia; msitinjak@binus.edu
* Correspondence: pingkan_rumondor@binus.ac.id

† Presented at the 2024 IEEE 4th International Conference on Electronic Communications, Internet of Things and Big Data, Taipei, Taiwan, 19–21 April 2024.

Abstract: Urban couples spend much time working, which poses challenges in their daily life. These challenges can cause stress, affecting relationship quality and an individual's well-being. We identified and described stressors and explored the use of technology to manage their stress. The participants consisted of three couples living in the Greater Jakarta area. A focus group discussion was used to collect the data, and inductive thematic analysis was used to analyze it. Urban couples experienced relationship stress, parenting stress, financial stress, work-related stress, and daily hassles. Couples can manage stress by using digital media and smart communication technology to provide entertainment and communication, as well as to search for information.

Keywords: dual-earner; urban couples; relationship quality; dyadic coping; stress

Citation: Rumondor, P.C.B.; Lim, S.L.O.; Zahit, R.A.; Julianto, A.F.; Xessa, C.; Pramesti, K.N.; Sitinjak, M.F. Thematic Analysis of Technology Use by Urban Couples in Stress Management. *Eng. Proc.* **2024**, *74*, 43. https://doi.org/10.3390/engproc2024074043

Academic Editors: Shu-Han Liao, Teen-Hang Meen and Cheng-Fu Yang

Published: 3 September 2024

1. Introduction

Women started working in Indonesia in 1932, with the movement of Suwarni Pringgodigdo [1]. In Indonesia, the modernization of society is changing the roles of husbands and wives within a marriage. Both the husband and wife often have jobs to sustain the family's living situation in urban areas. This trend is obvious in the Indonesian National Workforce Survey, which stated that 38.9% of workers in Indonesia were women and 61.0% were men [2]. The proportion of women in the workforce is increasing, which is a common characteristic of urban couples.

On average, workers in Jakarta spend more than 40 h/week, at 8 h/day, working. According to the National Force of Workers Survey, 70.3% of citizens in Indonesia at the productive age reported working more than 35 h [2]. This estimation does not include the time it takes to commute. Tomtom.com [3] estimates that, on average, Jakarta citizens spend around 214 h/year only commuting in traffic, and within those hours, it is estimated that 106 h are spent waiting in traffic jams. The overcrowded traffic and long working hours create a unique characteristic of everyday life in urban cities, unlike rural areas. Thus, we focused on the unique life experiences of urban couples in the Greater Jakarta area in dealing with daily hassles.

Stress is a condition or a demand from the environment typically greater than a person's normal capacity, requiring an additional response that can impact a person physically and psychologically [4,5]. Stress is conceptualized as stressors, which are any event, force, or condition that results in physical or emotional stress [6]. In this study, stress was viewed from a relational perspective to identify and describe daily stressors that contribute to urban couples' relationship quality.

Randall and Bodenmann formulated a stress typology to understand stress's impact on relationship quality [7]. Stressors are differentiated into (1) internal versus external stress. Internal stressors originate from within the relationship (such as conflicts, tensions, attitudes, needs, desires, and habits of one partner that disturb the other; a lack of compatibility among partners). In contrast, external stressors are the stressors that originate from outside of a relationship (such as stress in the workplace, financial stress, social stress in the neighborhood, or stress about the extended family, including siblings, parents-in-law, and other relatives); (2) major and minor stresses are defined by how intense the experience or condition felt by people within a relationship; and (3) acute versus chronic stresses are defined by the duration of the stress [7]. Randall and Bodenmann suggested that the experience of external, minor, and chronic stress impacts relationship quality the most [7]. Therefore, describing and identifying the external stressors are essential to minimize the adverse effects of stress on the marital quality of urban couples [8].

Relationships and marital quality are essential in shaping a happier and more prosperous life. Marital satisfaction is associated with higher life satisfaction and momentary happiness. This correlation is found in both men and women [9]. Meta-analysis study results showed that higher marital quality is associated with higher individual well-being [10]. These results support previous findings that higher marital quality is linked to a higher score on a self-rated health scale [11]. Thus, an intervention is needed to improve marital quality.

Couples need coping strategies to maintain their marital quality. In a romantic relationship, the coping strategies practiced by romantic partners are known as dyadic coping. The systemic transactional model (STM) explains that the dyadic coping process emphasizes the interdependence and mutuality among partners, meaning that the stress of one partner affects the other but also that the resources of one partner expand the resources of the other [12]. Stress-related function in STM can reduce stress from the spillover effect experienced by both partners (we-stress).

Many meta-analyses show that the conventional intervention method positively impacts marriage quality through education, such as a Relationship Education program [13]. Aside from conventional methods, various interventions for improving couples' relationship quality using modern information systems and technology are available [14]. Smartphones have also been used to maintain marital relationships [15]. However, no studies have focused on finding and identifying specific coping mechanisms for couples to manage stress using information and communication technology.

We explored the role of digital media and smart communication as tools for couples' coping mechanisms. Das [16] defined digital media as follows: "Digital media refers to the media encoded in machine-readable formats. Digital media can be created, viewed, communicated, modified, and preserved on digital electronic devices such as software, digital images, videos, web pages, websites, social media, digital data, digital audio, and E-books". Digital-based stress management is expected to reduce divorce risks among married couples [17,18]. For example, couples use smartphones to communicate with their partners, maintain relationships, share information, and perform specific tasks.

This research aims to answer the following: (1) What stressors can reduce the quality of marriage relationships among urban couples? (2) What coping strategies and mechanisms do urban couples use to manage and reduce stress? (3) How do urban couples utilize information systems and technology advancements such as digital media and smart communication to reduce and manage stress?

2. Material and Methods

We used qualitative methods, specifically inductive thematic analysis. A focus group discussion (FGD) was conducted to collect participants' data using interview questions.

2.1. Participants

Two dual-earner couples and one single-earner couple were recruited using the convenient sampling method (Table 1).

Table 1. Demography of participants.

	1st Couple	2nd Couple	3rd Couple
		Husband	
Code	PAR 1B	PAR 2B	PAR 3B
Age	42 years old	34 years old	48 years old
Job	Employee	Lecturer	Debt collector
		Wife	
Code	PAR 1A	PAR 2A	PAR 3A
Age	34 years old	34 years old	46 years old
Job	Employee	Housewife	Employee
Marriage	13 years	11 years	16 years
Children's age	9 and 6 years old	10, 3, and 1.7 years old	15 and 8 years old
Work/Home	Jakarta/Jakarta	Jakarta/Jakarta	Jakarta/Bekasi

2.2. Measures

Data were collected during the focus group discussion, which was conducted via a Zoom meeting, and experts on the topic were also interviewed. Participants were asked questions during the focus group discussion. See the Supplementary Materials from https://bit.ly/FGD-IQ (accessed on 27 July 2023).

2.3. Design and Procedures

We used a qualitative approach (i.e., FGD) as the data collection method and inductive thematic analysis to analyze the results. Participants were recruited by distributing flyers around Binus University, Greater Jakarta area. See the Supplementary Materials from https://bit.ly/FGD-IQ (accessed on 27 July 2023).

2.4. Data Analysis

Thematic analysis was used to identify, analyze, and report patterns within data, as well as to organize and describe the data [19].

3. Results

The thematic analysis results are presented in 141 highlights, which are organized into 88 themes. These themes are then reduced to 26, as illustrated in Figure 1.

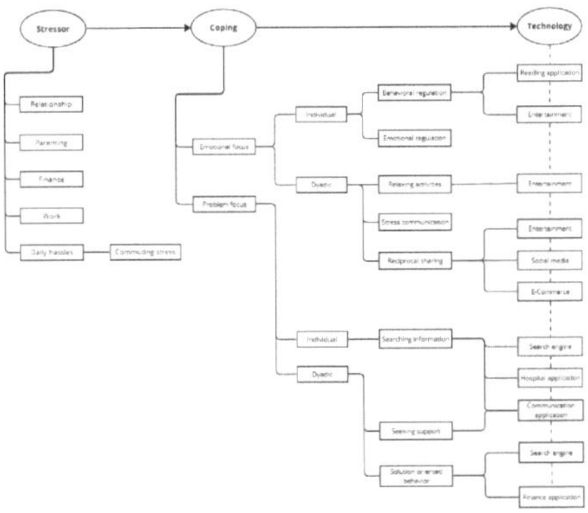

Figure 1. Stressors, coping strategies, and technology used to manage stress in urban couples.

The model consisted of the following three main parts: stressors, coping, and technology use. Each of these steps was correlated with the research question. First, the thematic analysis yielded five themes related to stressors that reduce the quality of marital relationships, as follows: (1) relationship stress, (2) parenting stress, (3) financial stress, (4) work-related stress, and (5) daily hassles.

3.1. Couples' Stressors

Relationship stress came from relationships with co-workers and family. Stressors also came from work supervisors:

> *"The supervisor asks to do something as if someone is eating red pepper. Once they order something, it's harsh and must be done right at the moment".* (48 years old, male, debt collector)

Family relationship stress came from relationships with in-laws. Although in-laws can function as a support system, asking for help from in-laws can be a challenge:

> *"Probably asking parents-in-law to take care of the kids. Sometimes, I feel bad or something like that. Sometimes, I feel like a burden to them. But, it is a better option rather than hiring strangers when no one is at home".* (42 years old, male, school finance department employee)

3.1.1. Parenting Stress

Parenting was challenging for urban couples, especially when their children experienced health issues:

> *"Since I was alone and had no one to help, it was unbelievable every day, especially one thing that usually causes stress when children get sick, and it continued in the same circle. It could happen around a week to the second child, then the next few days for a week to the third child. So, the doctor knew very well they got sick with a similar pattern".* (34 years old, female, housewife)

3.1.2. Financial Stress

Financial stress was not mentioned directly, but indirectly presented:

> *"Not only transferring money, but there is also an additional IDR 6.500 admin fee".* (34 years old, male, lecturer)

This implies that, in addition to regular financial stressors, fees caused additional stress for urban couples.

3.1.3. Work Stress

Work-related stress consists of stressors related to demands in the workplace. These demands are specific depending on the occupation:

> *"Usually, it's the pressure from work for me. The challenge or any kind of thing we need to keep up with the deadline for export shift things, we must know when the goods come in. That's all my problem in the workplace".* (34 years old, female, logistic employee)

3.1.4. Daily Hassles

The final stressor involves daily hassles, as follows: the challenges, responsibilities, and conditions that urban couples face daily. These stressors are considered minor and chronic due to their low intensity levels but occur daily [20]:

> *"Oh yes, it was because I was on the road during a traffic jam that caused stress".* (48 years old, male, debt collector)

3.2. Couples Stress Management

Couples' stress management is categorized into problem- or emotional-focused coping individually or dyadically.

3.2.1. Emotion-Focused Dyadic Coping

The emotion-focused dyadic coping is divided into the following two groups: individual behaviors and dyadic behaviors. Individual behaviors include behavioral and emotional regulation and relaxing activities. These activities are performed individually with information and communication technologies.

Emotional-focused coping, especially individual strategies, are behavioral and emotional regulation. Aside from passive behaviors, such as waiting for their partner to calm down, behavioral regulation also covers applications for reading and accessing the Internet. The following participant claims that their partner regained their composure before conducting stress communication:

> *"Waiting for my wife to be in a calm state, if she is not even in a calm state, then it will be unhelpful to vent"*. (34 years old, male, lecturer)

> *"We each read on our own"*. (34 years old, male, lecturer)

Participants explained how they use gadgets to calm themselves:

> *"Yes, using the gadget by ourselves"*. (42 years old, male, school's finance department employee)

Participants also waited for the right moment to control their emotions:

> *"... and wait for the right moment. I will wait for the right moment until I can think clearly about 'why does it happen?' and how can I make it logically sound"*. (34 years old, male, lecturer)

One of the participants mentioned that the only thing that he could do after experiencing a stressful situation was to be patient and not be triggered or angered by the situation. He stated that getting angry brought him nothing:

> *"Well, the only thing I could do was be patient. If I get fed up as well, the result will not do any good. So, just be patient"*. (48 years old, male, debt collector)

The following quote shows that a participant held their emotions back until they felt better, were more composed, and could talk about it:

> *"For me, I usually settle my emotions first and wait for the right moment... When I have felt better, I will then talk about it"*. (34 years old, male, lecturer)

The same thing happened to the following working mother, where she sometimes experienced a sense of yearning or missing her son, and the only thing she could do was be patient:

> *"I can only hold back my longing emotions because I know my first child is far from me. I mean, I am far from him and he has been with his grandma since kid"*. (46 years old, female, school finance department employee)

The following participant mentioned when she used social media, she was very happy, and it calmed her emotions when she saw content of someone playing the piano:

> *"I like the most.. What is it? Usually, like someone was playing piano. That's the kind of music I like"*. (46 years old, female, school finance department employee)

Dyadic behaviors include relaxing activities, stress communication, and reciprocal sharing. The following couple had the same hobby, and they often talked to each other and shared their feelings and experiences while watching a drama series together:

> *"We both liked it because we have the same hobby of watching drama. We were having a conversation while watching a Korean drama. Just like that, we were talking to each other"*. (34 years old, female, logistic employee)

The couples usually watched movies/series with the same title, but they progressed through the stories at different paces, making it feel like they were racing against each other:

> *"We often will watch the same title, but a lot of the time, she can progress through the series quicker, which can sometimes feel like a race between us two".* (34 years old, male, lecturer)

The couples liked to share stories about the problems they had, and it helped them feel better after venting out their stress on each other:

> *"As for me, mostly I talked it out. If there are any problems in my office, I would like to spill it out to (Participant 1B). Just like that, but I felt better when I let out everything".* (34 years old, female, logistic employee)

Lastly, couples mentioned using social media to share entertainment content even when they are in the same room:

> *"Mmmm... for this Ma'am, usually we use social media to share reels even when we are sitting next to each other"* (34 years old, male, lecturer)

3.2.2. Problem-Focused Dyadic Coping

The problem-focused dyadic coping mentioned by the participants consisted of individual and dyadic behaviors. Individual behavior focuses on solving a problem by searching for information, utilizing information and communication technologies (e.g., search engines and hospital applications), and communication applications such as WhatsApp:

> *"Usually, I look up my child's symptoms so I can ask and search it using Google and then look through an application. In Hermina, there is an application where you can see the doctor's availability and which day at which time. Later, I will contact my partner about what time he (Participant 2B) is going home, the doctor will be available during this time, can he make it? Just like that. If it's possible then okay. If not, is there availability during this time? That way".* (34 years old, female, housewife)

Similarly, dyadic behaviors include seeking support and solution-oriented behavior. The couples sometimes needed support and help from their families to care for their kids:

> *"Probably asking parents-in-law to take care of the kids..".* (42 years old, male, school finance department employee)

Participants also used features included with a financial application called Flip. The transfer feature from Flip allowed participants to save costs on admin fees, which suggests that finance-related issues do, indeed, cause stress among urban couples:

> *"Using m-banking really helps. On the other hand, I'm happy with the Flip features".* (34 years old, male, lecturer)

3.3. Technology Utilization for Couples' Stress Management

The thematic analysis results reveal the utilization of information systems and technology by couples to manage stress, as follows: entertainment applications, search engines, social media, e-commerce, and finance applications. Entertainment applications can take many forms, but the ones mentioned by the participants are streaming, reading, and gaming/leisure applications. The couples mentioned using streaming applications to watch entertaining content together, chat, and share:

> *"We both liked it because we have the same hobby of watching* [drama]. *We were having a conversation while watching a Korean drama. Just like that, we were talking to each other".* (34 years old, female, logistic employee).

The participants mentioned the application Webtoons, which they liked to use to read comics:

The participants mentioned Webtoon, an application for reading comics:

> *"Probably Webtoon, it's because I like to read comics".* (34 years old, female, housewife)

Couples also used search engines to find relevant information to solve their problems as effectively and efficiently as possible and hospital applications to search for information about medical check-up schedules and doctors' schedules:

> *"Usually, I look up my child's symptoms so I can ask and search for them using Google and then look through an application. In Hermina (hospital), there is an application where you can see the doctor's availability on which day and at which time..."* (34 years old, female, housewife)

The participants mentioned that for emotional regulation, they used ICT mainly to access entertainment and socializing apps. The couples did not use psychology-related applications:

> *"Usually, it's a streaming application for me than social media. But I don't use any psychologist thing application".* (34 years old, male, lecturer)

The couples used the social media application Instagram:

> *"Same. A social media* [application] *maybe. Social media like Instagram as well".* (34 years old, male, lecturer)

One of the participants mentioned Facebook as their favorite social media application:

> *"I personally liked Facebook the most".* (46 years old, female, school finance department employee)

The couples mentioned that they often used e-commerce applications to regulate their emotions by doing some online shopping. The e-commerce applications mentioned were Shopee and Tokopedia:

> *"Shopee, Tokopedia, and the likes of it".* (34 years old, male, lecturer)

The participants mentioned that Flip helped solve problems related to financial stress, specifically, the stress of high admin fees for mobile banking transactions:

> *"Using m-banking really helps. On the other hand, I'm happy with the Flip features".* (34 years old, male, lecturer)

4. Conclusions

The results of this research reveal how urban couples manage stress, especially using information and communication technology, such as digital and social media. Urban couples' daily stressors align with those of previous research. According to the literature, these stressors include parenting, relationships, traffic jams, and others [21,22]. Couples also experience stress related to their own, their partner's, or their child's health [23].

The findings of this research suggest that dual-earner urban couples often experienced stress associated with work and childbearing, since both couples work and raise their children as well as manage the household. The increasing number of working wives positively impacted the family preparedness for the potential absence of one's spouse's income in the case of spousal death, divorce, or layoff, as well as an increase in a wife's understanding of her husband [24]. Quality of life can be increased with the financial stability of a family. According to the STM, partners' well-being is strongly intertwined, and their happiness depends on one another [12]. Alternatively, couples experience the same stressful events, which affect each spouse individually [25]. If their partner is not in a good emotional state to conduct stress communication (e.g., their partner is in a bad mood), then they suppress their emotions momentarily and wait for the right moment to engage in stress communication after their partner has recovered to a more optimal state. Interestingly, one of the couples stated that the wife tends to keep things to herself instead of sharing because of concerns that the husband is angry. This is in line with previous research regarding spillover, which refers to the transmission of problems across domains [26–28].

The coping strategies used by urban couples to reduce and manage stress align with dyadic coping strategies. Each of these forms of dyadic coping was divided into emotional-focused and problem-focused ones, which indicate which aspect couples focused on when using dyadic coping to solve problems or manage negative emotions elicited by stress [8]. Another common emotion-focused coping strategy used individually and dyadically is humor.

Moreover, technology helped manage the stress of urban couples in terms of relationship maintenance [15]. Couples used technology to manage emotions individually or together with partners. There were differences between the coping strategies of husbands toward wives and wives toward husbands. Couples consumed the same entertainment content alone and then discussed it together. Interestingly, communication between partners using information and communicational technologies occurred even when both partners were in the same place.

In contrast, several coping strategies did not need technology's help. The couples regulate their emotions and are patient. Aside from this, one person chose to regulate their emotions with the help of their partner by engaging in stress communication. However, another person waited for the right moment and considered the state and condition of their partner before engaging in communication of stress. However, sophisticated technology did not replace the ability to manage one's behavior.

The devices at work were not considered as stress management tools by the participants, which is contrary to previous research [15]. This technology use was not seen in the data because the FGD session did not ask about it. Financial problems were not mentioned explicitly by the participants, whereas based on previous findings/research [29], financial problems must be a significant stressor.

There are limitations regarding the scope and the procedures in this research. Firstly, participants were limited to three couples. Even though there were enough participants to conduct an FGD, this number of participants is not enough to represent urban citizens. Future studies are necessary to recruit more participants and interview them, considering that FGDs are not effective if the number of participants is greater than eight. We did not distinguish participants from formal and informal work backgrounds because the previous study found differences in stress sources among families with work backgrounds [30]. Thus, it is necessary to consider work backgrounds and control for participants' socioeconomic statuses such as adding minimum wage and specific jobs.

Supplementary Materials: The following supporting information can be downloaded at: https://bit.ly/FGD-IQ (accessed on 27 July 2023).

Author Contributions: Conceptualization, P.C.B.R. and M.F.S.; methodology, P.C.B.R. and M.F.S.; software, A.F.J., C.X., and K.N.P.; validation, P.C.B.R. and M.F.S.; formal analysis, A.F.J., C.X., and K.N.P.; investigation, P.C.B.R. and M.F.S.; resources, S.L.O.L. and R.A.Z.; data curation, P.C.B.R., M.F.S., A.F.J., C.X., and K.N.P.; writing—original draft preparation, P.C.B.R., A.F.J., C.X., and K.N.P.; writing—review and editing, S.L.O.L. and R.A.Z.; visualization, A.F.J., C.X., and K.N.P.; supervision, P.C.B.R.; project administration, A.F.J., C.X., and K.N.P.; funding acquisition, P.C.B.R. and M.F.S. All authors have read and agreed to the published version of the manuscript.

Funding: This work is supported by the Research and Technology Transfer Office, Bina Nusantara University, as a part of Bina Nusantara University's International Research Grant entitled "Couples Retreat: Relationship Enhancement Intervention to Increase Relationship Quality in Urban Couples", with contract number: 029/VRTT/III/2023 and contract date: 1 March 2023.

Institutional Review Board Statement: The study was conducted in accordance with the Declaration of Helsinki and approved by the Institutional Review Board of Bina Nusantara University (LSET062022-24, 19 April 2023).

Informed Consent Statement: Informed consent was obtained from all subjects involved in the study.

Data Availability Statement: The data presented in this study are available upon request from the corresponding author due to privacy reasons.

Conflicts of Interest: The authors declare no conflicts of interest.

References

1. Janti, N. Perempuan Bekerja Dulu dan Kini. Available online: https://historia.id/politik/articles/perempuan-bekerja-dulu-dan-kini-DWeqe/page/1 (accessed on 25 July 2023).
2. Statistik, B.P. *Statistik Indonesia 2023*; Badan Pusat Statistik: Jakarta, Indonesia, 2023.
3. Jakarta Traffic. Available online: https://www.tomtom.com/traffic-index/jakarta-traffic/ (accessed on 29 March 2023).
4. Lazarus, R.; Folkman, S. *Stress, Appraisals, and Coping*; Springer: New York, NY, USA, 1984.
5. Bamuhair, S.S.; Al Farhan, A.I.; Althubaiti, A.; Agha, S.; Rahman, S.U.; Ibrahim, N.O. Sources of Stress and Coping Strategies among Undergraduate Medical Students Enrolled in a Problem-Based Learning Curriculum. *J. Biomed. Educ.* **2015**, *2015*, 575139. [CrossRef]
6. APA Dictionary of Psychology. Available online: https://dictionary.apa.org/coping-strategies (accessed on 28 April 2023).
7. Randall, A.K.; Bodenmann, G. The Role of Stress on Close Relationships and Marital Satisfaction. *Clin. Psychol. Rev.* **2009**, *29*, 105–115. [CrossRef] [PubMed]
8. Bodenmann, G. The Influence of Stress and Coping on Close Relationships: A Two-Year Longitudinal Study. *Artic. Swiss J. Psychol.* **1997**, *56*, 156–164.
9. Carr, D.; Freedman, V.A.; Cornman, J.C.; Schwarz, N. Happy Marriage, Happy Life? Marital Quality and Subjective Well-Being in Later Life. *J. Marriage Fam.* **2014**, *76*, 930–948. [CrossRef]
10. Ledermann, T.; Bodenmann, G.; Rudaz, M.; Bradbury, T.N. Stress, Communication, and Marital Quality in Couples. *Fam. Relat.* **2010**, *59*, 195–206. [CrossRef]
11. Proulx, C.M.; Snyder-Rivas, L.A. The Longitudinal Associations between Marital Happiness, Problems, and Self-Rated Health. *J. Fam. Psychol.* **2013**, *27*, 194–202. [CrossRef]
12. Bodenmann, G.; Randall, A.K.; Falconier, M.K. CHAPTER 1 Coping in Couples: The Systemic Transactional Model (STM). In *Couples Coping with Stress: A cross-cultural Perspective*; Routledge: New York, NY, USA, 2016; pp. 5–22.
13. Stanley, S.M.; Carlson, R.G.; Rhoades, G.K.; Markman, H.J.; Ritchie, L.L.; Hawkins, A.J. Best Practices in Relationship Education Focused on Intimate Relationships. *Fam. Relat.* **2020**, *69*, 497–519. [CrossRef]
14. Doss, B.D.; Roddy, M.K.; Nowlan, K.M.; Rothman, K.; Christensen, A. Maintenance of Gains in Relationship and Individual Functioning Following the Online OurRelationship Program. *Behav. Ther.* **2019**, *50*, 73–86. [CrossRef]
15. Rumondor, P.C.B. Is There an Application for Improving Marital Satisfaction? An Overview of Smartphone Usage in Urban Young Adults' Marital Interactions. *Makara Hum. Behav. Stud. Asia* **2019**, *23*, 97. [CrossRef]
16. Das, A. Impact of digital media on society. *Int. J. Creat. Res. Thoughts* **2020**, *8*, 2742–2748.
17. Aditya, Y.; Magno, C. Factors Influencing Marital Satisfaction among Christian Couples In Indonesia: A Vulnerability-Stress-Adaptation Model Facilitating Academic Self-Regualtion Using a Learning Mnagement System View Project Knowledge Channel View Project. *Int. J. Res.* **2011**, *7*, 11–32.
18. Falconier, M.K.; Jackson, J.B.; Hilpert, P.; Bodenmann, G. Dyadic Coping and Relationship Satisfaction: A Meta-Analysis. *Clin. Psychol. Rev.* **2015**, *42*, 28–46. [CrossRef] [PubMed]
19. Braun, V.; Clarke, V. Using Thematic Analysis in Psychology. *Qual. Res. Psychol.* **2006**, *3*, 77–101. [CrossRef]
20. Kanner, A.D.; Coyne, J.C.; Schaefer, C.; Lazarus, R.S. Comparison of Two Modes of Stress Measurement: Daily Hassles and Uplifts versus Major Life Events. *J. Behav. Med.* **1981**, *4*, 1–39. [CrossRef]
21. Demsky, C.A.; Ellis, A.M.; Fritz, C. Shrugging It off: Does Psychological Detachment from Work Mediate the Relationship between Workplace Aggression and Work-Family Conflict? *J. Occup. Health Psychol.* **2014**, *19*, 195–205. [CrossRef] [PubMed]
22. Useche, S.A.; Marin, C.; Llamazares, F.J. "Another (Hard) Day Moving in the City": Development and Validation of the MCSS, a Multimodal Commuting Stress Scale. *Transp. Res. Part. F Traffic Psychol. Behav.* **2023**, *95*, 143–159. [CrossRef]
23. Muscara, F.; Burke, K.; McCarthy, M.C.; Anderson, V.A.; Hearps, S.J.C.; Hearps, S.J.; Dimovski, A.; Nicholson, J.M. Parent Distress Reactions Following a Serious Illness or Injury in Their Child: A Protocol Paper for the Take a Breath Cohort Study. *BMC Psychiatry* **2015**, *15*, 153. [CrossRef]
24. Desmayanti, S. *Hubungan Antara Resolusi Konflik Dan Kepuasan Pernikahan Pada Pasangan Suami Istri Bekerja Pada Masa Awal Pernikahan*; Universitas Indonesia: Depok, Indonesia, 2009.
25. Timmons, A.C.; Arbel, R.; Margolin, G. Daily Patterns of Stress and Conflict in Couples: Associations with Marital Aggression and Family-of-Origin Aggression. *J. Fam. Psychol.* **2017**, *31*, 93–104. [CrossRef]
26. Almeida, D.M.; Wethington, E.; Chandler, A.L. Daily Transmission of Tensions between Marital Dyads and Parent-Child Dyads. *J. Marriage Fam.* **1999**, *61*, 49. [CrossRef]
27. Bolger, N.; DeLongis, A.; Kessler, R.C.; Wethington, E. The Contagion of Stress across Multiple Roles. *J. Marriage Fam.* **1989**, *51*, 175. [CrossRef]
28. Repetti, R.L. Effects of Daily Workload on Subsequent Behavior during Marital Interaction: The Roles of Social Withdrawal and Spouse Support. *J. Pers. Soc. Psychol.* **1989**, *57*, 651–659. [CrossRef] [PubMed]

29. Friedline, T.; Chen, Z.; Morrow, S.P. Families' Financial Stress & Well-Being: The Importance of the Economy and Economic Environments. *J. Fam. Econ. Issues* **2021**, *42*, 34–51. [CrossRef] [PubMed]
30. Fala, M.; Sunarti, E.; Herawati, T. Sources of Stress, Coping Strategies, Stress Symptoms, and Marital Satisfaction in Working Wives. *J. Ilmu Kel. Dan. Konsum.* **2020**, *13*, 25–37. [CrossRef]

engineering proceedings

MDPI

Proceeding Paper

Exploring Personalized Gamified Learning by Computer Software: Enhancing the Effects of Learning-Style Adaptation †

Chien-Hung Lai * and Cheng-Yueh Lin

Department of Information and Computer Engineering, Chung Yuan Christian University, Taoyuan 320, Taiwan; linek0820@gmail.com

* Correspondence: soulwind@cycu.org.tw

† Presented at the 2024 IEEE 4th International Conference on Electronic Communications, Internet of Things and Big Data, Taipei, Taiwan, 19–21 April 2024.

Abstract: The adaptability of learning styles to gamified learning models was explored to better understand the needs and advantages of students in different educational environments. Learning styles reflect the preferences and habits of each student, which are influenced by their upbringing and experienced educational methods. The findings of this study indicate variations in the adaptability of students with different learning styles in gamified learning models. For instance, active, intuitive, and visual learners generally are less suited to solitary learning modes as they prefer interactive and diversified learning approaches. Conversely, these students are better suited to competitive learning modes due to their competitive spirit and desire for challenges. Additionally, reflective, intuitive, intuitive, visual, sequential, and holistic learners are adaptable to collaborative learning modes, with visual learners being particularly adept at learning from others' perspectives. These students enjoy collaborative efforts and tend to achieve better learning outcomes in such environments. Linguistic learners may be less inclined toward gamified learning with graphic user interfaces, as they gravitate toward language and text-based learning methods and have less interest in graphical interfaces. The results of this study underscore the significance of individual learning styles in gamified learning and guide educators and designers to create effective learning environments tailored to students' needs and styles and enhance students' motivation for and effectiveness in learning. This contributes to personalized education to ensure that each student can fully unleash their potential.

Keywords: learning style; learning motivation; learning effectiveness; gamified learning model; adaptability

Citation: Lai, C.-H.; Lin, C.-Y. Exploring Personalized Gamified Learning by Computer Software: Enhancing the Effects of Learning-Style Adaptation. *Eng. Proc.* **2024**, *74*, 44. https://doi.org/10.3390/engproc2024074044

Academic Editors: Shu-Han Liao, Teen-Hang Meen and Cheng-Fu Yang

Published: 2 September 2024

1. Introduction

The operational mode of game-based learning is variable. For instance, in role-playing games, learners engage in the game by assuming one or multiple roles to solve problems or complete tasks in a virtual world according to game objectives [1]. Alternatively, computer simulations of real-life environments and scenarios provide learners with opportunities to grasp concepts. For instance, 'Stop Disasters' employs disaster simulations to help learners recognize the potential risks of natural disasters and learn how to effectively prevent and mitigate their impact on people and the environment [2]. The impact of game-based learning on students can vary depending on the specific game-based learning modes.

Various modes of game-based learning and their impact on student learning achievements and motivation were researched. The game modes encompass 'Single-Player Mode' and 'Multiplayer Mode'. In 'Single-Player Mode'. Individuals act as the primary agents of the game, unaffected by peers, and complete game objectives based on their performance. For instance, Papastergiou's research on single-player games incorporates memory-related knowledge from computer science courses into the game. This approach allowed learners to acquire course content through problem-solving and gameplay. To enhance the effectiveness of this approach, learners were required to embark on adventures throughout the game map, defeating monsters to progress to the next learning stage. This adventure-based approach facilitated course reviews and heightened learner interest [3].

The 'Multiplayer Mode' is divided into 'Competition Mode' and 'Collaborative Mode', both of which leverage peer influence as a motivational factor for learners. For example, Burguillo indicated that, over the past decade, the same course had employed different learning activities for competitive learning. The outcomes demonstrated that incorporating competitive elements into the game-based learning system stimulated learners' competitiveness during gameplay. This indicates that motivating students' learning motivation and performance can be achieved through peer competition [4]. Jong et al. integrated game elements with course content, creating online multiplayer cooperative learning games. In the study, students selected roles with different skills and collaborated with peers in teams. The findings revealed that students encountering difficult questions during the game had discussions in small groups or used their character's skills to provide an answer. Even if incorrect responses occurred, they could continue playing. The post-game analysis allowed students to identify the knowledge they lacked and reinforce their understanding. Consequently, the measured learning achievements in the game-based collaborative learning approach were significantly superior to traditional collaborative learning, demonstrating the positive impact of online multiplayer cooperative learning games on student learning effectiveness and their learning journey [5].

While prior research presented the enhanced effects of game-based learning on learning effectiveness, motivation, and even cognitive improvement [6], most studies have focused on specific game modes. There has been limited exploration into which game-based learning mode is appropriate for students. Previous results showed positive effects on students' learning behaviors, and not every student was keen on the game's mode of operation. Given the multitude of factors influencing learning behaviors [7], Chen and Macredie pointed out that key factors influencing learning include prior knowledge, gender, and cognitive style. Their experimental results demonstrated that different factors lead to variations in learning performance, even when the same learning strategy is employed [8,9]. Students' preferences in learning are a significant factor affecting learning effectiveness. Learning preferences were investigated from three dimensions: cognitive style, thinking style, and learning style. Regardless of the specific style, each impacted individual learning outcomes [10].

Based on the previous research, we developed a game-based learning system with three distinct game modes: 'Single-Player Mode', 'Competition mode', and 'Collaborative Mode'. The experimental course focused on 'Operating Systems', with students enrolled in this course as the experimental subjects. These students were grouped based on their learning styles. To compare different game modes and determine the most appropriate game-based learning mode for students, personalized and adaptive learning effects were investigated in this study.

2. Literature Review

2.1. Learning Style

Matching teaching methods to students' learning styles improves students' learning outcomes [11]. Felder and Soloman pointed out that students have their unique learning styles. However, learning styles are not inherently good or bad; they simply reflect how learners acquire information. As a result, learners possess multiple learning styles in their learning process. To enhance students' learning motivation and effectiveness, individual differences must be understood to provide tailored teaching methods that cater to different learning styles. This allows students to acquire knowledge according to their learning habits [12]. Thus, many researchers integrated learning styles into game design and investigated their impact on learning outcomes [13,14]. However, there has been no research analyzing game-based learning modes that suit a learner's learning style. Based on the previous results, we analyzed the compatibility of three game-based learning modes with students' learning styles to guide students to acquire knowledge during the gaming process and improve learning performance.

2.2. Gamified Learning Model

We categorized various digital game-based learning modes, including the single-player mode and multiplayer mode. The multiplayer mode was divided into competitive and cooperation modes.

1. Single-player mode

When learners lack peer stimulation in this mode, they need to engage in strategic thinking and methods to progress in the game. The process of investing time and effort generates intrinsic motivation, encouraging learners to strive for the mission's accomplishment or the achievement of stage goals [15]. Even when a game demands more than learners' current abilities, such as continuous training to overcome challenges, learners stick to their desire for achievement [16]. Therefore, the single-player mode in digital game-based learning enhances learners' motivation and willingness to learn independently. Repetitive practice and strategy adjustments improve learning outcomes. However, the absence of peer influence in the single-player mode leads to negative effects if the game design fails to stimulate learner motivation or lacks proper guidance. These negative effects include diverting learners' attention from learning to the game or confusing the simulation of virtual-world scenarios with real-life situations, neglecting the prerequisite of establishing the virtual environment. Therefore, the investigation of learning styles for learners in the single-player mode is important.

2. Competition mode

The digital game-based learning mode with competition enhances learning motivation [17] and promotes learning and focusing [18]. The effectiveness of the competition mode in digital game-based learning, in terms of improving learning performance, stems from establishing activity norms within this mode. Students can compete with each other within established rules to achieve goals and learn knowledge through the competitive process, which improves learning effectiveness [19,20] and encourages learners to outperform their peers due to their desire for winning or rewards. However, competitive learning has drawbacks. For instance, if learners become overly fixated on the competition, they may overlook the essence of learning [21]. In addition, competitive learning uses rankings, levels, glory, or victory as indicators of success, which leads to negative emotions, such as frustration or disappointment, especially for learners to compete. These negative emotions impact the overall learning experience. Therefore, as most studies support competitive learning to enhance learning motivation and improve learning outcomes, competition may not be appropriate for every learner. Thus, we explored which types of learning styles suit competitive learning.

Cooperative learning enables learners to construct knowledge through group discussions [22]. With the integration of information technology and cooperative learning, computer-assisted cooperative learning allows learners to overcome time and location constraints. Even when learners are in different places at different times, they can engage in collaborative activities, such as group discussions or practice exercises [23]. In Popov's study, students from different cultural backgrounds were grouped, and their perspectives on cooperative learning were investigated. The results showed that students with individualistic cultural backgrounds had more negative views of cooperative learning, suggesting that learners with a strong sense of individualism were not appropriate for collaborative learning [24]. Therefore, the appropriateness of cooperative learning requires further investigation. Therefore, we analyzed the type of learners for the cooperation mode in game-based learning to provide a personalized game-based learning environment.

3. Experiments

The subjects of this study were 122 students taking an operating system course majoring in information engineering. The students were grouped according to their learning styles. The learning-style questionnaire of the Felder–Soloman Learning Style Test was used in this study [25]. The questionnaire consists of 44 questions in 4 sets, with each set of two opposing types. Each question has two options, 'a' and 'b', representing the two opposing types. The experimental material was the content of the operating system course, which was divided into 8 concepts and assessed in three different game stages. Before the experiment, the students filled out questionnaires for motivation and learning style. The questionnaire for motivation was used for collecting pre-test data. Based on the questionnaire results, students were categorized into different style groups for an exploration of the effects of diverse game-based learning modes with different learning styles. The experiment consisted of three stages, each involving a different game-based learning mode. Each stage lasted for two weeks, and the entire experiment spanned six weeks. At the end of each stage, student performance was assessed using tests, and system usage data were collected. After completing all three stages of the experiment, students filled out a motivation questionnaire as post-test data.

Three types of game-based learning modes (single-player, competition, and cooperation) were tested. In the gameplay, the students were instructed on island adventures (Figure 1). Players can increase the mission completion rate of the islands by defeating monsters (answering questions). There are six islands: Flame Island, Desert Island, Ghost House, Starlight Tower, Forest Island, and Whale Cave. To distinguish each student who logs into the system, all the students, regardless of the game-based learning mode, registered before logging into the system with a student ID and password. The system used this registration information to identify students' performance in different game-based learning modes. Additionally, to allow students to track their learning progress, personal information was added to the system to view their current game progress and understand their learning situation. Teachers monitored students' progress through game-based learning activities.

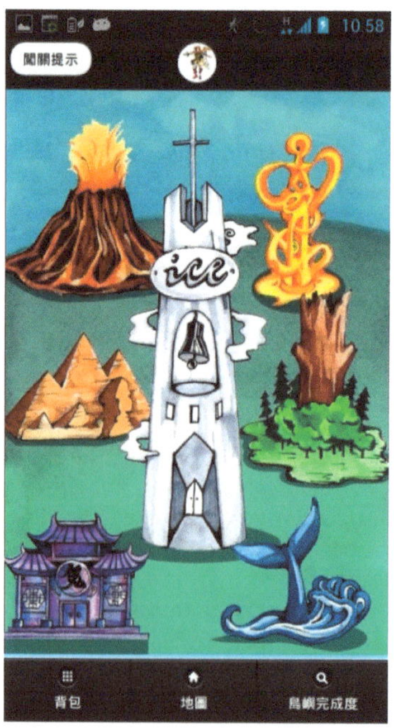

Figure 1. Interface of the game in this study.

3.1. Single-Player Mode

The single-player mode is designed with a mission-oriented approach, allowing students to explore the islands and complete the course content. When a student enters an island in the single-player mode, the system presents the game's storyline and provides relevant system operation instructions, such as the game's opening narrative. After reviewing the story content and system instructions, the student can begin the game. The adventure mode varies depending on the platform the player is using: shaking the phone or continuous mouse clicks. When the system detects that the student is shaking the phone or clicking continuously, it randomly generates questions, indicating an encounter with a monster. At this point, the student must answer the questions presented by the system. The results of these answers not only represent the student's familiarity with the topic, but also determine the rewards and penalties within the game. If a student answers a question correctly, they receive new equipment or items, while incorrect answers result in a reduction in the in-game character's health points. Due to the presence of many monsters (questions) on each island, the system randomly selects a monster (question) for students to battle (answer) when they enter an island. The questions are designed as multiple-choice questions, and students must reach a specified threshold for defeating the monsters on the island to consider the adventure completed. A successful battle indicates that the student's familiarity with the chapter has reached the system's predefined threshold. As each island is populated with a variety of monsters (questions), students entering an island engage in battles (answering questions) with these randomly selected monsters (questions).

The questions were created as multiple-choice questions, and students were required to reach a system-defined threshold for defeating the island's monsters to complete the adventure. If a student succeeds, the student reaches the level of familiarity with the content specified by the system for that chapter. To address the concerns of large quantities and prolonged answering times potentially causing student fatigue, we employed the Sequential Probability Ratio Test (SPRT) for threshold detection. To reduce the response time and the number of questions, the SPRT+ testing approach was used [26]. This method selects a probability model with high confidence. Recognizing that high confidence does not rely on students' self-assessment; the probability of answering correctly for unfamiliar concepts (Pn) is reduced from 0.75 to 0.6 in SPRT++ [27]. This means that, for each island adventure challenge, the system randomly generates ten monsters (questions). A student needs to complete the challenge by answering four questions correctly in a row, while continuous incorrect answers to four questions in a row result in challenge failure. Additionally, answering seven out of nine questions correctly is regarded as a successful challenge.

Because the single-player mode developed in this study was designed for students to complete independently, the students rely on themselves to pass each level in the game. They cannot have assistance from peers or other external support to complete these challenges. Within this framework, the impact on students with different learning styles was explored in this research to analyze the learning styles for the single-player mode in game-based learning.

3.2. Competition Mode

Based on the differentiation of various game-based learning modes using islands in the system development, students can choose the corresponding island to engage in the competition mode of game-based learning. Previous research results showed that competitive learning has positive effects on students, and incorporating competitive elements into game-based learning increases students' motivation and interest in learning. In many game-based learning studies with competitive elements, leaderboards are commonly used. For example, Hwang developed a competitive game-based learning system with a chessboard as the central theme, where players advanced a certain number of steps by rolling dice and encountered corresponding game tasks at each location. Solving these tasks earned them points. He incorporated leaderboards as a competitive element, allowing students to check their current rankings. The results of this study showed that such a competitive element improved students' learning attitudes and enhanced their interest in learning. Considering that an excessive number of competitive elements can complicate subsequent analysis in identifying specific sources of impact, the competition mode in this study adopted a leaderboard mechanism.

When students enter an island belonging to the competition mode, they can participate in island adventures similar to those in the single-player mode. They accumulate correct answers by attacking monsters (answering questions) and can check their current scores and peer rankings through the player leaderboard. This real-time leaderboard stimulates sound competition among peers. Since the course chapters corresponding to the single-player mode and competition mode are different, the progress and achievements accumulated by the students in the single-player mode are not carried over. In other words, students need to accumulate correct answers again when they switch to the competition mode, and the leaderboard in the competition mode presents activities within that mode as the basis for ranking.

3.3. Cooperation Mode

The cooperation mode is differentiated by islands in the game-based learning system. Students can choose the corresponding island for cooperative game-based learning. In the cooperation mode, when students enter an island, a level list is displayed. Each level accommodates up to 3 students. When a student chooses to enter any level, they see other students at the level. Students can view each other's equipment and status. If a student is ready to proceed, they can press the option to prepare for battle. When a student presses the ready-for-battle option, their status changes to ready. When three students in that level are ready for battle, they enter the question-answering screen. Each student takes turns to answer questions and attack monsters. When the monster's health reaches zero, they win. If there are errors in the answering process, students experience monster attacks, reducing the team's health. When the team's health reaches zero, the challenge fails. In the cooperation mode, the number of correct answers and question difficulty must be higher than in the competition mode. When students have questions at various levels, they can increase their chances of completing the challenge by discussing the questions with their team members in discussion.

4. Results and Discussion

4.1. Learning Motivation

To explore the changes in the learning motivation of students of different learning styles, we conducted a pre-test and post-test using an in-group one-way ANOVA test (Table 1). Except for linguistic learners, students with other learning styles improved their learning motivation after the experiment. F-values did not exceed the threshold, indicating that the increase in learning motivation did not have statistical significance. Though game-based learning employed a graphical user interface for visual effects, this design was less appealing to linguistic learners who preferred text and verbal modes. They may not be attracted to the visually oriented learning approach as students with other learning styles. Therefore, we observed a decrease in learning motivation among linguistic learners in the post-test.

Table 1. ANOVA test results of learning motivation for students with different learning styles pre-test and post-test.

Learning Style	Stage	N	Mean	Standard Deviation	F	Threshold
Active	Pre	12	154.083	28.659	0.389	4.301
	Post	12	160.75	23.661		
Reflective	Pre	17	159.941	33.346	0.071	4.149
	Post	17	162.588	23.529		
Sensing	Pre	21	154.857	12.444	0.135	4.085
	Post	21	158	12.570		
Intuitive	Pre	17	167.941	12.959	0.001	4.149
	Post	17	168.235	12.971		
Visual	Pre	61	155	23.776	3.76	3.92
	Post	61	162.885	21.060		
Verbal	Pre	4	172.75	52.449	0.072	5.987
	Post	4	163.75	41.788		
Sequential	Pre	10	162.6	33.738	0.227	4.414
	Post	10	168.9	24.718		
Global	Pre	21	166.238	26.717	0.152	4.085
	Post	21	169.143	21.256		

The α value is 0.05.

4.2. Learning Achievement

To understand the extent to which students with different learning styles exhibit noticeable improvements in learning achievements in various game modes, inter-group one-way ANOVA was used to analyze learning achievements before and after the experiment for each learning-style group. The results indicate the differences in learning achievements with different learning styles in different learning modes. Active learners showed significant improvements in learning achievements in the single-player and competition modes, but no significant difference was observed in the cooperation mode. Active learners performed better in competition modes, as they enjoyed challenges and competition, which stimulated their learning motivation. Reflective learners exhibited better learning achievements in the cooperation mode, whereas their performance was normal in the single-player and competition modes. Reflective learners preferred learning from other's perspectives in the cooperation mode. Intuitive learners performed well in competitive and cooperation modes, but showed less improvement in the single-player mode, indicating that intuitive learners enjoy challenging and interactive learning methods. Sensory learners demonstrated learning achievements in both competitive and cooperation modes, but their performance was less impressive in the single-player mode. Sensory learners preferred challenges and interactions. Visual learners achieved better learning outcomes in both competitive and cooperation modes, but performed less effectively in the single-player mode. Visual learners may require more visual stimuli to enhance their learning motivation.

Students with different learning styles exhibited various adaptability to different game-based learning modes. Active, intuitive, and visual learners were not suited to the single-player mode. The ANOVA results show a significant decline in these learning styles. While the students were interested in individual learning, they were inclined toward competitive and cooperation modes, which need more interaction and challenges and stimulate their learning motivation. Active, intuitive, reflective, visual, sequential, and global learners were well-suited to the competition mode. The ANOVA test results for learning achievements before and after the competition mode show significant improvements. The students performed better in competition modes because they enjoyed challenges and competition and enhanced their learning motivation.

Reflective, intuitive, sensory, visual, sequential, and global learners were well-suited to the cooperation mode, with visual learners particularly excelling in this mode. The ANOVA test results show a significant improvement for the students. Visual learners exhibited higher adaptability to the cooperation mode, possibly because they preferred teamwork and learning from others' perspectives. Verbal learners were less suited to game-based learning with a graphical user interface. These students were less interested in graphical interface game-based learning without significant improvement. In the experiment, the graphical interface was a challenge for verbal learners, who tended to learn through language and text-based learning. Active learners were not appropriate for the single-player mode but for the competition mode. Reflective learners were good at the cooperation mode, and they did not prefer the single-player mode, though their performance was acceptable. Active learners exhibited a significant decline in the single-player mode but improved in the competition mode, indicating they were better fitted to the competition mode. Reflective learners achieved better learning outcomes in the cooperation mode, and despite their lower preference for the single-player mode, their performance in this mode was acceptable.

5. Conclusions

We explored the adaptability of students with different learning styles in different learning modes in a game-based learning environment. Through the analysis of the experimental results, the following conclusions were obtained.

There were differences in the adaptability of students to different learning styles in the game-based learning modes. Active, intuitive, and visual learners were not good at the single-player mode. These students decreased their learning achievements in the single-player mode, possibly because they were inclined toward competition and cooperation for interaction and challenges. Therefore, in the design of game-based learning courses, educators must avoid the application of a single mode for students of various learning styles. Active, intuitive, reflective, visual, sequential, and global learners were good in the competition mode. These students improved their learning achievements in the competition mode, indicating their higher demand for challenges and competition. The competition mode stimulated their learning motivation and motivated them to engage in learning. Therefore, when designing competitive game courses, integrating elements of different learning styles must be considered to attract a broader range of students. Reflective, intuitive, sensory, visual, sequential, and global learners were good in the cooperation mode, with visual learners being adaptable to this mode. These students improved their learning achievements in the cooperation mode because they preferred teamwork and learning from others' perspectives. The cooperation mode cultivated students' collaborative abilities and provided a conducive environment for knowledge-sharing. Therefore, in the design of cooperative game courses, we must consider how to guide students to collaborate better, especially visual learners. Verbal learners were less appropriate for game-based learning with a graphical user interface. These students were less interested in graphical interface game-based learning, and there was no significant improvement observed in the learning achievements. They were challenged and preferred language and text-based learning. Therefore, it is necessary to provide diverse interface options to meet the needs of students with different learning styles.

The results of this study underscore the importance of learning styles in game-based learning modes and provide the basis for the design of personalized learning environments.

The results contribute to enhancing students' learning motivation and achievements and can be used for the development of education. Personalized education is the future of education as it ensures that every student realizes their potential in game-based learning. The needs of students with different learning styles need to be understood to offer adaptive learning environments for innovation in education.

Author Contributions: Conceptualization, C.-H.L.; methodology, C.-H.L.; software, C.-Y.L.; validation, C.-H.L.; resources, C.-H.L.; data curation, C.-H.L.; writing—original draft preparation, C.-H.L.; writing—review and editing, C.-H.L.; visualization, C.-H.L.; supervision, C.-H.L. and C.-Y.L. All authors have read and agreed to the published version of the manuscript.

Funding: This research received no external funding.

Institutional Review Board Statement: Not applicable.

Informed Consent Statement: Not applicable.

Data Availability Statement: Data are not available due to school privacy policies.

Conflicts of Interest: The authors declare no conflicts of interest.

References

1. Schmitz, B.; Schuffelen, P.; Kreijns, K.; Klemke, R.; Specht, M. Putting yourself in someone else's shoes: The impact of a location-based, collaborative role-playing game on behaviour. *Comput. Educ.* **2015**, *85*, 160–169. [CrossRef]
2. Pereira, G.; Prada, R.; Paiva, A. Disaster prevention social awareness: The stop disasters! case study. In Proceedings of the 2014 6th International Conference on Games and Virtual Worlds for Serious Applications (VS-GAMES), Valletta, Malta, 9–12 September 2014; pp. 1–8.
3. Papastergiou, M. Digital game-based learning in high school computer science education: Impact on educational effectiveness and student motivation. *Comput. Educ.* **2009**, *52*, 1–12. [CrossRef]
4. Burguillo, J.C. Using game theory and competition-based learning to stimulate student motivation and performance. *Comput. Educ.* **2010**, *55*, 566–575. [CrossRef]
5. Jong, B.S.; Lai, C.H.; Hsia, Y.T.; Lin, T.W.; Lu, C.Y. Using game-based cooperative learning to improve learning motivation: A study of online game use in an operating systems course. *IEEE Trans. Educ.* **2012**, *56*, 183–190. [CrossRef]
6. Hussein, M.H.; Ow, S.H.; Cheong, L.S.; Thong, M.K. A digital game-based learning method to improve students' critical thinking skills in elementary science. *IEEE Access* **2019**, *7*, 96309–96318. [CrossRef]
7. Zimmerman, B.J. Self-efficacy and educational development. *Self-Effic. Chang. Soc.* **1995**, *1*, 202–231.
8. Chen, S.Y.; Macredie, R.D. Cognitive modeling of student learning in web-based instructional programs. *Int. J. Hum.-Comput. Interact.* **2004**, *17*, 375–402. [CrossRef]
9. Chen, S.Y.; Macredie, R. Web-based interaction: A review of three important human factors. *Int. J. Inf. Manag.* **2010**, *30*, 379–387. [CrossRef]
10. Zhang, L.F. Further investigation thinking styles and psychosocial development in the Chinese higher education context. *Learn. Individ. Differ.* **2010**, *20*, 593–603. [CrossRef]
11. Smith, P.; Dalton, J. Accommodating learning styles: Relevance and good practice in VET. *Teacher* **2005**, *159*, 26–27.
12. Felder, R.M.; Silverman, L.K. Learning and teaching styles in engineering education. *Eng. Educ.* **1988**, *78*, 674–681.
13. Steck, L.W.; Engler, J.N.; Ligon, M.; Druen, P.B.; Cosgrove, E. Doing poverty: Learning outcomes among students participating in the community action poverty simulation program. *Teach. Sociol.* **2011**, *39*, 259–273. [CrossRef]
14. Toni Mohr, A.; Holtbrügge, D.; Berg, N. Learning style preferences and the perceived usefulness of e-learning. *Teach. High. Educ.* **2012**, *17*, 309–322. [CrossRef]
15. Orvis, K.A.; Horn, D.B.; Belanich, J. The roles of task difficulty and prior videogame experience on performance and motivation in instructional videogames. *Comput. Hum. Behav.* **2008**, *24*, 2415–2433. [CrossRef]
16. McCauley, C.D.; Van Velsor, E. (Eds.) *The Center for Creative Leadership Handbook of Leadership Development*; John Wiley & Sons: Hoboken, NJ, USA, 2004; Volume 29.
17. Hwang, G.J.; Chang, S.C. Effects of a peer competition-based mobile learning approach on students' affective domain exhibition in social studies courses. *Br. J. Educ. Technol.* **2016**, *47*, 1217–1231.
18. Chen, Z.H.; Liao, C.; Chien, T.C.; Chan, T.W. Animal companions: Fostering children's effort-making by nurturing virtual pets. *Br. J. Educ. Technol.* **2011**, *42*, 166–180. [CrossRef]
19. Chen, C.H.; Law, V.; Chen, W.Y. The effects of peer competition-based science learning game on secondary students' performance, achievement goals, and perceived ability. *Interact. Learn. Environ.* **2018**, *26*, 235–244. [CrossRef]
20. Sung, H.Y.; Hwang, G.J. Facilitating effective digital game-based learning behaviors and learning performances of students based on a collaborative knowledge construction strategy. *Interact. Learn. Environ.* **2018**, *26*, 118–134. [CrossRef]

21. Van Eck, R.; Dempsey, J. The effect of competition and contextualized advisement on the transfer of mathematics skills a computer-based instructional simulation game. *Educ. Technol. Res. Dev.* **2002**, *50*, 23–41. [CrossRef]
22. Shukor, N.B.A.; Tasir, Z.; van der Meijden, H.A.T.; Harun, J. Exploring students' knowledge construction strategies in computer-supported collaborative learning discussions using sequential analysis. *Educ. Technol. Soc.* **2014**, *17*, 216–228.
23. Balakrishnan, V. Using social networks to enhance teaching and learning experiences in higher learning institutions. *Innov. Educ. Teach. Int.* **2014**, *51*, 595–606. [CrossRef]
24. Popov, V.; Noroozi, O.; Barrett, J.B.; Biemans, H.J.; Teasley, S.D.; Slof, B.; Mulder, M. Perceptions and experiences of, and outcomes for, university students in culturally diversified dyads in a computer-supported collaborative learning environment. *Comput. Hum. Behav.* **2014**, *32*, 186–200. [CrossRef]
25. Felder, R.M.; Soloman, B.A. Index of Learning Styles Questionnaire. Available online: https://learningstyles.webtools.ncsu.edu/ (accessed on 30 January 2024).
26. Halpern, D.F. Assessing the effectiveness of critical thinking instruction. *J. Gen. Educ.* **2001**, *50*, 270–286. [CrossRef]
27. Lai, C.H.; Lee, T.P.; Jong, B.S.; Hsia, Y.T. Using SPRT+ to Reduce Measure Time on Student Learning Efficiency by Pre-defined Student's Confidence Indicator. *Int. J. Emerg. Technol. Learn. (iJET)* **2014**, *9*, 55–58. [CrossRef]

engineering proceedings

Proceeding Paper

Digital Diplomacy: A Case Study of Foreign Relations of Mongolian and India in Social Media by Big Data Analysis and Computation †

Shinetsetseg Jargalsaikhan, Shu-Chin Huang and I-Tung Shih *

Department of Business Administration, College of Management, Chaoyang University of Technology, Taichung 411310, Taiwan; shinee.jargalsaikhan@gmail.com (S.J.); schuang2@gm.cyut.edu.tw (S.-C.H.)
* Correspondence: itungshih99@gmail.com

† Presented at the 2024 IEEE 4th International Conference on Electronic Communications, Internet of Things and Big Data, Taipei, Taiwan, 19–21 April 2024.

Abstract: We explored digital diplomacy, an evolving field, focusing on the digital engagement strategies of India and Mongolia from 2012 to 2022 through a quantitative analysis of secondary data sourced from social media platforms. We investigated how these countries utilized digital tools to shape their international relations, highlighting the impact of digital diplomacy on traditional diplomatic practices and the potential for enhancing public diplomacy. By examining parameters such as post frequency and engagement rates, significant differences were determined to suggest strategic improvements for Mongolia. The findings offer the basis for the adoption of digital diplomacy, emphasizing its role in reshaping global interactions in the digital era.

Keywords: information and technology; international relations; public diplomacy; soft power; digital diplomacy

Citation: Jargalsaikhan, S.; Huang, S.-C.; Shih, I.-T. Digital Diplomacy: A Case Study of Foreign Relations of Mongolian and India in Social Media by Big Data Analysis and Computation. *Eng. Proc.* **2024**, *74*, 45. https://doi.org/10.3390/engproc2024074045

Academic Editors: Shu-Han Liao, Teen-Hang Meen and Cheng-Fu Yang

Published: 3 September 2024

1. Introduction

The rapid evolution of Information and Communication Technology (ICT) has significantly transformed diplomatic practices, enhancing the efficiency and innovation of global interactions [1]. This technological progression has strengthened both bilateral and multilateral relations, providing diplomats with advanced tools that facilitate active participation in international negotiations. This engagement helps them understand diverse perspectives and complex policies profoundly. The development of digital diplomacy strategies has revolutionized how nations engage, utilize social media and various digital platforms, and connect with global stakeholders and advocate their values and priorities effectively [2]. Recent exponential growth in the ICT sector highlights the increasing importance of digital tools in diplomacy. Diplomats are now required to master these technologies to stay competitive [3]. Many countries are investing heavily in digital diplomacy, recognizing its potential to transform traditional practices and significantly contribute to achieving foreign policy goals. The effective use of digital tools can enhance a nation's image, promote positive changes, and foster successful international cooperation [4].

Previous research has examined digital diplomacy's role across different nations. Researchers [5] explored digital tools and applications of Western Balkans' Foreign Ministries, explaining their strategic use. Antwi-Boateng [6] noted the challenges faced by the UAE, such as media regulations that balance the empowerment provided by digital tools against potential security risks. Listyowati [7] emphasized Indonesia's engagement with digital advancements to strengthen its regional influence and international collaborations.

Consequently, we scrutinized case studies of successful practitioners of digital diplomacy in India and Mongolia, focusing on these digital nations within the Asian continent.

The study result bridges the gap by using a quantitative methodology by analyzing secondary data retrieved from social media platforms including Facebook and Twitter and evaluating the activities and interactions of both nations over a decade from 2012 to 2022. By integrating Constructivist Theory and Actor-Network Theory, we explained digital diplomacy to understand digital diplomatic practices and offered practical implications for policymakers and diplomats to enhance their countries' diplomatic efforts on digital platforms. The results can be used to guide strategies for countries to improve their digital diplomacy practices, aiding in their engagement, public relations, and soft power efforts on the global stage.

2. Literature Review

2.1. Constructivist Theory

Constructivist Theory, advocated by Alexander [8], emphasizes the role of prevailing ideas and identities in shaping state actions, focusing on social constructs over purely rational considerations. Martha [9], Peter [10], and Nicholas [11] expanded this theory, applying it to various facets of international relations, including norms and identities within the global political arena. Constructivist Theory is relevant to digital diplomacy. For instance, Yousef [12] showed how non-state actors such as new media significantly alter international behaviors, pushing the evolution of public diplomacy strategies and emphasizing the role of shared norms. Rus Shafinas [13] explored how communication processes and behavioral modeling influence digital diplomacy and international relations. This theory helps to understand how the platforms develop shared meanings and new diplomatic norms, influencing the creation of perceptions and the formation of diplomatic relationships in our digital age.

2.2. Actor-Network Theory

Originating from Science and Technology Studies, Actor-Network Theory (ANT) treats technological objects as equal to human agents, a perspective that gained traction in international relations due to its emphasis on materiality and the dynamic nature of technological and human interactions. Christian [14] discussed how ANT underscores the need for diplomatic representation tools and the inclusion of both professional and private actors in diplomacy. Huxley [15] revealed how digital transformation is shaped by cultural and political contexts, influencing global diplomatic practices in Finland's Ministry of Foreign Affairs using ANT. Almuftah [16] reviewed the necessity to explore e-diplomacy's various facets through theories like ANT. This theory provides a unique way to examine the intricate relationships and power dynamics among technological tools, government bodies, and public entities to enhance the understanding of how digital diplomacy is practiced between India and Mongolia.

2.3. Digital Diplomacy and Public Administration

Digital diplomacy has emerged as a crucial strategy in modern international relations to promote a country's interests and values globally without coercion. Implemented alongside traditional diplomatic channels, this strategy demands digital tools to foster dialog, cultural exchange, and economic cooperation, enhancing international relationships and shifting the power dynamics between states and citizens [3]. It involves various online platforms to engage international audiences, counter misinformation, and advance national agendas [17]. However, the impact of digital diplomacy can be elusive and often gauged by social media metrics such as followers and engagement levels [18]. The widespread adoption of digital platforms in diplomatic circles underscores the growing importance of digital engagement in maintaining global relationships [19,20].

3. Research Methods

We employed a comparative and big data analytical approach to assess the digital diplomacy strategies of India and Mongolia, focusing on their social media usage over the past decade. By analyzing data from platforms, including Facebook and Twitter, we explored the effectiveness of each nation's digital diplomacy efforts. For the analysis, a range of diplomatic activities and metrics such as post frequency, content types, and engagement levels were analyzed to provide a view of their strategies and impact. This study adhered to high ethical standards, ensuring all data used are handled responsibly, reflecting the scholarly intent of this investigation.

4. Analysis Results

4.1. Digital Revolution of India

India has significantly advanced its digital diplomacy efforts by utilizing online platforms to amplify diplomatic operations amid resource constraints [20]. Initiated in 2010 by the Indian Ministry of External Affairs, this foray into digital diplomacy was adopted by Former Foreign Minister S.M. Krishna who began using Twitter in 2011 to address the concerns of Indians abroad. India's digital strategy includes using mobile apps, video conferencing, and high-speed internet to connect with both domestic and international audiences effectively [21]. Prime Minister Narendra Modi has been a pivotal figure in these efforts, advocating for a proactive digital diplomacy approach. As the Asian leader with the most Twitter followers, Modi uses these platforms to enhance India's global image as an environmentally conscious and development-oriented nation. His social media prowess was notably demonstrated during his 2014 election campaign, and he continues to engage with a global audience. Modi's Twitter account, established in 2009, has amassed 92.9 million followers, and his Facebook page, also started in 2009, boasts 48 million followers [22]. His posts typically receive widespread interaction, exemplifying the significant impact of his digital engagement [23]. The extent of his influence is illustrated in Figure 1, which charts the growth of his Twitter and Facebook followers.

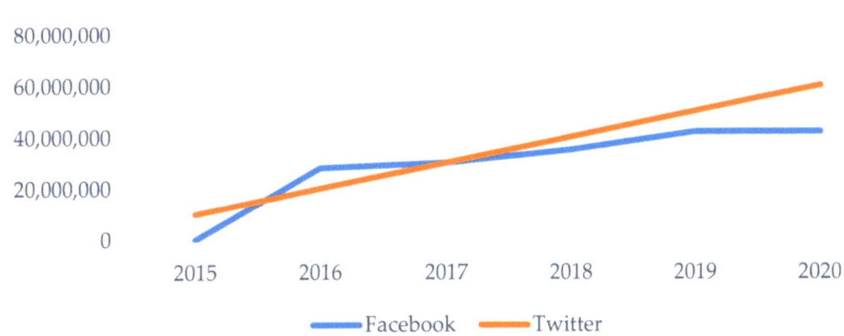

Figure 1. Growth of Narendra Modi's social media pages.

4.2. Embassy of India in Mongolia

Recognized globally for its effective use of social media, the Indian Ministry of External Affairs ranks among the top social media users. With substantial followings on digital platforms, the ministry engages with millions, setting a benchmark in digital diplomacy relations [20]. The embassy in Mongolia reflects this strategy by actively maintaining strong ties with the Indian government and its people and by managing a significant online presence. This proactive engagement on social media helps foster and sustain diplomatic relationships far beyond the Indian subcontinent [21].

4.3. *Impact of President of Mongolia on Digital Diplomacy*

Mongolia's adoption of digital diplomacy under President Khurelsukh Ukhanaa illustrates the potential of ICT in enhancing international relations, even among smaller nations [18,24]. Since joining social media in 2012, Ukhanaa has used these platforms sporadically, with notable increases in activity during certain years. His engagement has highlighted Mongolia's stance on international issues, as evidenced by his congratulatory tweet to Prime Minister Modi on India's vaccination milestone, which garnered significant attention. However, the engagement level of his accounts suggests room for increased consistency and broader strategic use of digital platforms. This is detailed in Figure 2, which shows the use of Facebook and Twitter by President Ukhanaa.

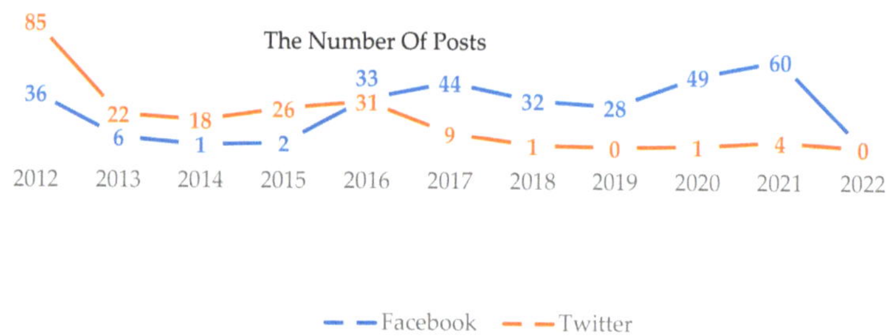

Figure 2. Use of Facebook and Twitter by U. Khurelsukh.

4.4. *Embassy of Mongolia in India*

Since its establishment on Facebook in 2012, the Embassy of Mongolia in India has used the platform to enhance bilateral relations and promote Mongolia's cultural and diplomatic initiatives. Despite a notable decrease in posting frequency and engagement from 2018 to 2021, the embassy's digital presence remains crucial for its diplomatic strategy. The absence of a Twitter account represents an opportunity for expansion to reach wider audiences and enhance digital engagement. This is reflected in Figure 3, which shows the embassy's Facebook usage and trends in engagement and post frequency over the years.

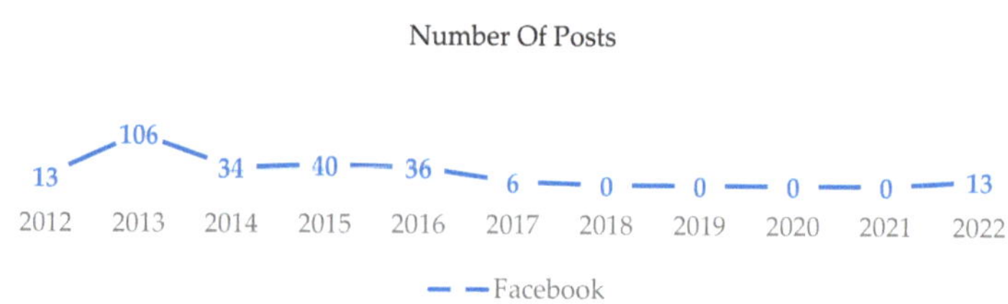

Figure 3. Facebook usage of Embassy of Mongolia in India.

Overall, both India and Mongolia demonstrate robust digital diplomacy efforts with varying degrees of emphasis and success. By leveraging social media effectively, these nations further enhance their international presence and diplomatic reach.

5. Conclusions

In modern diplomacy, digital diplomacy is a crucial tool for leveraging technology to enhance communication and collaboration rapidly and effectively. Digital diplomats play a key role in managing these interactions, ensuring that technology and information are used efficiently across policy development, government administration, and international relations. In this study, India as a leader in digital diplomacy, with Prime Minister

Narendra Modi driving the country was highlighted for a prominent global status. Over the past 14 years, India has skillfully used digital diplomacy to engage its citizens and a broad international audience, successfully promoting its cultural and developmental achievements.

However, the adoption of digital diplomacy varies significantly worldwide among wealthy and developing countries. Mongolia, for example, despite having a high number of internet users, shows limited implementation of digital diplomacy by its government officials. President Khurelsukh Ukhnaa has been relatively slow to adopt this modern approach. Nevertheless, the substantial populations of Indians in Mongolia and Mongolians in India—approximately 200 and 900, respectively—demonstrate significant potential for expanding digital diplomacy efforts between these two nations.

The result of this study emphasizes the ongoing need for effective digital diplomacy. It highlights the importance of the Constructivist Theory and the Actor-Network Theory, which provide frameworks for understanding the dynamic and transformative landscape of digital diplomacy. These theories reshape the conceptual framework of international relations in the digital era. By underscoring the critical role of technological advancements, the importance of digital diplomacy is reaffirmed in enhancing diplomatic practices and fostering stronger, more productive international relationships.

Author Contributions: Conceptualization, I.-T.S. and S.J.; Methodology, S.J.; Formal Analysis, S.J.; Investigation, I.-T.S.; Resource, S.-C.H.; Data Curation, I.-T.S.; Writing—Original Draft, S.J.; Writing and Review—Editing, S.-C.H.; Visualization, S.J.; Supervision, S.-C.H.; Project Administrator, I.-T.S.; Funding Acquisition, I.-T.S. All authors have read and agreed to the published version of the manuscript.

Funding: No external financial support was provided for this research.

Institutional Review Board Statement: Not applicable.

Informed Consent Statement: Not applicable.

Data Availability Statement: The information utilized to substantiate the outcomes of this research can be obtained by contacting the corresponding author via email at itungshih99@gmail.com.

Acknowledgments: The authors express their deep gratitude to Senior Lecturer P. Myagmardorj, Department of International Relations and Social Studies at the University of Humanities, whose valuable counsel and contributions regarding Mongolian insights significantly enhanced the content of this research.

Conflicts of Interest: The authors declare no conflicts of interest.

References

1. Ming'ala, M. The Role of 21St Century Communication Technology in Diplomatic Engagement. Doctoral Dissertation, University of Nairobi, Nairobi, Kenya, 2019.
2. Verrekia, B. Digital Diplomacy and Its Effect on International Relations. 2017. Available online: https://digitalcollections.sit.edu/isp_collection/2596 (accessed on 15 September 2023).
3. Bradshaw, S. *Digital Diplomacy-# Notdiplomacy*; Centre of International Governance Innovation: Waterloo, ON, Canada, 2015.
4. Hayden, C. Digital diplomacy. In *The Encyclopedia of Diplomacy*; JohnWiley & Sons, Ltd.: Hoboken, NJ, USA, 2018; pp. 1–13.
5. Justinek, G.; Carli, S.; Omahna, I. Digital Diplomacy in Practice: A Case Study of the Western Balkan Countries. In *Politics and Technology in the Post-Truth Era*; Visvizi, A., Lytras, M.D., Eds.; Emerald Publishing Limited: Bradford, UK, 2019; pp. 187–202.
6. Antwi-Boateng, O.; Al Mazrouei, K.A.M. The challenges of digital diplomacy in the era of globalization: The case of the United Arab Emirates. *Int. J. Commun.* **2021**, *15*, 19.
7. Listyowati, P.; Damayanti, C.; Dewi, U.N.M. Indonesia's Role in Digital Diplomacy Through the Regional Conference on Digital Diplomacy (RCDD). *Mandala J. Ilmu Hub. Int.* **2022**, *5*, 173–189.
8. Wendt, A. *Social Theory of International Politics*; Cambridge University Press: Cambridge, UK, 1999.
9. Finnemore, M. *National Interests in International Society*; Cornell University Press: Ithaca, NY, USA, 1996.
10. Katzenstein, P.J.; Keohane, R.O.; Krasner, S.D. International organization and the study of world politics. *Int. Organ.* **1998**, *52*, 645–685. [CrossRef]
11. Onuf, N.G. Constructivism. In *World of Our Making*; Routledge: Oxfordshire, UK, 2012; pp. 35–65.

12. Fassihi, Y.; Soorizadeh, A.; Nazerian, H. Investigating the Effect of Modern Diplomacy on Foreign Policy based on Constructivist Theory. *Int. J. Political Sci.* **2022**, *12*, 121–140.
13. Shafie, R.S. The Psychosemantic Realm of Social Media Warfare Affecting Public Diplomacy. *Proceedings* **2022**, *82*, 97. [CrossRef]
14. Bueger, C.; Stockbruegger, J. Actor-network theory. In *Technology and World Politics: An Introduction*; Routledge: Oxfordshire, UK, 2017; pp. 42–59.
15. Huxley, A. Discovering digital diplomacy: The case of mediatization in the Ministry for Foreign Affairs of Finland. 2014. Available online: https://www.diva-portal.org/smash/record.jsf?pid=diva2:747680&dswid=6878 (accessed on 15 September 2023).
16. Almuftah, H.; Weerakkody, V.; Sivarajah, U. e-Diplomacy: A systematic literature review. In Proceedings of the 9th International Conference on Theory and Practice of Electronic Governance, Montevideo, Uruguay, 1–3 March 2016; pp. 131–134.
17. Adesina, O.S. Foreign policy in an era of digital diplomacy. *Cogent Soc. Sci.* **2017**, *3*, 1297175. [CrossRef]
18. Rashica, V. The benefits and risks of digital diplomacy. *Seeu Rev.* **2018**, *13*, 75–89. [CrossRef]
19. Bjola, C.; Holmes, M. *Digital Diplomacy: Theory and Practice*; Routledge: Oxfordshire, UK, 2015.
20. Singh, S. Digital Diplomacy: India's Increasing Digital Footprints. *SSPC Res. Pap.* **2018**, *12*, 1–17.
21. Garud-Patkar, N. Is digital diplomacy an effective foreign policy tool? Evaluating India's digital diplomacy through agenda-building in South Asia. *Place Brand. Public Dipl.* **2022**, *18*, 128–143. [CrossRef]
22. Narendra Modi. 2023. Available online: https://twitter.com/narendramodi?s=11&t=D52L7aoTOTNATR--HFnqqA (accessed on 15 September 2023).
23. 2022. Available online: https://www.trackalytics.com/twitter/profile/narendramodi/ (accessed on 15 April 2022).
24. Digital Diplomacy Index. 2023. Available online: https://digital-diplomacy-index.com (accessed on 15 April 2022).

engineering proceedings

MDPI

Proceeding Paper

Hybrid Learning Effects on Indonesian Students Majoring in Industrial Engineering for Understanding and Performance: A Case Study with an Experimental Design †

Riana Magdalena Silitonga [1,2], Ferdian Aditya Pratama [3,*] and Ronald Sukwadi [1,4,*]

1 Department of Industrial Engineering, Atma Jaya Catholic University of Indonesia, Jakarta 12930, Indonesia; riana.magdalena@atmajaya.ac.id
2 Department of Industrial and Systems Engineering, Chung Yuan Christian University, Taoyuan City 32014, Taiwan
3 Data Science Department, Universitas Bunda Mulia, Jakarta 15143, Indonesia
4 Professional Engineer Program, Atma Jaya Catholic University of Indonesia, Jakarta 12930, Indonesia
* Correspondence: ferdian.aditya@outlook.com (F.A.P.); ronald.sukwadi@atmajaya.ac.id (R.S.)
† Presented at the 2024 IEEE 4th International Conference on Electronic Communications, Internet of Things and Big Data, Taipei, Taiwan, 19–21 April 2024.

Abstract: Due to the COVID-19 pandemic, most schools and colleges have adopted hybrid learning. Hybrid learning, also called "blended learning," mixes online and classroom instruction. Blended learning may become permanent as face-to-face and internet-based education become more accepted. We examined how hybrid learning affects the understanding of Indonesian students majoring in Industrial Engineering at Atma Jaya Catholic University. In this study, understanding matched learning efficacy. An experimental design was used to measure component influence. In strategic planning, strengths, weaknesses, opportunities, and threats (SWOT) analysis was used as an effective tool to examine an organization's internal and external variables with a learning methodology design. A questionnaire survey was conducted to measure the understanding of the SWOT analysis results and the related strategy. A total of 96 participants were involved in this study. The mixed learning method, using the weakness–opportunity or mini–maxi strategy with the divestment–investment principle, was found to be effective.

Keywords: experimental design; hybrid learning; learning method; SWOT analysis

Citation: Silitonga, R.M.; Aditya Pratama, F.; Sukwadi, R. Hybrid Learning Effects on Indonesian Students Majoring in Industrial Engineering for Understanding and Performance: A Case Study with an Experimental Design. *Eng. Proc.* **2024**, *74*, 46. https://doi.org/10.3390/engproc2024074046

Academic Editors: Shu-Han Liao, Teen-Hang Meen and Cheng-Fu Yang

Published: 3 September 2024

1. Introduction

Information technology is a means to disseminate collective knowledge for educational innovations. Innovative technology-based educational tools such as mobile devices, smartboards, Massive Open Online Courses (MOOCs), tablets, laptops, simulations, dynamic visualizations, and virtual laboratories have significantly transformed the educational landscape in schools and institutions [1]. In the last ten years, digitalization has influenced the global educational system, garnering attention from professionals, scholars, and policymakers in order to enhance educational progress [2]. While technological education covers various areas and is tailored to individual characteristics, there is a lack of studies on the selection of themes and career education during free semesters. Consequently, professors are hesitant to accept hybrid learning systems due to the extra burden they entail [3]. The current frameworks of technological knowledge derived from the philosophy of technology have not been widely utilized in technology education, particularly in the design of curricula. This is likely because most of these frameworks were not originally developed for technology education [4].

The hybrid learning system is anticipated to provide a resolution and combine in-person learning experiences by optimizing the utilization of technology when students are required to study remotely or online due to the pandemic [5]. The hybrid learning system has advantages such as fostering a productive and streamlined learning experience, providing easy accessibility and flexibility, reducing expenses and energy consumption in education, and enabling students to achieve optimal independent learning [6]. Implementing a hybrid learning system impacts students' metacognitive awareness [7]. Presently, there is significant progress in the advancement of hybrid learning, which is derived from the amalgamation of one or more models, methodologies, or media [8]. Indonesia is developing several hybrid learning methods, including face-to-face lectures, synchronous virtual collaboration, asynchronous virtual collaboration, and self-paced asynchronous learning [9].

There are several issues related to the quality of education in Indonesia. The main challenges faced in the education system include facilities, the inadequate quality of teachers, low student achievement, a lack of student interest in reading, the high cost of education, and the need for greater diversity tolerance (SARA) [10]. Hybrid learning has gained popularity in developed countries owing to the widespread availability of the internet. Extensive research has been conducted in developing countries, particularly in the ASEAN region. The disparity in the number of pupils and teachers occurs in developing and developed countries [11]. Indonesia's education system has been characterized by a large quantity of education but lacking in quality, failing to meet the country's aspirations for an education system at an international level. The causes for this are insufficient money, lack of human resources, flawed incentive systems, and ineffective management. However, the underlying cause is related to political dynamics and power struggles [12].

The Industrial Engineering Study Program of the Atma Jaya Catholic University of Indonesia has traditionally adhered to conventional learning methods known as teacher-centered learning until recently. Nevertheless, it has adjusted and adhered to the progress of education by using a student-centered learning approach. Consequently, the hybrid learning paradigm has been introduced in the Performance Measurement and Improvement course. Hybrid learning cultivates students to be engaged, self-reliant, accountable, creative, and proactive in their learning. In order to guarantee the effectiveness of the hybrid learning model, educational administrators must consider the following key factors: the integration of existing technologies, the provision of adequate student support facilities, motivation strategies, and the development of a well-designed and balanced online curriculum for students.

Currently, students in the Industrial Engineering study program at Atma Jaya Catholic University of Indonesia lack motivation and performance. This can be linked to the monotony associated with the traditional learning approach, which primarily emphasizes the role of professors. Consequently, a new instructional approach is needed to adopt hybrid learning. Hybrid learning is beneficial for stimulating students' curiosity and enhancing their efficiency by motivating them to be updated with campus improvements and changes. This learning strategy also encourages students to engage with the materials to actively acquire knowledge [13]. The hybrid learning model is anticipated to enhance students' motivation and performance, beyond the levels observed in the conventional learning paradigm. The effectiveness of implementing the hybrid learning paradigm has been confirmed by the results of multiple prior studies [14–18]. Hybrid learning is advantageous for students and their learning process. However, because of the diversity of the people involved, the outcomes of this program may vary.

We investigated the students' understanding of the learning process implemented through a hybrid learning approach. Utilizing the principles of experimental design and the True Experimental Design Nested Factorial Experiment, we conducted a SWOT analysis to develop strategies and establish a hybrid learning strategy. Such a hybrid learning approach can be used to enhance the learning outcomes of individual students with diverse personal backgrounds. We also explored how the hybrid learning model effectively enhanced students' academic performance and understanding.

2. Literature Review

2.1. Hybrid Learning

Virtual learning and hybrid learning facilitate learning and foster the development of digital literacy by promoting the utilization of digital resources as a means of communication [19]. In digital literacy, technology is the key to seeking and assessing resources and obtaining accurate and pertinent material for effective communication [20]. The authors of reference [21] examined how the combination of hybrid learning and critical thinking abilities affects the writing performance of undergraduate learners in Indonesia. The findings indicated that the implementation of hybrid Task-Based Language Teaching (TBLT) influenced the writing proficiency of the students.

Multiple researchers examined the influence of hybrid learning on digital literacy in language learning. The influence of hybrid learning on digital literacy was surveyed for fifteen undergraduate students enrolled in English Language Study Program Research [22]. Hybrid learning significantly enhanced the students' proficiency in digital literacy. Hybrid learning impacted grammar and digital literacy, too [23]. The findings indicated that the implementation of hybrid learning improved students' proficiency in grammar and digital literacy. In previous research, the effects of hybrid learning or the use of a single application on digital literacy in various academic fields were confirmed.

2.2. Experimental Design

The objective of the experimental research design is to ascertain the causal links between the independent and dependent variable(s). While there is ongoing discussion regarding the definition of a causal relationship [24], experts in organizational and behavioral sciences [25] agree that a cause–effect relationship is determined by three criteria: (a) a consistent relationship between the independent and dependent variables; (b) the independent variable changing before the dependent variable; and (c) ruling out other possible explanations for the observed relationship. Experimental study designs are crucial to reduce potential risks to internal validity. Internal validity refers to the level of confidence in the causal relationship between a spontaneous or manipulated change in the independent variable and the resulting change in the dependent variable [26].

2.3. Strengths, Weaknesses, Opportunities, and Threats (SWOT) Analysis

SWOT analysis was introduced in the early 1950s as a framework for examining organizational plans [27]. This framework has been extensively utilized in education for strategic planning and decision-making in complex situations that necessitate the perspectives of the talents of different individuals involved [28]. SWOT analysis offers a systematic framework for collecting information from different sources and presents a comprehensive assessment of the internal (strengths and weaknesses) and external elements (threats and opportunities) that may impact the incorporation of new technology in education [29]. SWOT analysis is employed to build plans based on internal and external elements that have the potential to impact decision-making within the business [30]. The advantages of using this method include the following: (a) providing a broad overview of the objective and establishing a framework for solving a problem by starting with a general approach and then moving to specific details; (b) being applicable at both the organizational and macroeconomic levels and addressing various decision subjects; and (c) highlighting opportunities and guiding decision-makers in addressing weaknesses and threats [31].

3. Methodology

3.1. Data Collection

We employed a probability sampling method (stratified random sampling) to recruit participants. Out of a population of 261 students majoring in industrial engineering at Atma Jaya Catholic University of Indonesia, aged between 18 and 23 years, 72 students were selected as participants. The example figures were calculated using the Slovin formula.

We gathered their performance data with factors using the Material Test, which was designed as part of the Measuring and Performance Improvement course material. The examination comprised 40 questions that were randomly organized with a variety of materials. For SWOT analysis, we collected data using qualitative and quantitative methods. The qualitative data were obtained by observing the learning activities of the participants. The quantitative data were gathered by a questionnaire on a 5-point Likert scale. The questionnaire consisted of items to measure the factors and indicators of learning approaches. The questionnaire responses in four sections were scored and weighted in SWOT analysis.

3.2. Research Variables

The dependent variable of this study was the efficacy of the learning method, while the independent variables were the aspects to influence the efficacy of the learning method. The independent factors including hybrid learning (M1), conventional learning (M2), and the performance rate (M3) were categorized into good (P1), average (P2), and poor (P3) groups. Gender was included as another independent variable.

3.3. Hypothesis

We employed an analysis of variance (ANOVA) and the F-value to assess the impact of the factor. Based on the computations, the null hypothesis (H0) and alternative hypothesis were tested at a certain significance level (α) (Table 1).

Table 1. Research hypotheses of this study.

Purposes	H0	H1
To test the effect of the influence of learning method factors	H0: Mi = 0 (There is no effect of i-level learning method factors on the learning effectiveness, which is measured by the level of understanding)	H1: Mi $\neq$ 0 (There is an effect of i-level learning method factors on the learning effectiveness, which is measured by the level of understanding).
To test the effect of the performance rate factor, the factor level is nested in the learning method factor	H0: Pj(i) = 0 (There is no effect of the j-level performance rate factor nested in the i-level learning method factor on the learning effectiveness, which is measured by the level of understanding)	H1: Pj(i) $\neq$ 0 (There is an effect of the j-level performance rate factor nested in the i-level learning method on the learning effectiveness, which is measured by the level of understanding).
To test the effect of the gender factor which is the factor level nested in the learning method and performance rate factors	H0: Gk(ji) = 0 (There is no effect of the k-level gender factor nested in the j-level performance rate factor and the first-level learning method factor on the learning effectiveness, which is measured by the level of understanding)	H1: Gk(ji) $\neq$ 0 (There is an effect of the k-level gender factor nested in the j-level performance rate factor and the i-level learning method factor on the learning effectiveness, which is measured by the level of understanding).

3.4. Data Analysis

A post hoc test or ANOVA and the Scheffe and Tukey tests were used to determine the impact of hybrid learning and identify the links between the factors and response variables. SWOT analysis was conducted to ascertain the necessary strategy and offer recommendations for the Performance Measurement and Improvement course. We reviewed any deficiencies, barriers, and challenges encountered in this study.

4. Results and Discussion

4.1. ANOVA

An ANOVA was conducted on the data of the learning method, performance rate, and gender factors. The criteria for a significant effect were a p-value less than 0.05 and an F-value greater than 1.95. The learning method and performance rate factors showed p-values of 0.002 and 0.000 and F-values of 9.33 and 19.33. However, gender had no significant impact on the knowledge level response (p-value of 0.126 and F-value of 1.67) (Figure 1).

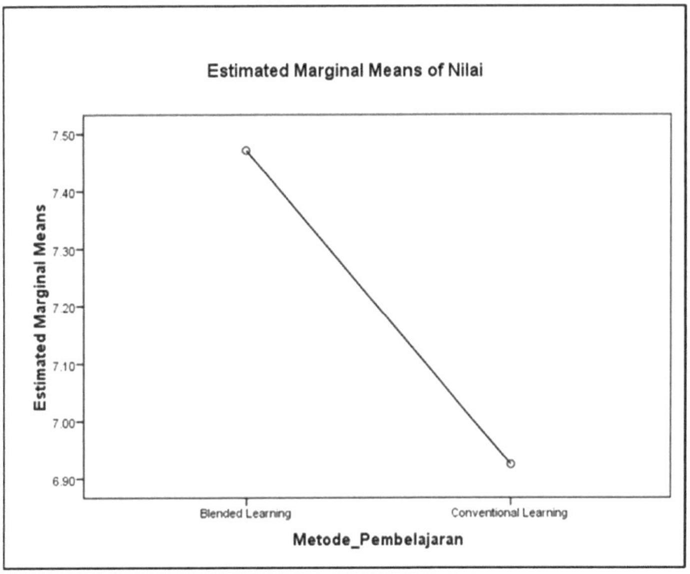

Figure 1. Effects of learning method factors on level of understanding.

To enhance understanding and learning efficacy, the learning approach and performance metrics are essential. Students must attain comparable levels of learning effectiveness. These findings align with earlier studies which found that the greater the interactivity of a learning approach, the higher the student's understanding of information. To optimize the advantage, a hybrid learning model needs to be deployed to attain all the learning objectives.

Figure 2 illustrates the division of the performance rate at three levels, each with its own categorization and values. These classifications and limits were determined based on the rating scale for all aspects of learning performance. A low performance rate was defined as a total value below 29, a medium rate as a value between 30 and 34, and a high rate as a value above 35. The performance rate component and the amount of knowledge demonstrated a direct correlation, whereby a greater performance rate corresponded to a better level of understanding and increased learning efficacy. Figure 2 also depicts the variations in the impact on the level of understanding at various levels of the performance rate. To obtain optimal learning effectiveness and understanding, students must have a high performance rate. Consistently attending learning sessions according to the directions and guidelines of the lecturer enhances the students' success rate. The consistent pattern results in excellent performance to attain the best possible outcome [32]. An individual with a high level of performance is more open to receiving feedback and effectively enhances their learning process without facing obstacles.

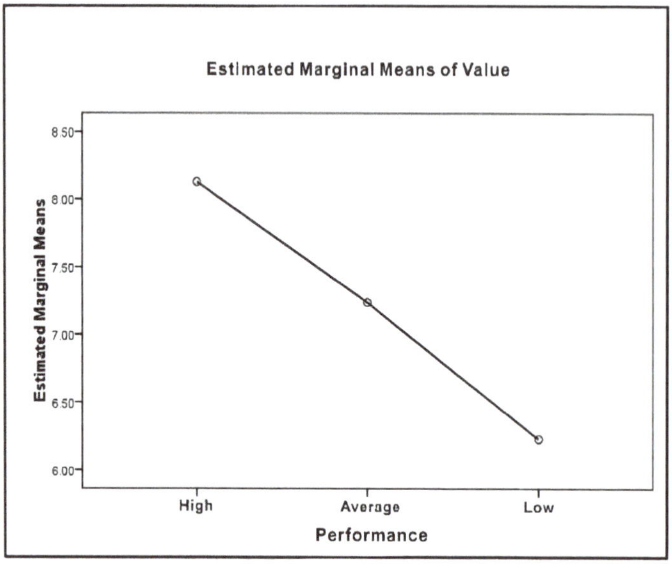

Figure 2. Relationship between performance rate factors and level of understanding.

Figure 3 depicts the correlation between the learning method and factors influencing the rate of performance. There is no interaction between them, as indicated by the lack of a line intersecting the two components. The impact created by the learning approach and performance were identical and varied with the level of understanding. Such results illustrated the efficacy of the mixed learning strategy with each learning method corresponding to an increased performance rate.

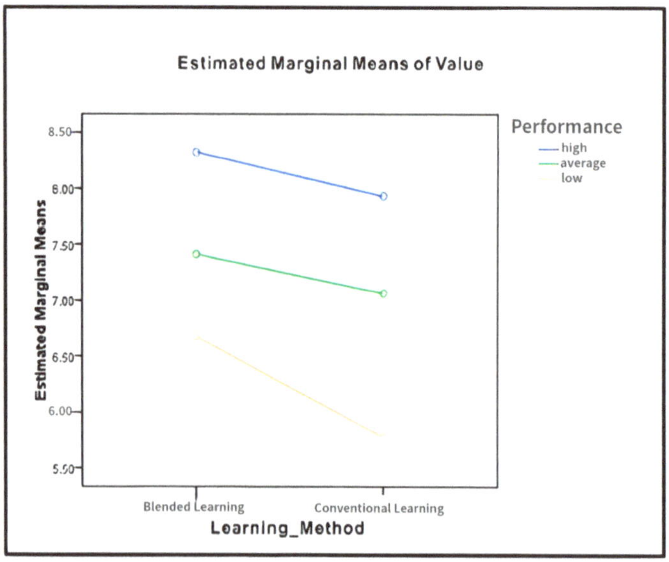

Figure 3. Relationship of interaction factors of learning methods and performance rate on level of understanding.

4.2. Post Hoc Test

Since the distinction between factors with less than three levels was evident, a post hoc test was conducted on variables that affected the response variable (i.e., the level of knowledge) at more than three levels, specifically the performance rate factor. A summary of the post hoc test results for the performance rate from the Scheffe and Tukey procedures is presented in Table 2.

Table 2. Recapitulation of post hoc test results for performance rate.

Treatment Comparison Pair	Average Difference	Conclusion
Low–Average	−1.0103	Real Different
Low–High	−1.9011	Real Different
Average–High	−0.8908	Real Different

Factors at all levels exhibited variations and impacts on the knowledge level. The average difference value represents the discrepancy between the mean values of the subsets within each factor level. The average performance rate was 1.0103, which was higher than the average low performance rate. The average high performance rate was 1.9011, which was higher than the average subset of the low performance rate. The high-performance rate was 0.8908, which was higher than the average performance rate. There was a positive correlation between the degree of understanding and performance rate. The related factors encompassed the cognitive abilities, level of engagement, proactivity, and receptiveness of pupils in the learning process.

4.3. Qualitative SWOT Analysis

The SWOT strategy was developed by analyzing the external and internal environments of the Industrial Engineering study program and synthesizing the relevant conditions. The strategic focal points were categorized based on the SWOT components. The approach was categorized as S-T, S-O, W-T, and W-O strategies. The factors in the SWOT strategy were used to create a robust and effective strategy that aligns with an organization's goals and fulfills its optimal requirements.

The S-O approach results in the maxi–maxi strategy. In this approach, the strategy is to be in equilibrium, where the organization's strengths may be effectively utilized to capitalize on every opportunity and enhance its position with ease. The S-T approach consists of the maxi–mini method. This strategy remains robust with the ideal capacity to effectively neutralize any current dangers. In the W-O approach, challenges are faced in capitalizing on opportunities due to its internal weaknesses. However, these weaknesses can catalyze transformation and be used to take advantage of existing chances. The W-T or mini–mini strategy is used to integrate weaknesses and threats. This strategy is ineffective due to unfavorable conditions within the corporation, and this approach needs to be revised.

4.4. Quantitative SWOT Analysis

The Industrial Engineering study program had the W-O approach as the mini–maxi strategy or divestment–investment principle. Thus, it was necessary to change the strategy. The coordinate of (−2.32, 0.39) indicated the combination of negative and positive values in quadrant III. Thus, when implementing hybrid learning, the Industrial Engineering study program had flaws to be addressed. Hence, it is imperative to modify the existing strategy to address the flaws and capitalize on emerging opportunities. Even with vulnerabilities, possibilities for divestment were found. Therefore, suggestions to adopt this integrated learning approach were made for immediately and in the long term. In the short term, it is necessary to enhance the preparedness of current resources, while long-term implementation is demanded to establish a learning system in online education.

5. Conclusions

A suitable educational approach leads to a productive educational setting, thereby fostering engaged and student-focused learning. Based on the results of this study, the hybrid learning method with the W-O or mini–maxi strategy based on the divestment–investment concept can be a successful approach to learning. For the introduction of hybrid learning, the Industrial Engineering Department must develop a performance-tracking tool for students and establish a website as a resource for literacy. Once hybrid learning is firmly established at Atma Jaya Catholic University of Indonesia, additional research can be conducted to assess the long-term impact on student performance and understanding.

Author Contributions: Conceptualization, R.M.S. and R.S.; methodology, R.M.S.; software, R.M.S.; validation, R.M.S., R.S. and F.A.P.; investigation, R.M.S.; resources, R.S.; data curation, R.M.S.; writing—original draft preparation, R.M.S., R.S.; writing—review and editing, F.A.P.; visualization, R.M.S.; supervision, R.S.; project administration, F.A.P.; funding acquisition, R.S. All authors have read and agreed to the published version of the manuscript.

Funding: This research received no external funding.

Institutional Review Board Statement: The study was conducted in accordance with the Declaration of Helsinki, and approved by the Institutional Review Board (or Ethics Committee) of Atma Jaya Catholic University of Indonesia for studies involving humans.

Informed Consent Statement: Informed consent was obtained from all subjects involved in the study.

Data Availability Statement: Data is contained within the article.

Conflicts of Interest: The authors declare no conflict of interest.

References

1. Haleem, A.; Javaid, M.; Qadri, M.A.; Suman, R. Understanding the role of digital technologies in education: A review. *Sustain. Oper. Comput.* **2022**, *3*, 275–285. [CrossRef]
2. Qureshi, M.I.; Khan, N.; Raza, H.; Imran, A.; Ismail, F. Digital Technologies in Education 4.0. Does it Enhance the Effectiveness of Learning? A Systematic Literature Review. *Int. J. Interact. Mob. Technol. (iJIM)* **2021**, *15*, 31–47. [CrossRef]
3. Park, W.; Kwon, H. Implementing artificial intelligence education for middle school technology education in Republic of Korea. *Int. J. Technol. Des. Educ.* **2023**, *34*, 109–135. [CrossRef] [PubMed]
4. Nordlöf, C.; Norström, P.; Höst, G.; Hallström, J. Towards a three-part heuristic framework for technology education. *Int. J. Technol. Des. Educ.* **2021**, *32*, 1583–1604. [CrossRef]
5. Zakaria, W.; Turmudi, T.; Pentang, J.T. Information and Communication Technology in Elementary Schools: A Comparison Between Hybrid and Face-to-Face Learning Systems. *Profesi Pendidik. Dasar* **2022**, *9*, 46–54. [CrossRef]
6. Bryan, A.; Volchenkova, K.N. Hybrid learning: Definition, models, implications for higher education. *Bull. South Ural. State Univ. Ser. Educ. Educ. Sci.* **2016**, *8*, 24–30. [CrossRef]
7. Hannula, J. Characteristics of teacher knowledge produced by pre-service mathematics teachers: The case of open-ended problem-based learning. *LUMAT Int. J. Math Sci. Technol. Educ.* **2019**, *7*, 55–83. [CrossRef]
8. Aristika, A.; Darhim; Juandi, D. Kusnandi the Effectiveness of Hybrid Learning in Improving of Teacher-Student Relationship in Terms of Learning Motivation. *Emerg. Sci. J.* **2021**, *5*, 443–456. [CrossRef]
9. Kashefi, H.; Ismail, Z.; Yusof, Y.M. Obstacles in the Learning of Two-variable Functions through Mathematical Thinking Approach. *Procedia—Soc. Behav. Sci.* **2010**, *8*, 173–180. [CrossRef]
10. Madhakomala, R.; Hakim, M.A.; Syifauzzuhrah, N. Problems of education in Indonesia and alternative solutions. *Int. J. Bus. Law Educ.* **2022**, *3*, 135–144. [CrossRef]
11. Gaol, F.L.; Hutagalung, F. The trends of blended learning in South East Asia. *Educ. Inf. Technol.* **2020**, *25*, 659–663. [CrossRef]
12. Rosser, A. *Beyond Access: Making Indonesia's Education System Work*; Lowy Institute For International Policy: Sydney, Australia, 2018.
13. Graham, C.R. Hybrid learning systems: Definition, current trends, and future directions. In *Handbook of Hybrid Learning: Global Perspectives, Local Designs*; Pfeiffer: Memmingen, Germany, 2006.
14. Wai, C.C.; Seng, E.L.K. Exploring the Effectiveness and Efficiency of Hybrid learning Tools in a School of Business. *Procedia Soc. Behav. Sci.* **2014**, *123*, 470–476. [CrossRef]
15. Inoue-Smith, Y. Designing And Implementing Mixed-Mode (Blended) Learning For College Students: A Case Study. In *Cognitive—Social, and Behavioural Sciences—icCSBs 2018*; Institute for Strategy of Education Development of the Russian Academy of Education: Moscow, Russia, 2019. [CrossRef]

16. Dai, J.; Li, Y. College Students' Acceptance and Willingness Towards Hybrid learning Experience. In *Lecture Notes in Computer Science*; Including Subseries Lecture Notes in Artificial Intelligence and Lecture Notes in Bioinformatics; Springer: Cham, Switzerland, 2018. [CrossRef]
17. Baragash, R.S.; Al-Samarraie, H. Hybrid learning: Investigating the influence of engagement in multiple learning delivery modes on students' performance. *Telemat. Inform.* **2018**, *35*, 2082–2098. [CrossRef]
18. Yigzaw, M.; Tebekaw, Y.; Kim, Y.M.; Kols, A.; Ayalew, F.; Eyassu, G. Comparing the effectiveness of a hybrid learning approach with a conventional learning approach for basic emergency obstetric and newborn care training in Ethiopia. *Midwifery* **2019**, *78*, 42–49. [CrossRef]
19. Alsowat, H.H. Hybrid Learning or Virtual Learning? Effects on Students' Essay Writing and Digital Literacy. *J. Lang. Teach. Res.* **2022**, *13*, 4. [CrossRef]
20. Shin, D.; Kwon, S.K.; Lee, Y. The effect of using online language-support resources on L2 writing performance. *Lang. Test. Asia* **2021**, *11*, 4. [CrossRef]
21. Tusino; Faridi, A.; Saleh, M.; Fitriati, S.W. The effect of hybrid task-based language teaching and critical thinking on writing performance in Indonesia. *New Educ. Rev.* **2020**, *61*, 109–118. [CrossRef]
22. Sutisna, E.; Vonti, L.H. Innovation development strategy for hybrid learning based English teaching and learning. *Engl. Rev. J. Engl. Educ.* **2020**, *9*, 103–114. [CrossRef]
23. Vonti, L.H.; Grahadila, L. Potentials and pitfalls of the implementation of hybrid learning in structure class in relation to the students' digital literacy and learning achievement. *JHSS J. Humanit. Soc. Stud.* **2021**, *5*, 17–21. [CrossRef]
24. Hitchcock, C.; Pearl, J. Causality: Models, Reasoning and Inference. *Philos. Rev.* **2001**, *110*, 639–641. [CrossRef]
25. Antonakis, J.; Bendahan, S.; Jacquart, P.; Lalive, R. On making causal claims: A review and recommendations. *Leadersh. Q* **2010**, *21*, 1086–1120. [CrossRef]
26. Podsakoff, P.M.; Podsakoff, N.P. Experimental designs in management and leadership research: Strengths, limitations, and recommendations for improving publishability. *Leadersh. Q* **2019**, *30*, 11–33. [CrossRef]
27. Benzaghta, M.A.; Elwalda, A.; Mousa, M.; Erkan, I.; Rahman, M. SWOT analysis applications: An integrative literature review. *J. Glob. Bus. Insights* **2021**, *6*, 55–73. [CrossRef]
28. Zhu, C.; Mugenyi, K.J. A SWOT analysis of the integration of e-learning at a university in Uganda and a university in Tanzania. *Technol. Pedagog. Educ.* **2015**, *24*, 1–19. [CrossRef]
29. Farrokhnia, M.; Banihashem, S.K.; Noroozi, O.; Wals, A. A SWOT analysis of ChatGPT: Implications for educational practice and research. *Innov. Educ. Teach. Int.* **2024**, *61*, 460–474. [CrossRef]
30. Stefan, D.; Vasile, V.; Oltean, A.; Comes, C.-A.; Stefan, A.-B.; Ciucan-Rusu, L.; Bunduchi, E.; Popa, M.-A.; Timus, M. Women entrepreneurship and sustainable business development: Key findings from a swot–ahp analysis. *Sustainability* **2021**, *13*, 5298. [CrossRef]
31. Gürel, E. SWOT Analysis: A Theoretical Review. *J. Int. Soc. Res.* **2017**, *10*, 994–1006. [CrossRef]
32. Chew, P.; Chrisochoides, N.; Gopalsamy, S.; Heber, G.; Ingraffea, T.; Luke, E.; Neto, J.; Pingali, K.; Shih, A.; Soni, B.; et al. Computational science simulations based on web services. In *Lecture Notes in Computer Science (Including Subseries Lecture Notes in Artificial Intelligence and Lecture Notes in Bioinformatics)*; Springer: Berlin/Heidelberg, Germany, 2003; Volume 2660. [CrossRef]

engineering proceedings

MDPI

Proceeding Paper

Turning Crises into Business Opportunities: An Exploratory Investigation of Customers' Pain Points in the Automobile Maintenance Industry Based on a Computer Database †

Shu-Chin Huang [1], Yen-Wen Chen [1], Hi-Ta Hsieh [2], Chih-Wen Hsiao [2] and Yi-Chang Chen [1,*]

1 Department of Business Administration, Chaoyang University of Technology, Taichung 413310, Taiwan; schuang2@gm.cyut.edu.tw (S.-C.H.); s10117083@gmail.com (Y.-W.C.)
2 Ph.D. Program of Business Administration in Industrial Development, Chaoyang University of Technology, Taichung 413310, Taiwan; a665885.boss@msa.hinet.net (H.-T.H.); chih1124@ms21.hinet.net (C.-W.H.)
* Correspondence: t2003151@cyut.edu.tw
† Presented at the 2024 IEEE 4th International Conference on Electronic Communications, Internet of Things and Big Data, Taipei, Taiwan, 19–21 April 2024.

Abstract: Companies need to decrease service failures through service recovery and by managing customers' emotions, which is important. Customer databases are vital to understand needs and service innovation. Utilizing data, companies can identify pain points and innovate services, reducing customer complaints. We examined 140 customer records from an auto maintenance company's database and found 602 failure descriptions. The main complaints include maintenance performance, service attitude, and professionalism. Employee behavior accounted for most failures. Pain points in the process were the most common, followed by support, financial, and productivity issues. Such results suggest that service innovation is needed.

Keywords: service failure; pain point; customer complaint; customer service database; service technology innovation

Citation: Huang, S.-C.; Chen, Y.-W.; Hsieh, H.-T.; Hsiao, C.-W.; Chen, Y.-C. Turning Crises into Business Opportunities: An Exploratory Investigation of Customers' Pain Points in the Automobile Maintenance Industry Based on a Computer Database. *Eng. Proc.* **2024**, *74*, 47. https://doi.org/10.3390/engproc2024074047

Academic Editors: Shu-Han Liao, Teen-Hang Meen and Cheng-Fu Yang

Published: 3 September 2024

1. Introduction

Scholars have identified customer flow as a revenue stream for enterprises, emphasizing that the effective management of customer complaints is pivotal for optimizing profit growth. Customer complaints encompass actions or inactions undertaken by consumers in response to unsatisfactory experiences following the purchase of goods or services [1]. In essence, customer complaints denote efforts by consumers to rectify dissatisfaction.

Singh [2] stated that when confronted with service failures, consumers typically exhibit various behaviors, including switching providers, directly addressing grievances with the service provider, seeking assistance from third parties or social networks, disseminating negative word of mouth (WOM) about their experiences, or passively accepting the situation. Day and Landon [3] classified dissatisfied consumer responses into two categories based on their proactive engagement: "non-action" and "action-taking". In the latter category, responses are delineated into "public action" and "private action". Public actions involve legal measures and complaints with consumer advocacy groups, while private actions entail boycotting products or sharing unsatisfactory experiences with acquaintances.

Numerous companies encounter challenges in effectively managing customer complaints, resulting in over half of customers harboring increased aversion towards the company following complaint resolution efforts. After a service failure, a secondary mishap engenders a "double deviation" phenomenon, amplifying customers' negative perceptions of the company, eliciting adverse reactions, and thereby exerting adverse impacts on the company's profitability and performance [4]. In food consumption, Dai and Wang underscored that heightened service quality provision by restaurant operators correlates with diminished customer complaints. Additionally, consumers emphasizing meal quality exhibited reduced satisfaction with service providers, consequently heightening the propensity for complaint behaviors.

However, customer complaints precipitate detrimental outcomes such as customer churn or compromised brand loyalty. Studies elucidated the potential for customer complaints to yield positive value for companies. For instance, Umashankar, Ward, and Dahl [5] posited that customer complaints serve as invaluable feedback mechanisms conducive to nurturing social bonds and thereby fostering enhanced brand loyalty. Similarly, Morgeson, Hult, Mithas, and Keiningham [6] claimed that the relation between service recovery and customer loyalty assumes heightened significance within economies characterized by elevated growth rates, intense competition, luxury market segments, and high levels of consumer satisfaction, as well as industries characterized by elevated expectations for tailored service provisions.

When service failure occurs, companies take service recovery actions [7]. In addition to solving the problems encountered by customers, they deal with the current negative emotions of customers to save potential losses. However, it is important to avoid service failure. Service innovation based on exploring customer complaints helps avoid the occurrence of the next customer complaint. Customer databases are an important source of information for smart business and brand marketing. The starting point of customer data mining is to discover the customer needs hidden in the data and make good use of the pain points to meet customers' needs for the innovation and development of service technology [8]. Such service innovation helps companies grow in the future.

Thus, we explored the reasons for customer complaints, the types of service failures that cause customer complaints, the customer pain points caused by service failure, and the relationship between service failures and pain points.

2. Research Method

2.1. Data Collection

The automobile maintenance service industry is mature and characterized by relatively low barriers to entry. The service is distinguished by a high degree of professionalism, intricacy, and technological sophistication. Variances exist between customers regarding satisfactory and unsatisfactory service outcomes. To understand customer failures, we selected 140 customer records from the database of an automotive maintenance enterprise. Subsequently, we investigated customer complaint records to unearth prevalent issues and dissatisfactions in the maintenance service. By understanding customer needs, companies can refine and innovate their service process.

2.2. Operational Definitions

The research variables of this study include customer complaints, service failure and its types, and functional pain points. Their definitions are presented in Table 1.

2.3. Analysis

We used a content analysis method to analyze customer complaint text. A content analysis was used to examine the information or content of written, symbolic materials [15]. The analysis steps are as follows: (1) propose research questions or hypotheses and review and examine the literature, (2) determine the scope of the research to determine the subject area of the research, (3) randomly select research samples, (4) establish category rules, (5) determine the unit of analysis, (6) code the data, and (7) conduct data statistics based on the research purpose.

2.4. Validity

The robustness of this research was validated using triangulation. Triangulation is a fundamental tool used in qualitative research, involving diverse methods or datasets to investigate the same phenomenon [16]. We analyzed customer complaints, observational records, and other pertinent datasets concerning automotive maintenance services. By harnessing multiple streams of evidence characterized by diverse data formats and contents and facilitating experts in the analysis and deliberation processes, the research results were presented in a comprehensive, nuanced, and realistic manner. Using the data sources and triangulation, the limitations inherent in a singular methodological approach were mitigated, and the potential for bias was reduced.

Table 1. Definitions of research concepts.

Variable	Dimension		Operational Definition
Customer complaints [2,9,10]	Reactions that customers have when faced with dissatisfaction after purchasing a product or service		
Reason for customer complaint	Work execution problems	Low reactivity	Unable to perform work correctly
		Low security	Not possessing the knowledge and abilities required to perform the services
	Professional performance problems	Low reliability	Service staff failed to demonstrate courtesy, consideration, and respect
		Poor competency	Service staff's credibility and honesty are low
	Service personnel problems	Poor manners	Customer was not served immediately
		Low reliability	Failure to help customers to avoid risky and unsafe situations
	Service resource planning problems	Low accessibility	Waiting time for receiving services is inappropriate or the work process is inconvenient
		Poor tangibility	Physical facilities for services, such as poor tools or equipment for services
	Failure to understand customer needs	Poor communication	Failure to listen to customers or communicate with them in a way that customers understand
		Low understanding	Not understanding customers' needs or asking about their special needs
Service failure [11–13]	Consumers' interactions during the service delivery process include interactions with personnel, the physical environment and facilities, and other intangible factors; once a mistake occurs and causes an unpleasant feeling to the customer, this phenomenon is called a service failure		
Types of service failure	Service delivery system failure		When errors occur in the provision of major services or products, policies, operating procedures, and other factors, errors that are subjectively determined by customers will affect their mood
	Customer need response failure		In normal delivery service behavior, the customer feels unhappy when the service staff is unable to meet the customer's order or special request
	Employee personal behavioral failure		The service attitude, skills, and professional knowledge of employees may affect customers' poor perception of the overall service, or the personal behavior of employees may cause customers to have unpleasant feelings
Functional pain point [8,14]	Financial pain point		Not obtaining value for money refers to pain points related to money and expenses
	Productivity pain point		No one rushes to help employees get work done; impact on productivity or time-related pain points
	Process pain point		Unable to smoothly complete all aspects of the service process
	Support pain point		No one can help when employees need help

3. Results

3.1. Reasons for Customer Complaints

To understand the reasons for customer complaints, we conducted a content analysis on the customer data. A total of 602 descriptions were analyzed for five reasons: work execution, professional performance, service personnel, service resource planning, and failure to understand customer needs (Table 2).

Table 2. Reasons for customer complaints.

Number	Complaints	Frequency	Percentage	Reason	Frequency	Percentage
1	Work execution problems	188	31.23%	low reactivity low security	106 82	17.61% 13.62%
2	Professional performance problems	161	26.74%	low reliability poor competency	143 18	23.75% 2.99%
3	Service personnel problems	138	22.92%	poor manners low reliability	38 100	6.31% 16.61%
4	Service resource planning problems	74	12.29%	low accessibility poor tangibility	66 8	10.96% 1.33%
5	Failure to understand customer needs	41	6.81%	poor communication low understanding	29 12	4.82% 1.99%
	Total	602	100.00%		602	100.00%

3.2. Service Failure Types

We divided the types of service failures into three categories. Employees' behavioral failures occurred the most (375 times, accounting for 62.29%), followed by customer demand response (157 times, accounting for 26.08%) and service delivery system failures (70 times, accounting for 11.63%) (Table 3).

Table 3. Analysis of service failures.

Order	Service Failure Type	Frequency	Percentage
1	Employees' personal behavioral failure	375	62.29%
2	Customer demand response	157	26.08%
3	Service delivery system failure	70	11.63%
	Total	602	100.00%

3.3. Pain Points

We divided functional pain points into four types: 49.50% were categorized as process, 24.42% as support, 18.44% as finance, and 7.64% as productivity (Table 4).

Table 4. Analysis of functional pain points.

Order	Functional Pain Point	Frequency	Percentage
1	Process pain point	298	49.50%
2	Support pain point	147	24.42%
3	Financial pain point	111	18.44%
4	Productivity pain point	46	7.64%
	Total	602	100.00%

3.4. Pain Points and Types of Service Failures

We conducted a crosstab analysis on the types of pain points and service failures. Employees' behavioral failures showed the highest rate (78.52%) in process pain point, followed by failures in responding to customer needs. Regarding to support pain point, the highest type was the service failure of responding to customer needs (68.71%). The most common financial pain points were employee behavioral failures (53.15%) and service delivery system failures (46.85%). The productivity pain points comprised employee behavioral failures (100.00%) (Table 5).

Table 5. Analysis of service failures with pain points.

		Service Delivery System	Employee Personal	Customer Demand Response	Total
Pain Point	Process	2.68%	78.52%	18.79%	100.00%
	Support	6.80%	24.49%	68.71%	100.00%
	Financial	46.85%	53.15%	0.00%	100.00%
	Productivity	0.00%	100.00%	0.00%	100.00%
Total		11.63%	62.29%	26.08%	100.00%

4. Conclusions

The causes of customer complaints included work execution problems, professional performance problems, service personnel problems, service resource planning problems, and failure to understand customer needs. Work execution problems occurred most frequently, with nearly one-third of customer complaints being related to the ineffective execution of service processes or the lack of professionalism of the service personnel. Therefore, it is important to improve service processes to deliver services efficiently and accurately. Additionally, the lack of professionalism of the service providers is also significant. Apart from standardized operating procedures, it is important to ensure the professional standards of each service provider and provide ongoing education and training.

The most frequently occurring type of service failure was "employee behavior". Consistent with the aforementioned findings, employees' service attitudes, skills, and professional knowledge impacted customers' negative perceptions and dissatisfaction. In automobile services, the professional competence of the service provider is important. Functional pain points were the most frequently occurring, accounting for nearly 50%. Process pain points were related to the effectiveness of completing the service process; thus, it is imperative for employees to assist other employees in completing or executing the service process.

The highest rates of process, support, financial, and productivity pain points were attributed to "failures in employee behavior", while the highest rate of support pain points was attributed to "failures in responding to customer needs". Additionally, the highest rate of financial pain points was linked to "failures in responding to customer needs", and the highest rate of productivity pain points was associated with "service delivery system failure".

Failure in employee behavior is associated with multiple pain points, including process, support, finance, and productivity. Car warranty service providers prioritize the cultivation of their employees' service attitudes, skills, and professional knowledge, as well as addressing their behaviors. By improving employees' behaviors, functional pain points can be removed.

Author Contributions: Conceptualization, S.-C.H., Y.-W.C. and Y.-C.C.; methodology, S.-C.H.; writing—original draft preparation, Y.-W.C. and Y.-C.C.; writing—review and editing, Y.-C.C., H.-T.H. and C.-W.H. All authors have read and agreed to the published version of the manuscript.

Funding: This research received no external funding.

Institutional Review Board Statement: Not applicable.

Informed Consent Statement: Not applicable.

Data Availability Statement: The raw data supporting the conclusions of this article will be made available by the authors on request.

Acknowledgments: All subjects' enthusiastic participation is greatly appreciated.

Conflicts of Interest: The authors declare no conflicts of interest.

References

1. Fornell, C.; Wernerfelt, B. Defensive marketing strategy by customer complaint management: A theoretical analysis. *J. Mark. Res.* **1987**, *24*, 337–346. [CrossRef]

2. Singh, J. Voice, exit, and negative word-of-mouth behaviors: An investigation across three service categories. *J. Acad. Mark. Sci.* **1990**, *18*, 1–15. [CrossRef]
3. Day, R.L.; Landon, E.L. Towards a theory of consumer complaining behavior. In *Consumer and Industrial Buying Behavior*; Woodside, A.G., Sheth, J.N., Bennett, P.D., Eds.; North-Holland: New York, NY, USA, 1977; pp. 425–437.
4. Hwang, I.S.; Wang, J.F. Customers' evaluations after service provider's complaint management: The relationships among perceived justice, anger, trait anger and behavioral intentions. *Commun. Manag. Q.* **2009**, *10*, 117–143.
5. Umashankar, N.; Ward, M.K.; Dahl, D.W. The benefit of becoming friends: Complaining after service failures leads customers with strong ties to increase loyalty. *J. Mark.* **2017**, *81*, 79–98. [CrossRef]
6. Morgeson, F.V.; Hult, G.T.M.; Mithas, S.; Keiningham, T.L. Turning complaining customers into loyal customers: Moderators of the complaint handling–customer loyalty relationship. *J. Mark.* **2020**, *84*, 79–99. [CrossRef]
7. Van Vaerenbergh, Y.; Orsingher, C. Service recovery: An integrative framework and research agenda. *Acad. Manag. Perspect.* **2016**, *30*, 328–346. [CrossRef]
8. Kranzbühler, A.M.; Kleijnen, M.H.; Verlegh, P.W. Outsourcing the pain, keeping the pleasure: Effects of outsourced touchpoints in the customer journey. *J. Acad. Mark. Sci.* **2019**, *47*, 308–327. [CrossRef]
9. Yoo, J.J.E.; Kim, T.T.; Lee, G. When customers complain: The value of customer orientation in service recovery. *Cornell Hosp. Q.* **2015**, *56*, 411–426. [CrossRef]
10. Zhan, F.; Luo, W.; Luo, J. Exhibition attachment: Effects on customer satisfaction, complaints and loyalty. *Asia Pac. J. Tour. Res.* **2020**, *25*, 678–691. [CrossRef]
11. Colgate, M.; Norris, M. Developing a comprehensive picture of service failure. *Int. J. Serv. Ind. Manag.* **2001**, *12*, 215–233. [CrossRef]
12. Hess, R.L., Jr.; Ganesan, S.; Klein, N.M. Service failure and recovery: The impact of relationship factors on customer satisfaction. *J. Acad. Mark. Sci.* **2003**, *31*, 127–145. [CrossRef]
13. Van Vaerenbergh, Y.; Orsingher, C.; Vermeir, I.; Larivière, B. A meta-analysis of relationships linking service failure attributions to customer outcomes. *J. Serv. Res.* **2014**, *17*, 381–398. [CrossRef]
14. Stein, A.; Ramaseshan, B. Towards the identification of customer experience touch point elements. *J. Retail. Consum. Serv.* **2016**, *30*, 8–19. [CrossRef]
15. Downe-Wamboldt, B. Content analysis: Method, applications, and issues. *Health Care Women Int.* **1992**, *13*, 313–321. [CrossRef] [PubMed]
16. Thurmond, V.A. The point of triangulation. *J. Nurs. Scholarsh.* **2001**, *33*, 253–258. [CrossRef] [PubMed]

engineering proceedings

MDPI

Proceeding Paper

Empirical Research on Regional Revitalization: A Case of Old Urban Railways †

Wen-Bor Lu *, Hsien-Wen Kuo and Chuan-Cheng Wang

Landscape and Urban Design, Chaoyang University of Technology, Taichung City 41349, Taiwan; k88021987654@gmail.com (H.-W.K.); as7307.3132@gmail.com (C.-C.W.)

* Correspondence: fisher27@hotmail.com

† Presented at the 2024 IEEE 4th International Conference on Electronic Communications, Internet of Things and Big Data, Taipei, Taiwan, 19–21 April 2024.

Abstract: Historically, railway facilities have been intertwined with daily life, communities, geography, and history, contributing to a rich cultural heritage and collective memory. However, current research on railway reuse primarily focuses on converting railway architecture into artistic displays, with limited exploration of urban railway revitalization. Addressing the challenges of urban railroads requires reevaluating space reuse models. Therefore, local revitalization has emerged as a key driver of society. We empirically explored the benefits of reusing urban old railroads from the perspective of local revitalization using the SMART Ecological Innovation Framework in revitalizing old railroads. We identified five forces: storytelling, market sensibility, aesthetics, regeneration, and local cultural design. Measurement items for these concepts were assessed using a five-point Likert scale, ranging from 1 (Strongly Disagree) to 5 (Strongly Agree). With a solid theoretical foundation, we employed confirmatory factor analysis to affirm the reliability and validity of these concepts, ensuring their stability. This study aimed to delve into regenerating old railways in Taichung City and explore the reuse benefits of urban railways to offer valuable insights for similar cases. The confirmatory factor analysis result revealed that storytelling, market perception, aesthetics, regeneration capability, and local design significantly contributed to the benefits of railway revitalization. Furthermore, the concept of local revitalization was effectively applied through these five forces in planning and design, stimulating economic development in idle areas.

Keywords: regional revitalization; railway reuse

Citation: Lu, W.-B.; Kuo, H.-W.; Wang, C.-C. Empirical Research on Regional Revitalization: A Case of Old Urban Railways. *Eng. Proc.* **2024**, *74*, 48. https://doi.org/10.3390/engproc2024074048

Academic Editors: Shu-Han Liao, Teen-Hang Meen and Cheng-Fu Yang

Published: 4 September 2024

1. Introduction

Vacant spaces, a result of major industrial changes, pose challenges such as resource waste and negative urban impact [1,2]. Despite their drawbacks, these spaces embody rich historical heritage and are transformed into cultural hubs, nurturing emerging industries and attracting cultural tourism [3]. In Europe, such spaces have successfully evolved into sustainable, people-centric environments and cultural districts, activating creativity and consumer functions [4]. Taiwan's urban evolution, driven by different eras, uncovers historical, cultural, and artistic values within vacant industrial sites [5]. Railways, vital indicators of social change, hold cultural significance, becoming part of collective memory [3].

Chang and Chen (2020) explored why tourist railways in Taiwan struggle to vitalize regions [6]: (1) limited thinking on tourism, emphasizing transportation, (2) insufficient tourism planning, and (3) ineffective resource linkage, leading to potential vacant space crises post-revitalization [7]. Existing studies focus on economic benefits and business models post-railway reuse, neglecting urban railway renewal. To understand this, the mutual relationship between urban structure and railway vacant space reuse needs to be explored, especially in cities with diverse characteristics, necessitating a context-specific reassessment.

Placemaking, addressing vacant spaces, emphasizes local cultural industry cultivation. Governments support this with technology and human resources for sustainable local economic growth, regional identity promotion, and heightened awareness of environmental protection [8]. Local development strategies integrate industry, geography, and talent to add value to local resources, reviving urban and rural areas, populations, and industries [9]. Taiwanese towns, possessing unique resources and challenges, can foster local identity through local support, simplified issue resolution, and resource integration from various sectors. David and Linda (2008) stressed the psychological importance of cultural identity, making placemaking's core lie in in-depth planning aligned with local culture, establishing identity, motivating collaboration, and achieving "sustainable operation" [10].

Placemaking is pivotal for a sound society. Addressing urban railway homogeneity demands reevaluating vacant space reuse models, using the SMART placemaking innovation forces proposed by [11,12]. After the renewal of an old railway, urban landmarks can expand, forming an industrial chain. The Taichung Green Space Corridor aligns with local cultural characteristics. Therefore, we explored the urban old railway reuse process and its benefits from a placemaking perspective.

2. Literature Review

2.1. Reuse of Idle Space

Shao and Liu (2018) categorized "Idle Space" into two main types: areas consistently excluded in city development and those previously used but abandoned due to uncontrollable factors [13]. The term "vacant space" in this study has evolved with time and history, arising from changes in functions and purposes during economic and industrial transformations [14]. When the original space loses its function or purpose, it presents positive reuse possibilities and latent development potential [15]. Huang (2003) viewed vacant spaces, especially transportation facilities such as railways, sugar factories, and distilleries, as "lost spaces" in urban development [16]. The concept of "reuse" is inspired by ideas about preserving historical buildings, encompassing renovation, rehabilitation, remodeling, recycling, retrofitting, environmental reshaping, extended use, and rebirth [17]. When the original space's function is updated, it rekindles vitality, offering development potential for the building and its surroundings. "Vacancy" is a condition, with "reuse" being the transformative means. Researchers noted the clustering of cultural and creative industries in urban areas to explore the factors stimulating this clustering and its impact on regional and economic development [18,19]. Vacant spaces cover excluded and abandoned areas, with reuse being crucial for revitalization [19,20]. It extends beyond buildings to enhance the vitality and development potential of the environment, contributing to urban regeneration, spatial sustainability, development, and increased space value [5,12,18,21].

2.2. Regional Revitalization

"Regional revitalization" traces its roots back to the Japanese colonial period, where it emerged to tackle challenges like the aging and depopulation of rural areas resulting from urban migration [22]. Taiwan confronts analogous issues, including economic deceleration, an aging demographic, diminishing birth rates, and an imbalance in urban–rural populations [23]. The current global economic climate further underscores the urgency for viable solutions [24–27].

On a global scale, there is a growing emphasis on preserving cultural heritage and repurposing unused spaces. Governments are increasingly directing their efforts toward urban renewal, aiming to breathe new life into central areas, generate additional value, and attract both industry and population to foster regional prosperity [28]. This collaborative endeavor necessitates the integration of various sectors and underscores the importance of grassroots participation [29].

Place shaping involves the interplay between people's perceptions and the inherent characteristics of spaces [30]. According to Hsu (2018), local revitalization involves crafting not just products but people's "life experiences" and fostering "cultural innovation". Key elements encompass food, housing, clothing, agriculture, health, environment, rehabilitation, art, entertainment, and community gatherings [23]. Lu (2019) identifies three regenerative DNAs—memory, culture, and industry—as crucial components for inventorying resources in the pursuit of local revitalization [31]. Local brands, as proposed by Evan et al. (2017) [32], serve as tools to establish a sense of place and drive economic development. Hong (2021) introduced the "local entrepreneurship study" with five SMART local innovation forces: storytelling, market perception, aesthetics, regeneration, and local design. Local revitalization is a multifaceted approach that delves into the intricacies of a locality, uncovering development elements often overlooked but pivotal for local progress.

Local revitalization is a diverse and multifaceted concept. "Local entrepreneurship study" encompasses the perspectives of multiple scholars. Therefore, referring to SMART local innovation and its five forces [11] and using them as scale indicators, we analyzed local revitalization, encompassing the following [11]:

- Story: Residents and visitors can tangibly experience elements that evoke emotions and create memories.
- Market Sense: By adopting the perspective and considering the latent needs and desires of residents and visitors, one can propose content that meets and exceeds their expectations.
- Aesthetic: The interpretation and imagination of sensory experiences, coupled with personal engagement in learning and the experiential process, are essential for transforming and presenting experiences that resonate deeply with residents and visitors.
- Re-: Through methods such as revitalization, redefinition, and recycling, existing resources can be reorganized into new content, imbuing them with fresh meaning.
- Terroir Design: Transforming local resources into experiential products or content becomes possible through a thoughtful design approach.

2.3. Railway Reuse

Railways are considered important indicators of social change [3]. In terms of architecture, industry, and labor culture, the development of railways possesses unique and irreplaceable value. Alessandra and Stefania (2023) pointed out that engaging in new activities with existing railway structures positively impacted the urban and regional environment and socio-economic development [30]. Railways are closely tied to the daily lives of people as a part of a generation's collective memory. With the transformation of railway systems, they become objects of preservation and nostalgia, passed down and revitalized through cultural creative methods [33]. Additionally, Giacomo et al. (2017) emphasized that railway design should be preserved based on specific circumstances and regional characteristics [34].

We reviewed recent (from 2018 to 2023) research related to railways, which primarily focused on the economic benefits assessment of cultural landscapes, studies on business models for reuse, and preservation modes [35]. However, there is limited research on the renewal and reuse of urban old railways, failing to adequately reflect the changes in contemporary society, industry, entertainment, and economic conditions. This gap is also acknowledged in the study by Zhang and Chen (2020) on tourist railways [29].

Therefore, a thorough investigation into the interrelationship between urban structure and the reuse of abandoned railway spaces is crucial for urban development, especially for cities with different population structures and urban characteristics. These cities need to adopt context-specific approaches based on their unique features and reevaluate the multi-faceted influencing factors involved in abandoned space reuse policies, which is the focus of this research.

3. Methodology

3.1. Research Framework

The main concept of this study involves an investigation into the urban old railway in the context of local revitalization, utilizing the SMART Cultural Innovation Pentad as a set of indicators. Through Confirmatory Factor Analysis (CFA), we validated its theoretical framework, establishing the practical applicability of the SMART Cultural Innovation Pentad as an indicator for local revitalization (Figure 1).

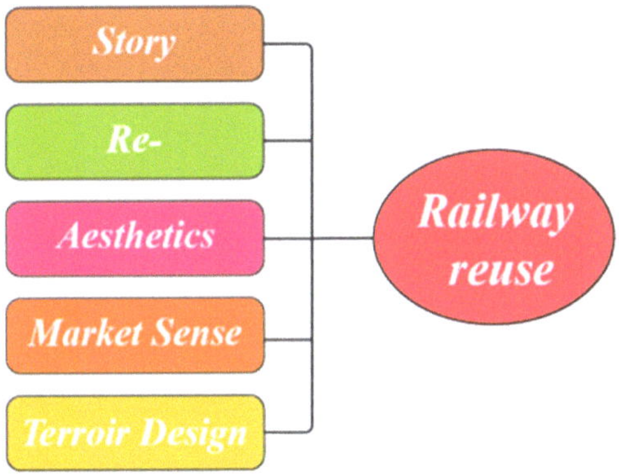

Figure 1. Research framework.

3.2. Pioneering Studies

In the context of local revitalization, we explored the introduction of the concept of repurposing old railways to understand the strength of influencing factors and assess whether the spatial design outcomes of reusing old railways maximize the potential for repurposing railway idle spaces. We selected the Greenway Railway in Taichung City as the research site, with Taichung Train Station as the starting point, as the surrounding space holds unique historical significance. We referred to Hong (2021) for the SMART local innovation pentagon as the evaluation indicator [11]. Through convenience sampling, open-ended interviews were conducted with visitors and local residents of the Taichung Greenway Railway with the interviews recorded for content analysis, having coded the interview content.

The results of the study indicated that design elements of railway reuse, such as elevated railway bridges and railway signals, successfully blend modern and retro elements. This allows for contemporaneity while evoking connections to Japanese history and preserving local historical narratives. These design elements significantly influence the reuse of old railways, transforming them into catalysts for local vibrancy. They closely connect previously dispersed roads, provide more convenient transportation, enhance pedestrian safety, and simultaneously preserve cultural heritage. The integration of past historical buildings and stories with modern design creates a cohesive experience. These findings serve as substantial references for the future planning of old railway areas in other regions, contributing to a more comprehensive understanding of the overall history of the area.

3.3. Confirmatory Factor Analysis, CFA

CFA was used to examine the reliability and validity of the measurement variables. Hair et al. (1998) proposed that the fit indices for assessing the adequacy of the hypothetical model include χ^2/df (<5), RMSEA (<0.08), and CFI, NNFI, and GFI (>0.9). The analysis results of this study demonstrated that all indicators of the research model were well fitted ($\chi^2 = 119.73$, df = 55, $\chi^2/\text{df} = 2.17$, RMSEA = 0.065, CFI = 0.95, NNFI = 0.97, GFI = 0.98), indicating the excellent overall fit of the assumed model [36].

4. Research Results

We conducted a sample survey on the socio-economic background of tourists and local shop owners along the Taichung Greenway (Table 1). The basic information included gender, marital status, age, education level, occupation, average monthly income, and place of residence. The majority of the respondents were male, accounting for 63.5% (179 people). A total of 63.8% (180) were married. The age group of 30 to 39 years old was the most common, representing 27.7% (78). As for education level, the majority had a college degree, constituting 56.7% (160). The most common occupation was "other", with 29.1% (82), followed by professional/service personnel at 23.8% (67). Regarding average monthly income, 42.2% (119) earned less than 30,000, and the majority resided in the central region, accounting for 77.3% (218 people).

Table 1. Five innovation forces, interview script.

Innovation Capability	Interview Questions
Story	1. In light of the current transformations in the old railway, what elements resonate with you? 2. Based on your personal impressions, what cultural characteristics do you observe in this old railway? 3. Are there specific places along this old railway that evoke emotions and memories for you?
Market Sense	4. Why did you choose to experience this old railway for leisure? 5. Regarding your experience with the old railway, what needs do you think should be addressed?
Aesthetics	6. Do you believe there is an aesthetic requirement for tourism or revitalization of the old railway? If so, what aesthetic elements do you consider important?
Re-	7. How effective do you think the current repurposing of the old railway is? Which revitalization elements do you find most beneficial?
Terroir Design	8. In your opinion, what local design elements are present in this old railway area?

The CFA model in this study was examined using common parameter estimation procedures and adhering to the assumption of multivariate normality. The skewness and kurtosis of the five SMART innovation forces ranged from −0.54 to −1.27 and from −0.100 to 1.197, indicating a normal distribution of the measurement variables. All variables had t-values ranging from 8.55 to 16.23, all exceeding the absolute value of 1.96, demonstrating statistically significant correlation coefficient estimates. Finally, according to the standards proposed by Hair et al. (1998) [36], the standardized factor loadings should exceed 0.5. However, in the "Re-" dimension, the standardized factor loading of the measurement variable "Having many locally native plant designs (planting)" was 0.2, and the measurement invariance was insufficient for a10 "Distinctive art installations" and a11 "Stitching together urban old spaces fragmented spaces". Therefore, it is recommended to remove these measurement variables to ensure the integrity of the model. The standardized factor loadings for the five latent constructs were as follows: "Story" at 0.82, "Market Sense" at 0.69, "Aesthetics" at 0.72, "Re-" at 0.73, and "Terroir Design" at 0.77. This indicates that the five SMART innovation forces have good compositional reliability (Table 2).

Table 2. Parameter estimation summary.

Latent Constructs and Measurement Variables	Standardized Factor Loadings	t-Value	Standard Errors	R^2	Composite Reliability
Story (s)					0.82
Old industrial cultural space (a1)	0.85	16.17	0.04	0.72	
Spaces of past life memories (a2)	0.66	11.54	0.06	0.42	
Integration with surrounding historical architectural spaces (a3)	0.81	15.11	0.05	0.66	
Market Sense (m)					0.69
Enhance human–environment safety measures (a4)	0.51	8.44	0.05	0.26	
Improve the connectivity of corridor spaces (a5)	0.66	11.61	0.04	0.46	
Provide cultural and educational environmental venues (a6)	0.63	10.84	0.05	0.40	

Table 2. *Cont.*

Latent Constructs and Measurement Variables	Standardized Factor Loadings	t-Value	Standard Errors	R^2	Composite Reliability
Revitalize social interaction spaces (a7)	0.60	10.35	0.05	0.34	
Aesthetics (b)					0.72
Old railway elements (a8)	0.80	14.66	0.04	0.58	
Old railway elements (a9)	0.70	12.43	0.05	0.49	
Re- (r)					0.73
Increase the number of visitors (a12)	0.73	12.37	0.05	0.41	
Enhance the functionality of the surrounding environment (a13)	0.78	13.08	0.05	0.46	
Terroir Design (w)					0.77
Integrate local historical context (a15)	0.81	14.96	0.04	0.66	
Preserve past characteristics (a16)	0.78	14.27	0.04	0.61	

Regarding discriminant validity, based on the analysis results in Table 3, the confidence intervals for the latent constructs do not include the value of 1.00, indicating that the "Story", "Market Sense", "Aesthetics", "Re-", and "Terroir Design" latent constructs of the five SMART innovation forces have discriminant validity. Combining the above results, the revised measurement model of the five SMART innovation forces is presented in Figure 2.

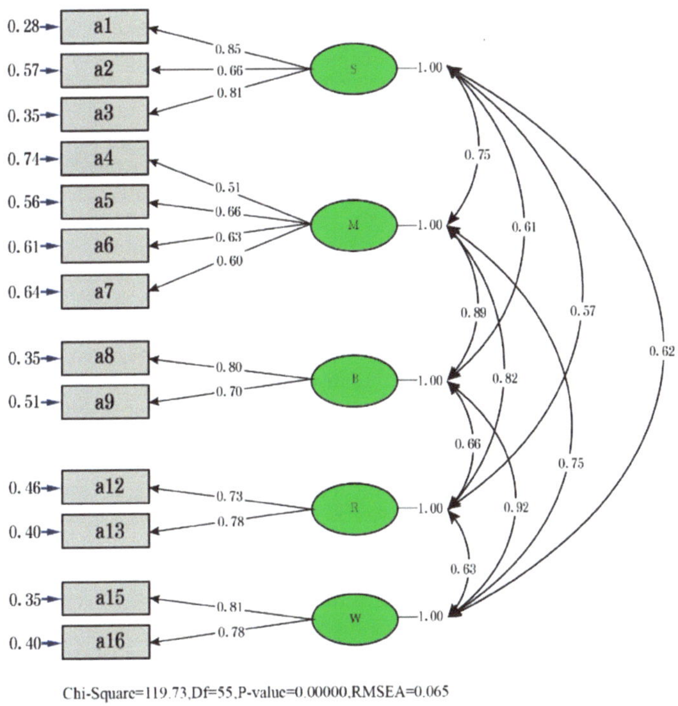

Figure 2. Standardized parameters of revised smart measurement model for innovation forces.

Table 3. Validity testing.

Latent Construct	Correlation Coefficient	Standard Error	Confidence Interval	Discriminant Validity
Story(s) and Market Sense (m)	0.75	0.05	0.85–0.65	Support
Story (s) and Aesthetics (b)	0.66	0.05	0.73–0.49	Support
Story (s) and Re- (r)	0.64	0.06	0.69–0.45	Support
Story (s) and Terroir Design (w)	0.62	0.05	0.72–0.52	Support
Market Sense (m) and Aesthetics (b)	0.93	0.04	0.98–0.79	Support
Market Sense (m) and Re- (r)	0.93	0.04	0.92–0.72	Support
Market Sense (m) and Terroir Design (w)	0.75	0.05	0.85–0.65	Support
Aesthetics (b) and Re- (r)	0.88	0.05	0.78–0.54	Support
Aesthetics (b) and Terroir Design (w)	0.93	0.04	0.98–0.84	Support
Re- (r) and Terroir Design (w)	0.77	0.05	075–0.51	Support

Note: Discriminant validity = Correlation coefficient ± (Standard error × 1.96).

5. Conclusions

We clarified the conceptual composition of "Story", "Market Sense", "Aesthetics", "Re-", and "Terroir Design" within the five SMART innovation forces and explored the interrelationships among these five latent constructs in the model. Using CFA, we validated the compositional model of the five SMART innovation forces: "Story", "Market Sense", "Aesthetics", "Re-", and "Terroir Design". In the "Aesthetics" dimension, the measurement variable was "Distinctive art installations", and in the "Re-" dimension, the measurement variables "Having many locally native plant designs (planting)" and "Stitching together urban old spaces fragmented spaces" did not meet the fit criteria. Therefore, we deleted these to ensure the integrity of the model. Other dimensions and variables met the standards, demonstrating that the overall research measurement model is acceptable. Furthermore, the t-values of the retained variables ranged from 8.55 to 16.23, indicating that the estimated correlation coefficients are statistically significant. The compositional reliabilities of the latent constructs were "Story" at 0.81, "Market Sense" at 0.69, "Aesthetics" at 0.72, "Re-" at 0.73, and "Terroir Design" at 0.77. The five SMART innovation forces constructed from the five dimensions have relatively high compositional reliability.

We examined the factor structure of the SMART innovation pentagon. The sampling results of this study provided a socio-economic background of tourists, revealing the distribution in gender, marital status, age, education level, occupation, average monthly income, and place of residence. This information contributes to a better understanding of the characteristics and needs of the audience in practical applications. Regarding the factor structure of the SMART innovation pentagon, an overall acceptable model had relatively high composite reliabilities of the latent factors. This suggested the reliability of the five dimensions constituting the SMART innovation pentagon. Notably, the retained variables statistically showed significant correlations, and the overall measurement model was acceptable in most cases.

For applications, specific consideration needs to be added to the results of the narrative power (Story) dimension. In the design of local revitalization, a similar strategy can be employed by integrating historical elements into everyday spaces. This design approach promotes the display of local cultural characteristics and contributes to enhancing the psychological and physiological well-being of the population, thereby establishing a resonant emotional connection within the community. By harnessing the power of story, the design of local revitalization becomes more than shaping physical spaces; it becomes a process of integrating history and culture into contemporary life. This cultural integration can inspire a sense of identity within the local area, encouraging active participation of community members in the preservation and promotion of local traditional values. Additionally, it provides an opportunity to reflect on the past, present, and future, enabling people to comprehensively understand and cherish the evolution of their environment. Therefore, in local revitalization, the elements of storytelling from this research into design strategies can help to create spaces that are more meaningful and connected to the local community. This thoughtful and innovative application allows for new perspectives and possibilities, further enhancing community sustainability and quality of living.

Author Contributions: Writing—review—editing and methodology, W.-B.L.; software, H.-W.K.; investigation, C.-C.W. All authors have read and agreed to the published version of the manuscript.

Funding: This research received no external funding.

Institutional Review Board Statement: Not applicable.

Informed Consent Statement: Not applicable.

Data Availability Statement: Data are contained within the article.

Conflicts of Interest: The authors declare no conflict of interest.

References

1. Wang, C.H. Heritage formation and cultural governance: The production of Bopiliao Historic District, Taipei. *Int. J. Herit. Stud.* **2013**, *19*, 676–691. [CrossRef]
2. Zheng, J. 'Creative industry clusters' and the 'Entrepreneurial City' of Shanghai. *Urban Stud.* **2011**, *48*, 3561–3582. [CrossRef]
3. Wang, C.-H.; Gao, Y.-T. Cultural and Creative Transformation of Taiwan's Railway Infrastructure. *Taiwan Soc. Res. Q.* **2020**, *116*, 151–199.
4. Pantović, K.; Čukić, I. Transformation models of unused spatial resources: Research study of Cultural Center "Magacin" in Belgrade. *Serbian Archit. J.* **2016**, *8*, 360–387. [CrossRef]
5. Lee, W.-Y. Study on the Reuse of Taiwan Sugar Factory Vacant Spaces. *J. Taitung Univ. Humanit.* **2016**, *6*, 1–69.
6. Chang, S.; Chen, P. Sightseeing railway planning and design. *Zhongxing Eng.* **2020**, *146*, 15–25.
7. Huang, S.-M.; Chen, Y.-L. Study on the Motivation, Artistic and Cultural Lifestyle, and Leisure Experience of Visitors to the Railway Art Network. In Proceedings of the 5th Outdoor Recreation, Recreation, and Tourism Academic Symposium, Taichung, Taiwan, 6 September 2003.
8. Chiu, Y. The Relationship of Regional Revitalization and History Build Adaptive Reuse Taking KingMa Inns as an Example. Doctoral Dissertation, Asia University, Taichung, Taiwan, 2021. Unpublished.
9. Han, M.-Z. Results Presentation of 'Design Flip, Local Creation' Demonstration Project. *J. Land Public Gov.* **2017**, *5*, 124–126.
10. David, M.; Linda, J. *Culture and Psychology*, 6th ed.; Cengage Learning: Boston, MA, USA, 2008.
11. Hong, Z.-Y. *Territorial Entrepreneurship*; Distant Flow Publishing: Taipei, Taiwan, 2021.
12. Lu, W.-B.; Kuo, X.-W.; Wang, C.-C. Exploring the Benefits of Reusing Urban Old Railways from the Perspective of Local Creation. In Proceedings of the 19th Conference on Technology and Society, Hsinchu, Taiwan, 3–4 May 2023.
13. Shao, Y.; Liu, B. Local Identity Regeneration of Unused Urban Spaces. *Int. Rev. Spat. Plan. Sustain. Dev.* **2018**, *6*, 21–34. [CrossRef]
14. Chu, M.-H. Myth of the Reuse of Taiwan's 'Vacant Spaces' for Art Spaces after 1949. *Art Forum* **2005**, *2*, 175–192.
15. Wang, H.-C. Cultural Space Reconstruction. In Proceedings of the International Symposium on Cultural Space Recon-Struction, Taipei, Taiwan, 15–16 February 2001.
16. Huang, H.-M.; Shih, L.-S.; Chen, H.-J. *Operation Reference Manual for Promoting the Reuse of Vacant Spaces*; Council for Cultural Affairs: Taipei, Taiwan, 2003; pp. 203–214.
17. Fu, C.-C. Construction of Theoretical Framework for the Reuse of Vacant Spaces in Taiwan. In Proceedings of the 2001 International Symposium on the Reuse of Vacant Spaces, Taipei, Taiwan, 15–16 February 2001.
18. Power, D. Cultural Industries in Sweden: An Assessment of their Place in the Swedish Economy. *Econ. Geogr.* **2002**, *78*, 103–127.
19. Rantisi, N. The competitive foundations of localized learning and innovation: The case of women's garment production in New York City. *Econ. Geogr.* **2002**, *78*, 441–462.
20. Hutton, T.A. Spatiality, Built Form, and Creative Industry Development in the Inner City. *Environ. Plan. A Econ. Space* **2006**, *38*, 1819–1841. [CrossRef]
21. Pratt, A.C. The Cultural Industries Production System: A Case Study of Employment Change in Britain, 1984–1991. *Environ. Plan. A* **1997**, *29*, 1953–1974. [CrossRef]
22. Yeh, C.-Y. Application Thinking of Local Creation after the Activation of Public Areas. *Taiwan Econ. Res.Mon.* **2022**, *45*, 130–136.
23. Hsu, C.-J. Local Creation, Remaking a Happy Society. *J. Land Public Gov.* **2018**, *6*, 36–43.
24. Hutton, T.A. Postindustrialism, postmodernism, and the reproduction of Vancouver's central area: Retheorising the 21st century city. *Urban Stud.* **2004**, *41*, 1953–1982. [CrossRef]
25. Kim, H.; Kim, E.J. Tourism as a Key for Regional Revitalization? A Quantitative Evaluation of Tourism Zone Development in Japan. *Sustainability* **2021**, *13*, 7478. [CrossRef]

26. Kong, L. Culture, Economy, Policy: Trends and Developments. *Geoforum* **2000**, *31*, 358–390. [CrossRef]
27. Porter, E.; Barber, A. The meaning of place and state-led gentrification in Birmingham's Eastside. *City Anal. Urban Trends Cult. Theory Policy Action* **2006**, *10*, 215–234. [CrossRef]
28. Choi, J.W.; Lee, J.H. An Impact Analysis of Idle Space Regeneration Types on Regional Revitalization. *J. Korea Plan. Assoc.* **2016**, *17*, 478–489.
29. Zhang, S.-X.; Chen, P.-T. Tourist Railway Planning and Design. *Chin. J. Eng.* **2020**, *146*, 15–25. [CrossRef]
30. Bianchi, A.; De Medici, S. A Sustainable Adaptive Reuse Management Model for Disused Railway Cultural Heritage to Boost Local and Regional Competitiveness. *Sustainability* **2023**, *15*, 5127. [CrossRef]
31. Lu, C.-W. How to Inventory Local DNA and Create Exclusive Community Industries. Taiwan Community Pass. 2019. Available online: https://reurl.cc/WNxdRk (accessed on 30 January 2023).
32. Cleave, E.; Arku, G.; Sadler, R.; Gilliland, J. Is it sound policy or fast policy? Practitioners' per-spectives on the role of place branding in local economic development. *Urban Geogr.* **2017**, *38*, 1133–1157. [CrossRef]
33. Lu, J.-H.; Liu, B.-C. From 'Station' to 'Art Pavilion'—Public Governance of Cultural Aggregation and Spatial Exclusion. *Urban Plan.* **2017**, *44*, 399–422.
34. Di Ruocco, G.; Sicignano, E.; Fiore, P.; D'Andria, E. Sustainable Reuse of Disused Railway. *Procedia Eng.* **2017**, *180*, 1643–1652. [CrossRef]
35. Lu, J.-H.; Liu, B.-C. Reflection on the Development of Arts and Culture Industry in Urban Governance Utilizing Vacant Spaces—A Case Study of Hualien Railway Cultural Park. *J. Humanit. Soc. Sci.* **2020**, *16*, 317–343.
36. Hair, J.; Anderson, R.; Tatham, R.; Black, W. Multivariate Data Analysis, 5th ed.Prentice Hall: Hoboken, NJ, USA, 1998.

engineering proceedings

Proceeding Paper

Visual and Environmental Stimuli Preferences in Pediatric Spaces †

Anggra Ayu Rucitra [1], Purwanita Setijanti [1], Asri Dinapradipta [1,*] and Ruka Kosuge [2]

[1] Architecture Department, Institut Teknologi Sepuluh Nopember, Surabaya 60111, Indonesia; anggra@interior.its.ac.id (A.A.R.); psetijanti@arch.its.ac.id (P.S.)
[2] Architecture Department, Shibaura Institute of Technology, Tokyo 1358548, Japan; kosuge@shibaura-it.ac.jp
* Correspondence: asdina_p@arch.its.ac.id
† Presented at the 2024 IEEE 4th International Conference on Electronic Communications, Internet of Things and Big Data, Taipei, Taiwan, 19–21 April 2024.

Abstract: Interior design is considered and practiced as a visual discipline in architecture. The environment and buildings are appreciated through visual representations. We explored how sensory interactions shape a genuine multisensory experience with visual stimulation as a primary focus in architecture and interior design. It is important to consider different factors that contribute to visual stimulation when designing spaces. Visual stimulation is experienced differently, depending on the observer, and it is important to understand how children perceive stimuli. Therefore, we determined the visual factors captured by children. The embedded design method was used for qualitative mapping of visual factors and 3D animation creation for visualization. Eye-tracking experiments were conducted to examine the factors that captured the attention of children. Children were attracted to moving objects such as videos, followed by images on walls, playgrounds, windows, and furniture. Fostering positive distraction is important in designing spaces for children.

Keywords: visual factor; multisensory environment; interior for children

Citation: Rucitra, A.A.; Setijanti, P.; Dinapradipta, A.; Kosuge, R. Visual and Environmental Stimuli Preferences in Pediatric Spaces. *Eng. Proc.* **2024**, *74*, 49. https://doi.org/10.3390/engproc2024074049

Academic Editors: Shu-Han Liao, Teen-Hang Meen and Cheng-Fu Yang

Published: 4 September 2024

1. Introduction

Vision is a predominant sense that extracts information about the nature, location, and movement of objects through the eyes and subsequent cognitive processes [1]. As humans spend 95% of their time indoors, human-centric architecture prioritizes visual aspects, overshadowing sensitivity to hearing, smell, touch, and taste [2]. A doctrinal criticism by Attoe (1989), adapted by Juhani Pallasmaa, stated that architecture is not just a building, but a mediation of both the significant and the trivial because buildings have a specific meaning concerning the human body and emotions [3]. Architecture is created to be enjoyed through the lens of a camera or a sequence of eyes, referred to as ocular-centric or retinal architecture [4]. Multisensory experiences are inherent in architectural works. In this context, there is an interaction between users and architecture which activates all senses. The results of these sensory experiences provide cognitive information and also influence users' emotions, such as a sense of renewal or therapeutic relief [3,4].

Architecture has been considered, theorized, taught, and practiced as a visual discipline. Hence, environments and buildings are developed through images, means, and visual representations [5]. Vision is the sense that captures temporal information [6,7], and the visual information helps understand the meaning and evaluate the aesthetic value of the environment. The visual system largely operates with contrast values such as lighting and color, but not with absolute values. For example, when a product needs to attract attention, its contrast needs to be increased in comparison to its environment [6]. Guided by organizing laws such as the Gestalt Principles, the visual system aims to create an understanding of the surrounding environment, where visual images are organized into the simplest and most easily understood forms [6,8].

In a healthcare facility, the visual environment is important. In total, 30% of related research emphasized the benefits of the visual environment to users, followed by the audio environment (20%), patient rooms (20%), increased security (17%), wayfinding (17%), family support spaces (17%), staff support spaces (14%), and sustainability (9%) [9]. Such a result illustrates that the visual environment is related to human behavior, interior science, and aesthetics.

Architecture influences human psychology [10,11]. Thus, the connection between the architectural environment and human psychology has been extensively studied, specifically regarding human health [12–14]. A study on interior design elements and accessories in space showed that the more favored interior design elements and accessories, the lower the stress levels [12]. To explain the atmosphere of a space, three types of environmental characteristics are determined: ambient/atmosphere, architecture, and interior design [15,16]. Ambience is an intangible atmosphere, including elements like lighting, noise levels, and temperature. Meanwhile, the architectural aspects tend to be permanent in the physical environment, such as room layout, size, shape, and window placement. The interior design is not as entirely permanent as furniture, color, plants, and aesthetic elements. Hence, the most mentioned and analyzed variables are nature and its elements [17,18].

Interior design and aesthetic elements are captured by the eyes as visual stimulation. In a space, visual factors observed by users include aesthetic elements in the space, television, and a window view [15,17]. Therefore, in a room, visual factors include TV, furniture, windows, the presence of images on the walls, prominent facilities, and aesthetic elements [12,13,18].

2. Environment Planning for Children

Designing architecture and interior spaces requires understanding the needs of users, particularly children. In America and Europe, since the 1980s and 1990s, there has been an increasing concern in society about the vulnerability of children in public spaces. Researchers have explored the paradoxical meaning of home as a public space and the street as a private space for children. Since they are compelled to use facilities designed for adults, these areas become vulnerable [19]. Therefore, it is crucial to have architectural and interior planning that caters to the physical and psychological needs of children. It is necessary to create enabling environments from a child's perspective as space is significant for them. A space is experienced as comforting, becoming part of a child's memories and influencing their character [20]. Children spend much time playing indoors, coinciding with increasing mental health issues. A literature review was conducted to explore the relationship between access to green spaces and mental health in children. The results showed that access to open green spaces, such as nature, was associated with improved mental well-being, overall health, and cognitive development [21]. For this reason, a deeper analysis of the spatial needs of children, in both architectural and interior design contexts, is needed. One aspect to consider is the visual environment, which is most often perceived by children.

Therefore, we investigated how visual factors were perceived by children who were receiving medical treatment as architecture plays an important role in the patient's healing process through multisensory stimulation obtained from the spatial atmosphere [9,12,13,18].

Over the past decade, there has been a significant increase in psychosocial research on cancer patients in developed countries. However, many clinical and psychosocial needs remain unmet and unaddressed [22]. Improving the quality of life for pediatric cancer patients is currently an international priority. Thus, we analyzed visual sensors in space connected to patient recovery. Pediatric cancer patients were surveyed as they are vulnerable and their sensory responses are at a lower limit.

3. Methods

Embedded design is a combined qualitative and quantitative method [23]. Collecting and analyzing more than one data type is necessary for a framework associated with various data by incorporating qualitative strands into a quantitative experiment. Randomized controlled trials are experimental designs commonly used in evidence-based medicine, although adjustments may be necessary for specific cases [23]. The embedded design method is appropriate for extracting information from qualitative data and obtaining measurement results to find connections at each stage. In this study, a literature review was conducted to seek theoretical foundations and understand the related theories. Afterward, the spaces were defined visually based on identified visual parameters and tested for children through videos by measuring through eye tracking and reinforcing the results with Likert scale interviews.

Based on the literature review, it was found that space affected human psychology [9,11,14,17]. Thus, we explored visual factors and their effects on human psychology, visual factors captured by the human eye in space, and the visual factors preferred by children. The result can be used as a guide in designing children's spaces.

4. Results and Discussion

Visual elements, including color, aesthetics, and distractions such as TVs and windows, contribute to the overall interior design experience [15,17]. Visual factors include visual distractions through audiovisual elements in the space, and aesthetic elements [12,13,18]. After identifying these factors, experiments were conducted by incorporating all these factors in this study. The color factor was neglected in this study because the previous literature found that calming colors were preferred by children [24].

To create space visualizations, a study on the visualization of space was needed. Interior architecture is supported by immersive technology that facilitates design visualization to make virtual spaces real spaces [25]. Visual displays through video, virtual, or immersive experiences are categorized as positive distractions that help users, including patients, overcome pain and traumatic experiences during treatment. These are often combined with relaxation, imagery, and captivating visual compositions [25].

In research on health, randomized control groups or trials are commonly used to gather evidence to link certain features or interventions [25,26]. To enrich and deepen the analysis, experiments were conducted on healthy children and those who were receiving medical treatment (pediatric cancer patients) in this study. Pediatric cancer patients were selected due to their limitations in the sensory response. The result was compared using the embedded method and randomized control trial. Children who could express their opinions were selected and categorized into preschoolers aged 4–6 years, school-age children aged 7–10 years, and teenagers aged 11–17 years [25]. The number of participants was 15 healthy preschoolers, 15 healthy school-age children, 15 healthy teenagers, and 45 cancer patients with the same age classifications.

The visualization of the space in this study was the children's chemotherapy room at X Hospital in Surabaya. This room was selected to investigate the correlation between architectural environments and pediatric cancer patients. The healthy children observed visualizations of the chemotherapy room with TV, furniture, natural imagery on the walls, the other facilities in the room, and the window. Pictures of the original condition of the room before the redesign were shown to them to compare the original room and the one stimulated by visual factors. Interviews were conducted with the pediatric cancer patients who had undergone chemotherapy in that room to see whether they preferred to undergo chemotherapy in a newly designed room. Figures 1 and 2 display room visualizations, with circles representing screenshots from participants eye tracking.

Visual factors such as natural imagery were tailored to the children's characteristics. However, aesthetics was not included in the experiment because there were none in the existing building. According to the interior design theory, aesthetic elements can be substituted with natural imagery ornamentation. The need for health facilities in the space prohibits the presence of aesthetic elements, serving as a basis for consideration. Also, the positioning of windows above the room is a determining factor in the selection of visual factors.

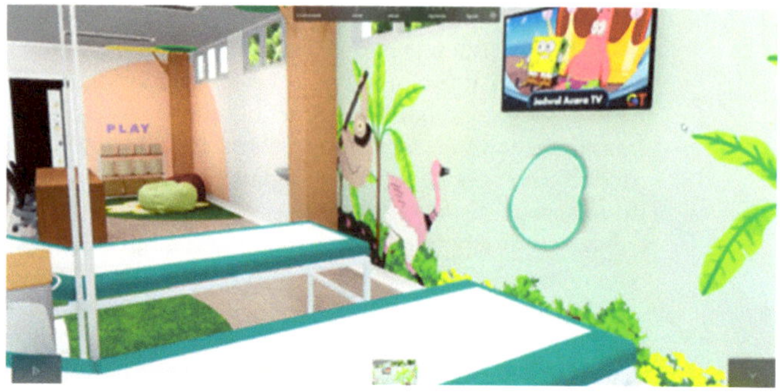

Figure 1. Room visualization and eye movement through eye tracking focus on natural imagery (Authors Analysis).

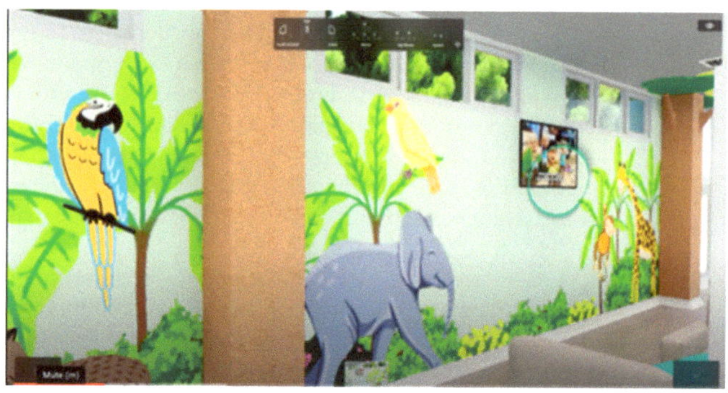

Figure 2. Room visualization and eye movement through eye tracking focus on Television (Authors Analysis).

A total of 90 children from each category were shown videos with eye-tracking equipment, and the results are shown in Table 1. These results were derived from the association of eye tracking with interviews during the experiment. The participants filled out a questionnaire on a five-point Likert scale (score of 1–5) based on their choices, showing what was most and least observed. The overall preference order for visual factors of the participants was (1) audiovisual elements, including both TV and handheld gadgets, (2) natural imagery such as murals on the walls, (3) other room facilities like the playground, (4) furniture such as chairs within the room, and (5) a view to the window.

Table 1. Experiment results.

		Children				Patients			
No	**Visual Factor**	**Preschool**	**School**	**Adolescent**	**Total**	**Preschool**	**School**	**Adolescent**	**Total**
1	Natural Imagery	51	62	63	176	48	63	66	177
2	Television	72	68	70	210	75	70	67	212
3	View to window	15	15	21	51	15	15	22	52
4	Furniture	30	37	46	113	30	37	40	107
5	Another Facility (Playground)	58	42	26	126	53	40	36	129

There were differences in preferences among preschoolers, school-age children, and teenagers in the prioritization of viewing other room facilities compared to the dominance of furniture. For teenagers, the dominance of furniture was more prominent than the playground. Also, there was no difference in visual preferences among children who are healthy and those diagnosed with cancer. The view from the window became the last preference not as a point of interest in the room. This showed the significant role of design elements, particularly the position and dominance of visual factors in the space, which need further investigation.

5. Conclusions

In this study, it was found that visual factors affected human psychology, and patients preferred the designed room to the original one. Visual factors were determined from the literature review, and an experiment was conducted to determine the preference levels of children. The existing conditions affected the space visualization. The order of visual preferences changed according to the existing conditions of the room. Hence, further study is needed on design principles related to visuals, such as proportion, dominance, and the positioning of visual factors. Health conditions do not show significant differences in the visual factor preferences of children. It is necessary to delve into children's needs before designing interior architectural facilities. Distractions from audiovisual elements are the primary preference because this stimulation is multisensory, and the presence of audio and visual elements can stimulate optimally. In a future study, audiovisual factors can be separated from visual factors. When planning interior architectural facilities for children, audiovisual factors need to be prioritized as they serve as positive distractions, specifically for child cancer patients during chemotherapy.

Author Contributions: Conceptualization, A.A.R., R.K and P.S.; methodology, A.A.R., P.S. and A.D.; software, A.A.R.; validation, P.S. and A.D.; formal analysis, A.A.R. and R.K; investigation, A.A.R.; data curation, A.A.R.; writing—original draft preparation, A.A.R. and P.S.; writing—review and editing, A.D.; visualization, A.A.R.; supervision, P.S and R.K. All authors have read and agreed to the published version of the manuscript.

Funding: This research received no external funding.

Institutional Review Board Statement: The study was conducted in accordance with the Declaration of Indonesia, and approved by the Institutional Review Board (or Ethics Committee) of RS. Dr Sutomo (protocol code 666/KEPK/V/2023, date of approval 5 May 2023).

Informed Consent Statement: Informed consent was obtained from all subjects involved in the study.

Data Availability Statement: The data that support the findings of this study are available on request from the corresponding author, psetijanti@arch.its.ac.id. Some of the data are not publicly available due to [restrictions, e.g., their containing information that could compromise the privacy of research participants].

Acknowledgments: Thanks to all parties involved in this research, including the Children's Cancer Foundation, Sepuluh Nopember Institute of Technology, as well as the hospital, all doctors, nurses, parents of patients, and pediatric cancer patients.

Conflicts of Interest: The authors declare no conflicts of interest. The data of all respondents are kept confidential and protected by the code of ethics. The funders had no role in the design of the study; in the collection, analyses, or interpretation of data; in the writing of the manuscript; or in the decision to publish the results.

References

1. Wade, N.; Swanston, M. *Visual Perception an Introduction*, 3rd ed.; Psychology Press: London, UK, 2012; p. 1.
2. Spence, C. Senses of place: Architectural design for the multisensory mind. *Cogn. Res. Princ. Implic.* **2020**, *5*, 46. [CrossRef] [PubMed]
3. Sabatini, S.N.; Kurniati, F.; Haristianti, V.; Sudrajat, I. Sumbangsih Juhani Pallasmaa dalam Teori Arsitektur. *J. RUAS* **2018**, *15*, 49–60. [CrossRef]
4. Pallasma, J. *The Eyes of the Skin: Architecture and the Senses*; Willey Academy, John Willey and Sons: Hoboken, NJ, USA, 2005.
5. Pallasma, J. Design for Sensory Reality: From Visuality to Existential Experience. *Archit. Des. J.* **2019**, *89*, 22–29. [CrossRef]
6. Nefs, H.T. On the visual appearance of objects. In *Product Experience*; Elsevier: Amsterdam, The Netherlands, 2018; pp. 11–39.
7. Schifferstein, H.N.J.; Spence, C. Multisensory product experience. In *Product Experience*; Elsevier: Amsterdam, The Netherlands, 2018; pp. 133–161.

8. Koffka, K. *Principles of Gestalt Psychology*, 2nd print. ed.; Harcourt, Brace: New York, NY, USA, 1936; pp. 1–14.
9. Rucitra, A.A.; Setijanti, P.; Dinapradipta, A. Healing Built Environment a Systematic Literature Review. *Seybold Rep. J.* **2023**, *18*, 5–29.
10. Sally, A. *Place Advantage: Applied Psychology for Interior Architecture*; John Willey and Sons: Hoboken, NJ, USA, 2009.
11. Kopec, D. *Environmental Psychology for Design*; Bloomsbury Publishing: New York, NY, USA, 2018.
12. Andrade, C.C.; Devlin, A.S.; Pereira, C.R.; Lima, M.L. Do the hospital rooms make a difference for patients' stress? A multilevel analysis of the role of perceived control, positive distraction, and social support. *J. Environ. Psychol.* **2017**, *53*, 63–72. [CrossRef]
13. Andrade, C.C.; Devlin, A.S. Stress reduction in the hospital room: Applying Ulrich's theory of supportive design. *J. Environ. Psychol.* **2015**, *41*, 125–134. [CrossRef]
14. Zhang, Y.; Tzortzopoulos, P.; Kagioglou, M. Healing Built-Environment Effects on Health Outcomes: Environment–Occupant–Health Framework. *Build. Res. Inf.* **2019**, *47*, 747–766. [CrossRef]
15. Dankner, S. Using Positive Visual Distractions and Color in Healthcare Settings to Reduce Patient Stress & Increase Patient Satisfaction. Master's Thesis, Philadelphia University, Amman, Jordan, 2017.
16. Harris, P.B.; McBride, G.; Ross, C.; Curtis, L. A Place to Heal: Environmental Sources of Satisfaction Among Hospital Patients. *J. Appl. Soc. Psychol.* **2002**, *32*, 1276–1299. [CrossRef]
17. Ulrich, R.; Zimring, C.; Zhu, X.; DuBose, J.; Seo, H.; Choi, Y.; Joseph, A. A Review of The Research Literature on Evidence-Based Healthcare Design. *Health Environ. Res. Des. J.* **2008**, *1*, 61–125. [CrossRef] [PubMed]
18. Dijkstra, K.; Pietrese, M.; Pruyn, A. Physical environmental stimuli that turn healthcare facilities into healing environments through psychologically mediated effects: Systematic review. *J. Adv. Nursing* **2006**, *56*, 166–181. [CrossRef] [PubMed]
19. Valentine, G. Children should be seen and not heard: The Production and Transgression of Adults Public Space. *Urban Geogr.* **1996**, *17*, 2005–2220. [CrossRef]
20. Slatter, B. *My Space: Creating Enabling Environment for Young Children*; Oxfordshire County Council: Oxfordshire, UK, 2007.
21. Mc Cormick, R. Does Access to Green Space Impact the Mental Well-being of Children: A Systematic Review. *J. Pediatr. Nurs.* **2017**, *37*, 3–7. [CrossRef] [PubMed]
22. Osborn, M.P.; Johnson, R.H. Worldwide benefits of improving cancer care for adolescents and young adults in LMICs. *Lancet Oncol.* **2020**, *21*, 487–489. [CrossRef] [PubMed]
23. Creswell, J.W.; Creswell, J.D. Research Design: Qualitative, Quantitative, and Mixed Methods Approaches. Scientific Research: Wuhan, China, 2018.
24. Rucitra, A.A.; Setijanti, P.; Dinapradiptra, A. Color Preferences Captured by Children in Space through Virtual Reality Simulation. An Analysis in the Pediatric Chemotherapy Room. In Proceedings of the 2022 IEEE International Conference on Industrial Engineering and Engineering Management (IEEM), Kuala Lumpur, Malaysia, 7–10 December 2022; pp. 0006–0010.
25. Van den Berg, M.; Hartmaan, T.; De Graaf, R. Supporting Design Reviews with Pre Meeting Virtual Reality Environments. *J. Inf. Technol. Constr.* **2017**, *22*, 305–321.
26. McCaul, K.D.; Monson, N.; Maki, R.H. Does distraction reduce pain-produced distress among college students? *Health Psychol.* **1992**, *11*, 210. [CrossRef] [PubMed]

engineering proceedings

Proceeding Paper

Perceptions of Using Online Evaluation Systems in Schools and Universities: A Case Study of Indonesian Educators †

Joice Yulinda Luke [1,*] and Shiyrah Theosebes Sela [2]

1 Digital Language Learning Center, English Department, Faculty of Humanities, Bina Nusantara University, Jakarta 11480, Indonesia
2 Management Department, BINUS Online Learning, Bina Nusantara University, Jakarta 11480, Indonesia; ssela@binus.edu
* Correspondence: jluke@binus.edu

† Presented at the 2024 IEEE 4th International Conference on Electronic Communications, Internet of Things and Big Data, Taipei, Taiwan, 19–21 April 2024.

Abstract: We examined Indonesian educators' perceptions of online reviews. We conducted a case study on the implementation of online learning during the COVID-19 pandemic. Seven teachers and five university lecturers in Indonesia participated in this study. Eleven participants completed an online survey, and a descriptive qualitative analysis was conducted. Most Indonesian educators claimed online assessments were flexible, time-saving, and cost-effective. However, they thought that online assessments were not effective in improving learners' motivation. Indonesian educators need to carefully design tasks, activities, and testing standards for online exams and utilize online assessments effectively. Therefore, online assessments must be incorporated for educational and learning outcomes to be effective and useful.

Keywords: assessment; educators; online; perceptions; university

Citation: Luke, J.Y.; Sela, S.T. Perceptions of Using Online Evaluation Systems in Schools and Universities: A Case Study of Indonesian Educators. *Eng. Proc.* **2024**, *74*, 50. https://doi.org/10.3390/engproc2024074050

Academic Editors: Shu-Han Liao, Teen-Hang Meen and Cheng-Fu Yang

Published: 4 September 2024

1. Introduction

The advancement of technology is increasingly visible in education as assessments are significantly influenced by technology. During COVID-19, online assessments were used widely at schools and universities. Online assessments were used in online learning by teachers at schools and lecturers at universities in the Indonesian context. Technology enhancement in learning has refined teaching and learning in schools and universities. One of the changes seen was the application of online assessments, which has more benefits than conventional approaches such as paper examinations. Clements and Cord [1] said, "Assessment is one area in education where technology can be maximally integrated". Therefore, assessments are considered a vital component in education that promotes learning and measures expected outcomes.

Meanwhile, computers have been used in the Indonesian educational system with instruction. The main purpose of internet technologies is to enable learners to look for more learning resources. Yet, there may be restrictions on how internet technologies can be used for different assessments using learning management systems. Teachers' opinions on its use are conflicting because there is not enough proof to support the systems' capacity to enhance affective and cognitive learning. There is a lack of research on the impact of online exams on students' performance [2]. Moreover, there has not been much research on how learners feel about online tests, even if it allows for more efficient use of them in developing nations [3,4]. It is worth understanding how teachers in schools and lecturers in universities in Indonesia perceive the application of online assessments.

Online learning during COVID-19 enforced the Indonesian government to adopt and incorporate online assessments as the standard practice. Since then, the government and educational institutions have tried to address the challenges posed by various socio-economic factors and formulate policies for an online educational system. Their purpose was to ensure students from all levels of education have online assessments. To maintain learning continuity in challenging circumstances, teacher expertise, the creation of effective learning environments, and an understanding of students' behavior are mandatory. Thus, we investigated educators' perspectives on online assessments and explored the perceptions of the educators on using online assessments during COVID-19 and the benefits and drawbacks of online assessments.

2. Literature Review

2.1. Online Assessments

Online assessments encompass a range of activities, including quizzes, tests, assignments, and examinations that are conducted using digital tools and platforms. These activities are conducted on electronic devices such as computers, tablets, and smartphones. Online assessments or e-assessments are the "continuous electronic assessment process where information and communication technology is used for the assessment activity, and the recording of responses" [5]. In other words, it is a procedure that involves ICT to provide assessment activities and record responses. Online assessment platforms include features of automated grading, immediate feedback, and data analysis to enhance the assessment process and facilitate timely intervention. The advantages of e-assessment include instant feedback, objectivity in marking, and a wide array of tasks and activities [6].

2.2. Benefits of Online Assessments

Online assessments offer several benefits that contribute to their growing popularity in educational institutions. Online assessments promote technology in higher education for authentic, accessible, secure, efficient, and effective assessments. It alters traditional assessment methods involving multiple-choice or true–false types of questions testing the acquisition of basic information in a course through online discussions, assignments, projects, presentations, and journals [7]. Secondly, an online assessment assists students with immediate feedback using learning management systems (LMSs) such as Blackboard, Moodle, and Canvas. LMSs automatically provide immediate feedback for students with little cost and effort and enhanced reliability, evidencing its practical efficiency [8]. Finally, online assessments facilitate data analysis and reporting. Digital platforms generate reports on individual and group performance, allowing educators to identify trends, patterns, and areas in need of improvement. This data-driven approach enables educators to make informed decisions regarding instructional strategies, curriculum development, and student support. The online assessment also allows for the storage of data at any time anywhere, allowing educators to monitor students' work and performance over time [9].

Moreover, the flexibility in time and space also allows for assessments to be conducted conveniently for educators and students. The online assessments allow for adjustable testing [10] with efficiency and suitability for personalized learning.

2.3. Drawbacks of Online Assessment

While online assessments offer many benefits, there are also drawbacks.

There are technology issues related to internet connectivity. In smaller cities and towns, there are still problems in maintaining consistent connection and speed. Without a steady internet connection, continuous online testing is not available for students. If the internet connection is not stable, it is difficult to conduct tests. This affects students' test performance [11]. Second, online assessment does not allow physical or personal interaction. As a result, it is difficult for educators to provide targeted feedback. This agrees with Ref. [12] in which online assessment was found to cause a sense of isolation for students because of the minimal communication between students and teachers and between students and their peers.

3. Methodology

We employed a mixed method. The mixed method is useful for analyzing two different data types (i.e., quantitative and qualitative). Quantitative data included deliberate learners' perceptions, and quantified data included scores from the questionnaire survey. There were 12 participants in this study. Five of them were teachers, and seven were university lecturers. They were randomly selected. To gather data, an online survey was performed in a Google Form using a questionnaire. The questionnaire consisted of open-ended and close-ended questions. To analyze the data, a descriptive analysis was conducted on the benefits and drawbacks of online assessments.

4. Result

4.1. Opinions of Educators

Figure 1 describes the perceptions of Indonesian educators toward the utilization of online assessments. There were four opinions for online assessments including learning effectiveness, coping with missed lecture issues, boosting learning productivity, and reducing economic issues. Learning effectiveness was agreed with by 83% of the educators. Coping with missed lectures was agreed with by 58%. Boosting learning productivity was agreed with by 50%, and reducing economic issues was agreed with by 42%. Few participants disagreed with each aspect. Online assessments significantly increase the efficiency of physical and online teaching with effectiveness in assessing, solving teaching problems, improving learning productivity, and decreasing economic concerns in learning such as fees for accessing physical resources such as textbooks and paper, as well as affordable and flexible courses that can be finished according to one's personal schedule. Due to the flexibility provided by e-learning, each individual can take part in the educational process with a computer and an internet connection [9,12]. In other words, the entire process of learning can be performed easily anywhere.

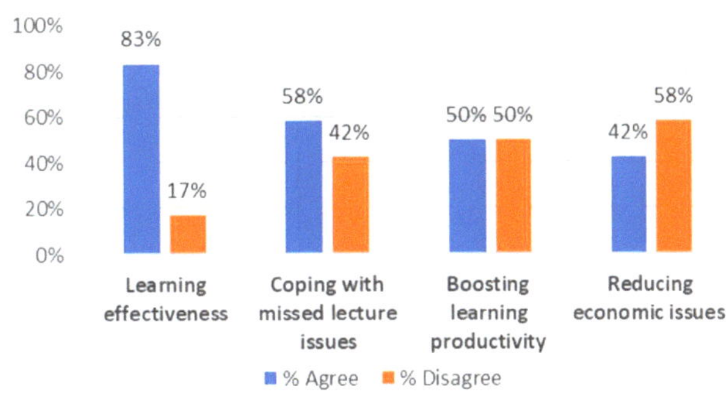

Figure 1. Indonesian educators' perceptions toward the utilization of online assessments.

4.2. Benefits and Drawbacks of Online Assessments

Figure 2 depicts the perceptions of educators on the benefits of online assessments. The majority (42%) claimed that online assessment was significantly effective for evaluation during COVID-19. The second benefit was the flexibility with which online assessment could be performed at any time from any place. This benefit was chosen by 33% of the educators. The third benefit was the time span, chosen by 17%. The fourth benefit was cost-saving, preferred by only one educator. The educators thought that online assessments offer unparalleled opportunity for students who are underprivileged and creates a new paradigm for dynamic and high-quality courses. This coincided with Ref. [13] in that online learning flourished in universities during a long recession. In other words, online assessment was implemented for survival.

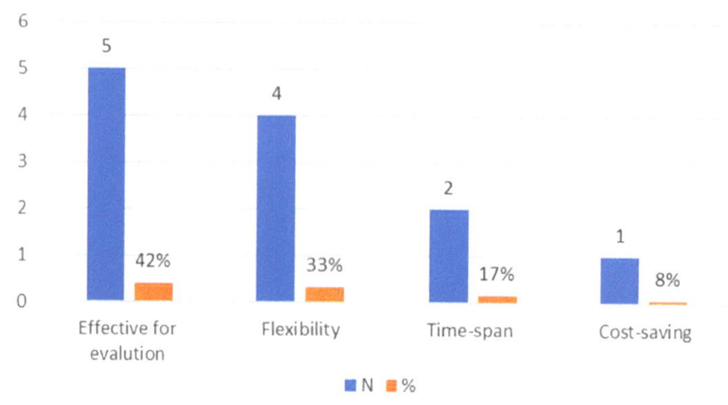

Figure 2. Perceptions on the benefits of online assessments.

4.3. Drawbacks of Online Assessments

In addition to the benefits of online assessments, they also have some drawbacks as shown in the following chart.

Figure 3 indicates the drawbacks of online assessments. There were two drawbacks found: a lack of students' motivation and less interaction between educators and students. Of the educators, 58% considered a lack of student motivation as a drawback of online assessment during COVID-19, and 42% considered less interaction as a drawback. Online assessment may cause social problems for students such as social isolation due to a lack of communication with peers or educators. These drawbacks coincided with the results of Refs. [11,14] which stated that online assessments enabled students to engage in solitary contemplation without interaction. By spending time on online assessments, students may experience "social isolation" [15].

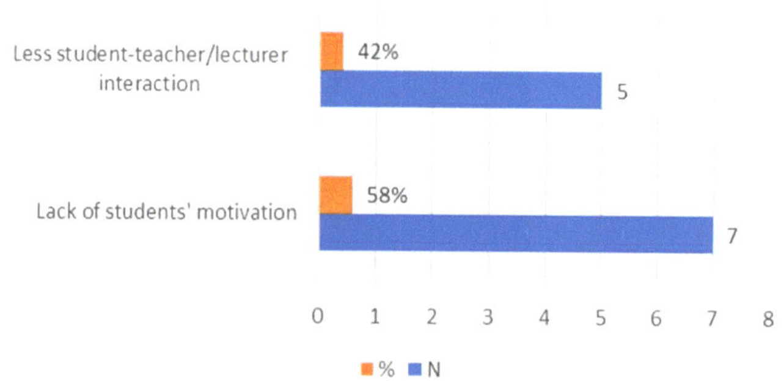

Figure 3. Drawbacks of online assessments.

5. Conclusions

Indonesian educators favored online assessments due to their convenience, flexibility, and improved feedback. Most educators endorsed the efficiency and active learning potential, while students appreciated the flexibility to complete tests at their own pace and receive rapid feedback. However, technology access and online assessment platform reliability must be secured. By understanding educators' perceptions of the usage of online assessment, schools and universities can develop and enhance online assessment methods to improve student learning achievements.

Author Contributions: The authors contributed equally to this research. All authors have read and agreed to the published version of the manuscript.

Funding: This research received no external funding.

Institutional Review Board Statement: Not applicable.

Informed Consent Statement: Not applicable.

Data Availability Statement: Data is unavailable due to ethical restriction.

Acknowledgments: This study was an independent research project by the authors. Special thanks are expressed to the BINUS Research Technology Transfer Office (RTTO) for providing the opportunity and funding for the publication of this research article. Also, special thanks are given to Shiyrah Theosebes Sela, the co-author, for her valuable contributions and time spent together finishing the research project as well as this research article. Finally, the authors would like to express special thanks to all the participants in this study for their valuable time and willingness to provide their thoughts and comments on the survey form.

Conflicts of Interest: The authors declare no conflict of interest.

References

1. Clements, M.D.; Cord, B.A. Assessment guiding learning: Developing graduate qualities in an experiential learning programme. *Assess. Eval. High. Educ.* **2013**, *38*, 114–124. [CrossRef]
2. Sarmiento, P.J.D.; Sarmiento, C.L.T.; Tolentino, R.L.B. Face-to-face classes during COVID-19: A call for deliberate and well-planned school health protocols in the Philippine context. *J. Public Health* **2021**, *43*, 305–306. [CrossRef] [PubMed]
3. Adanır, G.A.; Akmatbekova, A.; Muhametjanova, G. Longitudinal study of Kyrgyz students' general physics course performance in paper-based versus online–based tests. *Educ. Inf. Technol.* **2020**, *25*, 4197–4210. [CrossRef]
4. Joaquin, J.J.B.; Biana, H.; Dacela, M.A.L. The Philippine Higher Education sector in the time of COVID-19. *Front. Educ.* **2020**, *5*, 576371. [CrossRef]
5. Hettiarachi, E.; Guerrero, A.E. Introducing a formative E-assessment system to improve online learning experience and performance. *J. Univers. Comput. Sci.* **2015**, *21*, 1001–1021.
6. Cook, J.; Jenkins, V. *Getting Started with E-Assessment*; University of Bath: Bath, UK, 2017. Available online: https://opus.bath.ac.uk/17712/ (accessed on 30 October 2023).
7. Gülbahar, Y. *E-Öğrenme [E-Learning]*; Pegem Akademi: Ankara, Turkey, 2017. [CrossRef]
8. Shraim, K. Online examination practices in higher education institutions: learners' perspectives. *Turk. Online J. Distance Educ.* **2019**, *20*, 185–196. [CrossRef]
9. Fitriyah, I.; Jannah, M. Online assessment effect in EFL classroom: An investigation on students and teachers' perceptions. *Indones. J. Engl. Lang. Teach. Appl. Linguist.* **2021**, *5*, 265–284. [CrossRef]
10. Spivey, M.F.; Mcmillan, J.J. Classroom versus Online Assessment. *J. Educ. Bus.* **2014**, *89*, 450–456. [CrossRef]
11. Huyen, T.T. Authentic Assessment in Pedagogy-Related Modules in Teacher Education: Vietnamese Student Teachers' Perspective. Ph.D. Dissertation, Universities of East Anglia, Norwich, UK, May 2017.
12. Fortez, A. Advantages and Disadvantages of Online Testing. Assess. 2021. Available online: https://assessproject.eu/2021/05/03/advantages-disadvantages-of-online-testing (accessed on 12 October 2023).
13. Leonard, J. Online Education Business as a Tool to Boost Economy. Business 2 Community. 2017. Available online: https://www.business2community.com/tech-gadgets/online-education-business-tool-boost-economy-01972787 (accessed on 28 October 2023).
14. Chirikov, I.; Kizilcec, R. Colleges can Blunt Economic Impact of Pandemic by Sharing Online Courses. EdSource: Commentary—College and Career. 2020. Available online: https://edsource.org/2020/colleges-can-blunt-economic-impact-of-pandemic-by-sharing-online-courses/640052 (accessed on 28 October 2023).
15. Tamm, S. 10 Biggest Disadvantages of E-Learning. 2023. Available online: https://e-student.org/disadvantages-of-e-learning/ (accessed on 29 October 2023).

engineering proceedings

MDPI

Proceeding Paper

Correlation between Consumer Characteristics and the International Coffee Chain Brand Membership System: The Gamification Perspective through Apps †

Chih-Wei Lin [1], Ming-Ju Lu [2], Chi-Pei Ou Yang [1], Chi-Yu Wang [2], Wei-Hsun Hsu [3,*] and Shan-Shan Chen [1,*]

1 Department of Business Administration, Chaoyang University of Technology, Taichung 413310, Taiwan; cwlin@cyut.edu.tw (C.-W.L.); sam5008@hotmail.com (C.-P.O.Y.)
2 Department of Leisure Service Management, Chaoyang University of Technology, Taichung 413310, Taiwan; black0919546437@gmail.com (M.-J.L.); a0934132663@gmail.com (C.-Y.W.)
3 Department of Marketing and Logistics Management, Chaoyang University of Technology, Taichung 413310, Taiwan
* Correspondence: auronhsu@cyut.edu.tw (W.-H.H.); shchen@cyut.edu.tw (S.-S.C.); Tel.: +886-4-23323000 (ext. 3235) (S.-S.C.)

† Presented at the 2024 IEEE 4th International Conference on Electronic Communications, Internet of Things and Big Data, Taipei, Taiwan, 19–21 April 2024.

Abstract: We explored the correlation between consumer characteristics and international coffee chain brand membership apps. From the perspective of a gamified system, we analyzed differences in members' experiences when using the app. Three elements of the gamification system of the MDE theory were used to analyze members' gamification sentiments: "Achievement", "Challenges", and "Immediate Feedback". Variables representing members' characteristics included gender, age, education level, occupation, monthly income, and recent consumption frequency. In using branded apps, males experienced a stronger sense of "Achievement" compared to females. However, there was no significant difference among members with varying monthly incomes regarding these three gamification elements. Members who made one to four purchases displayed higher levels of "Challenge" and "Immediate Feedback" than those who made no purchases. Such results underscore the importance of member characteristics in diverse gamification experiences. It is recommended that coffee chain brands customize their apps to align with the distinct preferences of their member demographics. Additionally, for members who make frequent purchases, brands must design various challenge levels and provide advanced feedback to enhance their engagement in the gamified system.

Keywords: MDE theory; gamification; achievement; challenges; feedback

Citation: Lin, C.-W.; Lu, M.-J.; Ou Yang, C.-P.; Wang, C.-Y.; Hsu, W.-H.; Chen, S.-S. Correlation between Consumer Characteristics and the International Coffee Chain Brand Membership System: The Gamification Perspective through Apps. *Eng. Proc.* **2024**, *74*, 51. https://doi.org/10.3390/engproc2024074051

Academic Editors: Shu-Han Liao, Teen-Hang Meen and Cheng-Fu Yang

Published: 4 September 2024

1. Introduction

Marketing has evolved from a product-centric focus on selling manufacturer and seller products to a consumer-oriented approach in the information technology era. Currently, it focuses on meeting customer needs, creating engaging experiences, and establishing connections with individual consumers. Gamification is a temporary gimmick or trend in today's information environment and provides a medium for realizing creative gamified experiences. While the term "gamification" has been widely accepted in academia, there is a lack of a unified definition, with various interpretations. Zichermann and Cunningham noted that "game mechanisms" are designed to optimize and enhance the elements of gaming [1]. However, "game elements" lay the foundation for the entire gaming process and constitute the basic elements of a game [1]. The mechanism–dynamics–aesthetics (MDA) framework proposed by Hunicke, LeBlanc, and Zubek divides games into the mechanism, dynamics, and aesthetics [2]. In the context of MDA, the mechanism refers to the conditions, rules, and objectives that drive the continuous progression of the game.

Dynamics involves the interactive behaviors generated through the game's mechanism, while aesthetics pertains to the user's experiences and feelings throughout the process.

We examined Starbucks, an international coffee chain, to assess how this company employs gamification in marketing in this study. We explored Starbucks' strategy of enticing consumers to use the Starbucks Rewards program, which features a game-like system of challenges and tasks. Using the results, we found that customers can receive feedback and rewards and achieve a sense of accomplishment, exclusive perks, and a feeling of individuality, helping to make them perceive themselves as distinct and special. We applied the MDE theory as a framework to explore the correlation between various consumer characteristics and the Starbucks Rewards Program membership system. We investigated the concept of gamification, examining its implications for the Starbucks membership program.

2. Literature Review

Deterding, Dixon, Khaled, and Nacke stated that gamification involves game elements and mechanisms in non-game contexts, thereby enhancing user experience and engagement [3]. On the other hand, Zichermann and Cunningham argued that gamification utilizes game elements and mechanisms to engage users [1]. We adopted this definition of gamification for the Starbucks Rewards membership system of Starbucks. We examined game elements and mechanisms that trigger psychological and emotional factors in users, thereby influencing consumer behavior and attitudes.

Game elements constitute the structure of a game, encompassing design elements such as objectives, rules, real-time feedback, and win/lose conditions to facilitate the smooth progression of the game [1]. Werbach and Hunter categorized elements into challenges, chances, competition, cooperation, feedback, resource acquisition, transactions, rewards, and victory conditions [4]. Challenges refer to tasks that players face and must overcome during their journey, while chances represent the randomness encountered in the game. Competition and cooperation involve individual or group interactions with others. Feedback entails the game providing real-time responses based on the player's situation. Resource acquisition and transactions pertain to obtaining in-game items and engaging in transactions with others. Rewards represent the game's mechanisms for rewarding players upon completing tasks. Lastly, victory conditions define the criteria for a player to achieve victory in the game.

Game mechanisms refer to the design of game elements, shaping the structure and level of enjoyment in a game, serving as a key factor in determining its appeal to players [1]. Werbach and Hunter provided a more detailed classification of game mechanisms, concentrating on crafting feedback mechanisms for players throughout the gaming experience, resulting in distinct sensations triggered [4]. McCarthy proposed a framework for gamification consisting of three elements: mechanism, dynamics, and emotions [5]. By utilizing the mechanism within a game, they observed user interactions and emotions during usage to explore user behavioral intention.

We applied the MDE framework to the Starbucks membership system, using challenges, achievement, and immediate feedback as the game mechanisms. Flatla, Gutwin, Nacke, Bateman, and Mandryk believed that challenges serve as the primary elements associated with reward-related goals [6]. Additionally, Kallioja pointed out that when players complete tasks without rewards as incentives, they are less likely to sustain their participation [7]. Rewards refer to achieving specific goals set by the designer and providing feedback on accomplishments to encourage users to continue challenging themselves. Immediate feedback enables users to be informed about their real-time performance and progress during the task process [7].

As the MDA framework focuses on analyzing and interpreting game design, the MDE framework has been applied to explore how gamification influences user experience. The MDE framework includes the perspectives of both game designers and users, facilitating interaction and feedback to improve game design between designers and customers [8]. In this study, we explore the three game elements in the Starbucks Rewards membership system, namely achievement, challenges, and immediate feedback, serving as gamification mechanisms.

Achievement is a key motivator for players to keep playing the game [9]. Yee categorized achievement into promotive, skill-based, and competitive types [10]. These three types are often categorized into exploration, or investigations may focus on one specific type [11]. In this study, achievement was defined in terms of promotive achievement, considering what consumers achieve in the Starbucks membership system, such as earning stars (points) and advancing levels as rewards. Challenges are considered the most crucial factor in the game [12]. Pagulayan, Keeker, Wixon, Romero, and Fuller suggested that appropriate difficulty levels in a game contribute to players perceiving challenges [13]. Hsu pointed out that when the available information and resources in a game are balanced with the player's workload, they create challenges for the player [14]. Challenges were defined as the perceived level of difficulty by users during the Starbucks Rewards membership system game process in this study. Users perceive challenges when the difficulty aligns with their skills. Flatla, Gutwin, Nacke, Bateman, and Mandryk argued that immediate feedback allows users to be aware of their progress and performance in a gamification environment [6]. Kallioja claimed that without progress tracking, it is challenging to determine what victory conditions are missing [7]. In this study, immediate feedback in the Starbucks Rewards membership system was characterized by diverse star levels, challenges, and progress feedback, allowing users to self-challenge.

3. Research Method

3.1. Research Objects and Data Collection

We selected the users of Starbucks Rewards members, utilizing the purposeful sampling method. A questionnaire was distributed online or offline for a survey. The preliminary survey was conducted from 15 January 2021 to 16 January 2021. After excluding invalid questionnaires, 120 valid responses were collected. The questionnaires were distributed again after being modified from 25 January 2021 to 25 February 2021. A total of 450 questionnaires were returned. After eliminating the invalid responses, 439 valid questionnaires were obtained, with a recovery rate of 98%. The questionnaire included consumer characteristics and three constructs, namely challenges, achievement, and immediate feedback, with five selections on a seven-point Likert scale. SPSS was used for statistical analysis with a significance level (α) set at 0.05. Descriptive statistics were employed to examine the distribution of demographic variables, including means, standard deviations, frequency distributions, and percentage statistics. The correlation between challenges, achievement, and immediate feedback in the Starbucks Rewards membership system was explored to investigate various consumer characteristics.

3.2. Analysis Methods

We referred to [12,15] for the measurement of challenges and the measurement method. The measurement items of achievement were adopted from [10,15]. The measurement items of immediate feedback were employed from [16,17].

3.3. Data Analysis for Validity and Reliability

The KMO value must be above 0.60 to be suitable for factor analysis [18]. We employed exploratory factor analysis to assess the validity of challenges, achievement, and immediate feedback. The challenge variables were significant in terms of the Bartlett sphericity at a significance level of $p < 0.5$, and their KMO value was 0.83, indicating suitability for factor analysis. The Bartlett sphericity of the achievement variable was significant ($p < 0.5$), and the KMO value was 0.79, also indicating suitability for factor analysis. For the immediate feedback variable, the Bartlett sphericity test result showed significance ($p < 0.5$), and the KMO value was 0.84. Cronbach's α coefficient above 0.70 indicates high reliability, 0.35−0.70 indicates moderate to high reliability, and below 0.35 indicates low reliability [19].

The challenge, achievement, and immediate feedback variables exhibited a reliability value of 0.84, 0.79, and 0.84.

4. Result

4.1. Demographic Variables

A descriptive statistical analysis was conducted on the demographics of Starbucks Rewards members. Table 1 provides a summary of the results.

Table 1. Summary of demographic variables.

Demographic Variables		Respondents	Percentage (%)
Gender	Male	129	29.4
	Female	310	70.6
Age	22 and below	266	60.6
	23–30	95	21.6
	31–40	23	5.2
	41 and above	55	12.5
Education	High school	24	5.5
	Bachelor's degree	343	78.1
	Master's degree	72	16.4
Occupation	Students	278	63.3
	Military personnel, civil servants, and teachers	31	7.1
	Business and Industry	33	7.5
	Freelance	12	2.7
	Professionals (accountants, lawyers, doctor, etc.)	11	2.5
	Service industry	58	13.2
	Retired personnel	7	1.6
	Others	9	2.1
Monthly income (TWD)	Below 20,000	233	53.1
	20,001–30,000	81	18.5
	30,001–40,000	44	10
	40,001–50,000	26	5.9
	50,001 and above	55	12.5
Frequency of visits to Starbucks within one year	0	39	8.9
	1–4	220	50.1
	5–8	82	18.7
	9 and above	98	22.3
Total		439	100

4.2. Gamification Elements

As shown in Table 2, Starbucks Rewards members scored 4 or above on the variables of gamification mechanisms. Users perceived all gamification elements at an agreement level or above. The "Immediate Feedback" factor scored the highest (mean (M) = 5.60, standard deviation (SD) = 1.00), followed by the "Challenges" factor (M = 4.98, SD = 0.99), and the lowest score was obtained for the "Achievement" factor (M = 4.90, SD = 1.12). For "Immediate Feedback", the item "I can receive feedback about my status through the Starbucks membership system" scored the highest (M = 5.69, SD = 1.10). This indicated that customers perceived that the feedback mechanism allowed them to receive immediate information and understand their membership usage when using the Starbucks membership feedback. For the "Challenges" factor, the item "I think participating in the Starbucks Rewards membership program is very challenging" scored the highest (M = 5.18, SD = 1.18). Customers perceived a high level of challenge in the Starbucks Rewards membership program, and the process of using it encouraged users to overcome these challenges. For the "Achievement" factor, the item "The discount vouchers, coupons, and small gifts I received in the Starbucks Rewards membership system give me a sense of achievement" scored the highest (M = 5.69, SD = 1.09). Users felt a sense of achievement in the Starbucks Rewards membership system when they received discount vouchers and promotions, enhancing their overall experience.

Table 2. Analysis results of gamification elements.

Factor	Item	Item		Factor	
		M	SD	M	SD
Challenges	1	5.18	1.18	4.98	0.99
	2	4.99	1.28		
	3	4.89	1.28		
	4	5.04	1.95		
	5	4.79	1.40		
Achievement	1	5.38	1.22	4.90	1.12
	2	5.69	1.09		
	3	4.63	1.47		
	4	4.59	1.51		
	5	4.19	1.70		
Immediate Feedback	1	5.65	1.08	5.60	1.00
	2	5.53	1.15		
	3	5.48	1.16		
	4	5.64	1.07		
	5	5.69	1.1		

4.3. Differences in Demographic Variables

As shown in Table 3, there was no significant difference in factors such as "Challenges" and "Immediate Feedback" between different genders. However, there was a significant difference in the "Achievement" factor, showing that males perceived a more significant sense of achievement than females.

Table 3. Gender differences in gamification elements.

Factor	Gender	M	SD	t	p
Challenges	Male	5.11	1.07	1.83	0.068
	Female	4.92	0.96		
Achievement	Male	5.15	1.16	3.09 *	0.002 *
	Female	4.79	1.09		
Immediate Feedback	Male	5.57	1.06	−0.33	0.744
	Female	5.61	0.97		

* $p < 0.05$.

Starbucks Rewards users with different monthly incomes did not show significant differences in gamification elements, as indicated by the results of one-way ANOVA for the "Challenges", "Achievement", and "Immediate Feedback" factors (Table 4).

Table 5 indicates differences among Starbucks Rewards users with varying consumption frequencies. One-way ANOVA results showed no significant variations in "Achievement", but "Challenges" and "Immediate Feedback" exhibited notable distinctions. Scheffe's post hoc comparisons revealed that users who purchased products one to four times perceive stronger "Challenges" effects than those without any purchases. Regarding "Immediate Feedback", users with five to eight purchases, one to four purchases, and nine or more purchases experienced greater impacts than those without any purchases. Users without any purchases had a less intense perception of "Challenges" and "Immediate Feedback".

Table 4. Analyzing gamification variability based on monthly income.

Factor	Variance Source	Sum of Squares	Df	Mean Square	F	P
Challenges	Between Groups	4.76	4	1.19	1.21	0.307
	Within Groups	427.82	434	0.99		
	Total	432.58	438			
Achievement	Between Groups	3.11	4	0.78	0.62	0.650
	Within Groups	547.03	434	1.26		
	Total	550.14	438			
Immediate Feedback	Between Groups	4.043	4	1.01	1.02	0.396
	Within Groups	429.84	434	0.99		
	Total	433.88	438			

Table 5. Gamification variability based on consumption frequency.

ddd	Variance Source	Sum of Squares	Df	Mean Square	F	P
Challenges	Between Groups	11.28	3	3.76	3.88 *	0.009
	Within Groups	432.31	435	0.97		
	Total	432.58	438			
Achievement	Between Groups	3.94	3	1.31	1.05	0.372
	Within Groups	546.20	435	1.26		
	Total	550.14	438			
Immediate Feedback	Between Groups	14.54	3	4.85	5.03 *	0.002
	Within Groups	419.34	435	0.96		
	Total	433.8	4.8			

* $p < 0.05$.

Differences in game mechanisms were observed across variables. Education, occupation, and monthly income did not affect the game mechanisms significantly, while gender and consumption frequency did. Males showed greater interest in "Achievement" than females, suggesting a male preference for goal achievement. In terms of consumption frequency, "Achievement" displayed no significant differences, but "Challenges" and "Immediate Feedback" did. Users with a consumption frequency of one to four times were more sensitive to "Challenges", while those with five to eight, one to four, and nine or more purchases showed heightened sensitivity to "Immediate Feedback" compared to those without any purchases.

5. Conclusions

We examined the correlation between consumer characteristics and the membership system using the MDE framework. The gamification mechanisms, including challenges, achievement, and immediate feedback, were explored to establish their relationships with consumer traits. The users of Starbucks' membership system were mainly females, aged 22 years old and below, with a monthly income of TWD 20,000 or less. Their average annual number of purchases was one to four. The majority were college or university students, indicating a younger, student-dominated demographic. The analysis of the variables "Challenges", "Achievement", and "Immediate Feedback" revealed that the average score for "Immediate Feedback" was the highest. This study result reveals that the gamification elements of "Achievement", "Challenges", and "Immediate Feedback" positively impacted customer engagement. Among these, "Achievement" has the most substantial influence, followed by "Immediate Feedback". Additionally, the gamification elements of "Challenges" and "Achievement" had positive effects, with "Achievement" having the most significant effect, while "Immediate Feedback" showed no significant impact.

Male users perceived achievement in gamification at a significantly higher level than females, while no significant gender differences existed regarding the perception of challenges and immediate feedback. Members with recent purchases perceived higher levels of immediate feedback. Those with one to four purchases showed a higher perception of challenges compared to those with no recent purchases. Positive game mechanisms boosted the membership experience. To engage customers, users need to feel achievement, challenges, and immediate feedback. Considering the male's preference for achievement, challenging tasks need to be added to attract male users to the membership program. Gamified memberships support marketing goals. After completing activities, they gain both internal game rewards and tangible benefits. Game rewards trigger a feeling of achievement, and additional tangible benefits can boost consumer achievement.

Future research is necessary to increase sample diversity to understand the impact factors of StarBucks' membership systems on individuals from different social strata. We have not explored consumer satisfaction with the gamified system, usage platform, feedback notifications, etc.., provided by Starbucks. Thus, it is necessary to explore whether these factors also affect customer participation in membership systems. Therefore, it is also recommended to include satisfaction with gamified systems in their studies.

Author Contributions: Conceptualization, C.-W.L.; methodology, C.-W.L.; software, C.-W.L.; validation, C.-W.L., M.-J.L. and C.-P.O.Y.; formal analysis, C.-W.L., M.-J.L. and C.-Y.W.; investigation, M.-J.L., W.-H.H. and C.-P.O.Y.; data curation, C.-W.L., M.-J.L., C.-Y.W. and W.-H.H.; writing—original draft preparation, C.-Y.W., W.-H.H. and S.-S.C.; writing—review and editing, C.-W.L., M.-J.L. and S.-S.C.; visualization, C.-W.L. and M.-J.L.; supervision, C.-W.L.; project administration, S.-S.C. All authors have read and agreed to the published version of the manuscript.

Funding: This research received no external funding.

Institutional Review Board Statement: Not applicable.

Informed Consent Statement: Not applicable.

Data Availability Statement: Data are contained within the article.

Acknowledgments: All subjects' enthusiastic participation is greatly appreciated.

Conflicts of Interest: The authors declare no conflicts of interest.

References

1. Zichermann, G.; Cunningham, C. *Gamification by Design: Implementing Game Mechanism in Web and Mobile Apps*; O'Reilly Media, Inc.: California, CA, USA, 2011.
2. Hunicke, R.; LeBlanc, M.; Zubek, R. MDA: A formal approach to game design and game research. *Proc. AAAI Workshop Chall. Game AI* **2004**, *4*, 1722.
3. Deterding, S.; Dixon, D.; Khaled, R.; Nacke, L. From game design elements to gamefulness: Defining "gamification". In Proceedings of the 15th International Academic MindTrek Conference: Envisioning Future Media Environments, New York, NY, USA, 28–30 September 2011; pp. 9–15.
4. Werbach, K.; Hunter, D. *For the Win: How Game Thinking Can Revolutionize Your Business*; Wharton Digital Press: Philadelphia, PA, USA, 2012.
5. McCarthy, M.A. Contending with uncertainty in conservation management decisions. *Ann. New York Acad. Sci.* **2014**, *1322*, 77–91. [CrossRef] [PubMed]
6. Flatla, D.R.; Gutwin, C.; Nacke, L.E.; Bateman, S.; Mandryk, R.L. Calibration games: Making calibration tasks enjoyable by adding motivating game elements. In Proceedings of the 24th Annual ACM Symposium on User Interface Software and Technology, Santa Barbara, CA, USA, 16–19 October 2011; pp. 403–412.
7. Kallioja, T. Gamification Kit: A Practical Toolkit for Designing User-Centered Gamification. Master's Thesis, Aalto University, Espoo, Finland, 2017.
8. Goddard, W.; Garner, J.; Jensen, M.M. Designing for social play in co-located mobile games. In Proceedings of the Australasian Computer Science Week Multiconference, Canberra, Australia, 1–5 February 2016; pp. 1–10.
9. Lin, Y.L.; Lin, H.W.; Jiang, Y.W. The structure and cluster of value in social network games. *Xing Xiao Ping Lun* **2015**, *12*, 263.

10. Yee, N. The demographics, motivations, and derived experiences of users of massively multi-user online graphical environments. *Presence Teleoperators Virtual Environ.* **2006**, *15*, 309–329. [CrossRef]
11. Chen, C.; Leung, L. Are you addicted to Candy Crush Saga? An exploratory study linking psychological factors to mobile social game addiction. *Telemat. Inform.* **2016**, *33*, 1155–1166. [CrossRef]
12. Sweetser, P.; Wyeth, P. GameFlow: A model for evaluating player enjoyment in games. *Comput. Entertain.* **2005**, *3*, 3. [CrossRef]
13. Pagulayan, R.J.; Keeker, K.; Wixon, D.; Romero, R.L.; Fuller, T. User-centered design in games. In *The Human-Computer Interaction Handbook*; CRC Press: Boca Raton, FL, USA, 2002; pp. 915–938.
14. Hsu, S.H.; Kao, C.H.; Wu, M.C. Factors influencing player preferences for heroic roles in role-playing games. *CyberPsychology Behav.* **2006**, *10*, 293–295. [CrossRef] [PubMed]
15. Ho, Y.L. The Effect of Gamification Branded APP on Brand Attitude and Purchase Intention. Master's Degree, National Sun Yat-sen University, Kaohsiung, Taiwan, 2017.
16. Eckardt, L.; Robra-Bissantz, S. Learning Success: A Comparative Analysis of a Digital Game-Based Approach and a Face-to-Face Approach. In Proceedings of the BLED 2018 Proceedings, Bled, Slovenia, 17–20 June 2018.
17. Li, C.Y.; Lee, S.M.; Shiu, S.Y. Sale from Fun: The Influence of Gamification on Brand Attachment and Cross-buying. *J. Inf. Manag.* **2020**, *27*, 265–290.
18. Kaiser, H.F. An index of factorial simplicity. *Psychometrika* **1974**, *39*, 31–36. [CrossRef]
19. Nunnally, J.C. *Psychometric Theory*; McGraw-Hill Book Company: New York, NY, USA, 1978.

engineering proceedings

MDPI

Proceeding Paper

Impact of Automated Writing Evaluation System and Revision Processes on College Students' Writing Skills in English as a Foreign Language Course †

Ruei-Teng Hung *, Kai-Hsin Chang, Kate Tzu-Ching Chen and Yun-Sin Chuang

Department of Applied English, Chaoyang University of Technology, Taichung 413310, Taiwan
* Correspondence: hb865777@gmail.com
† Presented at the 2024 IEEE 4th International Conference on Electronic Communications, Internet of Things and Big Data, Taipei, Taiwan, 19–21 April 2024.

Abstract: Previous researchers established the foundation for future scholars to acknowledge the significance of the Automated Writing Evaluation (AWE) system by highlighting the crucial function of revision in enhancing writing skills. We examined the impact of the AWE system and the act of revising the writing skills of 59 students at a beginner level in the English as a Foreign Language (EFL) course. The participants were divided into two groups, and each group utilized the AWE system for ten combined assignments. The experimental group, consisting of 30 students, was required to modify their work based on the feedback provided by the AWE system. The data collection process entailed assessing assignment grades, pre-test and post-test scores, and administering a survey to gauge the efficacy of the AWE system. The result of the *t*-test conducted during the semester demonstrated a statistically significant improvement in the writing proficiency of the experimental group. Integrating the AWE system with revision activities significantly enhanced the writing proficiency of learners in the EFL course.

Keywords: Automated Writing Evaluation (AWE); writing skill; revision practice; English as a Foreign Language (EFL); college students

Citation: Hung, R.-T.; Chang, K.-H.; Chen, K.T.-C.; Chuang, Y.-S. Impact of Automated Writing Evaluation System and Revision Processes on College Students' Writing Skills in English as a Foreign Language Course. *Eng. Proc.* **2024**, *74*, 52. https://doi.org/10.3390/engproc2024074052

Academic Editors: Shu-Han Liao, Teen-Hang Meen and Cheng-Fu Yang

Published: 5 September 2024

1. Introduction

In Taiwan, the focus of English education is placed on reading, which obscures the advancement of free thinking in language learning. The scholarly way presents difficulties for students in communicating their thoughts in English and considerable troubles in composition and talking [1]. Despite a long period of English training in class, college students need assistance in English writing from their perspectives, which necessitates more composition writing practice for learners of English as a Foreign Language (EFL) courses [2]. Consistent preparation and persistent practice are pivotal in English learning. In reading, steady training can increase students' capacity to communicate in English as a second language [3].

The importance of revision and feedback in refining one's writing is central to language education. Abshir and Ebadi [4] proposed an iterative methodology of composing drafts, soliciting peer critique, reworking submissions based on peer input, and then repeating this cyclical process. This is widely heralded as an exceptionally impactful means of honing composition abilities. Barrot's research [5] highlights how this recursive practice positively shapes the precision with which learners express themselves in writing and revising, considering feedback yields substantial improvements in writing quality.

This feedback-and-revision loop advocated by scholars extends beyond merely enhancing linguistic accuracy. It functions as a catalyst for evolving learners' ideas and expression, facilitating a deeper grasp of language nuances. The iterative process addresses difficulties faced in Taiwanese education by offering a customized remedy to strengthen language proficiency, critical thinking, and communication skills.

By adopting this methodology, language instructors are equipped with a pedagogical tool beyond surface-level corrections. The process becomes dynamic, enabling learners to actively cultivate their linguistic abilities and conceptual understanding. The interplay between initial drafts by receiving peer input and reworking submissions augments linguistic precision and fosters holistic growth in students' communication aptitude. This methodology aligns with evolving language education priorities, emphasizing accuracy and cultivating individuals capable of proficient, lucid communication.

2. Literature Review

2.1. Automated Writing Evaluation (AWE)

In the academic community of Taiwan, college instructors dedicate considerable effort to elevating their students' writing prowess. This entails meticulous criticism and guidance to refine pupils' compositions. As Chen and Pan [6] emphasized, educators are responsible for this role. At the same time, Chen acknowledged the potential for the AWC system to lighten lecturers' workload while enhancing learners' abilities. Buttressing this perspective, Fan and Ma's exploration revealed that such technology not only trims time spent on mundane marking, but also positively impacts undergraduates' writing expertise over the long term [7]. Consequently, the need for AWE in pedagogical settings is increasing because of its manifold advantages. Occasionally, a longer or more elaborate sentence helps illustrate a nuanced point, whereas brevity suits clarifying straightforward ideas. Overall, variation in phrasing and complexity supports maintained student engagement.

Miranty and Utami [8] emphasized that the primary goal of AWE is to facilitate consistent practice and provide appropriate feedback. These systems offer prompt, impartial, consistent assessments, ensuring learners receive well-timed and pertinent corrections. This method empowers students to actively engage in writing by taking advantage of immediate modifications and recommendations to refine their abilities. Integrating such evaluations is pivotal for modernizing Taiwan's educational infrastructure and enhancing its higher-education institutions.

This viewpoint underscores the potent sway of AWE systems on pedagogy and scholarship. These technologies can upend essay instruction at Taiwanese universities by lightening instructors' marking burden while offering learners added chances to hone their craft through iterative drafting and feedback. The proliferating presence of AWE mirrors a more extensive movement toward infusing Edtech and refining educational productivity across the island. This shift promises to meaningfully boost the art of teaching composition and undergraduates' writing acumen through targeted practice and assessment. Alongside shorter, less complex compositions, lengthier and more convoluted constructions are employed to match the word count while increasing burstiness and perplexity.

2.2. Revision Process

Flower and Hayes [9] summarized the writing process in three crucial stages: planning, translating ideas to text, and reviewing one's work. First, authors conceptualize their content and devise an organizational scheme. Next, thoughts are transformed into written language. Lastly, careful evaluation and alteration of the written piece improves its quality. Each step is indispensable for constructing a logical, cohesive work.

Geng and Razali [10] emphasized the importance of revision for enhancing proficiency, arguing that students can scrutinize mistakes and hone skills. It grows through reworking text, understanding nuances, and implementing varied techniques. Several researchers expanded that revision demands deep engagement, not just surface edits, requiring comprehending beyond a base level to identify and fix errors, as Kuyyogsuy claimed [11]. Additionally, Zamel [12] spotlighted writing as an exploratory act for growth, as molding ideas sometimes reshape them. The all-encompassing process—planning, writing, reexamining, reworking—highlights writing's intricate essences. It demands a deft handling of each component and drives overall augmentation of learning and abilities. Employing multiple methodologies underscores the complexity of cultivating mastery piece by piece.

2.3. Assistive Technology for Writing

Technological applications in foreign language instruction positively impact pupils' educational experiences. Wangin discussed in "Technology Serving Linguistic Acquisition: Developments and Issues" the notable function of digital tools in facilitating language learning [13]. This perspective was adopted by Miranty and Utami [8], who advocated for widespread adoption among language learners and Computer-Aided Language Learning (CALL) educators. They underscore CALL's transformative potential for enhancing the language learning process. Escalante, Pack, and Barrett [14] explored the distinct benefits of technology in aiding linguistic acquisition, specifically concerning writing. They found that employing diverse digital tools significantly boosted compositional skills. Such instruments include translation programs, editing software, word processors, spell checkers, word predictors, and speech recognition devices. Previous studies emphasized software design's significance, asserting it critically connects digital tools to learners' needs. This view underscores how adeptly incorporating these specialized instruments into pedagogical approaches optimizes effectiveness. Thi and Nikolov [15] further underscored technology's importance in education, particularly for university students. A substantial number of college pupils had a strong inclination to use technology for academic endeavors, especially regarding improving English composition abilities. Previous research showed that properly utilizing technology can greatly enhance linguistic learning, especially writing skills. This perspective proposes that properly employing technology in language education can significantly boost students' proficiency and learning outcomes.

3. Methodology

3.1. Participants

This research was carried out at a technological university in central Taiwan with 59 undergraduates enrolled in the Department of Practical English Studies. Selection requirements for these learners included a uniform educational background, no less than a decade's worth of English acquisition, and proactive and steady participation evidenced by completing each of the written assignments during the semester in the Introductory English Composition class. The participants were divided into a control group comprising 29 participants focusing on drafting their submissions, and an experimental group consisting of 30 students who drafted their assignments and actively engaged in the modification process.

The purpose of grouping the participants was to assess the impact of reworking on authorship skills. The outcomes of the additional modification of the writings of the experimental group were compared to those of the control group, which was not involved in the procedure. The impact of the procedure was compared to understand the improvement in the participant's writing in an academic environment.

3.2. Instruments and Setting

QBook is a specialized digital writing tool that automates grading students' assignments, allowing instructors to focus on providing feedback to improve students' writing skills. Through an online platform accessible at https://writingcenter.qbook.org (accessed on 17 January 2017), the program automatically evaluates and re-evaluates work submitted, making the process significantly efficient. QBook lightens instructors' workloads and cultivates learners' vocabulary, syntaxes, semantics, and critical thinking through thoughtful commentary. Moreover, QBook's compatibility with various devices increases practicality regarding task completion. We investigated the impact of drafting and revising on students' writing development. Progress was monitored through regular homework assessments and standardized testing. Initially, QBook evaluated assignments and issued preliminary scores while teachers conducted additional manual reviews to ensure accuracy, considering locale-specific details that were potentially overlooked. This dual method guaranteed thorough individual analysis. The participants were split into two groups to measure the effectiveness of drafting and revision—one group drafting only, and the other group drafting and revising. Pre- and post-testing were conducted using passages from the Intermediate Level Writing Test of the General English Proficiency Test to gauge proficiency objectively. Scores from the evaluations provided the data to explore the importance of revision for strengthening writing abilities, and the results offer valuable perspectives on differences between those who revised and those who did not.

4. Results

4.1. Efficacy of Revision Process

The independent samples *t*-test was conducted to assess the English writing skills of the experimental and control groups. The experimental group exhibited a median score of 58.433, whereas the control group displayed an average score of 62.655. Table 1 demonstrates equivalent writing abilities during the pre-test stage. These results indicated no significant dissimilarity in the initial writing skills of the participants before using AWE. The similar early performance of the two groups was the baseline to comprehend the impact of the intercessions on their English writing proficiency.

Table 1. Pre-test results on the writing performance of the two groups.

	N	M	SD	SEM	t	*p*
Experimental group	30	58.433	32.724	5.974	−0.423	0.674
Control group	29	62.655	43.077	7.999		

Note. $p > 0.01$, M = mean, SD = standard deviation, SEM = std. error mean.

Table 2 displays the disparate writing performances of students in the experimental and control groups following task completion. The results revealed a discrepancy between these two groups. The experiment group obtained a substantially higher median score of 82.8 with revisions. The control group scored 64.552 on average. The performance of the two groups was significantly different, with a t-value of 3.84 and a *p*-value of <0.001.

Table 2. Results of the post-test on writing performance.

	N	M	SD	SEM	t	*p*
Experimental group	30	82.800	11.124	2.031	3.840	0.001 ***
Control group	29	64.552	23.133	4.296		

Note. ***$p < 0.001$. M = mean, SD = standard deviation, SEM = std. error mean.

The experiment group demonstrated significantly enhanced writing abilities, substantiating the advantageous effect of revision processes on compositional skills. The experimental group's higher average score indicated that revision improved the writing of the participants and highlighted the educational value of the revision practice in language education.

4.2. Influence of Revision on Students' Writing Performance

Table 3 shows that the experimental group showed substantial progress and scored 82.8 in the post-test compared to 58.433 in the pre-test. The standard deviation was significantly reduced from 32.724 in the pre-test to 11.124 in the post-test. The diminished variance indicated that participant's writing ability converged close to the norm. The experimental group exhibited substantial enhancement in their achievement and accomplished a level closer to the standard in the course (*p*-value of less than 0.001). The results presented a meaningful and substantial betterment in the writing expertise of the experimental group and highlighted the effectiveness of the revision process in cultivating individual skill progress and facilitating the advancement of writing in English.

Table 3. The results of the pre- and post-test results of the experimental group.

	N	M	SD	SEM	t	*p*
Pre-test	30	82.433	32.724	5.975	−4.558	0.000 ***
Post-test	30	82.800	11.124	2.031		

Note. *** $p < 0.001$. M = mean, SD = standard deviation, SEM = std. error mean.

Table 4 summarizes the decline in writing mistakes, an increased number of words completed by individuals in the experimental group, and a substantial decrease in errors from the pre-test to the post-test, underlining the advantageous influence of the training method. There was a significant reduction in the average number of mistakes, which was diminished from 22.70 in the pre-test to 9.67 in the post-test. The decrease in errors demonstrated a noteworthy improvement in the writing abilities of the experimental group. The average number of words in the experimental group fluctuated between 240.77 and 273.3. The increase in the number of words illustrated a significant advancement in writing productivity (a *p*-value of 0.00). Such outcomes emphasized the positive effect of the revision process on decreasing mistakes and increasing vocabulary, resulting in overall enhancements in the writing abilities of the experimental group.

Table 4. The pre-test and post-test results of the experimental group on writing errors and number of words.

	Pre-Test M	Pre-Test SD	Post-Test M	Post-Test SD	t	*p*
Writing errors	22.70	20.012	9.67	6.645	−4.588	0.000***
Number of words	240.77	51.753	273.3	25.163		0.001***

Note. ***$p < 0.001$. M = mean, SD = standard deviation, SEM = std. error mean.

5. Discussion and Conclusions

We explored the impacts of revision practices and AWE systems on the English writing proficiency of learners. The results presented the pivotal role of integrating AWE into English learning and enhancing students' writing abilities. The participants engaged in composition assignments to reduce repetitive errors. While AWE helped correct mistakes, the clarity of interpreting machine feedback is still required. This underscores the role of educators in guiding learners, highlighting the necessity of combining technological aids with conventional teacher-led instruction in teaching English writing. Similar to the result of Batchelor and King [16], the results of this study emphasized the significance of revision in increasing writing skills, thereby leading to a noticeable advancement in writing abilities. This advancement is attributed to the revision by AWE and timely feedback. This aligns with previous research results indicating the advantages of AWE in the revision stage [17,18]. AWE helps learners correct mistakes, thereby streamlining the revision process. Coinciding with the results of Geng and Razali [9], a preference for immediate feedback and the intricate interplay between AWE tools, student preferences, and the overall effectiveness of writing instruction were also proven in this study. AWE systems can meaningfully enhance the writing abilities of students. Educators must guide students to use automated feedback in the learning process. The participants in this study improved their compositions, indicating that while automated tools offer notable benefits, human intuition remains irreplaceable. By balancing between technology and instruction, effective composition competence can be achieved to maximize the efficiency of writing education in EFL courses in a technologically augmented learning environment.

Author Contributions: Conceptualization, R.-T.H. and K.-H.C.; methodology, R.-T.H.; software, K.T.-C.C.; validation, R.-T.H., K.-H.C. and Y.-S.C.; formal analysis, K.-H.C.; investigation, R.-T.H.; resources, K.-H.C.; data curation, K.T.-C.C.; writing—original draft preparation, R.-T.H.; writing—review and editing, K.-H.C.; visualization, K.T.-C.C.; supervision, R.-T.H.; project administration,

R.-T.H.; funding acquisition, K.-H.C. All authors have read and agreed to the published version of the manuscript.

Funding: This research received no external funding.

Institutional Review Board Statement: Not applicable.

Informed Consent Statement: Informed consent was obtained from all subjects involved in the study.

Data Availability Statement: Data sharing is not applicable to this article as no datasets were generated or analyzed during the study.

Conflicts of Interest: The authors declare no conflict of interest.

References

1. Cotos, E. Potential of AWE feedback. *Calico J.* **2011**, *28*, 420–459. [CrossRef]
2. Chen, K.T.-C. Identifying barriers faced by university EFL instructors in integrating mobile-assisted language learning. *Contemp. Educ. Technol.* **2023**, *15*, ep467. [CrossRef] [PubMed]
3. Alharbi, W. AI in the foreign language classroom: A pedagogical overview of automated writing assistance tools. *Educ. Res. Int.* **2023**, 4253331. [CrossRef]
4. Barrot, J.S. Integrating technology into ESL/EFL writing through Grammarly. *RELC J.* **2022**, *53*, 764–768. [CrossRef]
5. Chen, H.; Pan, J. Computer or human: A comparative study of automated evaluation scoring and instructors' feedback on Chinese college students' English writing. *Asian-Pac. J. Second Foreign Lang. Educ.* **2022**, *7*, 34. [CrossRef]
6. Fan, N.; Ma, Y. The Effects of AWE (AWE) Feedback on Students' English Writing Quality: A Systematic Literature Review. *Lang. Teach. Res. Q.* **2022**, *28*, 53–73. Available online: https://cyut.idm.oclc.org/login?url=https://www.proquest.com/scholarly-journals/effects-automated-writing-evaluation-awe-feedback/docview/2860855474/se-2?accountid=10048 (accessed on 15 May 2023). [CrossRef]
7. Miranty, D.; Utami, W. An AWE (AWE) in higher education. *Pegem J. Educ. Instr.* **2021**, *11*, 126–137. [CrossRef]
8. Flower, L.; Hayes, J.R. A cognitive process theory of writing. *Coll. Compos. Commun.* **1981**, *32*, 365–387. [CrossRef]
9. Geng, J.; Razali, A.B. Effectiveness of the AWE Program on Improving Undergraduates' Writing Performance. *Engl. Lang. Teach.* **2022**, *15*, 49–60. [CrossRef]
10. Kuyyogsuy, S. Promoting Peer Feedback in Developing Students' English Writing Ability in L2 Writing Class. *Int. Educ. Stud.* **2019**, *12*, 76–90. [CrossRef]
11. Zamel, V. The composing processes of advanced ESL students: Six case studies. *TESOL Q.* **1983**, *17*, 165–188. [CrossRef]
12. Wang, Q. The use of semantic similarity tools in automated content scoring of fact-based essays written by EFL learners. *Educ. Inf. Technol.* **2022**, *27*, 13021–13049. [CrossRef]
13. Escalante, J.; Pack, A.; Barrett, A. AI-generated feedback on writing: Insights into efficacy and ENL student preference: Revista de Universidad y Sociedad del Conocimiento. *Int. J. Educ. Technol. High. Educ.* **2023**, *20*, 57. [CrossRef]
14. Wang, C.; Mirzaei, T.; Xu, T.; Lin, H. How learner engagement impacts non-formal online learning outcomes through value co-creation: An empirical analysis. *Int. J. Educ. Technol. High. Educ.* **2022**, *19*, 32. [CrossRef] [PubMed]
15. Thi, N.K.; Nikolov, M. Effects of teacher, automated, and combined feedback on syntactic complexity in EFL students' writing. *Asian-Pac. J. Second Foreign Lang. Educ.* **2023**, *8*, 6. [CrossRef]
16. Batchelor, K.E.; King, A. Freshmen and five hundred words: Investigating flash fiction as a genre for high school writing. *J. Adolesc. Adult Lit.* **2014**, *58*, 111–121. [CrossRef]
17. Nunes, A.; Cordeiro, C.; Limpo, T.; Castro, S.L. Effectiveness of AWE systems in school settings: A systematic review of studies from 2000 to 2020. *J. Comput. Assist. Learn.* **2022**, *38*, 599–620. [CrossRef]
18. Parra, G.L.; Calero, S.X. AWE tools in the improvement of the writing skill. *Int. J. Instr.* **2019**, *12*, 209–226.

engineering proceedings

MDPI

Proceeding Paper

Building Design for Daycare Center and Group Home for Elderly Persons with Dementia †

Yen-Liang Lin and Sheng-Jung Ou *

Department of Architecture, Chaoyang University of Technology, Taichung 41349, Taiwan; yla.archi@gmail.com
* Correspondence: sjou@cyut.edu.tw

† Presented at the 2024 IEEE 4th International Conference on Electronic Communications, Internet of Things and Big Data, Taipei, Taiwan, 19–21 April 2024.

Abstract: We studied the impact of well-designed dementia care environments for people with dementia and how such environments reduce anxiety, alleviate fear, and slow the progression of the disease. The "group home" model has been particularly successful, as it emphasizes "home-like", family-oriented, and personalized care. A case study of the Yunlin County Elderly Long-Term Care Association showed that this model fostered a sense of belonging and serenity in residents, with high levels of satisfaction and effective design outcomes. The environments researched were found to enhance the well-being and quality of life of people with dementia in Taiwan.

Keywords: super-aging society; dementia care; elderly care; group-home model; dementia daycare centers; spatial design principles

Citation: Lin, Y.-L.; Ou, S.-J. Building Design for Daycare Center and Group Home for Elderly Persons with Dementia. *Eng. Proc.* **2024**, *74*, 53. https://doi.org/10.3390/engproc2024074053

Academic Editors: Shu-Han Liao, Teen-Hang Meen and Cheng-Fu Yang

Published: 5 September 2024

1. Introduction

Taiwan is expected to be a super-aging society in 2025. By 2051, the proportion of people aged over 65 in Taiwan will constitute 38.1% of the total population [1]. The Ministry of Health and Welfare has estimated that in 2022, the number of people with dementia in Taiwan exceeded 300,000, with seniors aged over 65 constituting 96% of this population [2]. Therefore, there is an urgent need to care for elderly persons with dementia. Numerous previous studies have shown a connection between environmental design factors and the behavior of individuals with dementia [3]. Improving the design factors has the potential to promote the more positive behaviors of the residents [3]. Consequently, the development of a care environment customized to the needs of elderly persons with dementia has become an issue of paramount importance in Taiwan.

2. Literature Review

Dementia is a complex neurodegenerative disease with certain defined symptoms. Behavioral characteristics worsen as the dementia progresses.

2.1. Care Environments for Dementia Patients

In recent years, research related to the living environments of elderly persons with dementia has garnered significant attention and has been published in *The Gerontologist*, *Research on Aging*, and the *Journal of Gerontology*. Research on dementia care published in journals such as *Alzheimer's Disease* and *Associated Disorders* and studies on applied psychology published in the *International Journal of Geriatric Psychiatry* have provided insights for related research. The development of dementia care environments and the factors influencing them have been discussed widely [4]. The study of care environments for elderly persons with dementia has found that building designs for the practice of environmental therapy enhance caregiving functionality [4]. Existing research also indicates that the living space plays a crucial role in significantly ameliorating the aberrant behaviors exhibited by dementia patients [5].

2.2. Types of Care for Elderly Persons with Dementia

There are various long-term care models available for individuals with dementia.

1. Home-Care: This model provides care for dementia patients within the familiar environment of their own homes. It typically includes in-home caregivers, nurses, and support services to help individuals continue living at home.
2. Community-Based Care: This includes daycare centers and "group homes". Daycare centers offer structured activities and supervision during the day, allowing caregivers a period of rest. Group homes, on the other hand, create a "home-like" atmosphere and provide professional care and support to residents in a community.
3. Institutional care: This model provides care in nursing homes and specialized care units specifically tailored for individuals with dementia. Institutional care is usually considered when individuals require more intensive medical and caregiving support.

2.3. Group Home

In the context of a group home, the primary focus is on creating a nurturing and "home-like" environment. The group home enhances the quality of living spaces and meets the need of elderly persons for independence. Notable examples from different regions highlight the importance of the living-space design in dementia care centers. In Columbia, Canada, the building code for dementia care centers mandates that living room be primarily designed as single occupancy to prevent interference [4]. In Virginia, in the U.S.A., there is a specific requirement that the living spaces for people with dementia must be self-contained and independent [4]. Group homes are characterized by a family-like atmosphere, a focus on individualized care, and small-scale, personalized care units. Each person with dementia is provided with a personal room, open shared spaces for group activities, and accessible shared facilities, including bathrooms and laundry, to ensure a comfortable and supportive environment [6]. The service model of dementia group homes offers holistic, "people-centered" care, encompassing both the physical infrastructure and the operational planning [7].

3. Research Methods

We conducted a case study of the care of elderly persons with dementia in Taiwan to investigate the "behavioral characteristics" and "spatial needs" of these elderly persons. The research methodology involves the following key steps.

3.1. Theory and Literature Review

A thorough examination of the existing theories and literature was conducted. We searched the comprehensive reviews of behavioral characteristics exhibited by elderly persons with dementia and classified relevant theories in spatial design to gain a theoretical foundation. We identified daycare centers and group homes as the two primary modes of environmental care for elderly persons with dementia. The care services offered at group homes and the spatial requirements of the existing environment were explored as the background and basis for the subsequent research.

3.2. Case Study

The Yunlin Elderly Long-Term Care Association was selected as a case study for an in-depth examination of the design and utilization of the space of the daycare center and group home. We collected information regarding the spatial design principles in these facilities to understand how these spaces were designed and utilized to meet the needs of elderly residents.

3.3. Proposal for Localization

Based on the findings from the case study, we made a proposal tailored to the context of Taiwan. This proposal serves as a reference for the future design of group home care facilities in the region. The proposal addresses local factors, cultural considerations, and the unique needs of elderly persons in Taiwan in order to ensure relevant and effective design recommendations.

3.4. Evaluation Framework

The evaluation of the environmental design of care facilities for elderly persons with dementia was conducted based on the following sources: "A Study of Building Plans and Design Guidelines for Care Institutions for the Dementia" [8] and "Contemporary Environments for People with Dementia" [9], which were used as the design guidelines. These design guidelines were designed to meet the requirements of individuals with dementia and create spaces to enhance their well-being and quality of life. We compiled 18 environmental design principles for elderly persons with dementia. The evaluation framework was used to assess the design of care environments for elderly persons with dementia. The framework can be used as a valuable tool for assessing and guiding the environmental design of care facilities for elderly persons with dementia.

3.5. Introduction to the Living Space of the Yunlin Elderly Long-Term Care Association

The Yunlin Elderly Long-Term Care Association was established in 2009 and provides care for elderly persons with dementia. The facility includes a daycare center and a group home to cater to the needs of these individuals. An overview of the building space configuration is set forth as follows.

- The ground floor serves as a hub for daily activities, programs, and care services for elderly residents with dementia. This space is designed to provide a supportive and engaging environment. The ground floor includes a group home with seven single rooms. This living arrangement emphasizes a "home-like" atmosphere, individualized care, and support in a communal setting. The ground floor features a dining room and a kitchen used to serve meals and provide communal dining experiences to the residents (Figure 1).
- The second floor is used as a multi-functional activity center. This space hosts activities and programs aiming to enhance the physical, mental, and social well-being of the elderly persons. The second floor serves as administrative and office spaces where a staff of 20 can manage and coordinate the various programs and services.
- The third floor includes classrooms for vocational training. These spaces are used to offer opportunities for skill development and engagement, contributing to the residents' independence. A service center on the third floor is a central point for the initiative to address the needs and concerns of elderly persons. It provides services and resources to enhance their quality of life. The third floor features a rooftop terrace designed as a healing garden. This outdoor space provides a peaceful and therapeutic environment for residents to enjoy nature, relaxation, and outdoor activities.

The space configuration of the Yunlin Elderly Long-Term Care Association reflects a holistic approach to caring for elderly persons with dementia and offering a range of services and environments to support their physical, emotional, and social well-being. The daycare center, group home, activity spaces, and outdoor garden spaces create a supportive and engaging living environment.

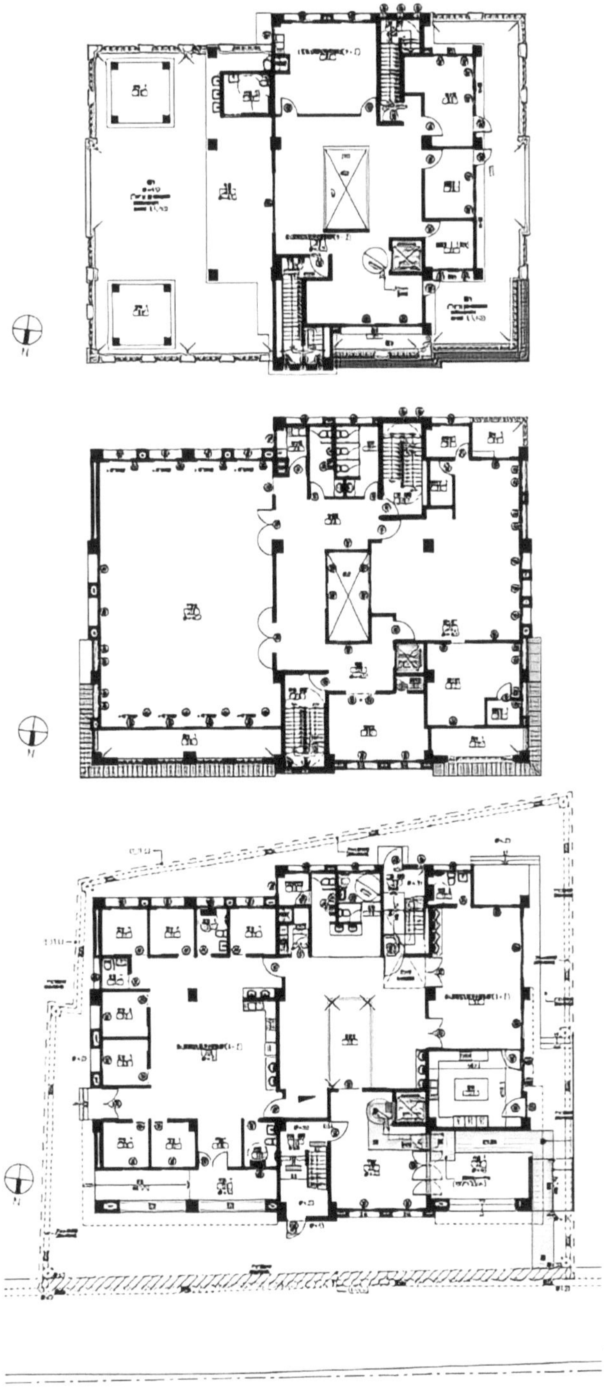

Figure 1. Floor plan of the Yunlin Elderly Long-Term Care Association.

4. Space and Environmental Design

The environmental design and spatial characteristics of the Yunlin Elderly Long-Term Care Association characterize the space as a nurturing and functional environment for the needs of elderly persons with dementia. The key aspects of its space and environmental design are as follows.

1. Location and environment of the building: The building is easily accessible with mass transportation, being just a ten-minute drive from the downtown railway station and close to the Yunlin Branch of the National Taiwan University Hospital. This location ensures easy access to medical facilities. In addition, it offers scenic views of rural agricultural areas, specifically, rice paddies (Figure 2).

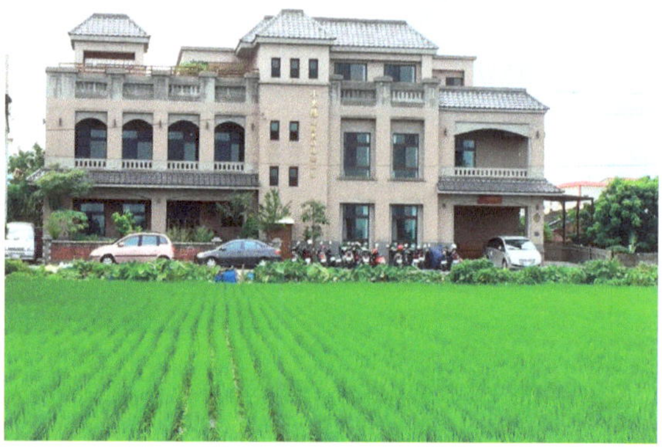

Figure 2. Adjacent scenery, with rural agricultural areas and rice paddies.

2. Space organization and zoning plan: The building has thoughtfully organized floors, as described below.
    - Ground floor: Dementia daycare center, group home with seven single rooms, and a central kitchen;
    - Second floor: Offices, multi-functional activity centers, vocational training venues, and pantry;
    - Third floor: A rooftop terrace used as a healing garden, home service support centers, and flexible space for community care attendants.
3. Architectural pathway system: The pathway system is designed for safety and convenience. It separates spaces for elderly persons and office workers and incorporates zones for the group home and the daycare center. The pathways are straightforward, well-illuminated, spacious, and free of elevation changes, ensuring the safety of the elderly persons. Multiple entrances and exits are equipped with security devices and electronic door locks, allowing for effective access control management.
4. Outdoor activity space: The ground floor includes outdoor garden areas with lounge seats and a balcony corridor, offering a serene environment for elderly persons to enjoy the outdoors and natural light (Figure 3a).
5. Walking path: Multiple indoor and outdoor walking paths connect various living and activity spaces for physical activity, relaxation, and a restful night's sleep (Figure 3b).

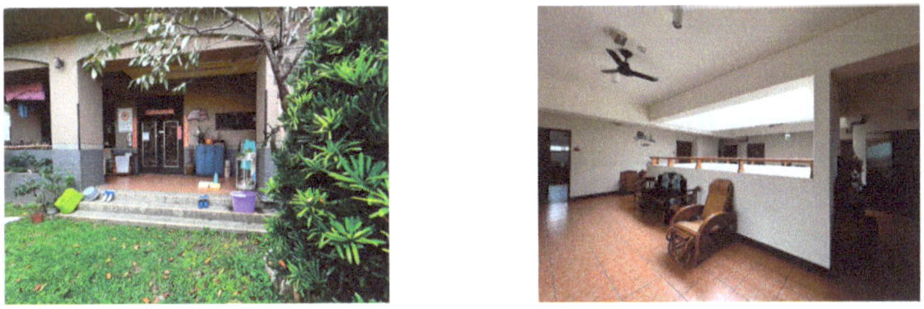

(**a**) (**b**)

Figure 3. (**a**) Outdoor activity space and (**b**) indoor walking path.

6. Central hall activity area: The area comprises three social spaces, namely, a central hall activity area with a daylight patio, open living rooms of the group home, and the entrance foyer, which serves as a welcoming hall (Figure 4).

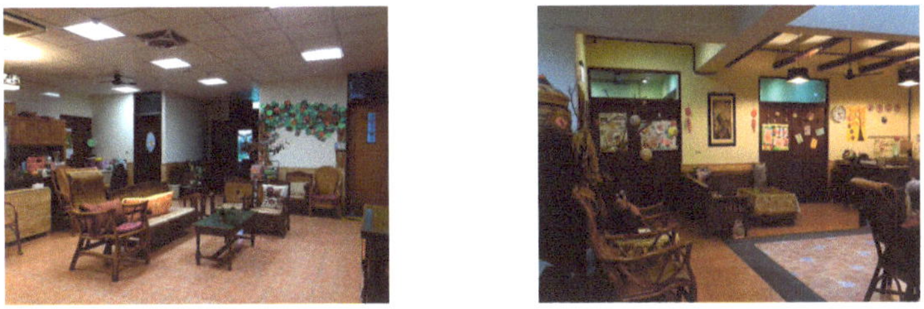

Figure 4. Central hall activity area.

7. Dining room and kitchen: The dining room is designed to promote a welcoming atmosphere, with six small dining tables and adjacent outdoor garden spaces. The design helps the constant population of dining companions to enhance memory and reduce feelings of alienation. Adequate meal preparation and kitchen facilities are available, ensuring a clean and safe environment for food preparation (Figure 5).

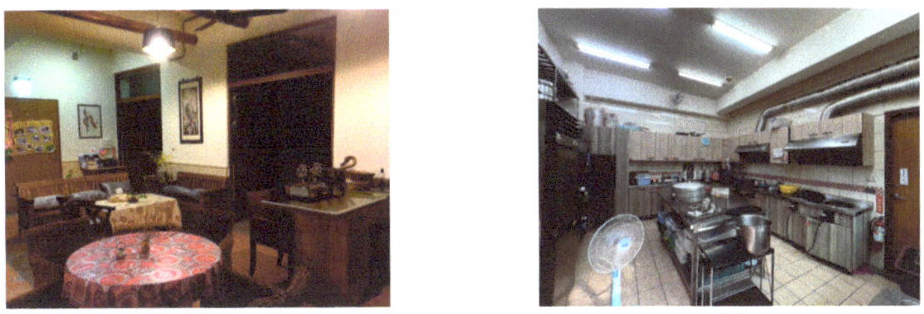

(**a**) (**b**)

Figure 5. (**a**) Dining room and (**b**) kitchen.

8. Bedrooms in the group home: The group home's living spaces on the first floor are designed to provide a "home-like" atmosphere, with seven single rooms and shared barrier-free bathroom facilities. The layout is centered around a central living space, with an emphasis on privacy and personalization (Figure 6a).
9. Bathroom and toilet: Barrier-free shared bathrooms are available throughout the facility, with vivid signage and easy-to-use sliding doors. The materials used are non-reflective, anti-slip, and easy to clean. These spaces feature windows for ventilation, heating, and exhaust equipment for comfort and safety (Figure 6b).

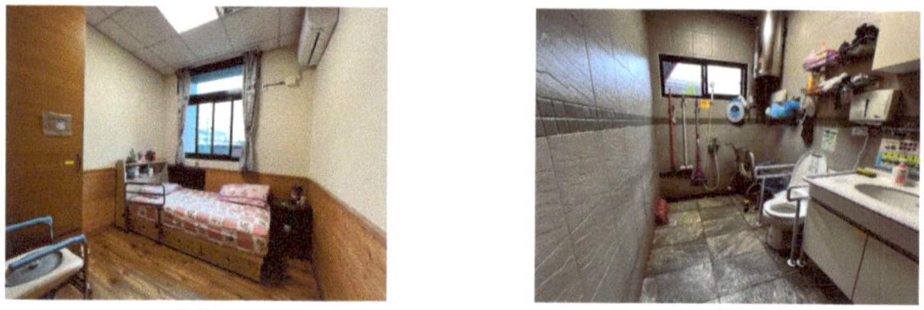

(**a**) (**b**)

Figure 6. (**a**) Bedroom and (**b**) toilet.

10. Nursing stations: Small tables near the nursing stations provide convenient locations from which the staff can observe and assist the elderly persons, avoiding an institutionalized feel (Figure 7a).
11. Office: The second floor is dedicated to office space for staff, accommodating up to 20 people, with additional areas for data archives and equipment (Figure 7b).

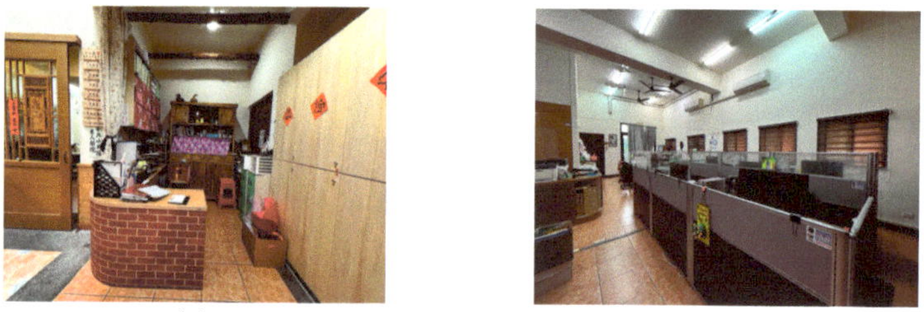

(**a**) (**b**)

Figure 7. (**a**) Nursing station and (**b**) office.

12. Pantry: A pantry is located adjacent to the office on the second floor.
13. Waste treatment room: There is a room for the treatment of domestic and medical waste for recycling and safe storage. It effectively prevents the spread of diseases.
14. Reception room: A reception room for family members and meetings, located on the second floor.
15. Multi-functional activity center and rehabilitation room: On the second floor, a multi-functional activity center and rehabilitation area which facilitates indoor activities, lectures, entertainment, and events (Figure 8).

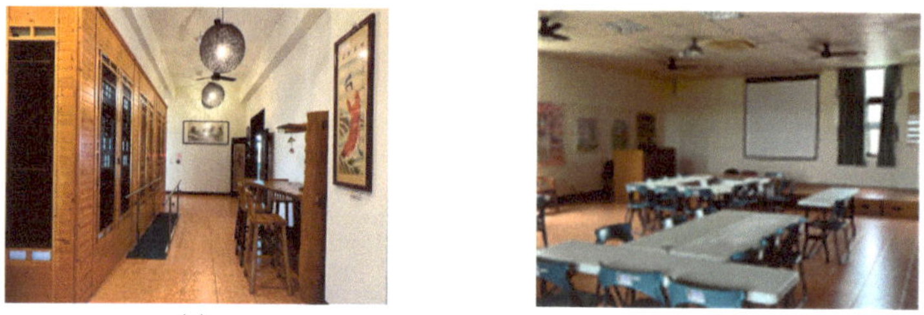

(**a**) (**b**)

Figure 8. (**a**) Rehabilitation room and (**b**) activity center.

16. Staff dormitory: The third floor is designated for care and management staff to use as rest areas (Figure 9a).
17. Religious space: A religious space on the third floor provides solace for the elderly persons (Figure 9b).

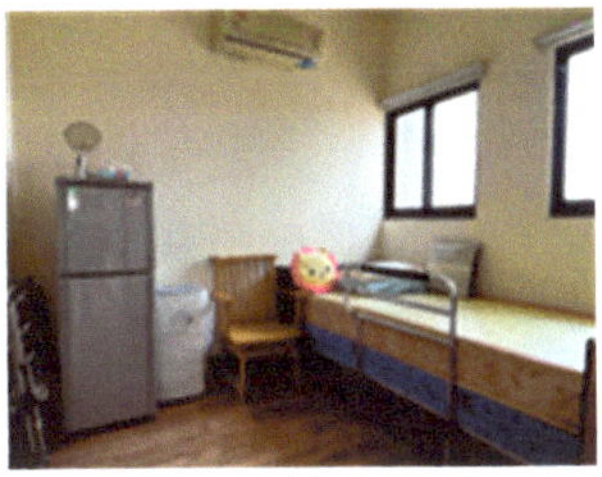

(**a**)

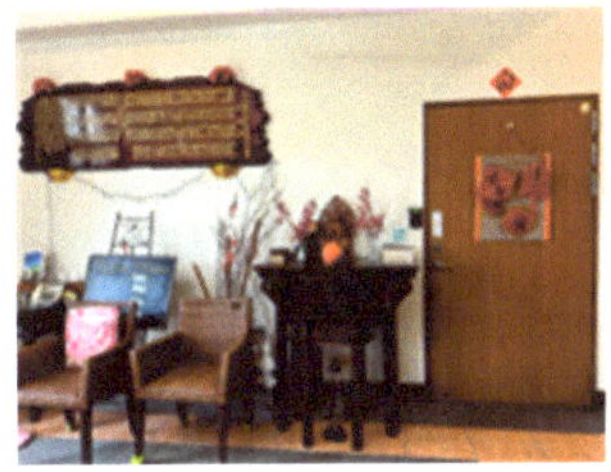

(**b**)

Figure 9. (**a**) Staff dormitory and (**b**) the religious space.

18. Other facilities: The third floor features a vocational training classroom, a care and attendant service center, and a rooftop-terrace healing garden (Figure 10).

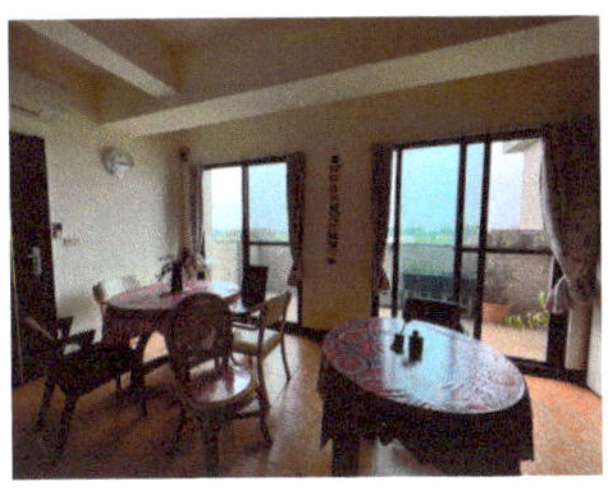

(**a**)

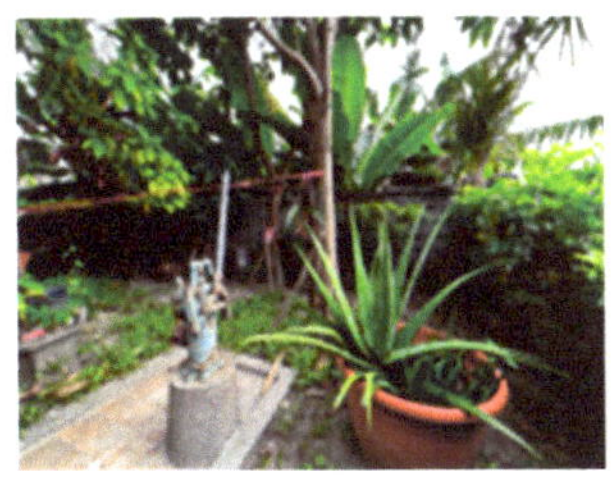

(**b**)

Figure 10. (**a**) Service center and (**b**) healing garden.

The group home's careful planning and the consideration of each space ensure that the Yunlin Elderly Long-Term Care Association provides a nurturing, safe, and supportive environment for elderly persons with dementia, focusing on their comfort and well-being.

5. Conclusions and Suggestions

This space for the Yunlin Elderly Long-Term Care Association highlights the significant impact of well-designed environmental spaces on elderly persons with dementia. A properly designed living environment helps to reduce anxiety, alleviate fear, and significantly slow down the progression of the disease. The implementation of the group home concept emphasizes a "home-like" atmosphere, aligns with the principles of small-scale, family-oriented, and individualized care, and creates a familial atmosphere. The utilization of the group home model enhances the quality of care, fostering a sense of belonging and peace of mind among elderly residents in a familiar setting. This building for the Yunlin Elderly Long-Term Care Association demonstrates the effectiveness of the group home model in achieving a high level of satisfaction and successful environmental design.

To introduce a model of environmental care for elderly persons with dementia, the dementia daycare center and group home residences of the Association can be referred to. Essential information about other construction facilities needs to be further analyzed by conducting field investigations of the environmental design and spatial utilization to understand the environments within these facilities and explore the connection between the "behavioral patterns" of elderly persons with dementia and the "built environment design" of care institutions. Based on the existing building layout, 18 spatial design elements for environmental facilities can be determined. These elements can serve as a future reference for creating environments tailored to the needs of elderly persons with dementia.

Challenges associated with caring for elderly persons with dementia have increased in complexity. Thus, an environmental space design is needed to accommodate various factors, including the topographies of different locations, environmental conditions, and evolving care patterns. Therefore, adjustments and changes to environmental design must be studied in order to meet the changing needs of elderly persons. The success of the group home model for the Yunlin Elderly Long-Term Care Association reveals the importance of continuously improving and customizing care environments to ensure the well-being of elderly persons with dementia in Taiwan.

However, further architectural design research is necessary to improve the well-being of elderly persons with dementia, including collaborations between caregivers and architectural experts in the design of dementia care facilities. There is an urgent need for standardized guidelines concerning the environmental design of dementia care facilities. These guidelines would be a valuable and essential reference for meeting the specific needs of elderly persons with dementia in Taiwan.

Author Contributions: Conceptualization, Y.-L.L. and S.-J.O.; methodology, S.-J.O.; software, Y.-L.L.; validation, Y.-L.L.; formal analysis, S.-J.O.; investigation, Y.-L.L.; resources, Y.-L.L.; data curation, S.-J.O.; writing—original draft preparation, Y.-L.L.; writing—review and editing, S.-J.O.; visualization, Y.-L.L.; supervision, S.-J.O.; project administration, S.-J.O. All authors have read and agreed to the published version of the manuscript.

Funding: This research received no external funding.

Institutional Review Board Statement: Not applicable.

Informed Consent Statement: Not applicable.

Data Availability Statement: No new data were created.

Conflicts of Interest: The authors declare no conflicts of interest.

References

1. National Development Council. *Population Projections Report in Taiwan, 2020–2070*; National Development Council: Taipei, Taiwan, 2020.
2. Taiwan Alzheimer's Disease Association (TADA). 2022. Available online: http://tada2002.ehosting.com.tw/eng/about.html (accessed on 22 August 2024).
3. Tseng, C.Y. Relationships between Environmental Features and Behaviors of Dementia Residents—An Example of Long-term Care Facilities in Taipei. Master's Thesis, Taipei Medical University, Taipei, Taiwan, 2007.
4. Hwang, Y.R. The Existing Problems and Trend of Construction for The Special Care Unit of Dementia. *J. Long-Term Care* **2004**, *7*, 352–354.
5. Bellelli, G.; Frisoni, G.B.; Bianchetti, A.; Boffelli, S.; Guerrini, G.B.; Scotuzzi, A.; Ranieri, P.; Ritondale, G.; Guglielmi, L.; Fusari, A.; et al. Special care units for demented patients: A multicenter study. *Gerontologist* **1998**, *38*, 456–462. [CrossRef] [PubMed]
6. Chen, C.H. The New Living Type for Dementia Elder in Aged Society: Group Home. *Taiwan J. Gerontol. Health Res.* **2009**, *5*, 17–35.
7. Liu, C.Y.; Su, C.L. Group home Service Model for the Elderly with Dementia: Lessons from Japan's Experience. *J. Long-Term Care* **2018**, *22*, 53–65.
8. Tsai, S.-Y.; Li, M.-H.; Ho, M.-C.; Lee, M.-P.; Chen, T.-Y. The Research on Design Principle of Indoor Home Environment for Seniors with Dementia. *J. Archit. Archit. Assoc. Taiwan* **2016**, *97*, 87–98. [CrossRef]
9. Cohen, U.; Day, K. *Contemporary Environments for People with Dementia*; Johns Hopkins University Press: Baltimore, MD, USA, 1993.

engineering proceedings

Proceeding Paper

Filipino Meal Recognition Scale with Food Nutrition Calculation and Smart Application †

Andrew D. R. Demition *, Zephanie Ann L. Narciso and Charmaine C. Paglinawan

School of Electrical, Electronics and Computer Engineering, Mapúa University, Muralla St., Intramuros, Manila 1002, Philippines; zalnarciso@mymail.mapua.edu.ph (Z.A.L.N.); ccpaglinawan@mapua.edu.ph (C.C.P.)
* Correspondence: addemition@mymail.mapua.edu.ph
† Presented at the 2024 IEEE 4th International Conference on Electronic Communications, Internet of Things and Big Data, Taipei, Taiwan, 19–21 April 2024.

Abstract: Nutritional awareness is considered prevalent in today's society. In effect, more people have been inclined to perform food calculations in the food they eat to improve their physical fitness and balance the meals they eat. In this study, the Internet of Things was used through a mobile application with Filipino meal recognition that was integrated into a weighing scale to simplify meal recognition and food calculation without individually scaling and measuring the macronutrients of each food. An ESP32 was programmed to determine the weight of the food sample. Moreover, a TensorFlow Lite Model was created using Teachable Machine, whereas the dataset comprised three Filipino meal combinations of rice, pork adobo, and pork giniling; rice, ginataang kalabasa, and pork giniling; and rice, ginataang kalabasa, and pork adobo. The model identified the 15 samples of Filipino meals per combination. The precision was 91.26% for the first meal combination, 82.73% for the second meal combination, and 85.46% for the third meal combination. One-factor ANOVA was conducted to determine the similarities of the actual and predicted macronutrient contents of the food samples, whereas 10 weight values of successfully determined food meals for each combination were used. The model recognized each Filipino food combination with an overall accuracy of 93.33%. The predicted macronutrient contents were similar to the actual macronutrient contents of the meal based on the statistical analysis performed.

Keywords: food recognition; TensorFlow; machine learning

Citation: Demition, A.D.R.; Narciso, Z.A.L.; Paglinawan, C.C. Filipino Meal Recognition Scale with Food Nutrition Calculation and Smart Application. *Eng. Proc.* **2024**, *74*, 54. https://doi.org/10.3390/engproc2024074054

Academic Editors: Shu-Han Liao, Teen-Hang Meen and Cheng-Fu Yang

Published: 3 September 2024

1. Introduction

The Internet of Things (IoT) is a revolutionary technology that goes beyond simple functionality and highlights how deeply it affects people as a whole. Apps demand databases of nutritional data and algorithms to provide users with customized advice for better eating practices. In today's world, Apps are useful tools for people who want to maximize their nutrition and promote healthier living [1]. System security is essential because the IoT is used more and contributes significantly to the infrastructure of countries.

Security research on cyber-physical and IoT systems is guided by different principles. An "Internet Protocol" must be implemented on even the smallest devices. IoT devices' ability to process data quickly and efficiently is constrained by their limited computer process unit (CPU), memory, and power [2]. Image processing is capable of solving real-world problems [3] in different applications such as medicine [4], plants [5], and animals [6]. The deep learning framework TensorFlow simulates, trains, and classifies data with an accuracy of up to 90% and yields promising results [7].

Accurate methods for measuring energy and food intake are crucial in treating obesity [8]. By providing users/patients with considerate and useful tools, helping them track their food intake, and compiling nutritional data, the long-term prevention of obesity and successful treatment programs are allowed. The ability to recognize food is crucial for food choices and consumption, both of which are vital for human health and well-being. For this reason, it is significant to facilitate various food-related vision and multimodal tasks such as cross-modal recipe generation and retrieval, food detection, and segmentation [9]. The recommended approach is available on mobile phones, which allow the user to snap a photo of the food and determine its calorie content instantaneously. Deep convolutional neural networks (DCNNs) are used to classify food pictures to accurately recognize the meal. The technology is used to recognize food portions with great accuracy. Through the use of technology, the user places the meal within an enclosure and snaps a single photo for food detection [10]. The technology allows for calculating the food item's calorie content. After the technology is used to analyze the user's meal photograph and calculate their caloric intake, the name of the food item and how many calories it contains are displayed [11].

A well-balanced diet is essential for optimal tissue function, illness prevention, and improved health. To provide individualized advice for healthy eating practices, the databases of nutritional data and algorithms are integrated with Apps. The Apps allow for healthier living and are practical tools to optimize their nutrition [12]. The connection between nutrition and health and the relationship between diet and health are becoming important for people [13]. To determine the application of the technology and Apps, we analyzed the efficacy of various detection techniques and instruments and compared their advantages and disadvantages. Food identification systems were also explored concerning food safety and dietary recommendations for different groups of people. We also reviewed the latest developments in smartphone use in the food business to provide a foundation for the expansion of food-related businesses including fast food identification, food source tracking, and customized diets [14].

Based on previous studies, we identified a key research gap in food recognition, traceability, and dietary customization. While prior research was performed to explore the effectiveness of detection techniques and the feasibility of applications, there is a need to study such elements in a single framework to cover the technical aspects of food recognition and the practicality of implementation, user-friendly design, and the provision of dietary advice. Convolutional neural networks (CNNs) were used to deliver the information successfully. However, for efficient training, CNNs need a lot of labeled data, time, and effort to be applied to different food products for food recognition.

Thus, it is necessary to analyze how emerging technologies benefit food-related industries and improve individuals' dietary choices and overall health. Therefore, we integrated AI-based food recognition into a weighing scale with a mobile application to show the macronutrient content of the food. Using Teachable Machine, a food recognition scale with the integration of TensorFlow, a user-friendly system was developed for accurate food recognition with food nutrition calculation. We created the system to measure the weight of the food combinations using image recognition and developed an intuitive user interface with IoT connectivity to the device to determine the system's capability by comparing the predicted and the actual macronutrient content of the food combination. The system represents a significant advancement in nutritional tracking technology by combining precise weight measurement using a load cell HX111 with AI. The system helps people adopt healthier eating habits by offering precise and up-to-date information about the nutritional value of the food they eat. By fusing IoT connectivity with user-centric design, the system provides nutrition tracking and becomes more convenient for users. The system can be applied to various industries. Enhanced quality control and traceability are allowed to ensure compliance with safety and nutritional standards for processed foods and agricultural products. Consumers can also access real-time nutritional data for educated dietary choices.

2. Materials and Methods

2.1. Conceptual Framework

In the system, images are captured as the dataset of the macronutrient content of food samples for providing calorie intake for the user. Foods and combinations are classified by utilizing the captured images in the dataset, and nutrition is calculated to predict the macronutrient content and calories. On the device and the mobile device, the weight, total calories, macronutrient content, total calorie intake, and needed calories are displayed (Figure 1).

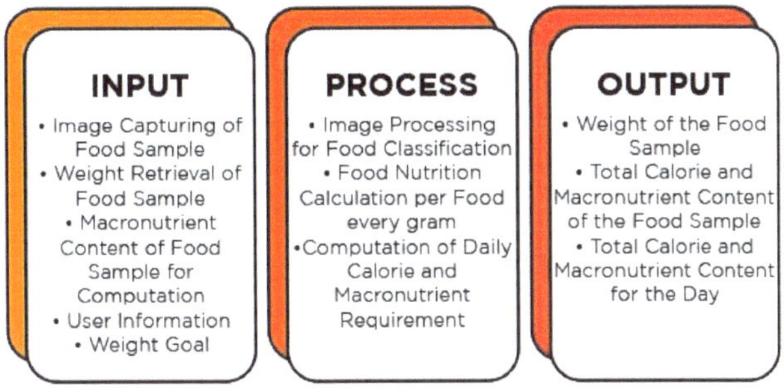

Figure 1. Conceptual framework.

2.2. Process Flowchart

In the system, the first process is logging in followed by the main menu to input the user profile including height, weight, age, gender, activity level, and target weight. Calculation is conducted using the food calculator menu based on foods captured. Macronutrient content is calculated based on the database of food samples and their weights. Foods and calories are deducted from the total calories needed for the day (Figure 2).

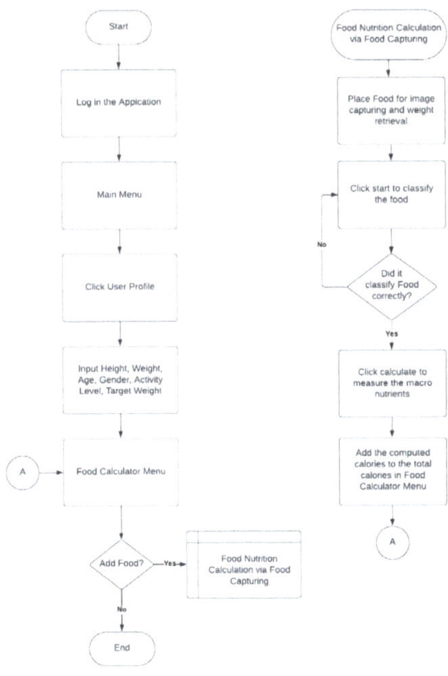

Figure 2. Process flowchart.

2.3. Hardware Development

In the system, a 12 V, 5 A, AC/DC power supply adapter was connected to the HW688 module to convert 12 to 5 V. Since the ring light and the ESP32 need 5 V, the HW688 supplies the right voltage needed. Components were connected to the ESP32 and the 16 × 2 I2C LCD to show the weight by utilizing the HX711 load amplifier (Figures 3–5).

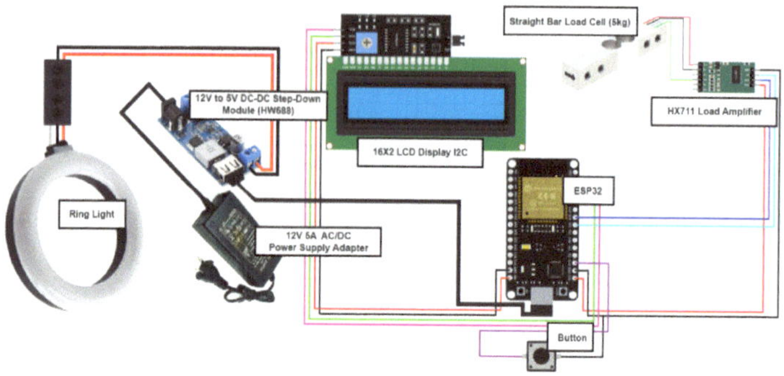

Figure 3. System hardware.

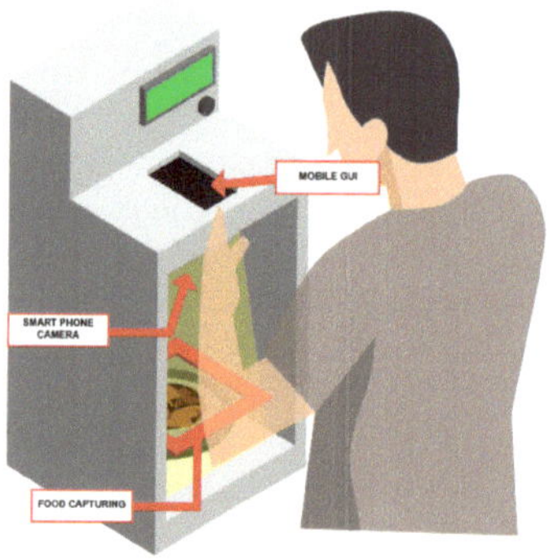

Figure 4. Experimental setup and prototype design.

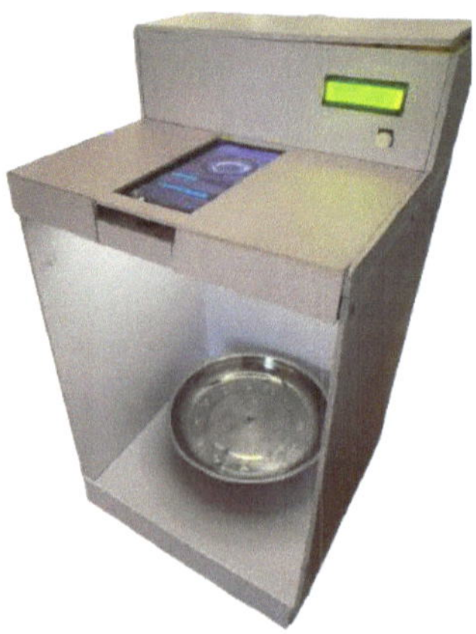

Figure 5. Prototype of developed system.

2.4. Software Development

The App was created using MIT App Inventor. The App includes a login page to create login credentials and the main menu for food calculation and a user profile where the user inputs their data for the computation of total calories needed per day. It also includes an interface for the weight output of the classified food combination (Figure 6).

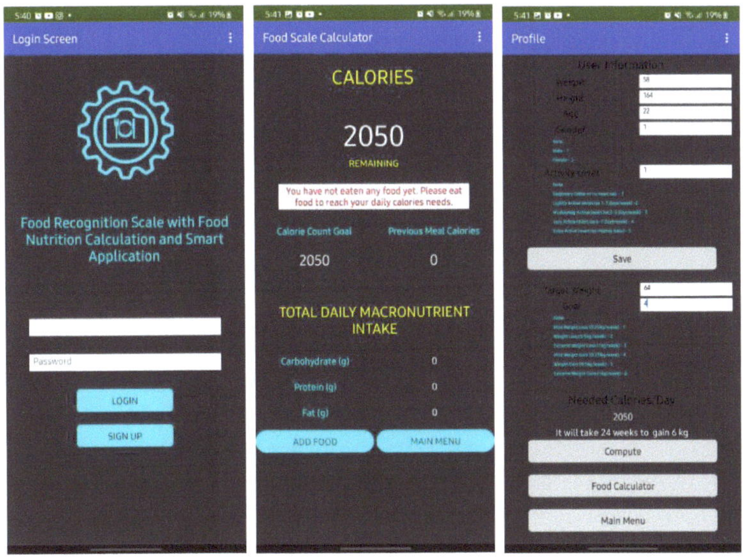

Figure 6. User interface of system.

2.5. Training and Food Nutrition Calculation

In the recognition model, the dataset or images of the sample are gathered. Figure 7 shows the different samples of food combinations to create the different food classification models.

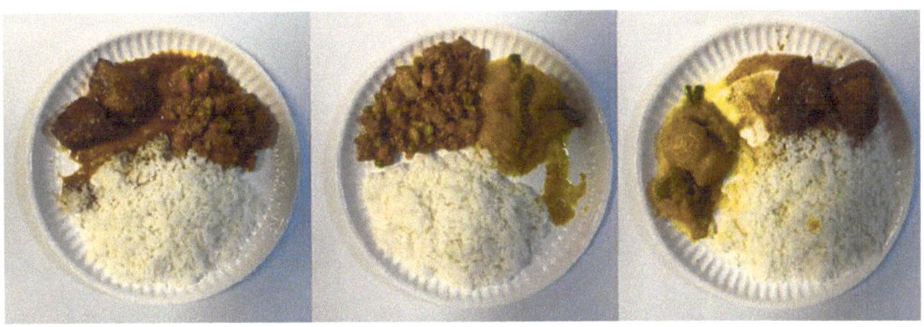

Figure 7. Samples of food combinations.

Figure 8 shows the interface of the Teachable Machine with the different food combinations. The Teachable Machine was utilized to train a TensorFlow model with the dataset and identify food combinations to determine the macronutrient content of the food combination. To calculate the actual calorie content per food sample, the calories of each food sample are multiplied by its conversion factor which is as follows.

$$TC_A = FV_1\left(\frac{TC_1}{S1}\right) + FV_2\left(\frac{TC_2}{S2}\right) + R\left(\frac{TC_3}{S3}\right) \tag{1}$$

where TC_A is the total actual calories of the food combination. FV_1 and FV_2 are the two Filipino viands on the plate, R is for Rice, TC_1 to TC_3 are the total calories in accordance with the food sample, and S_1 to S_3 are its serving size.

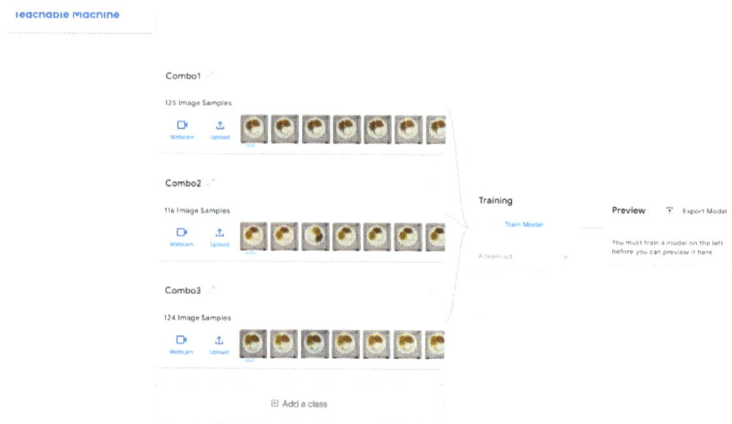

Figure 8. Dataset of food combination in Teachable Machine.

For predicting the total caloric and macronutrient content of the food combinations, the sample mean of each macronutrient was approximated. The total calories and macronutrient content for each parameter (AM_t) per serving size are equal to the sum of those of the listed food samples of the food combinations. The formula for the predicted caloric and macronutrient content per serving size is as follows.

$$AM_T = \frac{FV_1 + FV_2 + R}{3} \quad (2)$$

After gathering the total caloric content of the food combination per serving size AM_T, it is divided by the serving size (S) before multiplying by the total sum of each macronutrient content in grams of each retrieved food sample RF_1, RF_2, and RR in the food combination.

$$TC_P = \frac{AM_T}{S}(RFV_1 + RFV_2 + RR) \quad (3)$$

The macronutrient count is presented in Table 1. The information on the macronutrients is based on the values provided by the DOST-NFRI Food Exchange List for Meal Planning.

Table 1. Nutritional content of chosen Filipino foods.

Sample Menu	Quantity	Food Group	Carbohydrates (G)	Protein (G)	Fat (G)	Energy (Kcal)
Pork Adobo						
Pork Tenderloin	2 slices (70 g)	Low-Fat Meat	-	16	2	82
Potato	½ pc (85 g)	Rice B (Medium Protein)	11.5	1	-	50
Cooking oil	2 tsp (10 g)	Fat	-	-	10	90
		TOTAL	**11.5 g**	**17 g**	**12 g**	**222 kcal**

Table 1. *Cont.*

Sample Menu	Quantity	Food Group	Carbohydrates (G)	Protein (G)	Fat (G)	Energy (Kcal)
Pork Giniling						
Cooking oil	2 tsp (10 g)	Fat	-	-	10	90
Lean ground pork	1 slice (35 g)	Low-Fat Meat	-	8	1	41
Chicken egg	1 pc medium (55 g)	Medium-Fat Meat	-	8	6	86
Potato	½ pc (85 g)	Rice B (Medium Protein)	11.5	1	-	50
Carrots Green peas	1 cup (90 g)	Vegetable	6	2	-	32
Cooking oil	1 tsp (5 g)	Fat	-	-	5	45
		TOTAL	**17.5 g**	**19 g**	**12 g**	**254 kcal**
Ginataang Kalabasa						
Pork tenderloin	1 slice (35 g)	Low-Fat Meat	-	8	1	41
Squash String beans	1 cup (90 g)	Vegetable	6	2	-	32
Coconut cream	3 Tbsp (45 g)	Fat	-	-	15	135
Cooking oil	1 tsp (5 g)	Fat	-	-	5	45
		TOTAL	**6 g**	**10 g**	**21 g**	**253 kcal**
Rice						
White Rice	1 cup (160 g)	Rice B (Medium Protein)	46	4	-	200
		TOTAL	**46 g**	**4 g**	**0 g**	**200 kcal**

(Computed based on the values provided by the DOST-FNRI Food Exchanges Lists for Meal Planning).

3. Results and Discussion

Foods were classified and compared between the actual and predicted calories of the food combinations. *FC*1, *FC*2, and *FC*3 denote the food combinations of rice, ginataang kalabasa, and giniling. The average precision score for the food classification was calculated in the mobile application using the TensorFlow Lite model. For *FC*1, *FC*2, and *FC*3, the average precision score was 91.27, 82.73, and 85.47% (Table 2). The confusion matrix was constructed using 15 trials. For *FC*1, all were identified correctly, while for *FC*2 and *FC*3, one and two samples were misidentified. The computed overall accuracy was 93.33% (Table 3).

$$\text{Precision} = \text{TP}/\text{TP} + \text{FP} \tag{4}$$

$$\text{Recall} = \text{TP}/\text{TP} + \text{FN} \tag{5}$$

$$\text{Overall Accuracy} = \frac{\text{TP} + \text{TN}}{\text{TP} + \text{FP} + \text{TN} + \text{FN}} \times 100\% \tag{6}$$

$$\text{Overall Accuracy} = 93.33\% \tag{7}$$

Table 2. Average precision score of each food combination.

Number of Trials	Food Sample	Average Precision Score (%)
15	FC1	91.26666667
15	FC2	82.73333333
15	FC3	85.46666667

Table 3. Confusion matrix.

	FC1	FC2	FC3	Classification Overall
FC1	15	0	0	15
FC2	0	13	2	15
FC3	0	1	14	15
Truth Overall	15	14	16	45

Table 4 shows the different weights of *FC1*. The total calories of the sample were determined, too. For predicted total calories, the sum of the weights of each food sample was used and the computed macronutrient content per gram was used. The average actual total calories of *FC1* was 269.75 kcal, and the average predicted total calories was 270.40 kcal. The same process was conducted for *FC2* with different values because each food sample had a different macronutrient content. The average total calories was 319.95 kcal. The average predicted total calories was 323.70 kcal (Table 5). The average actual total calories of *FC3* was 284.79 kcal, and the average predicted total calories was 280.98 kcal (Table 6).

Table 4. Macronutrient content of *FC*1.

Food Combo			Actual			Predicted
Trial	Giniling (g)	Adobo (g)	Rice (g)	Sum (g)	Total Calories	Total Calories
1	37	47	125	209	254.29	246.35
2	54	56	88	198	236.15	233.39
3	84	52	123	259	302.74	305.29
4	84	63	78	225	261.29	265.21
5	95	55	106	256	295.87	301.76
6	60	50	93	203	239.97	239.28
7	57	62	105	224	268.29	264.04
8	94	80	67	241	279.82	284.07
9	81	69	87	237	277.79	279.36
10	86	57	99	242	281.34	285.25
			Average:		269.75	270.40

Table 5. Macronutrient content of *FC*2.

Food Combo 2			Actual			Predicted
Trial	Ginataang Kalabasa (g)	Adobo (g)	Rice (g)	Sum (g)	Total Calories	Total Calories
1	85	42	107	234	313.14	315.21
2	48	76	103	227	300.40	305.78
3	87	61	103	251	336.60	338.11
4	40	85	115	240	315.94	323.29
5	91	97	92	280	377.07	377.18
6	79	71	89	239	320.99	321.95
7	58	44	128	230	303.05	309.82
8	50	81	93	224	297.52	301.74
9	45	82	111	238	314.13	320.60
10	67	79	94	240	320.65	323.29
			Average:		319.95	323.70

Table 6. Macronutrient content of *FC*3.

Food Combo 2			Actual			Predicted
Trial	Ginataang Kalabasa (g)	Giniling (g)	Rice (g)	Sum (g)	Total Calories	Total Calories
1	85	42	107	234	313.14	315.21
2	48	76	103	227	300.40	305.78
3	87	61	103	251	336.60	338.11
4	40	85	115	240	315.94	323.29
5	91	97	92	280	377.07	377.18
6	79	71	89	239	320.99	321.95
7	58	44	128	230	303.05	309.82
8	50	81	93	224	297.52	301.74
9	45	82	111	238	314.13	320.60
10	67	79	94	240	320.65	323.29
			Average:		319.95	323.70

4. Conclusions

We developed a system for food classification using image classification and machine learning. A working prototype was fabricated, and the mobile application was developed to determine nutritional information on foods for a healthier lifestyle. The potential of image processing was confirmed in determining the macronutrient content of selected foods and meals. Nutrition and health monitoring using mobile applications can be further developed with technological advancements.

Author Contributions: Conceptualization, A.D.R.D. and Z.A.L.N.; methodology, A.D.R.D. and Z.A.L.N.; software, A.D.R.D.; validation, A.D.R.D., Z.A.L.N. and C.C.P.; formal analysis, A.D.R.D., Z.A.L.N., and C.C.P.; investigation, Z.A.L.N.; resources, Z.A.L.N.; data curation, A.D.R.D. and Z.A.L.N.; writing—original draft preparation, A.D.R.D. and Z.A.L.N.; writing—review and editing, C.C.P.; visualization, A.D.R.D.; supervision, C.C.P.; funding acquisition, A.D.R.D. and Z.A.L.N. All authors have read and agreed to the published version of the manuscript.

Funding: This research received no external funding.

Data Availability Statement: The data files generated and presented in this study are available upon request of the corresponding author.

Acknowledgments: The authors would like to thank Darwin Dormis, for providing the computation of nutritional content of the chosen Filipino viands based on DOST-NFRI Food Exchange List for Meal Planning.

Conflicts of Interest: The authors declare no conflicts of interest.

References

1. Abdelghani, W.; Zayani, C.A.; Amous, I.; Sèdes, F. User-centric IoT: Challenges and Perspectives. personales.upv.es. 2019. Available online: https://personales.upv.es/thinkmind/UBICOMM/UBICOMM_2018/ubicomm_2018_2_20_10049.html (accessed on 2 May 2024).
2. Mendoza, I.C.P.; Timbol, S.M.; Samonte, M.J.C.; Blancaflor, E.B. ImHome: An IoT for Smart Home Appliances. In Proceedings of the 2020 IEEE 7th International Conference on Industrial Engineering and Applications (ICIEA), Bangkok, Thailand, 16–21 April 2020. [CrossRef]
3. Paglinawan, C.C.; Hannah, M.; Frias, J.B. Medicine Classification Using YOLOv4 and Tesseract OCR. In Proceedings of the 2023 15th International Conference on Computer and Automation Engineering (ICCAE), Sydney, Australia, 3–5 March 2023. [CrossRef]
4. Ckyle, A.; Guillermo, D.M.; Paglinawan, C.C. Cassava Disease Detection Using MobileNetV3 Algorithm through Augmented Stem and Leaf Images. In Proceedings of the 2023 17th International Conference on Ubiquitous Information Management and Communication (IMCOM), Seoul, Republic of Korea, 3–5 January 2023. [CrossRef]
5. Galeno, P.C.; Sale, D.P.; Martin, M.B. SMS-Based Dog Detection in Residential Area Using YOLOv5 and ML.net. In Proceedings of the 2023 IEEE 11th Conference on Systems, Process & Control (ICSPC), Malacca, Malaysia, 16 December 2023. [CrossRef]

6. Perez, J.V.; Manangan, G.; Deveza, D.K.; Mendero, C.; Villaruel, H.V. Implementation of Convolutional Neural Network of Non-Biodegradable Garbage Classifier and Segregator Based on VGG16 Architecture. In Proceedings of the TENCON 2023 - 2023 IEEE Region 10 Conference (TENCON), Chiang Mai, Thailand, 31 October–3 November 2023. [CrossRef]
7. Abu, M.; Hazirah Indra, N.; Halim, A.; Rahman, A.; Sapiee, A.; Ahmad, I. A Study on Image Classification Based on Deep Learning and Tensorflow. *Int. J. Eng. Res. Technol.* **2019**, *12*, 563–569.
8. Kumar, R.D.; Julie, E.G.; Robinson, Y.H.; Vimal, S.; Seo, S. Recognition of Food Type and Calorie Estimation Using Neural Network. *J. Supercomput.* **2021**, *77*, 8172–8193. [CrossRef]
9. Min, W.; Wang, Z.; Liu, Y.; Luo, M.; Kang, L.-P.; Wei, X.; Wei, X.; Jiang, S. Large Scale Visual Food Recognition. *IEEE Trans. Pattern Anal. Mach. Intell.* **2021**, *45*, 9932–9949. [CrossRef] [PubMed]
10. Balbin, J.R.; Valiente, L.D.; Martin, K.; Olorvida, E.D.; Glenn, G.; Soto, M.L. Determination of Calorie Content in Different Type of Foods Using Image Processing. In Proceedings of the 2019 IEEE 11th International Conference on Humanoid, Nanotechnology, Information Technology, Communication and Control, Environment, and Management (HNICEM), Laoag, Philippines, 29 November–1 December 2019. [CrossRef]
11. Jijesh, J.J.; Jinesh, J.J.; Bolla, D.R.; Sruthi, P.V.; Dileep, M.R.; Keshavamurthy, D. Development of Food Tracking System Using Machine Learning. In Proceedings of the 2021 5th International Conference on Electrical, Electronics, Communication, Computer Technologies and Optimization Techniques (ICEECCOT), Mysuru, India, 10–11 December 2021. [CrossRef]
12. Gehlot, G. Dietexpert—Android Application for Personal Diet Consultant. *Int. J. Eng. Appl. Sci. Technol.* **2021**, *5*, 202–205. [CrossRef]
13. Mohanty, S.P.; Singhal, G.; Scuccimarra, E.A.; Kebaili, D.; Héritier, H.; Boulanger, V.; Salathé, M. The Food Recognition Benchmark: Using Deep Learning to Recognize Food in Images. *Front. Nutr.* **2022**, *9*, 875143. [CrossRef] [PubMed]
14. Ma, T.; Wang, H.; Wei, M.; Lan, T.; Wang, J.; Bao, S.; Ge, Q.; Fang, Y.; Sun, X. Application of Smart-Phone Use in Rapid Food Detection, Food Traceability Systems, and Personalized Diet Guidance, Making Our Diet More Health. *Food Res. Int.* **2022**, *152*, 110918. [CrossRef] [PubMed]

engineering proceedings

Proceeding Paper

Effects of Catalysts on the Structure and Piezoelectric Properties of PVDF/ZnO Nanowires for the Robotic Tactile Sensor †

Ming-Cheng Kao [1,*], Jun-Hong Weng [2], Chih-Hung Chiang [3], Kai-Huang Chen [4] and Tsung-Kuei Kang [5]

1 Department of Information and Communication Engineering, Graduate Institute of Aeronautics, Chaoyang University of Technology, Taichung 413310, Taiwan
2 Department of Electrical Engineering, Tunghai University, Taichung 407224, Taiwan; jhw@thu.edu.tw
3 Graduate Institute of Aeronautics, Chaoyang University of Technology, Taichung 413310, Taiwan
4 Department of Electronic Engineering, Cheng Shiu University, Kaoshiung 83347, Taiwan
5 Department of Electronic Engineering, Feng Chia University, Taichung 407102, Taiwan
* Correspondence: kmc@cyut.edu.tw
† Presented at the 2024 IEEE 4th International Conference on Electronic Communications, Internet of Things and Big Data, Taipei, Taiwan, 19–21 April 2024.

Abstract: Polyvinylidene fluoride (PVDF)-coated ZnO nanorod piezoelectric sensors were prepared on silicone-based polymer polydimethylsiloxane (PDMS) substrates using a hydrothermal method. The effects of catalysts (sodium hydroxide, ammonium hydroxide, and hexamethylenetetramine) on the lattice microstructure and piezoelectric properties of ZnO nanorods were analyzed. The piezoelectric properties of polyvinylidene fluoride-coated ZnO nanorods' tactile sensors with different catalysts were measured under different forces. ZnO nanorods with hexamethylenetetramine have a high c-axis (002)-preferred orientation hexagonal wurtzite crystal structure with a maximum length of 5800 nm and an aspect ratio of 72.5. The Polyvinylidene fluoride/ZnO nanorod sensor with hexamethylenetetramine showed an excellent linear response to external pressure in the range of 0.1~1.2 N, and the best sensitivity is 61.1 mV/N.

Keywords: ZnO; PVDF; nanorods; piezoelectric

Citation: Kao, M.-C.; Weng, J.-H.; Chiang, C.-H.; Chen, K.-H.; Kang, T.-K. Effects of Catalysts on the Structure and Piezoelectric Properties of PVDF/ZnO Nanowires for the Robotic Tactile Sensor. *Eng. Proc.* **2024**, *74*, 55. https://doi.org/10.3390/engproc2024074055

Academic Editors: Shu-Han Liao, Teen-Hang Meen and Cheng-Fu Yang

Published: 5 September 2024

1. Introduction

In recent years, there has been extensive research on tactile sensors for applications involving human skin, leading to their widespread adoption across various fields such as smart skin, wearable devices, the Internet of Things (IoT), and smart industries. Tactile sensors are categorized based on their physical mechanisms into piezoelectric, piezoresistive, capacitive, and photoelectric types. Among these, piezoelectric sensors have attracted considerable attention due to their numerous advantages, including high sensitivity, rapid response speed, low power consumption, and independence from external power sources [1–4]. The piezoelectric materials such as ZnO, $PbZr_xTi_{1-x}O_3$ (PZT), and polyvinylidene fluoride have been studied by many researchers and applied to tactile sensors due to their high piezoelectric and sensitivity properties [5–8]. However, PZT has limited applications because it contains lead. Polyvinylidene fluoride has good flexibility, high sensitivity, and softness properties, which are appropriate for wearable tactile sensors [9,10]. In addition, ZnO nanorods have gained widespread research interest due to their high sensitivity, good flexibility, and high piezoelectric coefficient [11,12].

Therefore, we combined ZnO nanorods and polyvinylidene fluoride for tactile sensor applications. The tactile sensors were prepared utilizing the high aspect ratio, large surface area, and excellent piezoelectric properties of ZnO nanorods and the high responsiveness and sensitivity of polyvinylidene fluoride to effectively convert the mechanical force into electrical signals. In this study, ZnO nanorods were synthesized on the flexible substrates using the hydrothermal method. The hydrothermal method is appropriate for preparing

ZnO nanostructures on polymer plastic substrates due to its simplicity, low cost, and low growth temperature. However, the crystal structure and morphology of ZnO nanorods are affected by processing parameters such as catalysts, solution concentration, temperature, and duration, which must be optimized. The crystal structure and morphology of ZnO nanorods can be improved by optimizing the conditions.

To further clarify the relationship between the microstructure and piezoelectric properties of ZnO nanorods and improve their piezoelectric properties, the effects of various catalysts (sodium hydroxide, ammonium hydroxide, hexamethylenetetramine) on the crystal structure and morphology of ZnO nanorods were analyzed. In this research, polyvinylidene fluoride was coated on the ZnO nanorod to form a polyvinylidene fluoride/ZnO nanorod tactile sensor. The effects of catalysts on the crystallization properties of the ZnO nanorods were studied, and the piezoelectric-sensing characteristics of polyvinylidene fluoride/ZnO nanorod tactile sensors with different catalysts were also investigated.

2. Materials and Methods

ZnO thin films were prepared as a seed layer on the polymer polydimethylsiloxane (PDMS) substrates using the sol–gel method. A homogeneous mixture of $Zn(C_2H_3O_2)_2 \cdot 2H_2O$ and $C_3H_8O_2$ was prepared at a concentration of 0.5 M and stirred at 60 °C for 3 h. The seed layer was then deposited onto the PDMS substrate using spin-coating at 3000 rpm for 30 s and was annealed at 600 °C for 2 min. ZnO nanorods were synthesized using the hydrothermal method using a zinc acetate solution (10 mM) mixed with sodium hydroxide (NaOH), ammonium hydroxide (NH_4OH), or hexamethylenetetramine ($C_6H_{12}N_4$) at 90 °C for 6 h. Subsequently, polyvinylidene fluoride films were deposited onto the ZnO nanorods using sol–gel and spin coating methods. PVDF powder was dissolved in N,N-dimethylformamide (DMF) solvent, and the solution was spin-coated onto the substrate surface. The polyvinylidene fluoride/ZnO nanorods were annealed at 90 °C for 1 h to remove the solvent and solidify the PVDF film. The copper electrodes adhered to both sides of the polyvinylidene fluoride film through conductive silver gel to form electrodes of the tactile sensor. Finally, the PDMS thin film with good flexibility was spin-coated on the PVDF thin film to complete the tactile sensor structure, as shown in Figure 1. The pressure was transferred to the piezoelectric layer using the PDMS thin film, protecting the sensor from damage by the external environment.

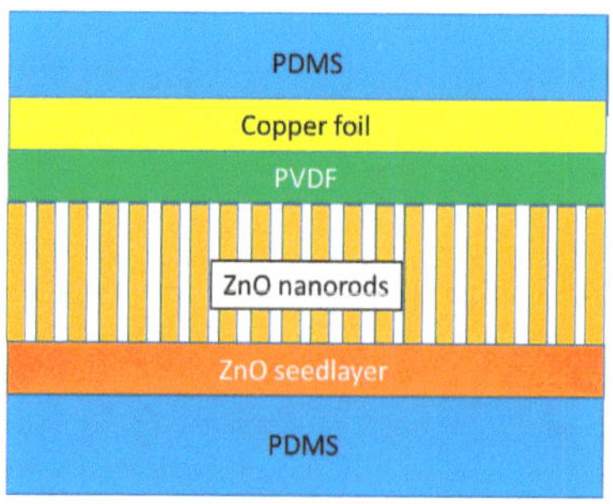

Figure 1. Structure of polyvinylidene fluoride/ZnO nanorod tactile sensor.

The lattice structure of ZnO nanorods was measured using an X-ray diffractometer (Rigaku Dmax 2200 X, Rigaku Corporation, Tokyo, Japan). The X-ray source is CuKα radiation (λ = 1.5418 Å), and the measurement angle range is 20–60°. The surface microstructure of ZnO nanorods was measured using a field emission scanning electron microscope (FE-SEM JEOL JSM-6700F, JEOL Ltd., Tokyo, Japan). The piezoelectric properties of PVDF/ZnO nanorod tactile sensors were measured using a charge amplifier to convert the pressure-generated charge signal into an output voltage. The experiment involved placing a polyvinylidene fluoride/ZnO nanorod tactile sensor on the measuring plate of a digital force gauge. When pressure was applied to the sensor with a finger, the force exerted was recorded using the digital force gauge. Simultaneously, the output voltage waveform of the tactile sensor was measured using a digital oscilloscope and was subsequently subjected to post-processing.

3. Results and Discussion

Figure 2 shows the X-ray diffraction crystallinity comparison of ZnO nanorods prepared with different catalysts (sodium hydroxide, ammonium hydroxide, and hexamethylenetetramine). All XRD patterns showed a hexagonal wurtzite structure and a strong c-axis orientation along the (002) plane (JCPDS card number 36-1451). ZnO nanorods with hexamethylenetetramine have the highest (002) diffraction peak intensity and exhibit excellent crystallinity compared with other samples. The catalyst impacted the crystallinity and structural properties of the ZnO nanorods. Hexamethylenetetramine promoted favorable nucleation and growth conditions for ZnO crystallization than sodium hydroxide and ammonium hydroxide catalysts.

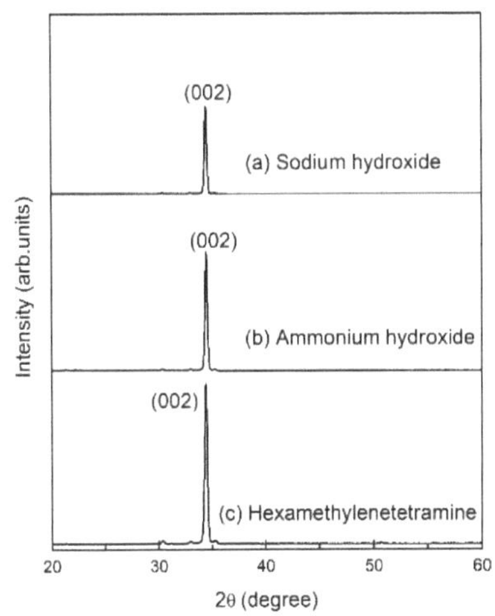

Figure 2. X-ray diffraction pattern of ZnO nanorods with catalysts of (**a**) sodium hydroxide, (**b**) ammonium hydroxide, and (**c**) hexamethylenetetramine.

Figure 3a–c shows the plane SEM images of the ZnO nanorods with sodium hydroxide, ammonium hydroxide, and hexamethylenetetramine, and Figure 3d presents the cross-sectional SEM image of ZnO nanorod with hexamethylenetetramine. The parameters of the average diameter, aspect ratio, and length of the ZnO nanorods are presented in Table 1. The average diameters of ZnO nanorods with sodium hydroxide, ammonium hydroxide, and hexamethylenetetramine catalysts are 40, 60, and 80 nm, respectively. The average lengths for sodium hydroxide, ammonium hydroxide, and hexamethylenetetramine were 1250, 3800, and 5500 nm, respectively. The average diameter, length, and aspect ratio of the ZnO nanorods with hexamethylenetetramine were the largest. This is because when hexamethylenetetramine was added to the aqueous solution, it was cleaved to form amines and provide OH groups to nucleate ZnO on the surface of the ZnO seed layer. Moreover, the amine cleavage rate of hexamethylenetetramine was slowed, and the pH value of the aqueous solution changed little, resulting in a low concentration of metal ion complexes [13]. Therefore, the nucleation reaction of ZnO was carried out at low supersaturation, which facilitated heterogeneous growth and made ZnO crystals easily grow into nanorods [14]. When sodium hydroxide and ammonium hydroxide catalysts were added to aqueous solutions, the pH of the solution changed significantly, resulting in high concentrations of metal complexes. ZnO enabled uniform nucleation, resulting in smaller diameters and lengths of nanorods [15].

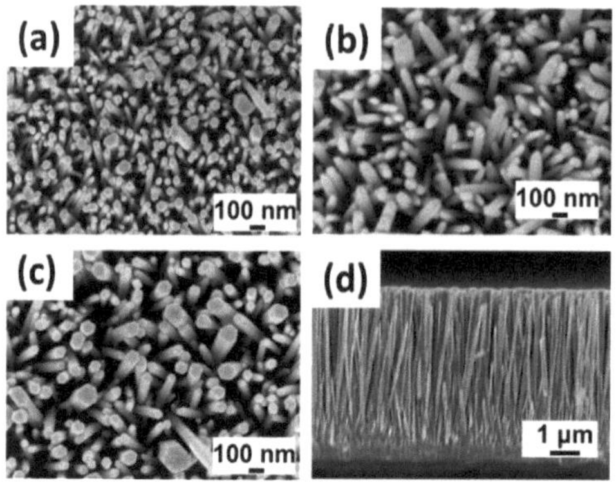

Figure 3. Plane SEM images of ZnO nanorods with the catalysts of (**a**) sodium hydroxide, (**b**) ammonium hydroxide, and (**c**) hexamethylenetetramine, and the cross-sectional SEM images of ZnO nanorods with hexamethylenetetramine (**d**).

Table 1. Structure parameters of ZnO nanorods with different catalysts.

Catalysts	Length (nm)	Diameters (nm)	Aspect Ratio
Sodium hydroxide	1250	40	31.3
Ammonium hydroxide	3800	60	63.3
Hexamethylenetetramine	5800	80	72.5

To measure the piezoelectric response of the nanorod tactile sensor, the charge signal generated by the sensor was converted into an output voltage using a charge amplifier, which was then captured and processed using a digital oscilloscope. Figure 4a–c shows the piezoelectric voltage of the PVDF/ZnO nanorod sensor with sodium hydroxide, ammonium hydroxide, and hexamethylenetetramine. The piezoelectric voltage peaks of the ZnO nanorod tactile sensors with sodium hydroxide, ammonium hydroxide, and hexamethylenetetramine were measured at 10, 35, and 53 mV, respectively, under a force of 1 N. The polyvinylidene fluoride/ZnO nanorod tactile sensor with hexamethylenetetramine showed a maximum voltage peak amplitude of 61 mV, as shown in Figure 4d, as the enhanced radial stress of ZnO nanorods with hexamethylenetetramine had the largest aspect ratio of 72.5 under the same pressure, resulting in enhanced piezoelectric displacement on the Z-axis of the nanorods [16]. In addition, when the piezoelectric polymer polyvinylidene fluoride film was coated on the ZnO nanorods, the voltage peak of the tactile sensor also increased. This was attributed to the fact that polyvinylidene fluoride is a piezoelectric material that can generate electrical charges in response to mechanical stress or pressure and increase the sensitivity of tactile sensors. ZnO nanorods enhanced the piezoelectric output of polyvinylidene fluoride films. This phenomenon has been reported in prior research, which the piezoelectric enhancement output of the polyvinylidene fluoride/ZnO nanorod structure was attributed to the synergistic effect of both polyvinylidene fluoride and ZnO nanorods [17–19]. The combination of ZnO nanorods and polyvinylidene fluoride film enhanced the overall responsiveness and performance of the tactile sensor when pressure is applied to the sensor [20].

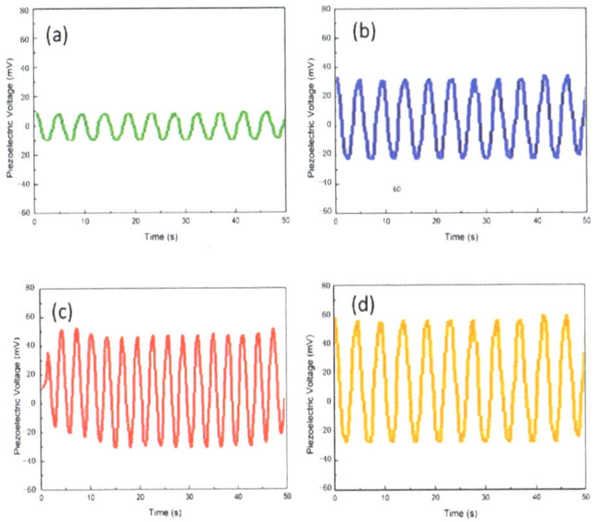

Figure 4. Comparison of piezoelectric sensing voltages of the ZnO nanorods tactile sensors with (**a**) sodium hydroxide, (**b**) ammonium hydroxide, (**c**) hexamethylenetetramine, which (**d**) is the polyvinylidene fluoride/ZnO nanorods with hexamethylenetetramine.

Figure 5 illustrates the influence of various catalysts on the voltage response of the polyvinylidene fluoride/ZnO nanorod tactile sensors across a range of external forces from 0.1 to 1.1 N. The corresponding voltage peak amplitudes in the dynamic piezoelectric response waveform of the tactile sensor are extracted upon the application of different forces. The voltage response of all tactile sensors exhibits a linear increase with rising pressure. The output voltages and sensitivities of the polyvinylidene fluoride/ZnO nanorods tactile sensors with different catalysts are shown in Table 2. The sensitivities of polyvinylidene fluoride/ZnO nanorod tactile sensors with sodium hydroxide, ammonium hydroxide, and hexamethylenetetramine are 31.8, 39.6, and 61.1 mV/N respectively. The polyvinylidene fluoride/ZnO nanorod tactile sensor with hexamethylenetetramine achieves a high sensitivity of 61.1 mV/N. Compared with sodium hydroxide, the sensitivity of ZnO nanorods with hexamethylenetetramine increased by about 2-fold. This was attributed to the significant aspect ratio c-axis orientation of ZnO nanorods with hexamethylenetetramine.

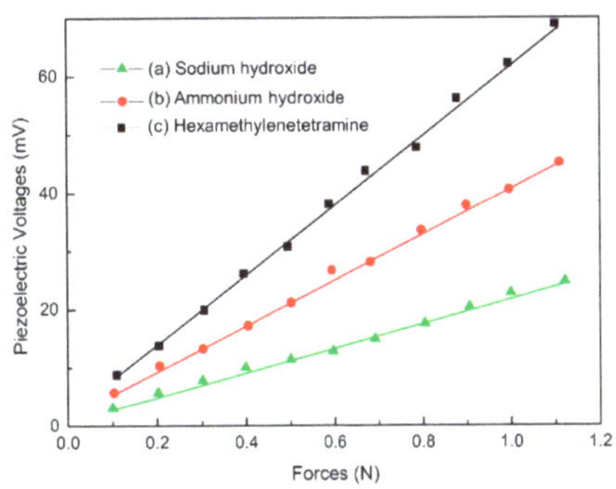

Figure 5. Piezoelectric sensing voltage of the polyvinylidene fluoride/ZnO nanorods tactile sensors with different catalysts under different pressures.

Table 2. Comparison of piezoelectric sensing voltage and sensitivity of the polyvinylidene fluoride/ZnO nanorods tactile sensors.

Catalysts	Piezoelectric Sensing Voltages (mV)	Sensitivity (mV/N)
Sodium hydroxide	22	31.8
Ammonium hydroxide	40	39.6
Hexamethylenetetramine	61	61.1

4. Conclusions

The polyvinylidene fluoride/ZnO nanorod piezoelectric tactile sensors were prepared on PDMS substrates using the hydrothermal method to study the effects of catalysts (Sodium hydroxide, Ammonium hydroxide, and Hexamethylenetetramine) on the lattice structure and surface microstructure of ZnO nanorods. The largest diameter, length, and aspect ratio of the ZnO nanorods were obtained using hexamethylenetetramine. The polyvinylidene fluoride/ZnO nanorod's tactile sensor with hexamethylenetetramine showed a maximum voltage peak of 61 mV and sensitivity of 61.1 mV/N, which was attributed to the high aspect ratio of the ZnO nanorod and the coating of polyvinylidene fluoride. The prepared polyvinylidene fluoride/ZnO nanorod piezoelectric tactile sensor has great potential for applications in robot tactile sensing and wearable devices.

Author Contributions: Conceptualization, M.-C.K. and C.-H.C.; methodology, M.-C.K. and C.-H.C.; formal analysis, M.-C.K., T.-K.K. and C.-H.C.; investigation, J.-H.W.; resources, K.-H.C.; data curation, M.-C.K.; writing—original draft preparation, K.-H.C. and C.-H.C.; writing—review and editing, T.-K.K.; visualization, M.-C.K.; project administration, M.-C.K.; funding acquisition, C.-H.C. All authors have read and agreed to the published version of the manuscript.

Funding: This research was funded by the National Science Council of the Republic of China under grant number NSC 111-2112-E-164-002.

Institutional Review Board Statement: Not applicable.

Informed Consent Statement: Not applicable.

Data Availability Statement: The data presented in this study are available on request from the corresponding author due to confidentiality agreement.

Conflicts of Interest: The authors declare no conflicts of interest.

References

1. Kumar, V.S.; Krishnamoorthi, C. Development of electrical transduction based wearable tactile sensors for human vital signs monitor: Fundamentals, methodologies and applications. *Sens. Actuators A Phys.* **2021**, *321*, 112582–112623. [CrossRef]
2. Tang, Z.J.; Wang, Z.; Lu, J.Q.; Ma, N.Q. Design of robot finger based on flexible tactile sensor. *Int. J. Adv. Robot. Syst.* **2019**, *16*, 1–10. [CrossRef]
3. Lepora, N.F.; Church, A.; de Kerckhove, C.; Hadsell, R.; Lloyd, J. From pixels to percepts: Highly robust edge perception and contour following using deep learning and an optical biomimetic tactile sensor. *IEEE Robot. Autom. Lett.* **2019**, *4*, 2101–2107. [CrossRef]
4. Wu, C.X.; Kim, T.W.; Park, J.H.; Koo, B.; Sung, S.Y.; Shao, J.J.; Zhang, C.; Wang, Z.L. Self-powered tactile sensor with learning and memory. *ACS Nano* **2020**, *14*, 1390–1398. [CrossRef] [PubMed]
5. Zhu, L.; Xiang, Y.; Liu, Y.; Geng, K.; Yao, R.; Li, B. Comparison of piezoelectric responses of flexible tactile sensors based on hydrothermally-grown ZnO nanorods on ZnO seed layers with different thicknesses. *Sens. Actuators A Phys.* **2022**, *341*, 113552. [CrossRef]
6. Misra, M.; Srivastava, A.K.; Kadam, A.N.; Salunkhe, T.T.; Kumar, V.; Nikalje, A.P.G. Substantial enhancement of optoelectronics and piezoelectric properties of novel hollow ZnO nanorods towards efficient flexible touch and bending sensor. *Colloids Surf. A Physicochem. Eng.* **2024**, *685*, 133232. [CrossRef]
7. Hari, M.A.; Karumuthil, S.C.; Rajan, L. Optimization of PVDF nanocomposite based flexible piezoelectric tactile sensors: A comparative investigation. *Sens. Actuators A Phys.* **2023**, *353*, 114215.
8. He, H.; Fu, Y.; Zang, W.; Wang, Q.; Xing, L.; Zhang, Y.; Xue, X. A flexible self-powered T-ZnO/PVDF/fabric electronic-skin with multi-functions of tactile-perception, atmosphere-detection and self-clean. *Nano Energy* **2017**, *31*, 37–48. [CrossRef]

9. Yang, J.; Chen, Q.S.; Xu, F.; Jiang, H.X.; Liu, W.L.; Zhang, X.Q.; Jiang, Z.X.; Zhu, G.D. Epitaxy enhancement of piezoelectric properties in P(VDF-TrFE) copolymer films and applications in sensing and energy harvesting. *Adv. Electron. Mater.* **2020**, *6*, 1–13. [CrossRef]
10. Siponkoski, T.; Nelo, M.; Palosaari, J.; Per¨antie, J.; Sobocinski, M.; Juuti, J.; Jantunen, H. Electromechanical properties of PZT/P(VDF-TrFE) composite ink printed on a flexible organic substrate. *Compos. B Eng.* **2015**, *80*, 217–222. [CrossRef]
11. Tan, Y.S.; Yang, K.; Wang, B.; Li, H.; Wang, L.; Wang, C.X. High-performance textile piezoelectric pressure sensor with novel structural hierarchy based on ZnO nanorods array for wearable application. *Nano Res.* **2021**, *14*, 3969–3976. [CrossRef]
12. Yang, T.; Pan, H.; Tian, G.; Zhang, B.; Xiong, D.; Gao, Y.; Yan, C.; Chu, X.; Chen, N.; Zhong, S.; et al. Hierarchically structured PVDF/ZnO core-shell nanofibers for self-powered physiological monitoring electronics. *Nano Energy* **2020**, *72*, 104706–104711. [CrossRef]
13. Govender, K.; Boyle, D.S.; Kenway, P.B.; O'Brien, P. Understanding the factors that govern the deposition and morphology of thin films of ZnO from aqueous solution. *J. Mater. Chem.* **2004**, *14*, 2575–2591. [CrossRef]
14. Greene, L.E.; Law, M.; Goldberger, J.; Kim, F.; Johnson, J.C.; Zhang, Y.; Saykally, R.J.; Yang, P. Low-temperature wafer-scale production of ZnO nanorods arrays. *Angew. Chem. Int.* **2003**, *42*, 3031–3034. [CrossRef] [PubMed]
15. Vayssieres, L.; Keis, K.; Hagfeldt, A.; Lindquist, S. Three-dimensional array of highly oriented crystalline ZnO microtubes. *Chem. Mater.* **2001**, *13*, 4395–4398. [CrossRef]
16. Deng, W.; Jin, L.; Zhang, B.; Chen, Y.; Mao, L.; Zhang, H.; Yang, W. A flexible fieldlimited ordered ZnO nanorod-based self-powered tactile sensor array for electronic skin. *Nanoscale* **2016**, *8*, 16302–16306. [CrossRef] [PubMed]
17. Bhunia, R.; Das, S.; Dalui, S.; Hussain, S.; Paul, R.; Bhar, R.; Pal, A.K. Flexible nano-ZnO/polyvinylidene difluoride piezoelectric composite films as energy harvester. *Appl. Phys. A Mater.* **2016**, *122*, 637. [CrossRef]
18. Lee, M.; Chen, C.Y.; Wang, S.; Cha, S.N.; Park, Y.J.; Kim, J.M.; Chou, L.J.; Wang, Z.L. A Hybrid Piezoelectric Structure for Wearable Nanogenerators. *Adv. Mater.* **2012**, *24*, 1759–1764. [CrossRef] [PubMed]
19. Ramadoss, A.; Saravanakumar, B.; Lee, S.W.; Kim, Y.S.; Kim, S.J.; Wang, Z.L. Piezoelectric-Driven Self-Charging Supercapacitor Power Cell. *ACS Nano* **2015**, *9*, 4337–4345. [CrossRef] [PubMed]
20. Fraleoni-Morgera, A.; Cesini, I.; Kumar, P.; Oddo, C.M. Hydrothermally grown ZnO nanorods as promising materials for low cost electronic skin. *ChemNanoMat* **2020**, *6*, 15–31. [CrossRef]

engineering proceedings

Proceeding Paper

Optimal Parameter Selection and Indicator Design for Technical Analysis Strategies by Computer Software: An Empirical Analysis of the Taiwan Futures Market †

Hsio-Yi Lin [1,*], Chieh-Yow ChiangLin [2] and Hsuan-Wei Tseng [2]

1 Department of Finance, National Pingtung University, Pingtung City 900, Taiwan
2 Department of Finance & Information, National Kaohsiung University of Science and Technology, Kaohsiung 824, Taiwan; clcy@nkust.edu.tw (C.-Y.C.); allenta109@gmail.com (H.-W.T.)
* Correspondence: hylin0907@mail.nptu.edu.tw

† Presented at the 2024 IEEE 4th International Conference on Electronic Communications, Internet of Things and Big Data, Taipei, Taiwan, 19–21 April 2024.

Abstract: In algorithmic trading, "overfitting" often arises during parameter optimization. To avoid scenarios where in-sample performance is excellent but out-of-sample performance fails to meet expectations, appropriate parameter combinations are crucial for enhancing the robustness of a strategy. To find the appropriate parameter combinations, we identified "parameter plateaus" in the three-dimensional space generated by strategy performance metrics. These plateaus represent parameter combinations where the surrounding performance metrics are relatively similar, reducing the risk of drastic performance drops. Utilizing the four parameter selection methods designed in this study (weighted selection, Standard Deviation Selection, Island Area Selection, and Island Volume Selection), we selected parameter combinations in-sample and validated them out-of-sample, complemented by "rolling window analysis" for long-term profitability stability. We used historical backtesting data from the Taiwan Stock Index Futures, covering the period from 1 January 2000 to 31 December 2022. The data were paired with trading strategies developed based on the moving average technical indicator. Through the four parameter selection methods and the system backtesting approach using rolling windows, we identified parameter combinations in-sample and then validated them out-of-sample. The results showed that the performance metrics improved by more than 50% over those generated using traditional optimal point selection methods, demonstrating the superiority of the parameter selection methods proposed in this study.

Keywords: program trading; walk forward analysis; parameter plateau

Citation: Lin, H.-Y.; ChiangLin, C.-Y.; Tseng, H.-W. Optimal Parameter Selection and Indicator Design for Technical Analysis Strategies by Computer Software: An Empirical Analysis of the Taiwan Futures Market. *Eng. Proc.* **2024**, *74*, 56. https://doi.org/10.3390/engproc2024074056

Academic Editors: Shu-Han Liao, Teen-Hang Meen and Cheng-Fu Yang

Published: 6 September 2024

1. Introduction

In algorithmic trading, when optimizing parameters for trading strategies, it is common to divide historical price data into two sets: in-sample and out-of-sample. The performance of a strategy applied to trading conditions often exhibits a phenomenon where the in-sample performance looks impressive, but the out-of-sample performance is significantly worse. This situation is referred to as "overfitting" in parameter optimization. Overfitting occurs due to various reasons such as excessive parameter optimization, insufficient sample size, or instability in the performance of parameter combinations.

To avoid overfitting in strategy development, it is crucial to choose appropriate parameter combinations. In a three-dimensional space created by parameter combinations and their performance, the performance of that combination differs significantly from those around it if the selected parameter combination is isolated. This leads to unstable profitability in real trading. Therefore, parameter plateaus or stability regions through appropriate parameter selection methods must be found.

There has been a lack of research proposing an objective strategy parameter selection method. Most studies have relied on systematic backtesting to determine the appropriate strategies for a particular asset. For example, Yan (2017) [1], Cheng (2018) [2], Lee (2019) [3], and Lin (2020) [4] have used plateau search algorithms to identify parameter plateaus and assess the strategy's applicability to assets. To address the issue of overfitting in parameter optimization, we proposed to use four parameter selection methods: "Weighted Parameter Combination Selection", "Standard Deviation Parameter Combination Selection", "Island Area Parameter Combination Selection", and "Island Volume Parameter Combination Selection". The purpose of using these methods is to avoid parameter isolation and identify parameter combinations within the in-sample dataset that belong to parameter plateaus. Each of these parameter selection methods is designed to cater to different characteristics of strategies and assets, aiming to find suitable methods for specific scenarios.

2. Literature Review

2.1. Parameter Optimization

In a strategy model, overfitting refers to the phenomenon where the parameters used in the strategy excessively memorize historical data, resulting in the poor generalization ability of the strategy [5]. In representing the performance indicators and parameters as a three-dimensional graph, high performance may be observed in certain parameter combinations where the performance significantly deviates from the surrounding parameters, resembling an isolated island. This is not desirable for a good strategy because, in real trading, the information about the traded asset is not historical but continuously updated. Therefore, a robust strategy must be used to avoid overfitting and strive to find stable parameter combinations (similar to plateaus) though they may not have the best performance and are not significantly different from neighboring parameter combinations [6]. To prevent the issue of overfitting, it is essential to avoid finding parameter combinations that form parameter islands and strive to discover what are known as parameter plateaus. At this point, it is challenging to define these parameter plateaus. In earlier research, the majority relied on visual judgment, meaning they subjectively determined whether a parameter combination constituted a plateau. However, Lee (2015) [7] introduced the concept of using the Regional Growth Algorithm to identify parameter plateaus. Subsequently, researchers such as Yan (2017) [1], Cheng (2018) [2], Lee (2019) [3], and Lin (2020) [4] also applied this algorithm to various technical indicators and assets. In this study, we used four parameter selection methods based on the literature mentioned above.

2.2. Walk Forward Analysis (Moving Window)

In validating the robustness of a trading strategy, it is common to split the backtesting period into in-sample and out-of-sample data sets based on a certain proportion. Assuming that the out-of-sample data represent unknown real market data, the optimization of parameter combinations is performed using historical data within the in-sample period. These optimized parameters are then tested on the out-of-sample data, simulating the performance of using the optimized parameter combination in a real market scenario.

The concept of "Walk Forward Analysis" was initially introduced by Robert Pardo [8]. This method involves dividing the backtesting period into multiple windows to examine how the optimized parameter combinations from the in-sample data perform in the out-of-sample period. If the strategy continues to yield profits in the out-of-sample period and consistently across different windows, the strategy possesses robustness. Conversely, if the strategy fails to perform well in the out-of-sample period, the strategy lacks robustness. To measure the robustness of a strategy in Walk Forward Analysis, the Walk Forward Efficiency (WFE) indicator is often used. This indicator is used to compare the performance of in-sample and out-of-sample data for each window by dividing the out-of-sample data by the in-sample data [6,8]. Through Walk Forward Analysis, it is assessed whether a strategy model is susceptible to overfitting. This method improves the strategy model or changes in parameter selection methods to avoid overfitting of strategy parameters [6].

3. Research Methodology

In this study, Taiwan Stock Index Futures (FITXN) was used as the trading asset, and a moving average-based trading strategy [9] was employed. Python's BackTrader external library was used for initial backtesting, while subsequent parameter search and strategy analysis were automated using Python. The BackTrader package in Python was used for optimization and backtesting. It generates daily profit and loss performance reports for all parameter combinations. Subsequently, Python was used for data processing and analysis, setting the in-sample and out-of-sample window sizes. Three performance indicators were evaluated using the four parameter selection methods designed in this study: "Weighted Parameter Combination Selection", "Standard Deviation Parameter Combination Selection", "Island Area Parameter Combination Selection", and "Island Volume Parameter Combination Selection". It was determined whether these methods outperform the "Single-Point Parameter Combination Selection" method in terms of out-of-sample performance. This assessment was used to determine the suitability of each parameter selection method for different combinations of assets and strategies.

1. Trading Backtest Asset and Data Source: The asset used for trading backtesting in this study was the Taiwan Stock Index Futures (FITXN), with data sourced from XQ Cai Pan Gao Shou's near-month futures daily data. The data from 1 January 2000 to 31 December 2021 comprised 2703 data points.
2. Trading Strategy Design (Moving Average Trading Strategy)
    (1) Indicator Introduction: The moving average is the arithmetic mean of the closing price over 'n' days.
    (2) Name Definitions: Two moving averages are defined, namely MA1 and MA2.
    (3) Entry Signals
        - Long Entry: When MA1 crosses above MA2 from below, and the position is flat (0), enter long at the next day's opening price.
        - Short Entry: When MA1 crosses below MA2 from above, and the position is flat (0), enter short at the next day's opening price.
3. Exit Signals
    a. Long Exit: When MA1 crosses below MA2 from above, and the position is long (1), exit at the next day's opening price.
    b. Short Exit: When MA1 crosses above MA2 from below, and the position is short (−1), exit at the next day's opening price.
    c. Indicator Parameters: MA1 and MA2 have lengths ranging from 1 to 60 with an interval of 1, resulting in 3600 parameter combinations.
4. Trading Basic Settings: The trading size for both entry and exit was fixed at 1 contract. The transaction cost was set at 50 units with a contract value of 200 units per point. The trading margin was 184,000 units.
5. Definition of Trading Performance Metrics
    (1) Net Profit: The total return is generated by the trading strategy over the entire backtesting period.

$$\text{Netprofit} = \text{Grossprofit} - \text{Grossloss}, \tag{1}$$

    (2) Maxdrawdown (MDD): The MDD is calculated as a risk of the trading strategy over the entire backtesting period.

$$\max\,(DD_1,\ DD_n), \tag{2}$$

    (3) Minimum Acceptable Return (MAR): The MAR index is a performance metric used to measure the risk-adjusted return of a trading strategy. It can be interpreted as the average annual return per unit of maximum risk. The formula for MAR includes a simple interest formula and a compound interest formula.

If the number of contracts traded varies with the size of the capital, the compound interest formula is used. In this study, the number of contracts traded was fixed, so the simple interest formula is employed as (3).

$$\text{MAR} = (\text{NetProfit}/\text{NumberofYears})/\text{MDD}, \quad (3)$$

(4) Walk Forward Efficiency (WFE): It is the annualized out-of-sample net profit divided by the annualized in-sample net profit, and this performance metric is used to measure the robustness of the trading system.

$$\frac{(\text{Out-of-sample Net Profit} - \text{Number of Years})}{(\text{In-sample Net Profit} - \text{Number of Years})}, \quad (4)$$

Figure 1 depicts a three-dimensional plot with the x-axis representing Parameter 1, the y-axis representing Parameter 2, and the z-axis representing the performance metric net profit. In order to avoid finding parameter combinations that may lead to performance peaks (where neighboring parameter combinations may not perform well, resembling isolated islands), parameter combinations that may not have the highest central performance but are robust (where neighboring parameter combinations also perform well, resembling plateaus) need to be identified. We used the four parameter selection methods to address this issue.

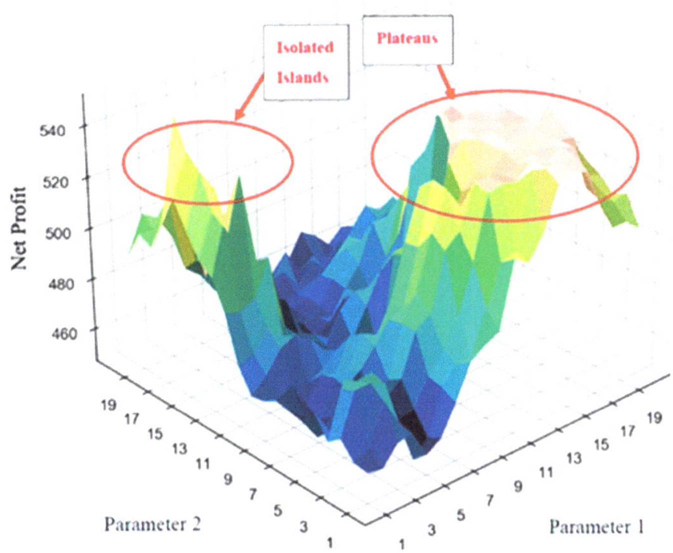

Figure 1. Parameter plateau and parameter island illustration.

In constructing the three-dimensional plot of parameters, we used net profit as the z-axis and two other performance metrics (MDD and MAR) separately to construct three-dimensional plots. We determined which performance metrics resulted in the most robust performance when combined with one of the parameter selection methods. If net profit is chosen as the filtering criterion, higher values are better. However, if the filtering criterion is MDD, since MDD is a risk indicator, lower values are preferable. If the chosen filtering criterion is MAR, higher values indicate better performance because MAR is the result of net profit divided by MDD.

The following is an explanation of the four parameter selection methods designed in this study.

3.1. Weighted Parameter Combination Selection Method

By taking a weighted average of the performance of each parameter combination and its neighboring parameter combinations, where neighboring parameter combinations are defined as those within one to three circles of expansion. The design of the weighting ratios adopts the concept of "inverse distance weighting", using the reciprocal of the distance between parameter combinations as weights (Equation (5)). The weight of the central parameter combination is 1. After weighting, parameter combinations that are farther away have a smaller influence.

$$w_i = \frac{1}{\sqrt{(x_i - x_{center})^2 + (y_i - y_{center})^2}}, \tag{5}$$

w_i: Weight of parameter combination i

x_i, y_i: Position of parameter combination i

x_{center}, y_{center}: Position of the central parameter combination

$x_i \neq x_{center}$ and $y_i \neq y_{center}$

If x_i, y_i are the central points, the formula's result would be infinite; in this study, the weight for this case is set to 1.

3.2. Standard Deviation Parameter Selection Method

The Standard Deviation Parameter Selection Method is used to identify parameter combinations within the in-sample dataset that exhibit relatively stable performance compared to their neighboring parameter combinations. This method begins by filtering out parameter combinations for each period in the in-sample dataset where the net profit is greater than the average net profit of all parameter combinations. It then calculates the standard deviation for each parameter combination concerning its neighboring parameter combinations. The standard deviation indicates the level of variation between the parameter combination and its neighbors; a higher standard deviation implies greater variation, while a lower standard deviation implies less variation. Finally, the method selects the parameter combination with the lowest standard deviation from all parameter combinations as the recommended parameter and evaluates its performance on the out-of-sample data. The formula for standard deviation is given by Equation (6).

$$\sigma_i = \sqrt{\frac{1}{N}\sum_{i=1}^{N}\left(Ind_i - \overline{Ind}\right)^2}, \tag{6}$$

σ_i: The standard deviation of the performance (net profit, MDD, MAR) of parameter combination i and its neighbors within two circles.

Ind_i: The performance value of parameter combination i (net profit, MDD, MAR).

$\overline{Ind}$: The mean of parameter combination i and its neighboring parameter combinations.

N: The number of parameter combinations i and its neighbors.

3.3. Island Area Parameter Selection Method

This method can be likened to comparing benchmark performance to sea level as illustrated in Figure 2. It examines the areas occupied by different islands located at sea level and selects the parameter point with the best performance from the largest island as the parameter choice. Regarding benchmark performance, we arranged the performance of all parameter combinations within the in-sample dataset from smallest to largest for each period. Subsequently, benchmark performance was determined by percentile ranks (PR). In this study, PR values were set at 90, 95, and 99.

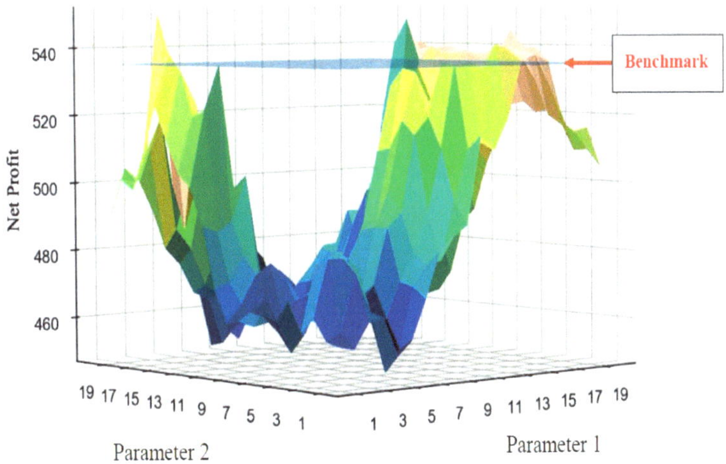

Figure 2. Three-dimensional illustration of island selection method.

3.4. *Island Volume Parameter Selection Method*

As shown in Figure 2, the approach involves examining the volumes (sum of performance) occupied by different islands located at sea level and selecting the parameter point with the best performance from the largest island as the parameter choice. Regarding benchmark performance, we arranged the performance of all parameter combinations within the in-sample dataset from smallest to largest for each period. Subsequently, benchmark performance was determined by percentile ranks (PR). As previously mentioned, PR values in this method were set at 90, 95, and 99.

4. Results

4.1. *Weighted Parameter Selection Method*

Table 1 presents the out-of-sample performance for the Weighted Parameter Selection Method. When filtering by net profit, 28 performance metrics outperformed the Best Point Selection Method, accounting for 62% of the total. Among these, one was statistically significant, and none were statistically inferior. When filtering by MDD, 28 performance metrics outperformed the Best Point Selection Method, making up 62% of the total. One was statistically significant, and none were statistically inferior. When filtering by MAR, 30 performance metrics outperformed the Best Point Selection Method, accounting for 67% of the total. Among these, seven were statistically significant, and two were statistically inferior.

Table 2 presents a comparison of in-sample and out-of-sample performance for the weighted selection method. When using net profit as the selection criterion, 10 WFE values were higher using the Best Point Selection Method, accounting for 67% of the total. When using MDD as the selection criterion, 10 WFE values were better than using the Best Point Selection Method, also accounting for 67% of the total. Finally, when using MAR as the selection criterion, 10 WFE values were better than using the Best Point Selection Method, constituting 67% of the total. As shown in Tables 1 and 2, the performance indicator ISNetProfit was measured in ten thousand units, and the shaded areas indicated that the performance of this indicator is superior to the "Best Point Parameter Selection Method".

Table 1. Out-of-sample performance for the weighted parameter selection method.

Window Proportion	Filtering Indicator / Benchmark \ Circles	NetProfit 0	NetProfit 1	NetProfit 2	NetProfit 3	MDD 0	MDD 1	MDD 2	MDD 3	MAR 0	MAR 1	MAR 2	MAR 3
11	NetProfit	68.16	62.13	58.32	−14.94	−2.24	−18.3	88.94	71.36	107.83	14	43.58	−7.98
	MDD	99.46	130.45	86.38	123.92	73.56	60.64	50.36	38.27	49.38	111.32	78.46	107.58
	MAR	0.033	0.023	0.032	−0.006	−0.001	−0.014	0.084	0.089	0.104	0.006	0.026	−0.004
21	NetProfit	10.8	−21.38	−43.62	−18.47	−34.23	−0.39	18.8	−16.38	−36.84	−76.8	−49.38	−18.4
	MDD	78.79	100.26	74.02	77.3	62.98	70.51	85.26	65.32	76.9	104.44	86.19	73.88
	MAR	0.007	−0.011	−0.029	−0.012	−0.027	0	0.011	−0.013	−0.024	−0.037	−0.029	−0.012
31	NetProfit	26.64	101.4	47.18	−0.98	16.34	−27.8	−34.82	−44.42	−93.81	5.46	75.72	−11.1
	MDD	153.29	84.54	96.09	104.72	48.33	76.46	102.55	98.2	119.66	63.26	70.25	90.55
	MAR	0.009	0.063	0.026	0	0.018	−0.019	−0.018	−0.024	−0.041	0.005	0.057	−0.006
41	NetProfit	10.89	168.6	165.46	81.19	−31.14	−15.58	11.85	47.13	−34.9	81.3	85.59	99.68
	MDD	154.26	70.96	74.78	46.14	51.23	75.88	37.9	40.04	70.92	66.32	46.14	46.14
	MAR	0.004	0.132	0.123	0.098	−0.034	−0.011	0.017	0.065	−0.027	0.068	0.103	0.12
51	NetProfit	133.34	217.8	183.62	165.8	−14.23	−18.96	25.02	42.59	−102.56	126.7	193.66	98.06
	MDD	112.62	73.17	57.29	61.82	54.38	34.36	36.8	30.2	159.68	64.51	59.84	62.5
	MAR	0.07	0.175	0.189	0.158	−0.015	−0.032	0.04	0.083	−0.038	0.116	0.19	

Table 2. Comparison of in-sample and out-sample performance for the weighted selection method.

Window Proportion	Filtering Indicator / Benchmark \ PR	NetProfit 0	NetProfit 1	NetProfit 2	NetProfit 3	MDD 0	MDD 1	MDD 2	MDD 3	MAR 0	MAR 1	MAR 2	MAR 3
11	ISNetProfit	1080.6	902.75	862.75	778.66	353.4	261.16	240.64	234.4	738.98	727.06	786.62	707.7
	WFE	0.063	0.069	0.068	−0.019	−0.006	−0.07	0.37	0.304	0.146	0.019	0.055	−0.011
21	ISNetProfit	1454.39	1184.47	1114.48	983.08	436.78	410.06	412.34	422.86	1261.32	1088.49	1032.11	1023.56
	WFE	0.014	−0.036	−0.078	−0.038	−0.156	−0.002	0.092	−0.078	−0.058	−0.142	−0.096	−0.036
31	ISNetProfit	1623.42	1421	1305.52	1193.8	550.28	488.21	473.56	475.6	1492.98	1207.53	1248.66	1035.88
	WFE	0.048	0.213	0.108	−0.003	0.09	−0.171	−0.222	−0.279	−0.189	0.015	0.183	−0.033
41	ISNetProfit	1819.73	1595.12	1420.3	1285.49	694.26	550.04	460.5	453.86	1538.33	1372.39	1266.86	1156.65
	WFE	0.024	0.424	0.464	0.252	−0.18	−0.112	0.104	0.416	−0.092	0.236	0.272	0.344
51	ISNetProfit	1989.32	1806.24	1611.88	1531.26	777.12	491.86	460.86	458.26	1799.66	1726.03	1689.72	1599.44
	WFE	0.335	0.605	0.57	0.54	−0.09	−0.195	0.27	0.465	−0.285	0.365	0.575	0.305

4.2. Standard Deviation Selection Method

The out-of-sample performance of the Standard Deviation Selection Method, using net profit as the selection criterion, showed that 34 performance indicators outperformed the Best Point Selection Method, accounting for 76% of the total. Among these, 11 indicators exhibited statistically significant outperformance, while none showed significant underperformance. When MDD was used as the selection criterion, 19 performance indicators outperformed the Best Point Selection Method, making up 42% of the total. Only one of these indicators was statistically significantly better, while five indicators were significantly worse. When using MAR as the selection criterion, 38 performance indicators with the Standard Deviation Selection Method were better, representing 84% of the total. Out of the 38 indicators, 12 indicators exhibited statistically significant outperformance, and 3 showed significant underperformance. Therefore, when comparing in-sample and out-of-sample performance for the Standard Deviation Selection Method, 12 WFE values that the Best Point Selection Method based on net profit, constituting 80% of the total. For MDD-based selection, seven WFE values were better than the Best Point Selection Method, accounting for 47%. Finally, when selecting based on MAR, 14 WFE values outperformed the Best Point Selection Method, making up 93% of the total.

4.3. Island Area Selection Method

The out-of-sample performance for the Island Area Selection Method with net profit as the filtering criterion showed that 30 performance indicators outperformed the Best

Point Selection Method, accounting for 67% of the total. Two were statistically significant improvements, and none exhibited significant deterioration. When using MDD as the filtering criterion, 19 performance indicators outperformed the Best Point Selection Method, constituting 42% of the total. Two showed statistically significant improvements, while one exhibited significant deterioration. With MAR as the filtering criterion, 38 performance indicators outperformed the Best Point Selection Method, representing 84% of the total. Among these, eight exhibited statistically significant improvements, and none showed significant deterioration. Furthermore, in the comparison of in-sample and out-of-sample performance for the Island Area Selection Method, 10 WFE outperformed the Best Point Selection Method when using net profit as the filtering criterion, accounting for 67% of the total. When using MDD as the filtering criterion, 12 WFE outperformed the Best Point Selection Method, constituting 80% of the total. Lastly, when using MAR as the filtering criterion, 10 WFE outperformed the Best Point Selection Method, representing 67% of the total.

4.4. Island Volume Parameter Selection Method

The out-of-sample performance for the Island Volume Selection Method with net profit as the filtering criterion showed that 32 performance indicators outperformed the Best Point Selection Method, accounting for 71% of the total. Among them, four were statistically significant improvements, and one exhibited significant deterioration. When using MDD as the filtering criterion, 24 performance indicators outperformed the Best Point Selection Method, constituting 53% of the total. One showed statistically significant improvements, and none exhibited significant deterioration. With MAR as the filtering criterion, 30 performance indicators outperformed the Best Point Selection Method, representing 67% of the total. Nine exhibited statistically significant improvements, and one showed significant deterioration.

When comparing in-sample and out-of-sample performance for the Island Volume Selection Method, 11 WFE outperformed the Best Point Selection Method, accounting for 73% of the total when using net profit as the filtering criterion. When using MDD as the filtering criterion, six WFE outperformed the Best Point Selection Method, constituting 40% of the total. Lastly, when using MAR as the filtering criterion, 10 WFE outperformed the Best Point Selection Method, representing 67% of the total.

5. Conclusions

We proposed using the Selection Method, Standard Deviation Selection Method, Island Area Selection Method, and Island Volume Selection Method in the Walk-Forward system backtesting approach. These methods identified appropriate parameter combinations within the in-sample data. These combinations were validated for the out-of-sample data using a trading strategy constructed based on the moving average indicator and applied to Taiwan Stock Index Futures from 1 January 2000 to 31 December 2022. The performance of the proposed parameter selection methods was compared with that of the traditional single-point selection method. Furthermore, the relationship between various parameters within each selection method (window ratio, extension cycles, or benchmark PR) and the MAR performance indicator was analyzed.

The performance indicators of the proposed four parameter selection methods exceeded those of the traditional single-point selection method by more than 50%. Therefore, compared to the traditional single-point selection method, the parameter selection methods proposed are effective in selecting robust out-of-sample strategy parameter combinations. Based on the relationship between the various parameters (window ratio, extension cycles, or benchmark PR) of each selection method and the MAR performance indicator, it was observed that superior performance tended to cluster around specific windows or extension cycles when combined with specific parameter selection methods. This phenomenon suggests that users can consider appropriately expanding the parameters (window ratio, extension cycles, or benchmark PR) of the selection methods in future research.

Author Contributions: Conceptualization, C.-Y.C. and H.-Y.L.; methodology, C.-Y.C. and H.-Y.L.; software, H.-W.T.; validation, C.-Y.C., H.-Y.L. and H.-W.T.; resources, C.-Y.C. All authors have read and agreed to the published version of the manuscript.

Funding: This research received no external funding.

Data Availability Statement: Data are contained within the article.

Conflicts of Interest: The authors declare no conflict of interest.

References

1. Yan, M.-C. Modeling and Design and Implementation of Profitability Evaluation of Automated Trading Strategies Using Data Mining. Master's Thesis, National Central University, Taoyuan, Taiwan, 2017.
2. Cheng, H. Design and Verification of an Automated Platform for Analyzing the Optimal Suitability of Multi-Commodity Primary and Secondary Strategies Using Distributed Computing. Master's Thesis, National Central University, Taoyuan, Taiwan, 2018.
3. Lee, H.-Y. Design and Implementation of an Automated Platform for Evaluating and Comparing Risk and Profitability in Multi-Commodity Multi-Strategy Trading. Master's Thesis, National Central University, Taoyuan, Taiwan, 2019.
4. Lin, H.-Z. Analysis and Comparison of Profit Stability in Multi-Commodity Correlations. Master's Thesis, National Central University, Taoyuan, Taiwan, 2020.
5. Tsai, Y.-L. Machine Learning—Overfitting and Underfitting That Cannot Be Ignored. IT Help. Available online: https://ithelp.ithome.com.tw/articles/10278254 (accessed on 3 September 2023).
6. Pardo, R. *The Evaluation and Optimization of Trading Strategies*, 2nd ed.; John Wiley & Sons Inc.: Hoboken, NJ, USA, 2008.
7. Lee, J.-W. Design and Implementation of a Multi-Dimensional Analysis Platform for Trading Program Optimization. Master's Thesis, National Central University, Taoyuan, Taiwan, 2015.
8. Ruggiero, R. Can Your System Do the Walk? Futuresmag. 2010. Available online: http://www.futuresmag.com/2010/03/31/can-your-system-do-walk (accessed on 10 September 2023).
9. Fernando, J. Moving Average (MA): Purpose, Uses, Formula, and Examples. Investopedia. Available online: https://www.investopedia.com/terms/m/movingaverage.asp (accessed on 23 September 2023).

engineering proceedings

Proceeding Paper

Online and Offline Hybrid Teaching System Based on Virtual Reality †

Hou Yu [1,*], Nurul Nadwa Zulkifli [1,*] and Nozieana Khairuddin [2]

1 Department of Science and Technology, Faculty of Humanities, Management and Science, Universiti Putra Malaysia Bintulu Sarawak Campus, Bintulu 97008, Malaysia
2 Institut Ekosains Borneo, Universiti Putra Malaysia Bintulu Sarawak Campus, Bintulu 97008, Malaysia; nozieana@upm.edu.my
* Correspondence: houyu0123@126.com (H.Y.); nurulnadwa@upm.edu.my (N.N.Z.)
† Presented at the 2024 IEEE 4th International Conference on Electronic Communications, Internet of Things and Big Data, Taipei, Taiwan, 19–21 April 2024.

Abstract: We describe in this article the current development status of virtual reality (VR) technology and its application prospects in education, and we describe the design and implementation process for a hybrid online and offline teaching system. This system utilizes VR devices and software to bring students into a virtual learning environment, to interact with virtual objects, and to perform practical operations. At the same time, the system provides online courses, learning resources, and social platforms to promote cooperation and communication among students. Compared with traditional teaching, this online and offline hybrid teaching system significantly improves students' learning interest and induces active participation. Students have positive experiences of using VR technology for learning and believe that the system provides rich and practical learning resources.

Keywords: online; offline; hybrid teaching system; virtual reality

Citation: Yu, H.; Zulkifli, N.N.; Khairuddin, N. Online and Offline Hybrid Teaching System Based on Virtual Reality. *Eng. Proc.* **2024**, *74*, 57. https://doi.org/10.3390/engproc2024074057

Academic Editors: Shu-Han Liao, Teen-Hang Meen and Cheng-Fu Yang

Published: 9 September 2024

1. Introduction

The application of virtual reality (VR) technology in teaching has been developing rapidly [1]. In teaching, VR technology has been widely applied in teaching English. By creating a simulated three-dimensional environment, VR technology enables students to gain experience and participate in the learning process [2] as shown in Figure 1. In English learning, VR technology provides an immersive language environment, enabling students to engage in dialogue and communication with virtual characters, thereby enhancing their oral expression and listening comprehension abilities [3,4].

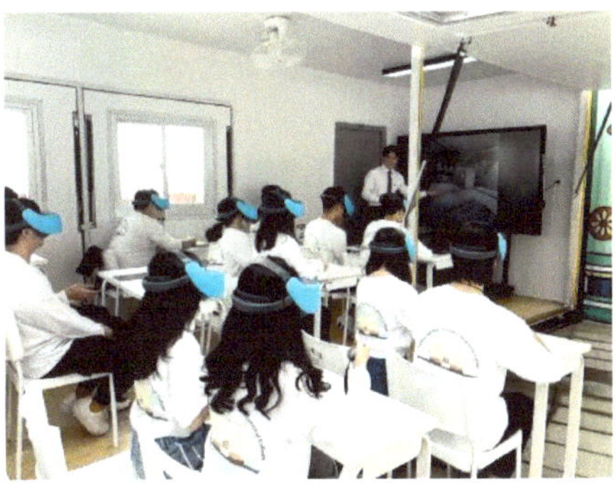

Figure 1. Example of a VR classroom.

VR technology can also be applied to English courses, in which students can experience cultural backgrounds through virtual travel and scene representation, thereby enhancing their memory and understanding of the English language [5,6]. Although VR technology has broad application prospects in teaching, it still faces challenges. Firstly, the high cost of VR devices limits their promotion in schools and educational institutions [7]. Secondly, teachers need to receive relevant training to effectively apply VR technology to teaching. The application of VR technology in teaching is actively advancing [8]. With the advancement of technology and the reduction of costs, the wider application of VR in education is expected, thereby providing students with a more diverse learning experience.

2. Design of Online and Offline Hybrid Teaching System Based on VR

2.1. System Design

A VR-based teaching platform system architecture is designed to provide a VR educational experience. The system combines VR technology and teaching methods to create an immersive and interactive learning environment for students. The core components of this system include hardware devices, software applications, and content resources. Hardware devices include VR headsets, joystick controllers, and other devices to place users in the virtual world and interact with its elements. The software is responsible for managing the entire system's operation and providing various functional modules such as course management and user authentication. The content is educational and is created by developers or teachers and uploaded to the platform as shown in Figure 2.

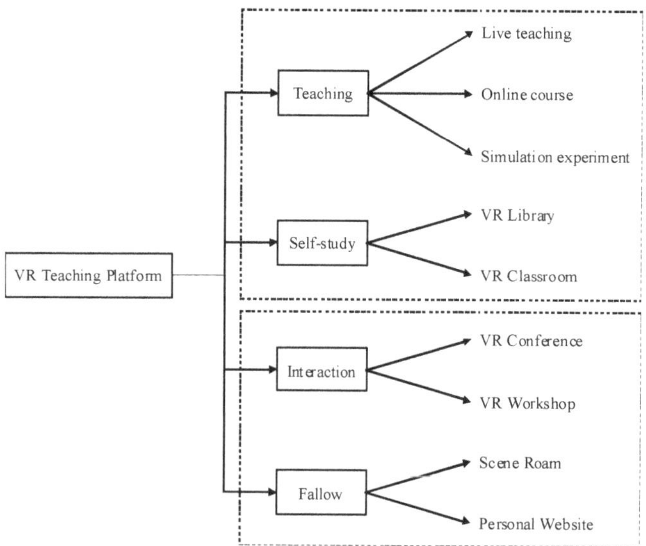

Figure 2. System architecture of the VR system.

2.2. Interactive Design in VR Teaching

VR technology has the potential to revolutionize the learning environment by providing learners with interactive modes that transcend the limitations of traditional teaching methods. Through the design of interaction-based tasks and feedback, interactive tasks and indirect metaphors effectively improve the user experiences of learners' by utilizing VR devices. The direct-metaphor design is associated with learners' existing experience levels so that learners can understand and master the task requirements quickly. For example, in education, direct metaphors can be used to transform mathematical problems into concrete object operations, thus allowing students to solve problems by touching, rotating, and so on. Indirect metaphor design guides learners to think and infer using suggestions or analogies and stimulates them to actively participate in the interaction process. This design increases interest and attraction and cultivates learners' independent thinking and creative thinking. For example, in language learning, indirect metaphors were used to help students understand abstract concepts or complex sentence structures (Table 1).

Table 1. Interaction mode of VR teaching.

Interaction Mode	Description
Free Exploration	By allowing users to explore the virtual environment freely, users can choose their areas of interest for learning. This approach can stimulate learners' curiosity and motivation, and increase their engagement.
Gesture Interaction	Use of gesture-recognition technology allows users to interact with virtual environments through hand movements and postures. For example, users can use gestures to select, drag, rotate, or zoom in and out of virtual objects to gain insight into related concepts.
Physical Interaction	A sensor-equipped controller allows users to touch, grasp, or manipulate virtual objects. This interactive approach helps users to more intuitively understand physics and solve problems, and it provides a more realistic experience.
Multi-Person Collaboration	Create virtual environments that support multi-person collaboration so that learners can work on tasks or learn with other users. This approach promotes cooperation and teamwork and provides opportunities to interact with others.
Visual Feedback	Provide timely feedback through visuals and animations to help learners understand whether their actions are correct. For example, when a user completes a task or performs an action, they can visually represent their success or failure.
Virtual Laboratory	The use of VR technology to create a simulation of a laboratory environment so that learners can carry out realistic practical operations. This approach reduces the need for resources, expenditure, and security provision that are required for actual operations, and provides more flexible learning opportunities.

Another important benefit of this approach to interactive task design is the reduction of additional cognitive load. As VR equipment requires high attention concentration and spatial perception ability, if there are complicated or non-logical operation instructions in the process of task execution, then it brings additional loads to users and reduces their understanding of task objectives and feedback information. Therefore, the interaction design must be created so as to avoid introducing too many irrelevant factors and to ensure that the instructions are concise and easy to understand. In summary, interactive tasks based on direct and indirect metaphor design are feasible on VR devices and enable the smooth, enjoyable, and efficient completion of tasks.

2.3. Hardware of VR Teaching System

The hardware of the VR teaching system includes equipment and components to support VR teaching (Figure 3).

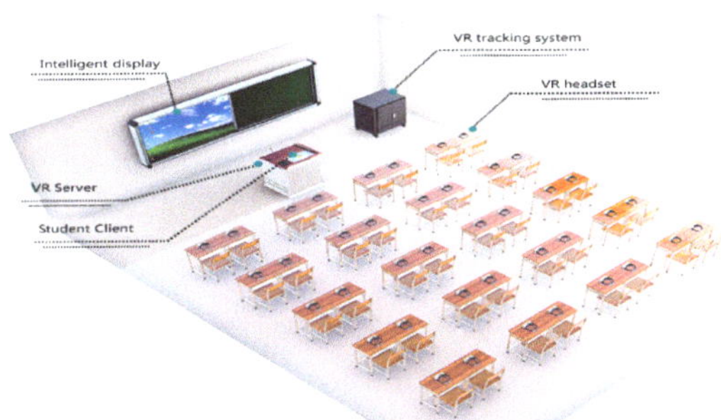

Figure 3. Hardware architecture of VR teaching.

1. VR headset: The VR headset is one of the core devices in VR teaching. It consists of a wearable device that is used to present VR content to the user's vision system. VR headsets typically include components such as high-resolution displays, sensors, and lenses to provide a realistic VR experience.
2. Tracking systems: Tracking systems are used to track a user's location and movements in a VR environment. These devices include external cameras, infrared sensors, gyroscopes, and laser trackers. Through the tracking system, teachers can understand the status of students in the virtual environment and give corresponding guidance.
3. Controller: The controller is the device through which the user interacts with the virtual environment. Controllers usually contain control elements such as buttons, joysticks, and triggers that simulate the user's hand movements or other operations. The controller allows students to perform various operations in a virtual environment, such as making selections, drawing, and operating virtual instruments.
4. Computing equipment: VR teaching requires powerful computing equipment that can handle a large number of graphics and computing tasks. These devices can be high-performance desktop computers, game consoles, or specialized VR all-in-one machines. Computing devices are responsible for rendering virtual environments in real time and transmitting them into VR headsets to deliver a smooth VR experience.
5. Interactive devices: In addition to controllers, VR teaching is realized with interactive devices such as gloves, motion-sensing devices, and haptic feedback devices to enhance the user's interactive experience with the virtual environment. These devices allow students to more intuitively feel the objects and actions in the virtual environment, further improving the teaching effect.

2.4. Three-Dimensional Modeling

The VR virtual experiment platform uses 3Dmax as a 3D engine, which has powerful functions and flexibility. By using 3Dmax, users can easily build a variety of parameters that match the physical object to create a realistic virtual scene. On the virtual experimental platform, users can carry out three-dimensional construction and mapping of objects. With simple steps, users can place objects of different shapes, sizes, and materials into a scene and adjust and position them. At the same time, elements are removed or added to improve the scene. In addition to the basic functions, the platform provides a variety of additional operational options. For example, in the model editing process, users can delete certain parts to achieve a specific effect; additional elements can also be added to enhance scene expressiveness. This flexibility allows users to create according to their needs as beginners or professionals.

The use of 3Dmax as a 3D engine on a VR virtual experiment platform allows for convenience and a range of possibilities. It is used to build parameters that meet the requirements of physical objects and provide a variety of operation options to meet the needs of users for three-dimensional construction, mapping, and other aspects. This makes the platform an ideal tool for applications in education, design, entertainment, and other fields. Designs of a student's perspective and a teacher's perspective is shown in Figures 4 and 5.

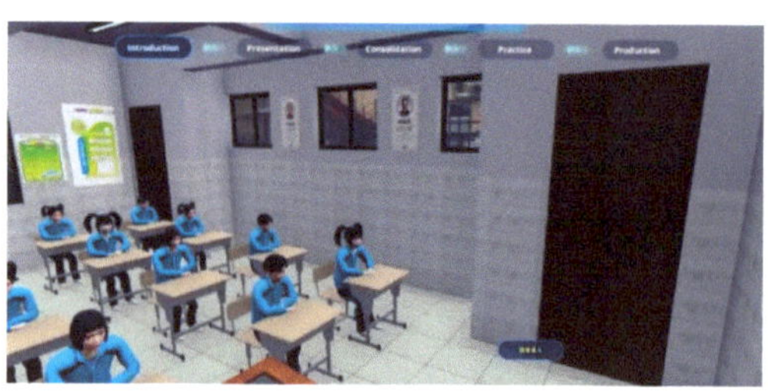

Figure 4. Student perspective in VR model.

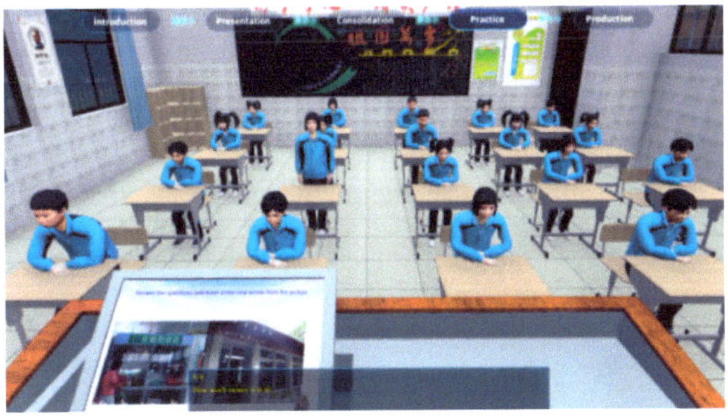

Figure 5. Teacher's perspective.

2.5. VR Teaching Scene

In VR teaching, VR technology is used to simulate a real teaching environment. Students wear specially designed VR headsets, enter a completely virtual environment, and learn in an immersive way. In VR teaching, a variety of real learning scenes such as historical scenes, science laboratories, and art exhibitions can be created. Students interact with objects in a virtual environment, observe details, experience hands-on operation, and receive immediate feedback and guidance. For example, in history lessons, students can experience historical events through VR teaching scenes, such as visiting ancient buildings and participating in major battles. They can move freely through virtual scenes, observe details, engage in conversations with historical figures, and learn about historical interpretations from different perspectives. This immersive learning style stimulates students' interest and improves their learning results. In science education, VR teaching scenarios are created to simulate a science laboratory's environment, including allowing students to conduct various experiments. Students can operate the virtual experimental equipment, observe the experimental results, and conduct experimental analysis with the guidance of a virtual tutor. This hands-on approach to learning develops students' experimental skills and scientific thinking. In addition, a new experience in art education can be obtained in VR teaching scenes. Students can visit the art exhibition hall, appreciate famous paintings, and understand the creative inspiration and skills of artists. They can also use VR tools for artistic creation, such as painting and sculpture, to cultivate their aesthetic ability and creativity. VR teaching scenarios provide an innovative way of delivering education to help students learn in an immersive way. It can broaden students' learning horizons, stimulate their learning interests, and promote the development of creative thinking. By combining virtual environments and reality, VR teaching scenarios will become an important part of education in the future.

3. Conclusions

This online and offline hybrid teaching system based on VR has significant advantages. The system overcomes the time and space limitations of the traditional teaching mode and provides students with an immersive learning experience. Students can participate in various simulation experiments, scene drills, and situational interactions through VR technology and enhance their sense of reality and participation in learning. At the same time, the online and offline hybrid teaching system can overcome the problems of human resources, material conditions, and time limitations faced by traditional offline classroom teaching, thus providing students with a more flexible and personalized learning mode. Secondly, the online and offline hybrid teaching system can effectively promote students' learning effectiveness. VR technology provides students with a new learning mode by stimulating students' learning interests and initiatives. Through virtual experiments, scene simulation, and interactive experiences, students can explore abstract concepts and gain knowledge to improve learning effectiveness. In addition, the online and offline hybrid teaching system can be used to adjust teaching strategies promptly through data analysis and feedback and enable the personalized tutoring of students to improve learning effectiveness. Thirdly, the online and offline hybrid teaching system based on VR faces challenges in application. Technical limitations may affect the stability and practicality of the system. The cost of system construction and maintenance is high, requiring sufficient investment and support. In addition, for non-technical disciplines, the application of VR technology may be subject to certain limitations. Therefore, in the promotion and application process, education resources, technical conditions, subject characteristics, and other factors need to be considered comprehensively. The online and offline hybrid teaching system based on VR has many prospects for use in education. The continuous innovation and improvement of VR technology will allow for more opportunities and challenges to be faced. By continuously optimizing the system's functions and teaching design, student participation and learning effectiveness can be improved. The system could play a greater role in higher education.

Author Contributions: Conceptualization, H.Y. and N.N.Z.; methodology, H.Y.; software, H.Y.; validation, H.Y., N.N.Z. and N.K.; formal analysis, H.Y.; investigation, H.Y.; resources, H.Y.; data curation, H.Y.; writing—original draft preparation, H.Y.; writing—review and editing, H.Y.; visualization, H.Y.; supervision, H.Y.; project administration, H.Y.; funding acquisition, N.N.Z. All authors have read and agreed to the published version of the manuscript.

Funding: This research received no external funding.

Institutional Review Board Statement: Not applicable.

Informed Consent Statement: Informed consent was obtained from all subjects involved in the study.

Data Availability Statement: Data sharing is not applicable to this article.

Conflicts of Interest: The authors declare no conflict of interest.

References

1. Żammit, J. Exploring the effectiveness of VR in teaching Maltese. *Comput. Amp; Educ. X Real.* **2023**, *3*, 100035.
2. Stam, D.; Jenkins, G.M.; Goettl, H.; Martinson, J.; Fondrick, A.; Lindahl, R.; Withrow, Z. Transforming the Heart of Student Learning and Engagement: A Randomized Crossover Trial for the Novel Application of Immersive VR in Teaching Electrocardiography Interpretation. *J. Acute Care Phys. Ther.* **2023**, *14*, 181–190. [CrossRef]
3. Isabel, T.; Vanessa, S.; Omar, C.; Buigues, C. Evaluating video VR teaching for nursing students. *Med. Educ.* **2023**, *57*, 1157–1158.
4. David, K.; Matthias, C.; Stephan, S. Immersive VR-based instruction in vocational schools: Effects on domain-specific knowledge and wellbeing of retail trainees. *Empir. Res. Vocat. Educ. Train.* **2023**, *15*, 9.
5. Kresge, C.; Justice, S.; Stanford, S.; McClerking, C. The Use of VR in Teaching Diagnostic Reasoning to Advanced Practice Registered Nurse Students. *Nurse Educ.* **2023**, *49*, 55–56. [PubMed]
6. Koucheki, R.; Lex, J.R.; Morozova, A.; Ferri, D.; Hauer, T.M.; Mirzaie, S.; Ferguson, P.C.; Ballyk, B. Immersive VR and Cadaveric Bone are Equally Effective in Skeletal Anatomy Education: A Randomized Crossover Noninferiority Trial. *J. Surg. Educ.* **2023**, *80*, 1028–1038. [CrossRef] [PubMed]
7. Álvaro, A.; Pablo, F.; Diego, V. Higher Education in the Pacific Alliance: Descriptive and Exploratory Analysis of the Didactic Potential of VR. *Multimodal Technol. Interact.* **2023**, *7*, 30.
8. Agbo, F.J.; Olaleye, S.A.; Bower, M.; Oyelere, S.S. Examining the relationships between students' perceptions of technology, pedagogy, and cognition: The case of immersive VR mini games to foster computational thinking in highe r education. *Smart Learn. Environ.* **2023**, *10*, 16. [CrossRef]

engineering proceedings

Proceeding Paper

Grammatical Gender Effect on Object Similarity Perception of Indonesian–German Bilinguals: Use of Big Data Analysis and Computation †

Feidora Nadia Putri * and Farah Mutiasari Djalal

Psychology Department, Bina Nusantara University, West Jakarta 11480, Indonesia; farah.mutiasari@binus.edu
* Correspondence: feidora.putri@binus.ac.id

† Presented at the 2024 IEEE 4th International Conference on Electronic Communications, Internet of Things and Big Data, Taipei, Taiwan, 19–21 April 2024.

Abstract: We investigated how grammatical gender affects the way bilinguals perceive the similarity of an object. We adopted the Sapir–Whorf hypothesis regarding the effect of language on a person's way of thinking. Different language characteristics allow for different ways of thinking when using other languages. Forty-six Indonesian–German bilinguals participated in this study to explore the perception of 112 pairs of object pictures. A pair of pictures of a person and an object or an animal were shown to the participants. Fourteen pictures of objects and animals were used, each of which was used with a masculine and feminine noun article. The language used in the study did not affect the similarity scores of the participants in different languages for the gender of objects shown.

Keywords: grammatical gender; perception; similarity; Sapir–Whorf hypothesis; bilingual; object similarity; big data analysis

Citation: Putri, F.N.; Djalal, F.M. Grammatical Gender Effect on Object Similarity Perception of Indonesian–German Bilinguals: Use of Big Data Analysis and Computation. *Eng. Proc.* **2024**, *74*, 58. https://doi.org/10.3390/engproc2024074058

Academic Editors: Shu-Han Liao, Teen-Hang Meen and Cheng-Fu Yang

Published: 10 September 2024

1. Introduction

Language is the communication means used by humans to exchange information. Language usage is an individual's experience, which has the most intense and continuous involvement [1] (pp. 233–262). When communicating with one another, individuals prefer to use their mother tongue [2] to ensure the information is easily grasped. However, communication can be difficult when carried out in different languages. Recently, the number of bilinguals is increasing. Being bilingual allows individuals to obtain information and communicate more broadly. Bilingualism impacts the brain structure and function, improving adaptive abilities in their lives [3,4] (pp. 7565−7574 in [3]). Differences in individuals' behavior in each language are related to grammatical capacity and affect individuals' perspectives on the language [5] (pp. 1−9). Each language has its characteristics, including systematic pronunciation patterns, word formation, and grammatical construction, that contribute to the development of different grammar [6]. Different language characteristics allow individuals to have different ways of thinking. An example of the influence on the way of speaking in language is the perception of its speakers [7,8] (pp. 928−933 in [8]). Perception is an evaluation process of an individual's performance toward specific objects [9]. The Sapir–Whorf hypothesis [10,11] explains that the language used by individuals influences how they think about reality [12] (pp. 13486−13490). Language influences and determines how individuals perceive their surroundings, including nature and their social environment [13] (pp. 1−5). The Sapir–Whorf hypothesis is used to examine how language influences how individuals think about reality and how they perceive objects.

The grammatical distinctions of each language can be seen in nouns. When naming an object, the gender article of the noun (i.e., masculine, feminine, or neutral) is taken into consideration. The determination of noun articles to grammatical gender is different in languages. In different languages, noun articles are assigned to objects differently, resulting in grammatical genders that do not correspond to their functions. For example, female genitals in French have the gender le, which is a masculine noun article; the skirt in German has a masculine noun article, der; and the moon in German has a masculine gender, whereas it is considered feminine in other languages. An understanding of the variations in the article assignment of grammatical gender and its impacts on speakers is needed.

The effect of grammatical gender on perception was conducted in Ref. [8] (pp. 928–933). The researcher discovered that speakers view an object as biologically female or male using grammatical gender, depending on the object's article. The Sapir–Whorf hypothesis was used to reveal that the language an individual uses affects how they think about something. Another influence is observed in speakers of languages with grammatical gender in the description of an object [14]. Spanish speakers describe "bridge" by giving adjectives related to masculinity, such as strong, big, towering, and solid, because the article "bridge" in Spanish is masculine. Meanwhile, German speakers associate "bridge" with feminine adjectives, such as elegant, fragile, and peaceful, because in German, "bridge" has a feminine noun article. This demonstrates that grammatical gender influences speakers in describing adjectives on an object according to its noun article.

Despite the grammatical differences between Bahasa Indonesia and German, many Indonesians are learning German. Since Bahasa Indonesia does not have grammatical gender, research on it has never been conducted in Indonesia. As many Indonesians are learning a second language that has grammatical genders, it is necessary to study the influence of grammatical gender on a person's way of thinking, especially the perception of daily.

2. Materials and Methods

This experiment was conducted to explore how the participants assigned similarities between female or male objects that have feminine and masculine noun articles. The participants were Indonesian–German bilinguals. They were randomly assigned to the Bahasa Indonesia version or the German language version of the test. The participants were shown pairs of colored pictures describing people and objects or animals. This study was a conceptual replication of Ref. [8] (pp. 928–933). We hypothesized that there were differences in the perceived similarity of objects in the gender in different languages. More specifically, the subject group tested in German showed a higher level of similarity between pairs of pictures with the same gender (pairs of images of women with objects or animals of feminine noun articles) compared to pairs of images with different gender references (different genders, for example, pairs of images of women with objects or animals with masculine noun articles). However, this similar pattern was not observed in the experiment group of Bahasa Indonesia.

2.1. Participants

We recruited 46 Indonesian–German bilingual participants aged 17–52 years (M = 26 years). There were 23 female and 23 male participants. Most participants had a high school diploma. Three randomly selected participants were rewarded for their participation in the study. Most participants rated their reading and speaking skills in Bahasa Indonesia at the C2 level. Then, most participants rated their German reading and speaking skills at the C2 level, too. On average, the participants had learned their second language for 6.7 years and had lived or were living in their second language country for an average of 6.3 years.

2.2. Materials

The measuring tool was adopted from Phillips and Boroditsky (2003), which consists of 8 pictures of people and 14 pictures of objects and animals [8]. Four female images (woman, ballet dancer, bride, and little girl) and four male images (man, king, giant, and little boy) were used in the experiment. Fourteen images of objects and animals were chosen according to their grammatical gender: seven images with feminine gender articles (sun, clock, toothbrush, fork, cat, mouse, and snail) and seven images with masculine gender articles (toaster, spoon, moon, broom, fox, whale, and frog) in German. The set of images of people, objects, and animals were paired in one picture, where the images of people were located on the left side and the images of objects and animals on the right side, resulting in 112 pairs of images. A total of 112 pairs of pictures were grouped into two: pairs of pictures with the same gender (feminine–feminine or masculine–masculine, Figure 1) and pairs of pictures with a different gender (feminine–masculine or masculine–feminine, Figure 2). The pictures were colored and original (except for the king and the giant). The rating scale in the similarity ranged from 1 (very unlikely) to 9 (very likely). To answer the questions, the participants writy/(aere not given a time limit. The order of the image pairs was different for each participant. The participants were split into two language groups: those tested with Bahasa Indonesia and those tested with German. There were no differences in the procedures and stages of the study between the two language versions.

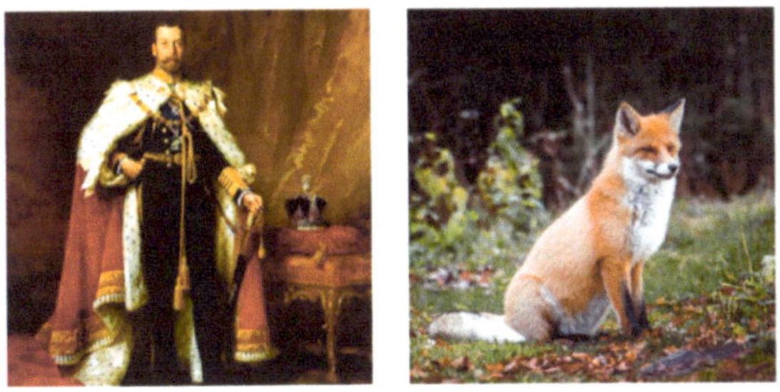

Figure 1. Same gender (masculine–masculine) items.

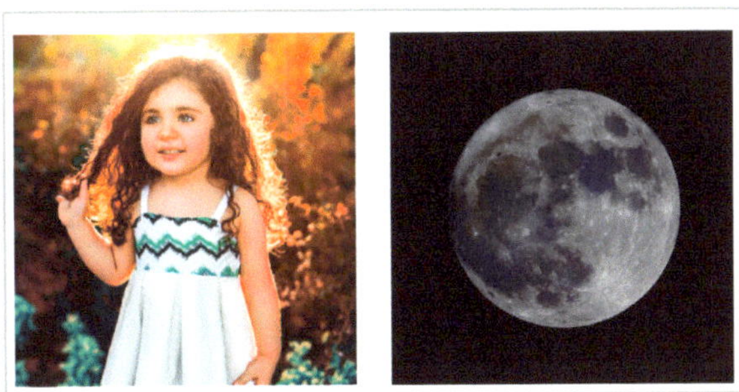

Figure 2. Different gender (feminine–masculine) items.

The group of participants tested in Bahasa Indonesia received the following research instructions: "Each time you will be shown a pair of pictures. We ask you to rate how similar the two pictures are. Choose the number 1 if you think the two pictures are VERY UNLIKELY and choose the number 9 if you think the two pictures are VERY LIKELY. There is no wrong answer, please choose the answer that suits you best. If you need a short break, you can close this page and continue by clicking on the following page address [https://binuspsy.limequery.org/392351?lang=id] and please save this page (e.g., by bookmarking this page)/do not close this page. Please try to complete this survey in one sitting. This survey takes approximately 20 min". The group tested using German was given the same instructions in the German language and was given a different survey link.

2.3. Procedure

The experiment was conducted using an online-based platform, LimeSurvey, which was disseminated through social media. Participants who fit the criteria received a randomly generated link to one of the language versions. The participants did not choose a particular language. After accessing the link, the participants were asked to fill out an informed consent before conducting the study. The research procedures and instructions before rating the level of similarity were explained to the participants. The participants proceeded to the next question if they rated the level of similarity in the previous question. After answering all questions, the participants rated their reading and speaking abilities in Bahasa Indonesia and German.

3. Results

We used an independent sample *t*-test to compare the mean of the similarity ratings of the two groups in Bahasa Indonesia and German instructions. To determine the interaction between the item types (same gender vs. different genders) of the two groups, we used mixed ANOVA in 2 × 2. Analyses were conducted using Jeffry's Amazing Statistics Program (JASP). Before comparing the similarity between language groups, the data obtained were analyzed using the chi-squared test and independent sample t-test to ensure that no other variables (i.e., gender, final education level, language proficiency, age, duration of stay in the second language country, active use of the second language, and length of second language acquisition) affected the research hypotheses. There were no extraneous variables that affected the results of the research hypotheses.

The two language version groups showed no difference in the mean scores in the similarity of image pairs (in Bahasa Indonesia: M = 2.14, SD = 1.79; in German: M = 3.09, SD = 1.68; t(44) = 1.86, p = 0.007, d = 0.55; Figure 3).

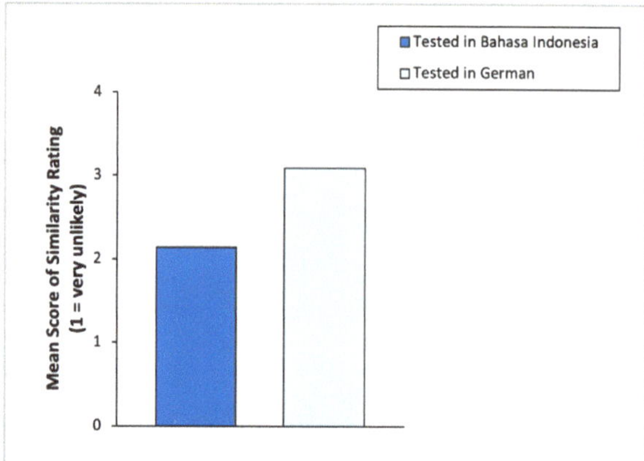

Figure 3. Comparison of mean scores in similarity.

The mixed ANOVA analysis result showed no significant interaction between the item types (same gender vs. different gender, Figure 4) in different groups. The German group rated similarity higher than the Bahasa Indonesia group (M = 3.11, SD = 1.72 in German; M = 2.15, SD = 1.82 in Bahasa Indonesia). The German group rated similarity higher than the Bahasa Indonesia group (M = 3.06, SD = 1.65 in the German group; M = 2.12, SD = 1.76 in the Bahasa Indonesia group). The interaction between item type and language version was not significant (F(1) = 0.05, p = 0.083, h2 < 0.05).

The results of the independent sample *t*-test and mixed ANOVA 2 × 2 showed no significant difference in the similarity context rated by the two groups.

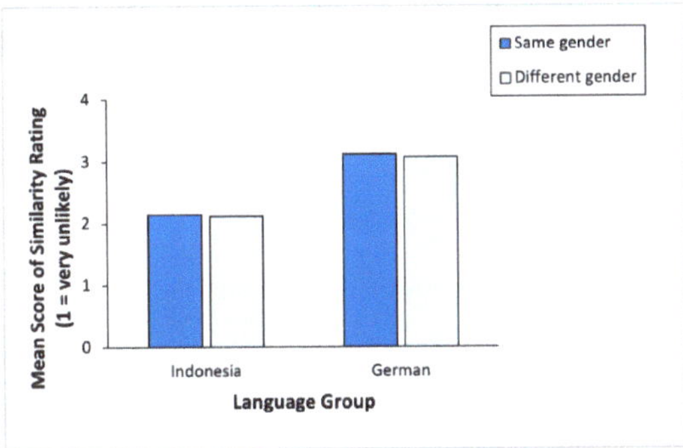

Figure 4. Comparison of mean of similarity (same gender and different gender) between groups.

4. Discussion

The difference in language did not affect the level of similarity of pairs of object images in this study. The Bahasa Indonesia and German groups showed no difference in the score for the similarity context for the same and different gender items. The result is different from that in Ref. [8] (pp. 928–933), which found that the language affected the assessment of the level of similarity in the gender of an object. The speakers of languages with grammatical gender perceived an object as biologically feminine and masculine based on the noun article (feminine and masculine). Differences in the results between the results of this study and the previous one may be due to different methods. The use of instruction in different languages is insufficient to change the perception of the participants. However, the language used in the instructions affected the experiment results [7].

The items used also affected the results. The images used in this study were different from those in previous studies [8] (pp. 928–933). The items used in the experiment of this study were the original images of the object (except for the pictures of a king and a giant) in color. Color is one of the elements that affect an individual's visual perception [15]. In addition, since the background in the image was not uniform, it influenced the ratings of the participants. One of the participants in this study thought that a resemblance was found between the items and the background, which hindered him from focusing on the item. As a result, it was likely for the participants in this study to estimate the resemblance of items based on other aspects of the image (e.g., color and backdrop).

Apart from the research procedures that affected the results, the number of participants might influence the results. A total of 46 participants took part in this study, while 55 participants were recruited in the previous study. The normality of the result also might affect the results. The results of this study did not support the Sapir–Whorf hypothesis, which argued that one's perception is influenced by the language one speaks [10,11].

5. Conclusions

The way bilinguals think or perceive cannot be manipulated by the second language they speak. In this study, it was found that the language instruction used in the research did not influence the bilingual perception of objects. Thus, the way of thinking is influenced mainly by the mother tongue. There were no significant differences between the Bahasa Indonesia and German groups. The participants in the groups' similarity scores were not significantly different. There were also no significant differences in the perception of the similarity of items of the same and different genders in the two language groups. The language used did not affect the ratings of the similarity of the images between objects by the two groups. Differences in perception might have occurred when a non-colored (black-and-white) line drawing was used in this study. This implies that the color and background of the object may influence the perception of the similarity of the object. In the previous study [8] (pp. 928–933), the Sapir–Whorf hypothesis was supported, revealing that language affects the assessment of the similarity of an object. More specifically, Phillips and Boroditsky found that the speakers of languages with grammatical gender perceive an object as biologically feminine and masculine based on the noun article (feminine and masculine).

Author Contributions: Conceptualization, F.N.P. and F.M.D.; methodology, F.N.P.; software, F.N.P.; validation, F.N.P. and F.M.D.; formal analysis, F.N.P.; investigation, F.N.P.; resources, F.N.P.; data curation, F.N.P.; writing—original draft preparation, F.N.P.; writing—review and editing, F.N.P. and F.M.D.; visualization, F.N.P.; supervision, F.M.D.; project administration, F.N.P. All authors have read and agreed to the published version of the manuscript.

Funding: This research received no external funding.

Institutional Review Board Statement: Not applicable.

Informed Consent Statement: Informed consent was obtained from all subjects involved in the study.

Data Availability Statement: The data and materials presented in this study are publicly available in the Open Science Framework at https://osf.io/c5x6b/. Most of the research materials were collected from a royalty-free license platform at https://unsplash.com.

Acknowledgments: This study was pre-registered in an open repository public platform (OSF) that can be reviewed here: https://osf.io/4m6qs/.

Conflicts of Interest: The authors declared no potential conflicts of interest with respect to the research, authorship, and/or publication of this article.

References

1. Bialystok, E. The bilingual adaptation: How minds accommodate experience. *Psychol. Bull.* **2017**, *143*, 233–262. [CrossRef] [PubMed]
2. Aini, N. Bahasa Indonesia Sebagai Media Komunikasi Sehari-Hari. Universitas Mitra Indonesia, Kota Bandar Lampung: Lampung, Indonesia, 2019, *to be submitted*. [CrossRef]
3. DeLuca, V.; Rothman, J.; Bialystok, E.; Pliatsikas, C. Redefining bilingualism as a spectrum of experiences that differentially affects brain structure and function. *Proc. Natl. Acad. Sci. USA* **2019**, *116*, 7565–7574. [CrossRef] [PubMed]
4. The Amazing Benefits of Being Bilingual. BBC Future. Available online: https://www.bbc.com/future/article/20160811-the-amazing-benefits-of-being-bilingual (accessed on 8 September 2020).
5. Athanasopoulos, P.; Bylund, E.; Montero-Melis, G.; Damjanovic, L.; Schartner, A.; Kibbe, A.; Riches, N.; Thierry, G. Two languages, two minds: Flexible cognitive processing driven by language of operation. *Psychol. Sci.* **2015**, *26*, 518–526. [CrossRef] [PubMed]
6. Akmajian, A.; Farmer, A.K.; Bickmore, L.; Demers, R.A.; Harnish, R.M. *Linguistics: An Introduction to Language and Communication*, 7th ed.; The MIT Press: Cambridge, MA, USA, 2017.
7. Boroditsky, L.; Ham, W.; Ramscar, M. What is universal in event perception? Comparing English & Indonesian speakers. In *Proceedings of the Twenty-fourth Annual Conference of the Cognitive Science Society*; Taylor & Francis Group: London, UK, 2002; Volume 24. [CrossRef]
8. Phillips, W.; Boroditsky, L. Can quirks of grammar affect the way you think? Grammatical gender and object concepts. *Proc. Annu. Meet. Cogn. Sci. Soc.* **2003**, *25*, 928–933.
9. Sutrisman, D. *Pendidikan politik, persepsi, kepemimpinan, dan mahasiswa*; Guepedia: Kabupaten Bogor, Indonesia, 2019.
10. Sapir, E. *Language: An Introduction to the Study of Speech*; Harcourt, Brace, and Company: New York, NY, USA, 1921.
11. Whorf, B.L. *Language, Thought, and Reality: Selected Writings of Benjamin Lee Whorf*; Carroll, J.B., Ed.; The MIT Press: Cambridge, MA, USA, 1956.
12. Lucy, J.A. Sapir-whorf hypothesis. *Int. Encycl. Soc. Behav. Sci.* **2001**, 13486–13490. [CrossRef]
13. Neuliep, J.W. Sapir-whorf hypothesis. In *The International Encyclopedia of Intercultural Communication*; Kim, Y.Y., McKay-Semmler, K.L., Eds.; John Wiley & Sons, Inc.: Hoboken, NJ, USA, 2017; pp. 1–5.
14. Grammatical Gender and the Effect on Perception. Medium. Available online: https://medium.com/@heiseras/grammatical-gender-and-the-effect-on-perception-2babe35bc4d7 (accessed on 4 April 2021).
15. Similarity Principle in Visual Design. Nielson Norman Group. Available online: https://www.nngroup.com/articles/gestalt-similarity/ (accessed on 10 May 2021).

engineering proceedings

MDPI

Proceeding Paper

Unlocking the Learning Potential: ChatGPT as a Virtual Platform for Cross-Interaction in English Language Learning †

Wen-Chi Hu and Radovan Škultéty *

Language Center, Chaoyang University of Technology, Taichung 413, Taiwan; winniehu@gmail.com
* Correspondence: skultety@gmail.com

† Presented at the 2023 SSIM IEEE 3rd International Conference on Social Sciences and Intelligence Management, Taichung, Taiwan, 15–17 December 2023.

Abstract: We explored how participants learning English as a foreign language (EFL) perceive the use of ChatGPT for English communication in combination with voice control for GPT, a Google Chrome extension, both of which are AI chatbot functionalities. A revised version of the ChatGPT Engagement and Perception Questionnaire (CEPQ) was distributed to 70 participants. The results indicated a generally positive response: participants recognized ChatGPT's beneficial effect on their confidence in English communication, their indirect interaction experiences with people from different cultural backgrounds, and their familiarity with the system. Overall, 66% of the participants had prior experience with ChatGPT, 65% noted an increase in curiosity, and 77% reported improved confidence in communicating in English. However, 33% experienced frustration due to ChatGPT's occasional misunderstandings, pointing to the need for enhanced natural language processing capabilities. While 31% expected easy communication with an AI chatbot, the same proportion struggled with pronunciation comprehension. The installation of the voice control extension was straightforward for 57% of participants. A notable challenge was time management, with 47% finding the time allotted for practice tasks insufficient, underscoring the importance of addressing this to improve student engagement and learning outcomes. These results provide a reference on user experiences with AI chatbots in the context of English language learning.

Keywords: ChatGPT; language learning technology; English as a foreign language (EFL); AI chatbot

Citation: Hu, W.-C.; Škultéty, R. Unlocking the Learning Potential: ChatGPT as a Virtual Platform for Cross-Interaction in English Language Learning. *Eng. Proc.* **2024**, *74*, 59. https://doi.org/10.3390/engproc2024074059

Academic Editors: Shu-Han Liao, Teen-Hang Meen and Cheng-Fu Yang

Published: 10 September 2024

1. Introduction

This study aims to explore the integration of artificial intelligence (AI) in English as a foreign language (EFL) teaching. By incorporating AI tools into language learning, we explored how to enhance communication skills in EFL. One such AI tool is ChatGPT, an AI chatbot designed to simulate human conversations and provide language practice opportunities. We investigated the perceptions of students of EFL regarding the use of ChatGPT with the voice control extension, a Google Chrome plugin, for English conversation purposes. The findings of this research contribute to the understanding of EFL students' perceptions of AI chatbot communication in English. By understanding the positive impacts, challenges, and usability aspects of ChatGPT, educators and developers can optimize the integration of AI technologies in language learning environments. Then, it is possible to enhance language proficiency and foster practical communication skills in EFL through innovative AI-driven tools such as ChatGPT.

Integrating AI into education demands a user-centered approach focusing on comprehending students' attitudes and customizing the functions accordingly [1]. Hence, when integrating AI into education, it becomes vital to consider students' perceptions to ensure user-oriented implementation and optimize its functionalities. This study provides pedagogical insights on leveraging ChatGPT, emphasizing critical considerations for users to harness its full potential. As the utilization of ChatGPT gains recognition as a promising method to enhance English acquisition, it becomes imperative to explore the sentiments and viewpoints of EFL learners regarding ChatGPT, thereby assisting researchers in gaining deeper insights into its efficacy in language learning given the scarcity of studies addressing the perceptions of Taiwanese university students regarding ChatGPT. We conducted a questionnaire survey to collect resource data to explore the following:

1. The participants' perceptions regarding the use of ChatGPT, an AI chatbot, for English communication purposes in EFL;
2. Frustrations or challenges that participants encounter when using ChatGPT, particularly regarding understanding and pronunciation comprehension.

2. Literature Review

We adopted two key educational theories: constructivist theory (CT) and autonomous learning theory (ALT). These theories provide a robust theoretical foundation for application. We fostered constructive and autonomous processes, enabling students to navigate their learning journey with the aid of ChatGPT.

2.1. CT

CT was proposed by Piaget and later expanded by Vygotsky, who posited that knowledge is constructed through active engagement with the world, rather than passive reception [2,3]. This theory was epitomized in this study as students interacted with ChatGPT, creating their understanding through problem-solving activities. Through problem-solving activities and dynamic interaction with ChatGPT, students constructed their understanding and embodied the essence of constructivist theory in their learning process. In this study, ChatGPT served as a facilitator of this active learning approach. By engaging with ChatGPT, students were encouraged to explore, question, and reflect—fundamental aspects of the constructivist learning paradigm. Through this dynamic interaction, students acquired specific knowledge and developed authentic language usage, improved their problem-solving skills, and engaged in conversations. The dialogs with ChatGPT encouraged students to actively construct meaning, fostering an enriched, personalized learning journey.

2.2. ALT

ALT suggests that when students assume responsibility for their learning, they are likely to develop effective learning strategies and become motivated as independent learners. The concept of autonomy, which originates from political and moral philosophy, is multifaceted and has been extensively discussed in academia [4]. Initially, learning autonomy focused on completely independent learning [5,6]. This approach advocates for learners to take full responsibility for decision making in their learning journey. According to Holec, teachers play a crucial role in closely monitoring and attending to the pedagogical aspects for their students [7]. This perspective highlights the shared roles of teachers and students within the autonomous learning model, with teachers acting as facilitators and students as experts in their learning process. Similarly, Lewis believed that fostering learner autonomy needs guidance and interdependence, as learners cannot develop autonomy alone [8]. In this context, ChatGPT and the teacher act as guides to assist students in their English learning journey.

Furthermore, autonomous learning offers EFL learners several advantages. Lu, Jiang, and Throssell suggested that autonomous learning improves language proficiency, critical thinking skills, lifelong learning habits, and adaptability to diverse learning contexts [9]. Additionally, Mehdiyev explored the advantages of autonomous learning as perceived by EFL students. These advantages include increased motivation, the opportunity for personalized learning experiences, greater flexibility, and enhanced empowerment in making decisions about their learning process [10]. Finally, computer technology facilitates autonomous learning by EFL university students, promoting their active engagement, self-directedness, and accountability in the learning process [11].

2.3. An AI Chatbot in an EFL Context

Technology continues to evolve and transform many aspects of our lives, and education is no exception. As a result, English teaching is also changing owing to technological advancements. One innovative approach that has garnered increasing interest is the use of ChatGPT. This tool is recognized as a promising solution for teaching English with greater efficiency and effectiveness [12]. Incorporating ChatGPT into oral and aural English teaching allows numerous significant advantages. These benefits heighten student engagement, improve confidence in English communication, enhance language skills, and increase student autonomy, creating an authentic and interactive language-learning environment that features intelligent communication.

2.3.1. Engagement

Tatsenko and Donik explored the impact of using ChatGPT in the classroom, specifically in English language learning [12]. Their findings indicated that incorporating ChatGPT into the learning process increased student engagement and equipped them with practical skills for future careers.

2.3.2. Confidence

Fryer and Carpenter found that ChatGPT reduced shyness among language learners [13]. Students expressed greater confidence in their English communication skills after using ChatGPT. Moreover, the chatbot provided a supportive environment where they could practice language skills without fear of judgment, leading to increased self-assurance [14].

2.3.3. Language Skill Enhancement

The thoughtful suggestions of the scholars help harness the full potential of ChatGPT for the expansion of EFL education. By integrating ChatGPT into the classroom, learners can enhance English language skills in fluency, comprehension, and communication skills. Vocabulary acquisition and pronunciation also improve through regular interactions with ChatGPT [14].

2.3.4. Student Autonomy

ChatGPT provides numerous benefits for EFL communication teaching, as it can function as a virtual assistant, simulate authentic conversations, and offer accessible language learning opportunities anytime and anywhere [12].

2.3.5. Authentic and Interactive Environment

Kohnke, Moorhouse, and Zou emphasized the significance of rich input in achieving successful second language acquisition [15]. They highlighted that AI-powered chatbots offer linguistic input, enable daily conversation practice, and create an authentic and interactive language-learning environment. ChatGPT facilitates an authentic and interactive language-learning environment [16].

2.3.6. Intelligent Communication

A notable benefit of using AI-powered chatbots for language teaching and learning is their ability to communicate intelligently, learn from prior interactions, and act as tireless language-learning assistants [15,17,18]. Ultimately, integrating ChatGPT into English language teaching provides benefits such as increased student engagement, enhanced confidence in English communication, improved language skills and learning autonomy, an authentic and interactive learning environment, and intelligent communication capabilities. These findings highlight the potential of ChatGPT as a valuable tool for practical and accessible language education in the digital era.

2.4. Authentic English Conversation

Speaking skills in language learning are difficult to acquire due to the need to integrate multiple language abilities [19]. Daily conversations are the most effective way to practice and enhance oral and aural skills. Students require meaningful conversation practice to enhance their language skills instead of simply reading aloud from textbooks. Meaningful conversation practice involves actively engaging in conversations where students can apply and develop their speaking abilities in authentic and relevant contexts [16]. Hwang, Guo, Hoang, Chang, and Wu emphasized the importance of authenticity in language learning [20]. In this approach, the value of offering learners opportunities to practice English in real-life situations is acknowledged as a way to engage in meaningful dialogues and interact with genuine language resources, which contributes to more effective language acquisition. Authentic material consist of spoken or written language data generated in real communication rather than created explicitly for language teaching purposes [21,22]. Hence, EFL teaching must be authentic, reflecting real-world language usage through sources. It must also be task-based, engaging learners in practical language use through role-plays, problem-solving, discussions, and simulations [21,23]. To improve EFL learners' English proficiency, it is essential to (1) prioritize speaking practice and provide opportunities for active participation through activities such as discussions, debates, role-plays, and presentations; (2) emphasize authentic communication by encouraging real-life conversations; and (3) utilize technology tools and multimedia resources to enhance oral English skills [24].

3. Research Methodology

To collect data, we distributed a revised version of the ChatGPT Engagement and Perception Questionnaire (CEPQ) to 70 participants. This questionnaire was designed to gather information on the participants' perspectives on diverse facets of using ChatGPT including the following aspects: the influence of ChatGPT on their confidence in communicating in English, their indirect experiences of interacting with native English speakers or people from different cultural backgrounds, the students' level of familiarity with the system, the challenges they faced, and the practicality of features such as the voice control extension.

3.1. Context and Participants

Seventy freshman EFL students enrolled in the Everyday English course reported general satisfaction with their speaking experiences using ChatGPT. The course's curriculum featured a conversation activity with ChatGPT as a key element of the language practice exercises. Throughout the course, students participated in a variety of English learning activities. These included installing the ChatGPT voice control extension for Google Chrome, engaging in casual conversations, participating in guessing games, completing problem-solving exercises, and posing daily questions to ChatGPT. The students participated in these activities either individually or in pairs. Upon completion of these activities, they engaged in a brief oral reflection session to share their experiences and insights from the conversations with ChatGPT.

3.2. Instruments

We utilized a modified version of the 13-item CEPQ, which was adapted from Seraj, Habil, and Hasan [25]. The modifications were made to better align the questionnaire with the goals and context of this study, ensuring its relevance and applicability. The value of Cronbach's alpha for the questionnaire items was 0.834, indicating a high level of internal consistency and supporting the reliability, validity, and overall robustness of the collected data (Table 1).

Table 1. Reliability of questionnaire survey.

Cronbach's Alpha	Lower Bound	Upper Bound	Number of Items
0.834	0.770	0.886	13

4. Results and Discussion

We adopted analysis of variance (ANOVA) to analyze the data of male and female participants. The results showed no significant difference between the two groups, indicating that gender did not play a significant role in the observed variables analyzed (Table 2).

Table 2. Top five items of CEPQ.

Items	Mean (Standard Deviation)			
	Male	Female	Total	Rank
6. This lesson helped me get more confident using English for communication.	4.13 (1.14)	4.13 (0.797)	4.13 (0.916)	1
13. I don't usually have a chance to talk to foreigners, but I could experience it indirectly through AI chatbots such as ChatGPT.	3.87 (0.815)	3.96 (0.955)	3.93 (0.906)	2
1. I tried ChatGPT before so I am familiar with the way how to use it.	3.96 (0.878)	3.87 (1.172)	3.9 (1.079)	3
2. This lesson aroused my interest in learning more about ChatGPT.	3.87 (0.920)	3.83 (0.842)	3.84 (0.862)	4
3. I didn't have any problems logging in to ChatGPT and installing the voice control extension.	3.91 (0.949)	3.72 (1.097)	3.79 (1.048)	5

The students' top five responses to the questionnaire demonstrated that most participants firmly acknowledged the positive impact of using ChatGPT in enhancing their English learning. It was found that the lesson significantly boosted the individuals' confidence in utilizing English to communicate effectively. The second-ranked response reflected the limited opportunities to engage directly with native English speakers or people from different cultural backgrounds, but the participants indirectly experienced such interactions through AI chatbots such as ChatGPT. The third-ranked response indicated that the participant had prior experience with ChatGPT, resulting in their familiarity with its usage and functionality. The fourth-ranked item in the questionnaire results indicated that the lesson sparked curiosity among the students, stimulating their desire to explore and delve deeper into the intricacies of ChatGPT. The fifth item indicated that students reported a seamless experience logging into ChatGPT and installing the voice control extension without any issues (Table 2).

The questionnaire data showed noteworthy results. First, 66% of participants reported having a prior experience with ChatGPT, showcasing their familiarity with the system's operations. Additionally, 65% of the participants acknowledged that the recent instructional session piqued their interest and motivated them to learn more about ChatGPT. Furthermore, 77% of the students felt that the session enhanced their confidence in using English for effective communication, suggesting a positive influence on their linguistic skills and overall confidence in English as a tool for interpersonal interaction. Most strikingly, 93% of the participants recognized that they lacked opportunities to converse with native English speakers or people from different cultural backgrounds, yet they were able to gain indirect exposure to such interactions through AI chatbots such as ChatGPT.

The results also indicated challenges faced by the respondents. For example, 33% of them experienced frustration when ChatGPT failed to understand them, emphasizing the need for ongoing improvement in natural language processing technologies for smoother and more accurate user interactions with AI-based language models. Concurrently, 31% of the respondents thought that engaging in a conversation with an AI chatbot such as ChatGPT was simple. However, the same percentage of participants reported difficulties with ChatGPT's ability to comprehend their pronunciation. Overall, 57% of the participants reported no issues in accessing ChatGPT and installing the voice control extension, indicating that a significant number of users found the platform user-friendly and the integration of the voice control feature straightforward. This suggests that the interface is intuitive and well-supported, aiding in easy installation and use. Such successful technical execution of ChatGPT ensures a seamless and efficient user experience, particularly in the integration of the voice control extension within the ChatGPT system.

Overall, 47% of participants indicated that the time allotted was insufficient to complete all the assigned practice tasks during the class. In contrast, 23% of respondents confirmed that the provided time was adequate to finish all the tasks. This variation in time management underscores the differences in students' availability and time allocation, which may affect their ability to engage with and complete the tasks. Educators must take these findings into account and mitigate potential time constraints to improve student participation and enhance learning outcomes. Consequently, the survey results presented important aspects such as the participants' familiarity with ChatGPT, the effectiveness of instructional sessions, the challenges faced, and the importance of managing time effectively. These are important in refining technological and teaching strategies to improve the utility of ChatGPT in educational contexts and catering to the varied needs of EFL learners (Table 3).

Table 3. Students' perception.

	Core				
Items	**1**	**2**	**3**	**4**	**5**
1. I tried ChatGPT before so I am familiar with the way how to use it.	3%	7%	24%	29%	37%
2. This lesson aroused my interest in learning more about ChatGPT.	0%	6%	29%	41%	24%
3. I didn't have any problems logging in to ChatGPT and installing the voice control extension.	1%	9%	33%	24%	33%
4. It was great to speak English whether my sentence was perfect or not.	1%	9%	34%	33%	23%
5. I think it's possible to speak comfortably to an AI chatbot such as ChatGPT.	1%	21%	46%	31%	0%
6. This lesson helped me get more confident using English for communication.	1%	3%	19%	36%	41%
7. I was frustrated when ChatGPT didn't understand me.	9%	14%	44%	19%	14%
8. ChatGPT often didn't understand my pronunciation.	13%	29%	27%	20%	11%
9. I didn't have enough time to finish all the practice tasks in this class.	21%	26%	30%	14%	9%
10. I didn't have enough time to explore all the possibilities the AI chatbot offers.	11%	20%	20%	29%	20%
11. I didn't feel like I was communicating with people, so I couldn't keep talking for long.	6%	31%	36%	16%	11%
12. AI often doesn't understand my pronunciation, so I think it would be better to do text-chatting.	6%	24%	40%	20%	10%
13. I don't usually have a chance to talk to foreigners, but I could experience it indirectly through AI chatbots such as ChatGPT.	0%	7%	23%	40%	30%

5. Conclusions

We examined the experiences of EFL learners using ChatGPT to practice English speaking. The findings enriched the existing findings on how users interact with AI chatbots in English language learning. These insights are valuable in guiding the development and refinement of AI chatbot technologies, ultimately enhancing their role in supporting student communication, engagement, and overall learning success in EFL teaching methodologies.

The experience of the participants was overwhelmingly positive. Thanks to their interaction with ChatGPT, they showed confidence in boosting their English communication after they became familiar with the system. A significant proportion of participants had prior experience with ChatGPT, indicating its prevalence. Meanwhile, several participants experienced frustration due to the chatbot's lack of understanding, which implies that improvements in natural language processing are essential. Additionally, pronunciation comprehension challenges were faced by several participants, highlighting the need for further attention. Nevertheless, the installation of the voice control extension was easy for a majority of the participants. Time constraints were another factor, with a substantial percentage of participants reporting insufficient time for completing practice tasks. The study's findings are consistent with prior scholarly research [14], showing that a majority of Taiwanese EFL students recognize the potential of AI tools, such as ChatGPT, in enriching their English learning experience. ChatGPT was recognized as a highly effective tool for their educational progress.

To maximize the benefits of using ChatGPT in education, Kohnke, Moorhouse, and Zou highlighted the need for teachers to acquire digital competencies, which include mastery of technology, alignment with teaching methods, and social consciousness [15]. This necessitates a thorough understanding of ChatGPT's features and their periodical updates, ChatGPT's operational mechanics, the design of practical activities, the ability to tackle challenges, and mindfulness of ethical issues. Additionally, Mohamed proposed strategies to foster professional development, curriculum design, and the application of effective teaching methods, all aimed at utilizing ChatGPT to improve EFL teaching quality [26].

Indeed, the effectiveness of ChatGPT in education depends significantly on the digital proficiency of both educators and students. Equipping both parties with essential technological know-how and an understanding of educational principles enables them to exploit the advantages of ChatGPT in enhancing the language teaching and learning experience.

Author Contributions: Conceptualization, W.-C.H. and R.Š.; methodology, W.-C.H.; validation, W.-C.H.; formal analysis, W.-C.H.; investigation, W.-C.H. and R.Š.; writing—original draft preparation, W.-C.H.; writing—review and editing, R.Š.; visualization, R.Š.; supervision, W.-C.H. All authors have read and agreed to the published version of the manuscript.

Funding: This research received no external funding.

Institutional Review Board Statement: Ethical review and approval were waived for this study due to the fact that the study only involved anonymous surveys with minimal risk to participants, which, according to the institution's guidelines, does not require IRB approval.

Informed Consent Statement: Inform consent was obtained in digital format.

Data Availability Statement: The data presented in this study are available on request from the corresponding author due to privacy and ethical considerations. The data are stored on university servers and are subject to institutional policies on data sharing.

Conflicts of Interest: The authors declare no conflict of interest.

References

1. Liu, B. Chinese University Students' Attitudes and Perceptions in Learning English Using ChatGPT. *Int. J. Educ. Humanit.* **2023**, 3, 132–140. [CrossRef]
2. Piaget, J. *Science of Education and the Psychology of the Child*; Coltman, D., Translator; Orion Press: New York, NY, USA, 1970.

3. Vygotsky, L.S.; Cole, M. *Mind in Society: Development of Higher Psychological Processes;* Harvard University Press: Cambridge, MA, USA; London, UK, 1978.
4. Holec, H. On Autonomy: Some Elementary Concepts. In *Discourse and Learning;* Holec, H., Ed.; Longman: London, UK, 1985; pp. 173–190.
5. Dickinson, L. *Self-Instruction in Language Learning;* Cambridge University Press: Cambridge, UK, 1987.
6. Gao, G.; Ting-Toomey, S. *Communicating Effectively with the Chinese;* Sage Publications: Thousand Oaks, CA, USA, 1998.
7. Holec, H. Training teachers to cope with the inherent variability of their Office. *Innov. Lang. Learn. Teach.* **2011**, *5*, 111–118. [CrossRef]
8. Lewis, H.A. A teacher's reflections on autonomy. *Stud. High. Educ.* **1978**, *3*, 149–159. [CrossRef]
9. Lu, J.; Jiang, H.; Throssell, P. Autonomous learning in tertiary university EFL teaching and learning of the People's Republic of China: Challenges and new directions. *Int. J. Learn. High. Educ.* **2013**, *19*, 111–121. [CrossRef]
10. Mehdiyev, E.M. Opinions of EFL students regarding autonomous learning in language teaching. *J. Lang. Linguist. Stud.* **2020**, *16*, 521–536. [CrossRef]
11. Aprianto, E.; Purwati, O. Multimedia-assisted learning in a flipped classroom: A case study of autonomous learning on EFL university students. *Int. J. Emerg. Technol. Learn.* **2020**, *15*, 114. [CrossRef]
12. Tatsenko, N.V.; Donik, I. Make teaching English easier with ChatGPT. In Proceedings of the X. All-Ukrainian Scientific Conference of Students, Postgraduates, Faculty Members, and Collaborators, Sumy, Ukraine, 27–28 April 2023; pp. 106–109.
13. Fryer, L.; Carpenter, R. Bots as language learning tools. *Lang. Learn. Technol.* **2006**, *10*, 8–14.
14. Ali, J.K.M.; Shamsan, M.A.A.; Hezam, T.A.; Mohammed, A.A. Impact of ChatGPT on learning motivation: Teachers and students' voices. *J. Engl. Stud. Arab. Felix* **2023**, *2*, 41–49. [CrossRef]
15. Kohnke, L.; Moorhouse, B.L.; Zou, D. ChatGPT for language teaching and learning. *RELC J.* **2023**, *54*, 537–550. [CrossRef]
16. Chiu, T.K.F.; Moorhouse, L.M.; Chai, C.S.; Ismailov, M. Teacher support and student motivation to learn with AI (AI) based chatbot. *Interact.Learn. Environ.* **2023**, 1–17. [CrossRef]
17. Fryer, L.K.; Nakao, K.; Thompson, A. Chatbot learning partners: Connecting learning experiences, interest and competence. *Comput. Hum. Behav.* **2019**, *93*, 279–289. [CrossRef]
18. Kim, N.Y. A study on chatbots for developing Korean college students' English listening and reading skills. *J. Digit. Converg.* **2018**, *16*, 19–26. [CrossRef]
19. Little, D. The Common European Framework of Reference for Languages: Content, purpose, origin, reception and impact. *Lang. Teach.* **2006**, *39*, 167–190. [CrossRef]
20. Hwang, W.Y.; Guo, B.C.; Hoang, A.; Chang, C.C.; Wu, N.T. Facilitating authentic contextual EFL speaking and conversation with smart mechanisms and investigating its influence on learning achievements. *Comput. Assist. Lang. Learn.* **2022**, 1–27. [CrossRef]
21. Nunan, D. *Designing Tasks for the Communicative Classroom;* Cambridge University Press: Cambridge, UK, 1989.
22. Mudawe, O.M.N. Enhancing EFL students' cultural awareness through *Friends* sitcom. *Int. J. Appl. Linguist. Engl. Lit.* **2020**, *9*, 76–84. [CrossRef]
23. Oura, G.K. Authentic task-based materials: Bringing the real world into the classroom. *Sophia Jr. Coll. Fac. Bull.* **2001**, *21*, 65–84.
24. Tang, W. How to Improve EFL Learners' Oral English Proficiency? In Proceedings of the 2nd International Conference on Social Sciences and Humanities and Arts (SSHA 2023); Sedon, M.F.B., Khan, I.N., Eds.; Atlantis Press: Paris, France, 2023; pp. 730–736. [CrossRef]
25. Seraj, P.I.; Habil, H.; Hasan, K. Investigating EFL learners' readiness of using smartphone and problems for learning oral English communication skills at tertiary level in an EFL context. *Int. J. Interact. Mob. Technol. (IJIM)* **2020**, *14*, 148. [CrossRef]
26. Mohamed, A.M. Exploring the potential of an AI-based Chatbot (ChatGPT) in enhancing English as a Foreign Language (EFL) teaching: Perceptions of EFL Faculty Members. *Educ. Inf. Technol.* **2023**, *29*, 1–23. [CrossRef]

engineering proceedings

Proceeding Paper

Sports Broadcasting: How Big Data Technology Impacts the Viewer Experience in Baseball Broadcasting †

Pi-Yun An

Department of Communication Arts, Chaoyang University of Technology, Taichung 41310, Taiwan; piyunan@gm.cyut.edu.tw

† Presented at the 2024 IEEE 4th International Conference on Electronic Communications, Internet of Things and Big Data, Taipei, Taiwan, 19–21 April 2024.

Abstract: Baseball is one of the most esteemed professional sports in Taiwan, and its broadcast production techniques are highly developed. Coupled with the sport's inherently statistical nature, the application of big data was explored in professional baseball broadcasting. Through systematic analysis and understanding of the data collection and utilization of big data in the USA and Taiwan, the results of this study provide the basis for the application and technical capabilities of big data analysis in Taiwanese baseball broadcasting in the future.

Keywords: big data; sport broadcasting; baseball

Citation: An, P.-Y. Sports Broadcasting: How Big Data Technology Impacts the Viewer Experience in Baseball Broadcasting. *Eng. Proc.* **2024**, *74*, 60. https://doi.org/10.3390/engproc2024074060

Academic Editors: Shu-Han Liao, Teen-Hang Meen and Cheng-Fu Yang

Published: 11 September 2024

1. Introduction

In the sports industry, data analysis is a longstanding practice. The precise measurement of a player's value enhances their athletic abilities and skills, consequently improving the efficacy of tactics and training programs. In recent years, big data applications have been used widely, diversifying their range. Sporting events are the critical domain for big data usage. It is utilized for player training and selection and for predicting individual athletic performances. Its significant impact is observed in professional sports teams or leagues in Europe and the United States. Advanced analytical systems are used to gather players' on-field performances, motion techniques, game results, and others, accumulating vast amounts of data for subsequent analysis. Apart from aiding teams and leagues in player training, selection, and performance prediction, broadcasters use these data to display real-time statistics during games, enabling commentators to provide deeper insights and increase the viewers' engagement and enjoyment.

2. Technology and Sports Events

Technology and sporting events have shared an inseparable relationship, especially during the Olympic Games, which serve as an excellent opportunity for host countries and companies to showcase their technological prowess. The 2012 London Olympics introduced data analysis technology into athletic competitions [1], while the 2016 Rio Olympics became the first to employ VR and 360-degree technology in event broadcasts [2]. The emergence of uncrewed aerial drones broke the constraints of traditional cameras limited by the venue. The 2018 PyeongChang Winter Olympics witnessed the deployment of 5G mobile broadband and high-speed broadcasting, significantly enhancing the quality of viewing experiences [3]. Additionally, uncrewed vehicles were introduced to transport athletes and spectators. The 2020 Tokyo Olympics, impacted by the COVID-19 pandemic, utilized innovative technologies to overcome restrictions on in-person attendance. Utilizing the high-speed transmission characteristics of 5G and specially positioned sports cameras, audiences were able to view the competitions from the athletes' perspectives. Virtual reality (VR) equipment allowed viewers to experience matches from a first-person viewpoint, cheering alongside virtual neighboring spectators. The use of 8 K/12 K high-resolution images enabled audiences to observe athletes' subtle facial expressions and muscle movements clearly on their screens [4]. The broadcast presentation was no longer confined to the singular perspective of television; the aforementioned technologies created an immersive and participatory viewing experience.

Apart from the Olympics, various sports events have used the application of technology, such as the Hawk-Eye system. Originally developed for cricket, the Hawk-Eye system was first used in televised cricket matches in 2001, providing commentators with data on ball speed, trajectory, and more. In 2002, the British Broadcasting Corporation (BBC) utilized Hawk-Eye technology during tennis broadcasts, enabling audiences to view the action in real time. The technology was then formally introduced into matches, allowing players to challenge line referee decisions. Hawk-Eye technology has been adopted in multiple sports, including badminton and volleyball, and used for sideline judgment challenges in 2014. In the 2013–2014 season, the English Premier League was using Hawk-Eye goal-line technology to determine whether a ball crossed the goal line for a valid goal.

Many groundbreaking technologies have emerged in the quadrennial FIFA World Cup as well. The Semi-Automated Offside Technology (SAOT), introduced in the 2022 Qatar World Cup, utilizes 12 tracking cameras installed in the stadium to track the ball and the positions of all players. These data were processed through big data algorithms to help referees confirm player positions for making offside decisions.

3. Big Data Cases in Sport: National Basketball Association (NBA) and Major League Baseball (MLB)

With the widespread availability of cloud storage devices and the proliferation of various sensors and smart devices, the wave of big data has swept through the sports domain. Data analysis in sports is no longer just about statistical analysis; big data analysis has become mainstream in professional sports. It impacts the operations and decision-making of all sports teams, transforming the operational landscape of professional sports leagues, including game formats, player trade management, and the overall game experience [5]. Among the major North American professional sports leagues, baseball and basketball exhibit the highest proportion of big data applications with Major League Baseball in the US reaching up to 97%, and the NBA at 80%.

Since the 1980s, the NBA has been utilizing data management technology, encompassing detailed records of game statistics such as player scores, rebounds, assists, blocks, steals, turnovers, fouls, and more, meticulously documented by sideline personnel. Upon analysis, these statistics not only reveal individual performances but can even illustrate players' offensive and defensive performances during matchups. During the 2010–2011 season, four NBA teams utilized the dynamic camera technology provided by SportVU, known as the Player Tracking System. Through six high-resolution tracking cameras stationed along the basketball court's catwalk at a frequency of 25 frames per second, these cameras generated thousands of images per minute, capturing athletes' subtle movements comprehensively for analysis. From 2013 onwards, SportVU became an official partner of the NBA, leading the NBA to instantly publish SportVU-derived data on the NBA's official website and NBATV. This enabled audiences to access more professional and reference-worthy basketball data, allowing each viewer to derive pleasure from watching games based on their understanding of the data.

In 2018, the NBA began collaborating with Sportradar and Second Spectrum, equipping all NBA arenas with multiple dynamic cameras recording players' in-game dynamics. Apart from utilizing image processing and machine learning models to analyze and apply vast databases, Second Spectrum employs machine learning to automatically detect and record various "meaningful" behaviors on the court, such as touches, shooting, passing, dribbling, screens, and more, and evaluates players' choices on the court through statistical methods, predicting the shooting accuracy of players at particular positions. SportVU and Second Spectrum have transformed NBA teams' decision-making, player training, tactics, player assessment criteria, and fans' viewing experiences, propelling NBA basketball games into another developmental stage.

In comparison to basketball, baseball's advanced data development commenced earlier. Due to the game's pace and on-field interactions, baseball places greater emphasis on various data sets than basketball. Baseball is appropriate for data analysis because it is a turn-based sport, where each game comprises a series of individual pitching and hitting matchups all of which serve as independent samples for analysis. Baseball is inherently a sport that reveals probabilities, utilizing metrics such as batting average, on-base percentage, slugging percentage, earned run average, and fielding percentage, among others, as references for pitching, offensive and defensive strategies, and tactical instructions from the coaching staff during games.

In the early stages of baseball development, only basic statistics such as game scores and hit counts were recorded. In 1858, sportswriter Henry Chadwick invented the box score to provide various game statistics. In 1964, Earnshaw Cook enabled people to understand the potential of using data to analyze baseball through his work "Percentage Baseball". Bill James in the 1970s conducted a series of analyses for the Society for American Baseball Research (SABR) concerning baseball statistical data and began writing "The Bill James Baseball Abstract" in 1977, published annually until 1984. This series of works introduced numerous new arguments based on data, initiating the wave of sabermetrics, and advanced baseball data research.

Since 2007, MLB has introduced advanced analysis systems such as the Pitchf/x system and Hitf/x. Approximately 20 data collectors are installed in each ballpark. The Pitchf/x system records various data such as the velocity, location, pitch type, release point, spin angle, and the outcome of pitcher–batter matchups for every thrown ball. This results in a substantial surge in baseball data, where a single game generates around 300,000 high-resolution photos, resulting in over 1 TB of data and potentially reaching a massive 7 TB [6,7]. Subsequently, MLB integrated systems capable of tracking players (ChyronHego) and tracking the ball (Trackman high-speed camera system), allowing for comprehensive spatial data collection introduced as Statcast, adopted by all MLB teams. The Statcast database collects intricate on-field events as data, presenting new metrics such as exit velocity, launch angle, spin rate, tunneling, and pop time, and later widely used derived data to evaluate player performance such as hard-hit rate and barrel rate as shown in Figures 1–3. These next-generation scientific data have started to be featured in in-game broadcasts, providing anchors and commentators with a basis for analyzing player athletic abilities and enhancing the professionalism and entertainment value of game reporting. These data have gradually become familiar to audiences, allowing fans to discuss star players' performances based on scientific data rather than speculation.

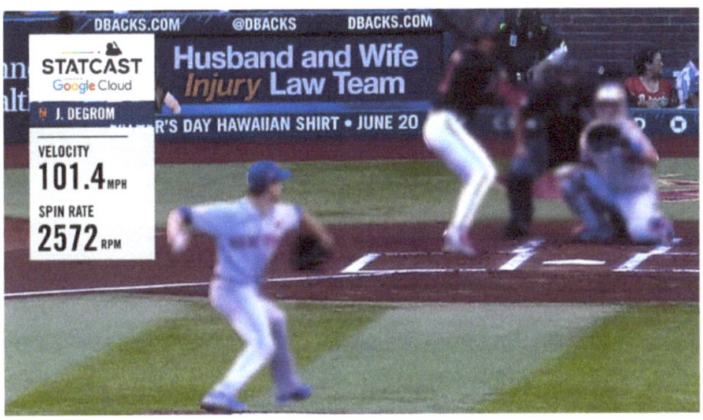

Figure 1. Statcast delves deep into pitchers' performance.

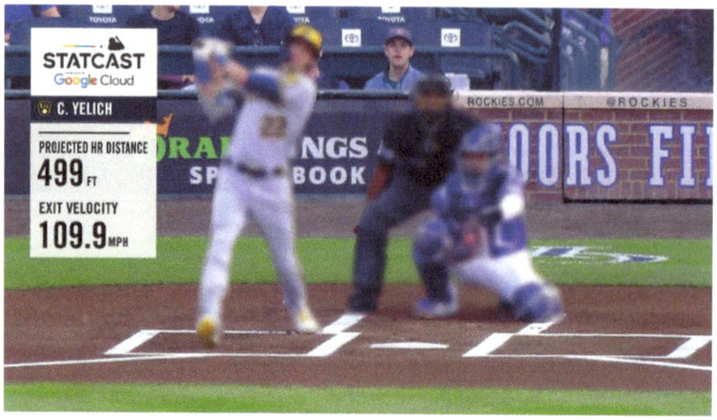

Figure 2. Statcast allows for exact measure of home run.

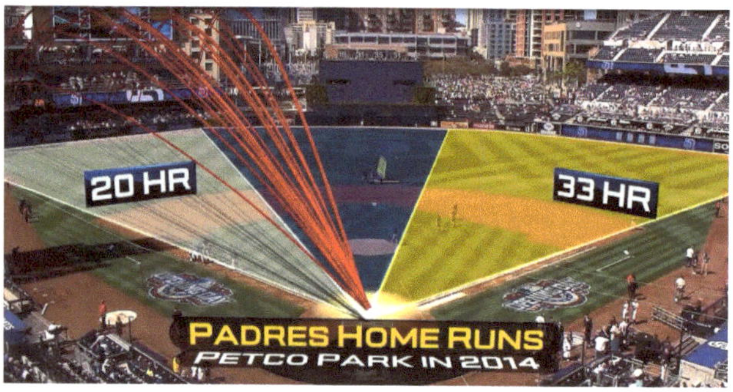

Figure 3. MLB hitter's spray chart.

In 2020, MLB replaced Trackman with Hawk-Eye, requiring the installation of 12 cameras in the ballpark. While Trackman could only track one fast-moving object, typically the ball, Hawk-Eye can track all moving objects within the frame, enhancing its precision in detecting the ball and players and capturing swing times and trajectories. The interconnection between the development of sports and television broadcasting indicates that this linkage not only enhances entertainment but also contributes to the promotion of a particular sport. Throughout the broadcast of games, leveraging technological advancements enables the display of various aspects of the game process and related information on screens. This includes the trajectory of pitches, K-Zone, Hawk-Eye, and other elements. By developing relevant technologies from an entertainment perspective, audiences are allowed to immerse themselves in the tension and excitement elicited by the game.

4. Big Data in Chinese Professional Baseball League (CPBL)

In the era of big data, the traditional statistics recorded in the box score, such as a player's runs, hits, errors, and other basic data, no longer suffice for the modern needs of data analysis in baseball. While CPBL and its associated teams have started exploring advanced statistics, the current CPBL broadcasts continue to display primarily basic, calculable statistics on the screen for viewers. These typically include batting average, earned run average, wins, runs batted in, and saves as shown in Figures 4 and 5.

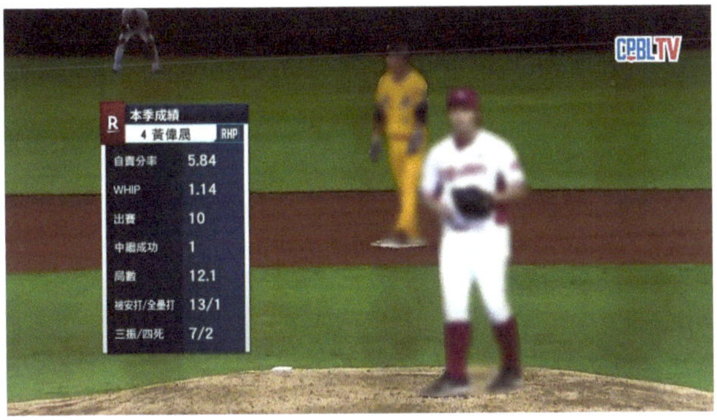

Figure 4. CPBL pitcher data. (ERA, WHIP, Games, Holds, IP, H, HR, K/B).

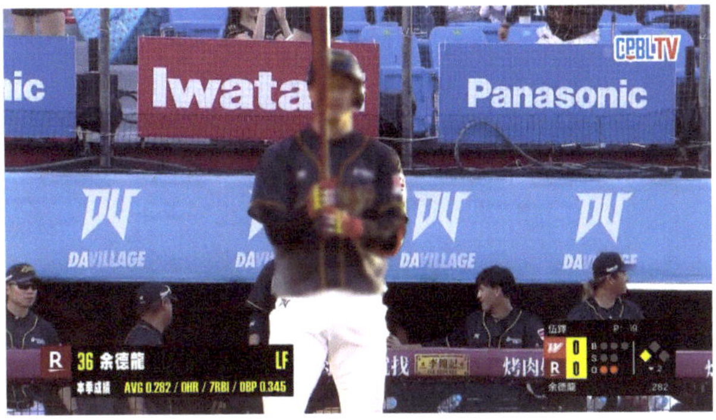

Figure 5. CPBL hitter data.

In 2018, the Fubon Guardians and the CTBC Brothers installed Trackman systems at their home stadiums in Xinzhuang and Taichung, respectively. In 2020, the Wei Chuan Dragons, which returned to the CPBL, also equipped their stadiums in Tianmu and Douliu with Trackman. Differing from these three teams that purchased the "Trackman" data analysis system used by MLB teams, the Uni-President 7-Eleven Lions opted for the portable Rapsodo system. The Taoyuan Monkeys collaborated with a local data analytics company, using eight high-speed cameras to measure the trajectory of pitches and hits, as well as players' movements, achieving automatic video recording and editing.

A research team in Taiwan developed the Karma Zone system in 2018. The system, consisting of six high-speed cameras, introduced two applications: an electronic strike zone and a 3D motion analysis system. Karma Zone utilizes images captured by two high-speed cameras positioned over the first base side and behind the home plate to calculate the coordinates in space. The results are displayed on the broadcast screen as a grid pattern of the strike zone as shown in Figures 6 and 7. It displays on the broadcast screen in less than a second after a pitcher throws the ball. This system provides data on hitting positions, ball speed, hitting velocity, and various other information in the future. The teams plan to release an app for fans to access these data by downloading the app.

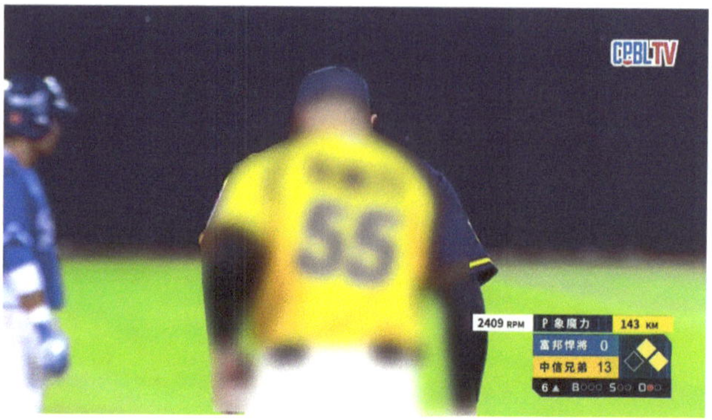

Figure 6. CPBL pitching spin rate. (First line: Pitcher's name. Left: Spin Rate. Right: Pitch Speed. Second: line: Score).

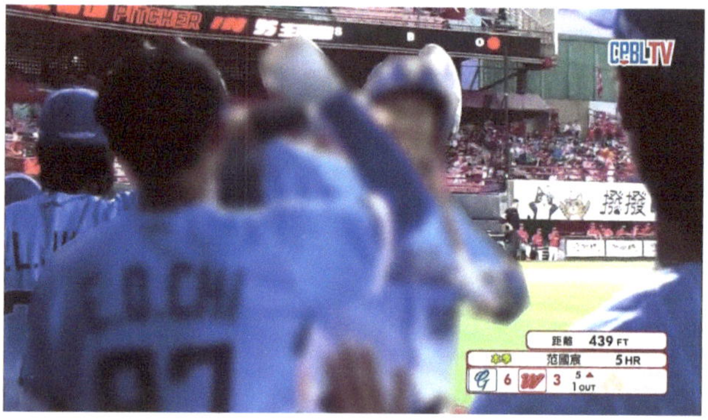

Figure 7. CPBL home run distance. (First line: Home Run Distance. Second line: Hitter's Name and HR).

In May 2020, the CTBC Brothers integrated the Trackman data mirroring system into their broadcasts, displaying data like the grid pattern, pitcher ball speed, ball rotation speed, initial hitting speed, and home run distances. This development brings Taiwanese baseball broadcasts closer to the trend of incorporating big data.

5. Discussion

The MLB has developed data-driven baseball for many years. However, Taiwan has only recently begun to focus on data analysis, utilizing technology to collect and record player statistics and continuing to establish a big data backend for analysis. The aim is to provide coaches and players with data-backed strategies in the field. This allows for in-game decision-making and tracking the developmental trajectory of young players, ensuring whether players are following the growth curve planned by the team. Nonetheless, the CPBL still has a considerable gap in terms of personnel in its team's data departments and investment compared to MLB.

There are several reasons why the concepts of using data analysis are not widespread in Taiwan's baseball industry or CPBL teams [5]. These include unfamiliarity with data analysis, lack of confidence in its accuracy, concerns over the increased operational costs associated with data analysis, and the concept of making decisions through data analysis not being widely accepted in Taiwan. In reality, data analysis requires capturing a vast amount of data through hardware equipment and then using software to conclude. Due to the substantial financial support required for hardware setup, database system establishment, and hiring of technical talent, CPBL's limited number of teams leads to insufficient data collection, and limited commercial interests, making it difficult to attract local and foreign scholars for research and related investments. Moreover, CPBL struggles to attract investment or create profits similar to sports big data technology and service companies including MLB Advance Media (MLBAM). In contrast, MLB teams are significantly concerned about baseball statistics due to the multimillion-dollar player market dynamics. However, apart from improving team performance and player athletic skills, there are no other compelling reasons to attract investment in the league.

Undeniably, the collection and analysis of sports data have already occupied a significant position in professional sports, with most discussions focusing on enhancing player performance. However, there has been scarce research on the impact of these data on audiences watching the game on screen. General viewers tend to concentrate their attention on the wins and losses of the teams rather than the statistics generated in professional sports. Only a few individuals with an interest in statistics seek to understand the meaning and implications of the data provided on the screen. Zheng and Chen pointed out that complex information poses a challenge to the audience's information-processing ability [8]. Sports data can create barriers among audiences with different experiences, making it difficult for fans with varying levels of experience to enjoy watching sports games. Their research revealed that in situations with less experience, statistical information does not assist low-engagement fans in understanding baseball events. However, visualizing player information allows for low-engagement fans to derive more enjoyment and meaning while making it easier to comprehend the game. On the other hand, high-engagement fans, due to their extensive baseball knowledge and experience, do not significantly benefit from any type of information provided during broadcast experiences.

6. Conclusions

Big data have brought about significant changes in various facets of daily life, bringing substantial transformations in business, daily living, and government governance. In sports, numerous research teams in Taiwan are utilizing precise technological tools to collect and analyze athletes' trajectories. Through the use of AI algorithms, these teams provide coaches and athletes with tailored and intelligent training suggestions, transitioning athlete training from conventional methods into an era of "intelligent training" through "scientific digital analysis". The immediate, voluminous, diverse, and long-term data characteristics on the sports field are essential for data science research teams, particularly in baseball, where countless events unfold in every game. In the future, all actions on the baseball field are bound to be covered by cameras, radars, and calculation software. However, research related to the application of big data in sports broadcasting remains scarce. Audience members have needs for media, sparking motivation and media usage behavior [9]. For audiences watching games on screen, the question arises as to whether the substantial amount of information brought about by big data can increase their motivation or enhance their viewing pleasure. Television was previously a passive form of entertainment with the primary motive for most programs being entertainment, while information-based viewing motives were more prevalent in news programs. However, with modern technological advancements, traditional television viewing experiences are no longer adequate to meet audience needs. The transformation of television media is inevitable to comply with these trends. It is needed to discuss how baseball broadcasts integrate new technologies to pique audience interest without adding burdens to viewers.

Funding: This research received no external funding.

Institutional Review Board Statement: Not applicable.

Informed Consent Statement: Not applicable.

Data Availability Statement: Detailed information about the presented study can be freely obtained by contacting the authors.

Conflicts of Interest: The author declares no conflict of interest.

References

1. Salmon, J.L.; Harrison, W.K. A Data Analytics Approach to Evaluation of Competition in the 2012 Summer Olympic. *J. Data Sci.* **2017**, *15*, 373–390.
2. Willie, K.; Risen, T. Rio 2016 Will Be the First Virtual Reality Olympics. *U.S. News*. 30 June 2016. Available online: https://www.usnews.com/news/articles/2016-06-30/rio-2016-will-be-the-first-virtual-reality-olympics (accessed on 25 April 2024).
3. Toh, M. 5G Is Helping Make Pyeongchang the Most High-Tech Olympics Ever. *CNN Business*. 19 February 2018. Available online: https://money.cnn.com/2018/02/19/technology/pyeongchang-winter-olympics-5g-intel/index.html (accessed on 25 April 2024).
4. Tiled Media. Watching the Tokyo 2020 Olympics in VR, April 2022. Available online: https://www.tiledmedia.com/watching-the-tokyo-2020-olympics-in-vr-an-insider-review/ (accessed on 25 April 2024).
5. Chang, C.H. Improving Taiwanese Baseball Data Analysis Goes Hand in Hand with U.S.A. *Sci. Educ. Mon.* **2018**, *407*, 2–17.
6. Granville, V. Beyond Moneyball: How Big Data Is Changing Baseball. *Analytikus*. 4 November 2016. Available online: https://www.analytikus.com/post/2016/11/03/beyond-moneyball-how-big-data-is-changing-baseball (accessed on 25 April 2024).
7. Woodie, A. Today's Baseball Analytics Make Moneyball Look Like Child's Play. *Datanami*. 24 October 2014. Available online: https://www.datanami.com/2014/10/24/todays-baseball-analytics-make-moneyball-look-like-childs-play/ (accessed on 25 April 2024).
8. Zheng, M.C.; Chen, C.Y. Types of Major League Baseball Broadcast Information and Their Impacts on Audience Experience. *Informatics* **2022**, *9*, 82. [CrossRef]
9. Palmgreen, P.; Wenner, L.A.; Rosengren, K.E. Uses and Gratifications Research: The past ten years. *Media Gratif. Res. Curr. Perspect.* **1985**, *11*, 37.

engineering proceedings

MDPI

Proceeding Paper

Factors Influencing Consumer Impulsive Buying Behavior regarding Mobile Game Purchase Intention †

Jen-Chieh Chung [1], Ying-Hsiao Lai [2,*] and Yu-Tzu Chang [1]

1 Department of Marketing and Logistics Management, Chaoyang University of Technology, Taichung 413310, Taiwan; jcchung@cyut.edu.tw (J.-C.C.); s10934032@gm.cyut.edu.tw (Y.-T.C.)
2 Department of Leisure Service Management, Chaoyang University of Technology, Taichung 413310, Taiwan
* Correspondence: ylai@cyut.edu.tw

† Presented at the 2024 IEEE 4th International Conference on Electronic Communications, Internet of Things and Big Data, Taipei, Taiwan, 19–21 April 2024.

Abstract: We explored impulsive buying behavior regarding mobile games and the factors influencing it. Data were collected from 389 participants. The results presented differences between different types of impulse buying. The findings contribute to the future study of consumer behavior and provide implications for commercial providers.

Keywords: impulsive buying behavior; purchase intention; mobile game

Citation: Chung, J.-C.; Lai, Y.-H.; Chang, Y.-T. Factors Influencing Consumer Impulsive Buying Behavior regarding Mobile Game Purchase Intention. *Eng. Proc.* **2024**, *74*, 61. https://doi.org/10.3390/engproc2024074061

Academic Editors: Shu-Han Liao, Teen-Hang Meen and Cheng-Fu Yang

Published: 11 September 2024

1. Introduction

According to the report from the Groupe Speciale Mobile Association (GSMA), the number of smartphone users reached 4.3 billion in 2022, comprising 54% of the total population [1]. Since the majority of consumers use smartphones, applications (APPs) are launched, and more categories are created. With smartphones, we can browse the internet, send emails, or download apps anywhere [2]. Also, we can play mobile games and watch videos. Therefore, playing video games is one a usual leisure activity.

Mobile games refer to games played on mobile handheld devices such as smartphones and personal digital assistants (PDAs) with wireless communication capabilities [3]. Newzoo announced that the number of global mobile gamers increased to 3.3 billion in 2023, and the market size reached USD 9.26 billion [4]. The majority of game players are from the Asia–Pacific region, approximately 53% of the global market. According to statistics from Sensor Tower, Taiwan ranked fifth in the global mobile game consumer market in 2022 [5]. This shows the importance of Taiwan's mobile game market in the global industry.

Research related to mobile games has been conducted on how mobile games can help college students relieve stress, release negative emotions, exchange ideas, meet social needs, improve academic achievements, etc., and help their physical and mental development through games. These are the positive impacts [6–8]. Chu indicated that college students are a high-risk group for mobile game addiction [9]. When mobile players spend more time playing, their degree of involvement will increase [10,11]. Also, mobile game use affects impulse buying [12]. Impulsive buying is a perceptual, strong, and urgent behavior that occurs when consumers suddenly feel emotionally excited and have a continued desire to buy [13]. On the other hand, previous studies have shown that when mobile players are highly involved, emotions are easily aroused [12,14]. Indeed, when mobile game players have more positive emotions while they play games, they usually engage in impulsive buying [15,16]. Emotion is a term related to the human body, a personal psychological state related to thoughts, feelings, and behaviors [17,18]. Therefore, involvement, emotion, and impulse buying behaviors are related to each other. The majority of college students play mobile games and are easily addicted. We explored impulsive buying behavior in mobile games, the degree of involvement, and positive emotions.

2. Methodology

The students from a university in Taiwan were selected as participants. To investigate the characteristics of the students, a stratified random sampling method was applied. In 2019, 11,317 students were enrolled at this university. Under the confidence level of 95% and the maximum error $d = 0.05$, the following equation was used to estimate the minimum sample size.

$$n = \frac{N}{N\left(\frac{2d}{Z_{\alpha/2}}\right)^2 + 1} \tag{1}$$

The minimum sample size was determined to be 372. Thus, 400 questionnaires were collected from students at the university, and 389 valid responses were collected (97.3%).

3. Results and Discussions

3.1. Descriptive Statistics

Since the stratified random sampling method was adopted, the chi-square test (goodness-of-fit test) was conducted to examine whether the sampling structure was fit for the normal distribution. All variables were fit to the population parameters. Among the respondents, there were 100 freshmen (25.7%), 73 sophomores (18.7%), 127 juniors (32.7%), and 89 senior students (22.8%). In total, 146 of the respondents were male (37.6%) and 243 were female (62.4%), 136 students majored in management (35.0%), 54 students majored in science and engineering (13.8%), 61 students majored in design (15.6%), 82 students majored in humanities and social sciences (21.2%), and 56 students majored in informatics (14.3%). Regarding monthly disposable income, 25.83% students had an income of NTD 3001–6000, 24.04% earned NTD 6001–9000, 17.90% earned less than NTD 3000, 11.76% earned NTD 9001–12,000, 11.25% earned more than NTD 15,001, and 9.21% earned NTD 12,001–15,000. A total of 99.74% of the participants played mobile games, and 41.43% spent money on mobile games. To understand the behavior of the participants regarding mobile games, the questionnaire was divided into two parts: positive emotions and impulse buying. We used a Likert 5-point scale [19]. To reduce the dimensions of the questionnaire, factor analysis was used [20].

3.2. Factor Analysis

The KMO value of the degree of involvement was 0.569, and two main factors were extracted. Factor 1 was named "Time and Energy" [10,11]; Factor 2 was named "Interest" based on the definition of "involvement is the consumer's perceived value of the product or purchase decision" [21] (Table 1). Table 2 shows that the KMO value of positive emotion was 0.784. Two main factors were extracted, named "Positive Behavior" and "Positive Feelings".

Table 1. Results of involvement.

Items	F1	F2	Factor Name
I spend a lot of time playing mobile games every week	0.781	0.136	Time and Energy
I spend a lot of time playing mobile games every time	0.644	0.071	
Most of my leisure and entertainment are related to technology products, such as playing TV consoles, online games, etc.	0.607	0.052	
I spend a lot of money on mobile games every month	0.263	0.770	Interest
I am fond of mobile games	0.303	0.709	
KMO value		0.569	

Table 2. Positive emotion.

Items	F1	F2	Factor Name
Spending in games makes me proud	0.826	0.084	Positive behavior
Spending in games makes me pleasantly surprised	0.789	0.136	
Spending in games makes me calm	0.737	−0.009	
Spending in games makes me glad	0.699	0.193	
Playing this game puts me in a good mood	0.160	0.854	Positive feelings
I think this is a fun game	0.131	0.810	
I feel very happy now	0.056	0.741	
I think the story of this game is very interesting	0.059	0.713	
KMO value		0.784	

Table 3 shows that the KMO value of impulse buying was 0.780. After rotating the axis, the component matrix extracts three factors. Factor 1 was named "Glad type"; Factor 2 was named "conflict type." Since consumers who bought mobile games impulsively usually lacked thoughtfulness and made reckless buying decisions, Factor 3 was named "Uncontrollable".

Table 3. Results of impulse buying.

Items	F1	F2	F3	Factor Name
I enjoy buying products on impulse	0.893	0.043	0.184	Glad type
I get a rush of pleasure when I buy something impulsively	0.925	0.119	0.109	
When I buy on impulse, I find myself joyful, happy, and fanaticism	0.914	0.110	0.141	
Sometimes I regret making impulsive buying	0.030	0.732	0.134	Conflict type
Sometimes I feel self-accusation for impulsively buying things	0.078	0.833	0.095	
I experience some emotional conflict when making impulse buying	0.129	0.811	0.089	
I experience mixed feelings of pleasure and guilt trip from impulse buying	0.254	0.782	0.031	
I tend to spend the money I make as quickly as possible	0.187	0.053	0.835	Uncontrollable type
I buy things even if I can't afford them	0.179	0.042	0.805	
I often buy things I don't need and by the time I know it, I have a little money left	0.030	0.211	0.756	
KMO value			0.780	

Pearson correlation coefficient analysis is used to explore the degree of linear correlation between factors [22]. Table 4 shows a highest positive correlation coefficient of 0.422 between positive feelings and the glad type, with a significant p-value of 0.05. The lowest positive correlation coefficient was between time and energy and the conflict type (0.121). A negative correlation was observed for positive behaviors and the uncontrollable type (−0.176). Most items were related to each other positively.

Table 4. Correlation coefficients matrix of factors.

	Time and Energy	Interest	Positive Behavior	Positive Feelings	Glad Type	Conflict Type	Uncontrollable Type
Time and Energy	1						
Interest	0.000	1					
Positive behavior	0.320 *	−0.002	1				
Positive feelings	0.172 *	0.149 *	0.000	1			
Glad type	0.122 *	0.202 *	0.181 *	0.422 *	1		
Conflict type	0.121 *	−0.090	0.089	−0.066	0.000	1	
Uncontrollable type	0.023	0.233 *	−0.176 *	0.230 *	0.000	0.000	1

Note: * $p < 0.05$.

It was found that Taiwanese college students spent more time and energy playing mobile games. In addition to having higher positive consumption behaviors and feelings, they also had feelings such as high pleasure, regret, and self-blame when impulsive buying happened. When consumers spent more money on mobile games, they had higher positive feelings, emotions for impulse buying, and irrational consumption behaviors.

4. Conclusions

The degree of involvement, positive emotions, and impulse buying behavior of Taiwanese college student players regarding mobile games were closely related. The popularity of mobile games has advantages and disadvantages for college students. Although people improve their physical and mental development through mobile games, they have negative problems due to addiction, which affects impulsive buying and emotions. The players' involvement in mobile games affected emotions and impulsive buying behavior, thus confirming the correlation between the three for Taiwanese college students' use of mobile games.

Author Contributions: Conceptualization, J.-C.C. and Y.-H.L.; methodology, J.-C.C., Y.-H.L. and Y.-T.C.; validation, J.-C.C., Y.-H.L. and Y.-T.C.; formal analysis, J.-C.C., Y.-H.L. and Y.-T.C.; resources, J.-C.C. and Y.-T.C.; data curation, J.-C.C., Y.-H.L. and Y.-T.C.; writing—original draft preparation, J.-C.C. and Y.-H.L.; writing—review and editing, J.-C.C. and Y.-H.L.; supervision, J.-C.C. and Y.-H.L.; funding acquisition, none. All authors reviewed and edited the manuscript. All authors have read and agreed to the published version of the manuscript.

Funding: This research received no external funding.

Institutional Review Board Statement: Not applicable.

Informed Consent Statement: Not applicable.

Data Availability Statement: No new data were created or analyzed in this study. Data sharing is not applicable to this article.

Conflicts of Interest: The authors declare no conflicts of interest.

References

1. Groupe Speciale Mobile Association. Smartphone Owners Are Now the Global Majority, New Gsma Report Reveals. 2023. Available online: https://www.gsma.com/newsroom/press-release/smartphone-owners-are-now-the-global-majority-new-gsma-report-reveals/ (accessed on 20 October 2023).
2. Kaya, S.; Argan, M. An Exploratory Qualitative Study on Mobile Leisure (M-Leisure): A Case of Mobile Phone Users in Turkey. *J. Internet Appl. Manag.* **2015**, *6*, 21–32. [CrossRef]
3. Jin, D.Y. *Mobile Gaming in Asia: Politics, Culture and Emerging Technologies*; Springer: Berlin/Heidelberg, Germany, 2017.
4. Newzoo. *Newzoo's Global Games Market Report 2023*; Newzoo: Amsterdam, The Netherlands, 2023.
5. The State of Mobile Gaming 2023. Sensor Tower. 2023. Available online: https://go.sensortower.com/state-of-mobile-gaming-2023 (accessed on 20 October 2023).

6. Pine, R.; Fleming, T.; McCallum, S.; Sutcliffe, K. The effects of casual videogames on anxiety, depression, stress, and low mood: A systematic review. *Games Health J.* **2020**, *9*, 255–264. [CrossRef] [PubMed]
7. Wang, P. Analysis on Advantages and Disadvantages of Playing Mobile Games among Colleges Students. *J. High. Educ. Res.* **2022**, *3*, 29–33. [CrossRef]
8. Li, F.; Zhang, D.; Wu, S.; Zhou, R.; Dong, C.; Zhang, J. Positive effects of online games on the growth of college students: A qualitative study from China. *Front. Psychol.* **2023**, *14*, 1008211. [CrossRef] [PubMed]
9. Chu, K.M. Related Research between College Students' Mobile Game Addiction, Mobile Self-Efficacy, and Academic Performance in Taiwan. *Psychol. Sch.* **2022**, *60*, 931–942. [CrossRef]
10. Stone, R.N. The marketing characteristics of involvement. *Adv. Consum. Res.* **1984**, *11*, 210–215.
11. Snodgrass, J.G.; Dengah, H.F., II; Lacy, M.G.; Bagwell, A.; Van Oostenburg, M.; Lende, D. Online gaming involvement and its positive and negative consequences: A cognitive anthropological "cultural consensus" approach to psychiatric measurement and assessment. *Comput. Hum. Behav.* **2017**, *66*, 291–302. [CrossRef]
12. Jones, M.A.; Reynolds, K.E.; Weun, S.; Beatty, S.E. The product-specific nature of impulse buying tendency. *J. Bus. Res.* **2003**, *56*, 505–511. [CrossRef]
13. Rook, D.W. The buying impulse. *J. Consum. Res.* **1987**, *14*, 189–199. [CrossRef]
14. Liao, C.; To, P.L.; Wong, Y.C.; Palvia, P.; Kakhki, M.D. The impact of presentation mode and product type on online impulse buying decisions. *J. Electron. Commer. Res.* **2016**, *17*, 153.
15. Adelaar, T.; Chang, S.; Lancendorfer, K.M.; Lee, B.; Morimoto, M. Effects of media formats on emotions and impulse buying intent. *J. Inf. Technol.* **2003**, *18*, 247–266. [CrossRef]
16. Andani, K.; Wahyono, W. Influence of Sales Promotion, Hedonic Shopping Motivation and Fashion Involvement Toward Impulse Buying through a Positive Emotion. *Manag. Anal. J.* **2018**, *7*, 448–457. [CrossRef]
17. Munezero, M.; Montero, C.S.; Sutinen, E.; Pajunen, J. Are they different? Affect, feeling, emotion, sentiment, and opinion detection in text. *IEEE Trans. Affect. Comput.* **2014**, *5*, 101–111. [CrossRef]
18. Poria, S.; Majumder, N.; Mihalcea, R.; Hovy, E. Emotion recognition in conversation: Research challenges, datasets, and recent advances. *IEEE Access* **2019**, *7*, 100943–100953. [CrossRef]
19. Likert, R. A technique for the measurement of attitudes. *Arch. Psychol.* **1932**, *22*, 55.
20. Kaiser, H.F. An index of factorial simplicity. *Psychometrika* **1974**, *39*, 31–36. [CrossRef]
21. Mittal, B.; Lee, M.S. A causal model of consumer involvement. *J. Econ. Psychol.* **1989**, *10*, 363–389. [CrossRef]
22. Pearson, K.V.I.I. Note on regression and inheritance in the case of two parents. *Proc. R. Soc. Lond.* **1895**, *58*, 240–242.

engineering proceedings

MDPI

Proceeding Paper

Residential Design for Future: Comparative Study on Benefits, Needs, and Characteristics of "Multi-Purpose Residential Architecture" Design Concept †

Ting-Yueh Chen [1,2,*] and Shu-Ying Tsai [1]

1 Department of Architecture, Faculty of Design, National Taipei University of Technology, Taipei 10608, Taiwan; tsaishuying0914@gmail.com
2 Department of Architecture, Faculty of Design, Chao-Yang University of Technology, Taichung 41349, Taiwan
* Correspondence: patrick52310@gmail.com; Tel.: +886-919426999

† Presented at the 2024 IEEE 4th International Conference on Electronic Communications, Internet of Things and Big Data, Taipei, Taiwan, 19–21 April 2024.

Abstract: As the population ages, the living environment for the elderly is receiving more attention. "Multi-Purpose Residential Architecture" is transforming the traditional ways of building horizontally to meet a person's daily activity and living needs. We surveyed 140 seniors over the age of 55 years to find their perspectives on building and expanding space vertically. Differences between the needs and expectations for living spaces between different ages of seniors were found. There are not enough facilities and space in Taiwan to meet the seniors' needs for their daily lives, social activities, care, and other support.

Keywords: living environment for the elderly; multiple-purpose residential architecture; expanding space vertically

Citation: Chen, T.-Y.; Tsai, S.-Y. Residential Design for Future: Comparative Study on Benefits, Needs, and Characteristics of "Multi-Purpose Residential Architecture" Design Concept. *Eng. Proc.* **2024**, *74*, 62. https://doi.org/10.3390/engproc2024074062

Academic Editors: Shu-Han Liao, Teen-Hang Meen and Cheng-Fu Yang

Published: 14 September 2024

1. Introduction

Many countries are impacted by aging. Having an aging society does not only mean changes to a community's composition but also the need to transform living spaces based on the changes between different generations, technologies, abilities, and environments [1]. The physical functions and abilities of humans deteriorate with age. However, through adequate social and physician activities, staying healthy can be achieved for a longer time and delay the aging process. There is a positive relation between the quality of life and our physical health [2]. Senior care policies set "aging in place" as one of the ideal goals. It is ideal for seniors to retire and age naturally in their original community to keep their abilities independent and be respected for their self-worth and privacy [3]. Seniors are used to "aging at home", believing that they must stay in the environment they are most familiar with as the existing living space is the most appropriate for their age and daily needs. According to statistics from the Ministry of Health and Welfare, 70% of seniors over the age of 65 live in inadequate living conditions such as living in apartments without an elevator or in a multi-story house [4].

2. Materials and Methods

2.1. Literature Review

2.1.1. Life Characteristics of the Elderly and Environmental Factors

With aging, physical conditions deteriorate. It also increases the risk of falling [5]. As the brain ages, mental and emotional changes are faced. With age, even if mental and emotional health remains, more time is needed to process and reflect thoughts, memories, and messages [6]. As people age, their physical and mental abilities change. Therefore, seniors need to stay active and engaged. Many seniors show a "grey strength" that influences public policies around living space and residential designs [7].

Statistics showed that approximately 40% of seniors found it difficult to leave their homes, 25% had challenges walking, 23% were worried about falling, 10% found it hard to cross the road, and 2% were worried about getting lost [8]. Seniors' daily and social activities influence their physical and mental health. If seniors engage in social activities actively, they tend to have higher satisfaction with their lives and a positive influence on their physical and mental health [9]. When a senior's physical abilities deteriorate, they tend to have smaller areas of activities [10]. Seniors may naturally withdraw from social life or reduce their social interactions when their physical condition deteriorates. This is why it is important to provide essential services from health care to social, financial, and entertainment facilities to meet seniors' needs within walking distance [11].

Seniors mentally withdraw from social interactions due to the change in their physical conditions. Their areas of activities are often smaller than they had when they were younger. Depending on a senior's physical health, it is ideal to access their daily needs within a 10 to 15 min walking distance, which is approximately 500 m [12].

2.1.2. Multiple-Purpose Residential Architecture for Elderly

Cohousing is an architectural design that originated in Denmark in the 1960s. It combines the characteristics of private, independent living with a network of public facilities and community support that are easily accessible. It also encourages members of the same community to actively participate and manage their space and community. It brings many social, economic, and environmental benefits to people living in the same community. Cohousing was later adapted into the "Senior Cohousing" concept to meet the unique needs of residents in their later years. It often adds an emphasis on universal design, accessibility, safety, co-caring and mutual support, or whatever else may emerge to meet the needs of residents. Senior Cohousing solves many issues facing seniors as they age. This type of new design concept changes how people perceive aging. It creates a new culture that helps to keep seniors staying active in their community through those transformative years [13]. This is a new concept to design condominiums to meet the needs of an aging society. It also differentiates the living space and prioritizes spaces to meet the needs of seniors and people with diverse abilities. For example, the "urban environment" concept is used to provide spaces for a person with diverse abilities (such as a person with vision problems, mobility issues, or a person in a wheelchair) that are easily accessible within a radius of 100 m, ensuring the "building entrance" meets the needs of individuals. It also includes areas such as the kitchen, bathroom, and bedrooms as accommodating and accessible areas. These can be easily modified or renovated for the future based on the needs of an individual [14].

The principles of Multi-Purpose Residential Architecture (MPRA) include the following.

1. Diverse: The residential space is not only designed for seniors but also for people of any age with diverse physical and mental abilities. The functionalities of the space can be commonly shared—meeting the diverse living needs of seniors and residents.
2. Independent: Safety is a must-have when it comes to the space and facility design. It also provides flexible design and functionality to support seniors to live independently.
3. Variety: We provide quality healthcare and senior care services with a variety of choices for food services and social and educational opportunities to better fulfill and support seniors' healthy living.
4. Meaningful: MPRA supports seniors' daily activities and needs, a healthy and independent environment, and respect to enjoy their everyday lives with fulfillment and meaning.
5. Network: MPRA is a service hub with the potential to build a network of hubs internationally so seniors can travel and reside in hubs and share the same principles and services. It is a franchise to be prompted globally [4].

2.1.3. Environmental Assessment Indicators of MRPA

Physical space impacts health and welfare. The World Health Organization has already determined that our physical space is a key element of the quality of life [15]. The National Design Guide of the United Kingdom indicates that environmental design impacts health, well-being, sense of security, level of tolerance, sense of belonging, and the level of community engagement. Environmental assessment indicators demonstrate the quality of life in different environments, identify issues, and improve the living environment [16]. In recent years, many studies assessed senior homes and facilities emphasizing the residents' quality of life [17]. Key principles of "Inclusive Design" for urban living include Familiarity, Easiness, Uniqueness, Accessibility, Comfortableness, and Safety. These principles are set to ensure that all users can enjoy, understand, and have easy access to community amenities and streets [8].

The Environmental Audit Tool (EAT) has been used previously to evaluate senior homes. It started in Australia and includes assessments of Safety; Appropriate Ratios; Visibility; Reduced Irritants; Supporting Positive Environment Simulations; Promoting Activities and Engagement; Familiarity; Community Privacy; Providing Community Connections; and Encouraging Independent Living. EAT was designed to help front-line workers and service providers improve services through physical space. It was later used by architects and designers as a tool to inspect and evaluate existing physical space to support patients, residents, and workers, utilizing the facilities to enhance the quality of services and provide a healing and comforting environment [18].

The Sheffield Care Environment Assessment Matrix (SCEAM) is used to evaluate senior homes and residences. It includes assessments of Safety/Health; Actual Support; Cognitive Support; Normalcy; Personalization; Choices/Control; Privacy; Level of Comfortableness and Environment; Attentiveness to Outdoor Space; and Community [19].

Evaluation of Older People's Living Environments (EVOLVE) is a design assessment tool developed by Sheffield College in 2010 to evaluate a variety of senior residences. It is based on the foundational principles of "SCEAM" in two major categories: General Needs and Senior Support Needs. General Needs include Personalization and Choices; Dignity and Privacy; Comfortableness and Control; Personalized Care; Social Support within the Building; and Outdoor Environment and Social Support. Senior Support Needs include Accessibility; Support for Independence; Sensory Stimulation; Dementia Support; Health and Safety; Security; and Care Work [20].

British Columbia, Canada, has a "Senior Guide" available, which includes environmental assessment tools that include home support, life choice, independence, community care, rehabilitation services, day services, temporary care for nursing staff, life support, home care, and small group nursing services (4–6 people) [21].

Since the concept of MPRA is new, there is no established assessment tool. Therefore, we compared popular environmental assessment tools to design the survey. Through observations and analysis, we listed the following categories based on the needs, environment utilization, and behaviors of seniors in Taiwan. The five categories for environmental factors and the explanations of their relations are as follows:

1. Safety: Characteristics of the maximum environmental safety protection.
2. Accessibility: Satisfy the needs of seniors to arrive, enter, unite, and access spaces.
3. Comfortableness: Ensuring people reach their destination smoothly while enjoying outdoor living space and public amenities.
4. Social support: Social activities and mental health support are available within the environment.
5. Independence/Privacy: Seniors can easily join a variety of activities available in various spaces and scales with their privacy protected.

2.2. Data Analysis

We designed the survey to assess the respondents' feedback on the MPRA for seniors referring to the previous research. The assessment indicators were selected for the seniors of the age of over 55 years. We divided the respondents into three different groups based on their age: 55–64, 65–74, and over 75 years old. We compared the answers from 140 responses of the three groups. We used SPSS20.0 to analyze the results.

2.2.1. Reliability Analysis

Reliability is tested to decide whether the results collected in a survey have consistency and stability. We used Cronbach's Alpha to evaluate the survey. If the analysis and assessment value is higher, the results are consistent with a smaller deviation. The value of Cronbach's Alpha was higher than 0.9 to confirm the reliability of the survey.

2.2.2. Basic Data Analysis

Among the 140 respondents, 37.9% were males and 62.1% were females. Moreover, 42.1% were 55–64 years old, while the rest were older than 65 years old. Furthermore, 9.3% had a junior high school education; 21.4% attended senior high school or career school; 55.1% had a junior college or university education; and 14.3% had a postgraduate degree. Regarding living situations, 48.6% lived in a house or townhouse; 2.9% lived in social housing; 36.4% resided in a condominium building with an elevator; and 11.4% lived in a condominium building without an elevator. Regarding cohabitation, 17.1% lived alone; 24.3% lived with a spouse; 24.3% lived with a spouse and at least a child; 17.1% had three generations living together; 5% lived with a caregiver; and 2.1% lived with at least a parent. These statistics were consistent with those of the Ministry of Health and Welfare showing that over 70% of seniors were in disadvantaged living conditions.

Furthermore, 60.7% were aware of MPRA, 79.3% were willing to live in a community utilizing the MPRA concept, 80.7% believed that their living space needed to be changed as they age, and 79% agreed that MPRA met the needs of seniors by transforming the traditional daily activity spaces into a network of services with buildings of a higher density. Regarding time spent away from their residence, 47.9% spent 10 min, 34.3% took 10 to 20 min, 8.6% took 20 to 30 min, and only 7.9% spent 30 min away. Regarding the number of residents in the MPRA community, 47.9% preferred having less than 10; 18.6% preferred 11 to 15; 25.7% preferred 16 to 30; and 7.9% preferred 30. This revealed the preference for living in smaller residential communities based on the residents' diverse needs. It also showed how it was important to build a higher-density facility for seniors in Taiwan, including outdoor spaces. Several seniors needed to take a longer commute time to the areas of activities.

2.2.3. Analysis of Multiple-Choice Questions

Seniors' needs for space and community environment change according to their physical and mental abilities were assessed. There are issues identified regarding improving the current environment and community amenities.

When being asked about preferred activities for social interactions, "arts and crafts" was required by 62.7% of the respondents followed by "volunteering" (54.2%); "weekend dining" (50.8%); "eco-farm visits" (50.8%); "community gatherings" (44.4%); "markets" (42.4%); and "theatre and performances" (39%). For preferred amenities in a community, "park and green space" was chosen by 87.9% with "convenient stores" (80.7%), "medical clinics" (77.9%), "exercise and gym space" (77.1%), "outdoor activity space" (77.1%), "community classes" (57.1%), "care hubs" (57.1%), "rehabilitation space" (27.1%), "senior care center" (57.1%), "religious space" (28.6%), "eco-farms" (33.6%), "community office" (27.1%), "child care" (23.6%), and "hotels and travel accommodation" (22.9%). For preferred services at a reasonable cost of MPRA, 86.4% believed that cleaning services were important. This was followed by "meal services' (71.4%), "assisted rehabilitation" or "assisted outdoor walk service" (70%), "assisted living" (52.1%), and "medina delivery" (45.7%). Regarding the benefits of MPRA, physical and emotional health was important for the respondents (79.3%) along with a safe living environment (76.5%), diverse interactions (75.7%), the quality of life with public facilities (66.4%), community participation rate (54.3%), and inheritance from generations of experience (33.6%).

2.2.4. Environmental Indicators

- Safety: The visibility of traffic signs, pedestrian walk time signals, and the accessibility of simple and proper traffic guidance scored low with 74.3% of the respondents agreeing.
- Social Support: Community healthcare and senior care sanitation scored low as 63.6% expressed dissatisfaction.
- Privacy: The functionality of existing public amenities was scored low as 36% of the respondents indicated dissatisfaction.
- Accessibility: The distance between home and service locations in the existing community and the density of public amenities scored low as 40% expressed dissatisfaction.
- Comfortableness: The availability of different sizes of activity spaces in communities was scored low as 47.9% indicated dissatisfaction.

2.2.5. Significance

We used environmental indicators to assess the community's inclusiveness for senior citizens to set five major indicators. We surveyed 140 respondents based on their individual needs, feedback, and level of satisfaction with their outdoor living environment. Analysis of variance (ANOVA) and independent t-tests were conducted to understand the diverse needs of seniors and the differences between their cognition and attitude (Table 1).

Table 1. Differences in environmental indicators.

Indicators	Question	Ages
Safety	The community environment makes people feel safe and secure	F = 4.910 p = 0.009 **
Independence/Privacy	Space with privacy and social functions	F = 7.298 p = 0.001 ***
Social support	Activities in the area where you currently live meet your needs	F = 4.391 p = 0.014 *
Social support	Nursing care and adult sunshine services in the current community	F = 3.855 p = 0.024 *

1 Source: compiled by this research. 2 statistically significant "*" as $p < 0.05$, statistically significant "**" $p < 0.01$, and statistically highly significant "***" as $p < 0.001$.

Regarding safety, 32.2% of the respondents aged 55–64 years strongly agreed, 17.2% of those aged 65–74 years disagreed, 5.9% aged over 75 years disagreed, and 8.5% of those aged 55–64 years, 12.5% of those aged 65–75 years, and 29.4% of those aged over 75 years strongly agreed. With independence and privacy, 34.9% of the respondents aged 55–64 years strongly disagreed, and 26.6% of those aged 65–74 years disagreed, while 70.6% of those aged 75 years disagreed. The respondents were dissatisfied with the availability of spaces and environments that encourage more social interactions while respecting their privacy. Thus, it is necessary to provide choices, diversity, and a variety of activities in space. Regarding social support, 45.8% of the respondents aged 55–64 years disagreed, while 31.3% of those aged 65–74 years and 23.5% of those aged 75 years also disagreed. Regarding day-care services, 16.9% of those disagreed, while 54.2% of the respondents aged 55–64 years, 4.7% of those aged 65–74 years, and 51.6% of those aged 75 years disagreed, too. Respondents aged over 75 years believed that there was a lack of services available for senior care, followed by those aged 65–74 and 55–64 years. It is necessary to improve the services available for senior care to make them feel confident about the availability of services (Table 2).

Table 2. Differences in cognitive attitude.

Question	Ages
The living environment needs to change as we are getting old	F = 4.910 $p = 0.009$ **
Time from home to most frequently used facilities?	F = 19.822 $p = 0.003$ **
Do you think transforming horizontal service to vertical service is more suitable for the elderly?	F = 12.605 $p = 0.050$ *

1 Source: compiled by this research. 2 statistically significant "*" as $p < 0.05$, statistically significant "**" $p < 0.01$.

Regarding the time spent commuting to the space for activities, 55.9% of the respondents aged 55–64 years wanted to spend less than 10 min while 30.5% needed 10 to 20 min; 6.8% needed 20 to 30 min and 6.8% needed longer than 30 min. For the respondents between the ages of 65 and 74 years, 50% needed less than 10 min, 35.9% needed 10 to 20 min, 12.5% needed 20 to 30 min, and 1.6% needed longer than 30 min. For the respondents aged over 75 years, 29.4% needed less than 10 min, 41.2% needed 10 to 20 min, and 50% needed longer than 30 min. Moreover, 11.8% of the respondents ages 55–64 years disagreed that MPRA was necessary to transform the traditional ways of accessing daily activity spaces in the building with more density, while 76.5% agreed and 11.8% strongly agreed. Furthermore, 8.3% of the respondents aged 65–74 years strongly disagreed and 4.2% disagreed while 66.7% agreed and 20.8% strongly agreed. Lastly, 14.3% of the respondents aged over 75 years strongly disagreed and 35.7% disagreed, while 50% agreed.

3. Results

3.1. Needs for Living Space and Mpra Design Concept

In total, 79.3% of the respondents showed their willingness to live in a community designed with the MPRA concept, and 80.7% wanted to change their living space as they age. Their areas of activity are reduced as their physical and mental health deteriorates. Moreover, 47.9% of the respondents preferred to spend less than 10 min to arrive at the space, and 79.3% wanted to have the space in a building with a high density. The respondents believed the MPRA design concept could provide a safer living environment (76.5%), improve diverse interactions (75.7%), maintain their physical and mental health (79.3%), improve their quality of life (75.7%), promote the sharing of more public amenities (66.4%), and increase the level of community engagement (54.3%). Most respondents had a positive attitude toward the MPRA design concept.

Dissatisfaction was observed in social support, comfortableness, accessibility, independence and privacy, and safety. Moreover, 63.6% of the respondents were dissatisfied with social support. Services available for senior care, day-care, and social support were insufficient to meet the needs of the respondents in Taiwan. Over 50% of the respondents preferred "park and green space" (87.9%), "convenient stores" (80.7%), "medical clinics" 77.9%), "exercise and gym space" (77.1%), "community classes" (57.1%), "care hubs" (57.1%), "rehabilitation space" (27.1%), and "senior care center" (57.1%).

In adopting the MPRA design concept, the needs of diverse users must be considered. Based on the needs of residents and their physical and mental abilities, a range of options and spaces must be available to meet their needs. Then, satisfaction with and ability to access social supports and independent living can be enabled to mitigate the deterioration of their physical and mental abilities.

3.2. Ages and Cognitive Attitudes and Spatial Needs for MPRA

In total, 74.6% of the respondents aged 55–64 years, 93.8% of those aged 65–74 years, and 47.1% of those over 75 years needed changes in their living space as their physical and mental abilities changed. Moreover, 88.3% of the respondents aged 55–64 years, 87.5% of those aged 65–74 years, and 50% of the respondents aged over 75 years had preconceptions about the MPRA design. The level of acceptance for a change in environment became lower with age. Therefore, it is necessary to apply the MPRA design concept as early as possible to provide familiarity with aging. Moreover, 55.9% of the respondents aged 55–64 years and 50% of those aged 65–74 years preferred 10 min regarding travel time to their activity areas, but 50% of those aged 75 years needed over 30 min of travel time.

Many necessities do not meet the needs of the respondents' regular activities. It is important to provide the respondents with a variety of space options and activities that meet their diverse needs.

4. Discussion and Conclusions

Neighborhood social capital and cohesion are important for the life and well-being of the elderly [22]. The loneliness of the elderly affects their health, well-being, and longevity [23]. Leisure activities and social support help people resist stress, reduce the incidence of diseases, and maintain physical and mental health [24]. Residents' participation, involvement, and dedication are positively correlated with well-being [25].

Most of the respondents in this study showed a positive attitude toward the MPRA design concept. They wanted their living space to be changed as they age because their areas of activities became more limited. By using the MPRA design concept, spaces can be vertically expanded to transform the traditional ways of expanding spaces horizontally. The new concept of the expansion allowed the respondents to be more engaged in social activities, delayed their aging process, and supported more positive and healthy interactions. It also promotes connections and relationships between residents, visitors, and MPRA residents.

The MPRA design concept must be used to provide a variety of housing options and services for the needs of the residents. In addition to adopting common design concepts and providing a therapeutic environment for residents, stronger connections between the residents and the local community and society must be provided for seniors to live independently with better accessibility. In the MPRA design concept, common design ideas and therapeutic design need to be integrated to connect it to the existing community and social welfare systems and the transportation network. This maximizes seniors' abilities to live independently in an inclusive and accessible environment in an aging society.

The results of this study show the following necessities for seniors:

- Safety: Indoor carpets to reduce the possibility of slipping, falling, injury, and noise.
- Accessibility: The destination reached by public transportation and connected to the local community service.
- Comfort: The design of assistive devices to increase the sense of dignity for the elderly, such as intelligent lift cabinets and handrails embedded into the interior wall design or combined with other art installations (Figure 1)
- Privacy/Independence: different room sizes and households and an intelligent identification system.
- Social support: Day-care and temporary-care facilities to increase activity space and care.

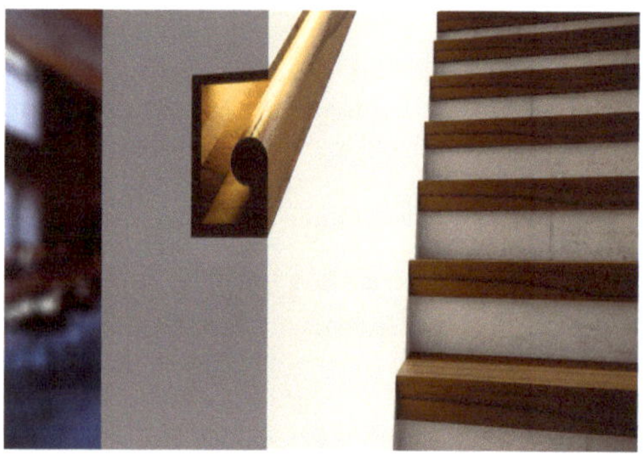

Figure 1. Handrails embedded into the interior wall design.

Author Contributions: Conceptualization, T.-Y.C. and S.-Y.T.; methodology, T.-Y.C. and S.-Y.T.; software T.-Y.C.; validation, T.-Y.C.; formal analysis, T.-Y.C.; investigation, T.-Y.C.; resources, T.-Y.C.; data curation, T.-Y.C.; writing—original draft preparation, T.-Y.C.; writing—review and editing, T.-Y.C. and S.-Y.T.; visualization, T.-Y.C.; supervision, S.-Y.T. All authors have read and agreed to the published version of the manuscript.

Funding: This research received no external funding.

Institutional Review Board Statement: This study did not require ethical approval.

Informed Consent Statement: Informed consent was obtained from all subjects involved in the study.

Data Availability Statement: Data are contained within the article.

Conflicts of Interest: The authors declare no conflict of interest.

References

1. Agata, W.; Magda, M.; Ewa, P. Designing Residential Architecture for Future Societies. The Central and Eastern European Context—On the Basis of the Example of Poland. In *Advances in Human Factors and Ergonomics in Healthcare and Medical Devices, International Conference on Applied Human Factors and Ergonomics*; Springer: Berlin/Heidelberg, Germany, 2021; Volume 263, pp. 337–344.
2. Godbey, G. *Leisure in Your Life: An Exploration*, 3rd ed.; Venture: State College, PA, USA, 1999.
3. Wu, W.; Chuang, K.Y. Aging in Place: The Direction of Taiwan Long-Term Care Policy in the 21st Century. *Taiwan J. Public Health* **2001**, *20*, 192–201.
4. Li, J.J. *HoChin Cohousing Compound: Happiness Senior's Life*, 3rd ed.; PA: Ce-MA: Taipei, Taiwan, 2020.
5. Paterson, D.H.; Jones, G.R.; Rice, C.L. Ageing and physical activity: Evidence to develop exercise recommendations for older adults. *Can. J. Public Health* **2007**, *98*, 69–108.
6. Patoine, B.; Mattoli, S. *Staying Sharp: Current Advance on Brain Research. Memory Loss and Aging*; AARP Andrus Foundation: Washington, DC, USA; The Dana Alliance for Brain Initiatives: New York, NY, USA, 2012.
7. Carvalho, A. On the importance of common spaces in housing: Social interaction for elderly living. *Territorio* **2018**, *86*, 136–145. [CrossRef]
8. Burton, E.; Mitchell, L. *Inclusive Urban Design: Streets for Life*; Elsevier: Oxford, UK, 2006.
9. Zastrow, C.H.; Kirst, A.; Karen, K.; Hessenauer, S.L. Understanding Human Behavior and the Social Environment. Brooks/Cole Pub Co.: Utah Salt Lake City, UT, USA, 2018.
10. Wang, J.P.; Qun, T. Study on the Walking Space Design of the Aged People. *Huazhong Archit.* **2009**, *27*, 49–50.
11. Lin, W. Outdoor Space Design of senior citizens living areas in urban. *Huazhong Archit.* **2005**, *2*, 77–78.
12. Chen, C.H. The Concept of Total Planning for Senior Housing. *Taiwan Gerontol. Geriatr.* **2006**, *1*, 122–139.
13. Senior Cohousing How-to Guide, How to Create Retrofit Cohousing: Applying the Principles of Senior-Cohousing to Existing Homes and Communities. Available online: https://communitycouncil.ca/wp-content/uploads/2020/01/HOW-TO-Create-Retrofit-Cohousing-2016.pdf (accessed on 10 February 2023).
14. Niezabitowska, E. Mieszkania dla ludzi starych i młodych w kontekście potrzeb i cyklu życia budynku mieszkalnego (Flats for the old and young in the context of their needs and useful life of a residential building). In *Przestrzenie Starościi*; Zrałek, M., Ed.; Publishing House Oficyna Wydawnicza Humanitas; Wyższa Szkoła Humanitas: Sosnowiec, Poland, 2012.
15. Ulrich, R.U.; Zimring, C.; Zhu, X.; DuBose, J.; Seo, H.B.; Choi, Y.S.; Quan, X.; Joseph, A. A review of the research literature on evidence-based healthcare design. *HERD* **2008**, *1*, 61–125. [CrossRef] [PubMed]
16. National Design Guide-Planning Practice Guidance for Beautiful, Enduring and Successful Places. Available online: https://assets.publishing.service.gov.uk/media/602cef1d8fa8f5038595091b/National_design_guide.pdf (accessed on 12 February 2023).
17. Ke, S.F.; Li, H. Environmental assessment tools for dementia patients: A review. *Chin. J. Nurs.* **2014**, *49*, 211–215.
18. Environmental Assessment Tool-High Care. Handbook. Available online: https://www.enablingenvironments.com.au/uploads/5/0/4/5/50459523/dta_resource3_digital.pdf (accessed on 2 March 2023).
19. Parker, C.; Barnes, S.; McKee, K.J.; Morgan, K.; Torrington, J.; Tregenza, P. Quality of life and building design in residential and nursing homes for older people. *Ageing Soc.* **2004**, *24*, 41–62. [CrossRef]
20. Lewis, A.; Torrington, J.; Barnes, S.; Darton, R.; Holder, J.; McKee, K.; Netten, A.; Orrell, A. EVOLVE: A tool for evaluating the design of older people's housing. *Hous. Care Support* **2010**, *13*, 36–41. [CrossRef]
21. Senior Cohousing How-to Guide. How to Create New-Build Cohousing. Available online: https://communitycouncil.ca/wp-content/uploads/2020/01/HOW-TO-Create-New-Build-Cohousing-2016.pdf (accessed on 10 February 2023).
22. Cramm, J.M.; Dijk, H.M.; Nieboer, A.P. The Importance of Neighborhood Social Cohesion and Social Capital for the Well Being of Older Adults in the Community. *Gerontologist* **2012**, *53*, 142–152. [CrossRef]
23. Paredes, A.M.; Lee, E.E.; Chik, L.; Palmer, B.M.; Palinkas, L.A.; Kim, H.C.; Jeste, D.V. Qualitative study of loneliness in a senior housing community: The importance of wisdom and other coping strategies. *Aging Ment. Health* **2020**, *25*, 59–566.

24. Santrock, J.W. *Life-Span Development*, 9th ed.; McGraw-Hill: New York, NY, USA, 2004.
25. Chen, M.F.; Chen, S.Y. A Study on the Degree of Community Participation of Organic Villagers and Its Influence on Happiness. *Agric. Ext. Anthol.* **2012**, *57*, 159–169.

engineering proceedings

Proceeding Paper

Use of Nearpod in Reducing Word Usage Errors in Chinese Lessons †

Mei Rianto Chandra [1,*] and Qian Kun [2]

1 Chinese Department, Bina Nusantara University, Jakarta 11480, Indonesia
2 School of Liberal Arts, Jiangsu University, Zhenjiang 212013, China; qkjon@ujs.edu.cn
* Correspondence: mei.chandra@binus.edu
† Presented at the 2024 IEEE 4th International Conference on Electronic Communications, Internet of Things and Big Data, Taipei, Taiwan, 19–21 April 2024.

Abstract: Nearpod is a learning platform that allows interactions between students in online learning so that students can have the opportunity to provide ideas and answers to questions given directly. We used qualitative methods to analyze the differences between students' understanding of learning material before and after using Nearpod. The objects were 30 students who studied teaching materials for three months. The test material was used for students to study. In 40−60% of learning, the materials were used. An examination was conducted by composing sentences and making sentences. The change in the increase in student's errors showed a significant difference. In conversation-solving questions, correct answers increased from 33 to 74%, and in sentence construction, that increased from 30 to 67%. This result presented students' positive responses to Nearpod with a satisfaction rate of 80%. Students who used Nearpod improved word memory but needed to pay attention to the choice of words when typing using pinyin input.

Keywords: language learning; Nearpod; memorize; Mandarin

Citation: Chandra, M.R.; Kun, Q. Use of Nearpod in Reducing Word Usage Errors in Chinese Lessons. *Eng. Proc.* **2024**, *74*, 63. https://doi.org/10.3390/engproc2024074063

Academic Editors: Shu-Han Liao, Teen-Hang Meen and Cheng-Fu Yang

Published: 18 September 2024

1. Introduction

Nowadays, in teaching Mandarin, PowerPoint materials are widely used. Interactive teaching supports are used more than before apart from using books and materials. Third-party applications provide a fun learning experience for students. Learning Mandarin is different from learning other foreign languages. Learning Mandarin requires an understanding of the characteristics of the Mandarin language, so this challenges learners [1].

Online learning demands collaboration between teachers and students. Nearpod can be useful for foreign students as they have challenges in using Mandarin every day. Students view online education as having a big impact. Student participation is essential to engage in the learning environment [2]. Student participation is crucial to enhancing the learning outcome [3]. The quality of online education needs to be improved to be at a similar level to traditional face-to-face classroom-based education [4].

2. Conceptual Background

2.1. Online Learning Platform

Electronic media is difficult to use but valuable in motivating students and the teacher to understand content, students, and technology [5,6]. It enables an integrated learning management for Chinese as a foreign language learning in Indonesia. It is necessary to continuously evaluate e-learning to ensure higher-quality teaching and learning [7]. A lack of collaboration between students negatively impacts this [8]. Learning through mobile devices allows students to search for data and communicate with material related to the available databases and the interactive environment in learning to increase learning interactions between participants [9,10].

2.2. Nearpod Platform Learning

Nearpod can be used to make presentations, provide instructors with knowledge, and engage students in a variety of ways. It also provides real-time assessments to make students learn in class actively [11–14]. Distance learning enhances effective learning and improves collaboration and interactions in teaching, including providing high-level cognitive tasks [15–17]. This Nearpod application also makes it easier for teachers to design online-learning, owing to its features. Using e-modules on science materials, "energy and change" can be available for students. Nearpod can be used in a teaching and learning process that is interactive, motivating, and interesting [14,18,19]. Nearpod is also used to explore content and activities and improve academic performance and student participation in educational resources [20,21].

2.3. Relationship between Technology and Learning

Game-based learning positively influences students. The effect of gamification stimulates students' cognitive processes and learning experiences [22]. Student learning engagement is lower in problem-based learning in writing classes with Augmented Reality than in traditional teacher-centered learning, partly due to the need for student involvement in learning [23]. There are other factors, such as limited resources and inappropriate administrative structure, which affect learning outcomes [24]. In mobile learning, techniques and learning theories are used to meet shifting demands [25]. Overall, technology can increase the learning effect and restore the essence of learning [26].

3. Research Method

A qualitative approach research method was used for 31 students to determine the effects of Nearpod before and after its use. The framework of this research is presented in Figure 1.

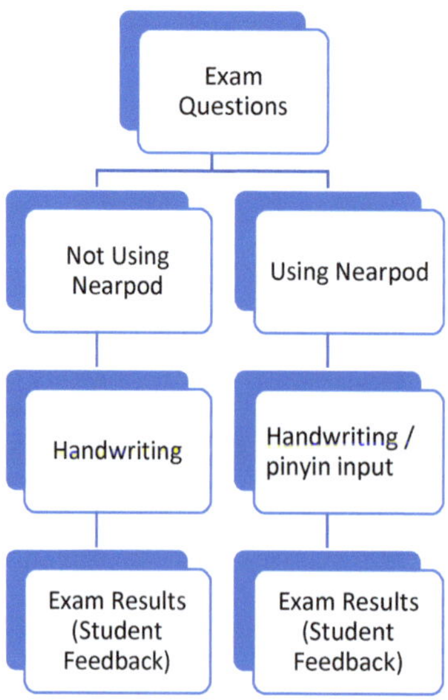

Figure 1. Framework of this research.

3.1. Nearpod

3.1.1. Main Function

Nearpod's interactive screen provides pages about lessons, profiles, reports, and sub-plans. Users are only given a quota of 100 Mb/account for a free account (Figure 2). The types of interactive media presented vary, ranging from video learning, VR field trips, matching pairs, wall-climb games, and others.

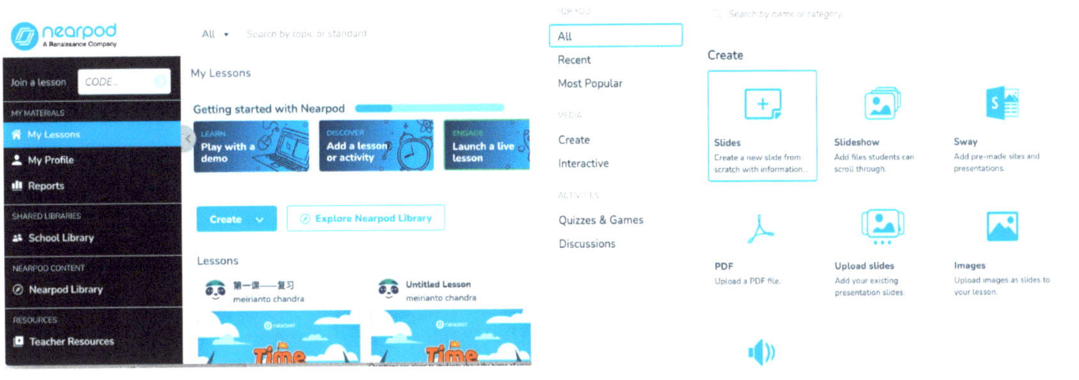

Figure 2. Main function of Nearpod.

3.1.2. Interaction Function

The functions of Nearpod allow users to answer on their respective boards, and the teacher can monitor what the students are wiring them in real-time (Figure 3).

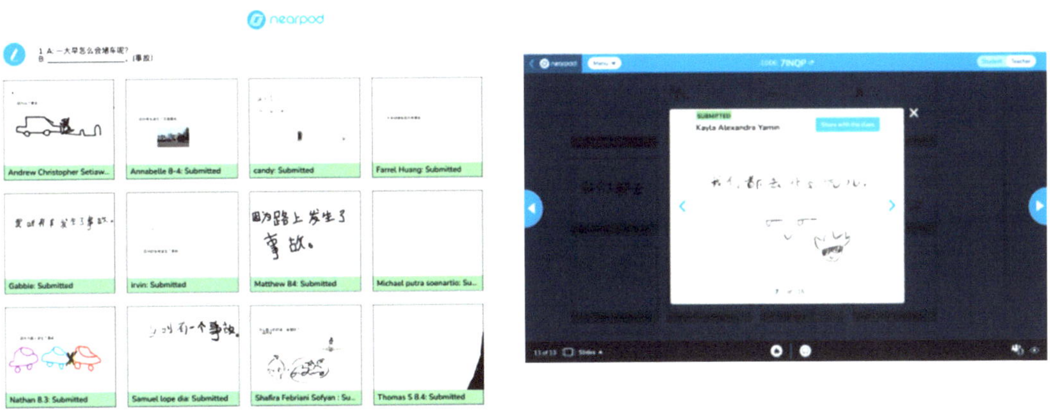

(a) (b)

Figure 3. (**a**) Interactive wall and (**b**) answers on it.

The answers for Figure 3a, 因为路上发生了事故 (Because there is accident in the street); 当时有一个(起)事故 (there is a accident at that time); Figure 3b 我们都去北京玩儿 (we go to Beijing to have fun).

4. Result and Discussion

4.1. Errors in Learning

Questions are given to students about the types of vocabulary and the review of the exercises on Nearpod (Table 1). Learners are asked to complete the sentences and make sentences using the words given (Table 1).

Table 1. Nearpod questions.

Complete the Dialogue:
1. A: 一大早怎么会堵车呢? (How could there be a traffic jam so early in the morning) B: ___________。(事故) (Accident)
2. A: ___________. (把)。(Preposition) B: 好的,我马上送过去。(Okay, I'll send it over right away)
3. A: ___________. (以前) (A long time ago) B: 真的假的? 看不出来哦。(Is that true or not? I can't tell.)
4. A: 这道题怎么会填错呢? (How could this question be answered incorrectly?) B: ___________。(马虎) (careless)
5. A: 你这周末都去哪儿玩了? (Where did you go this weekend?) B: ___________. (都) (all)
Making Sentences: 以前, 被, 什么… 也 …, 每隔, 送给 (a long time ago, auxiliary, whatever… also, every period, give)

Wrong answers from students included grammatical errors, including word order errors (syntax) and word meanings (semantics), and class errors in writing words, including words with the same meaning (Table 2).

Table 2. Correct and wrong answers.

Words	Using Nearpod		Ratio
	No	Yes	
Complete Dialogue	**Right Answers**		
事故 shìgu (accident)	50%	87%	+37%
把 bǎ (preposition)	43%	76%	+33%
以前 yǐqián (a long time ago)	23%	76%	+53%
马虎 mǎhu (careless)	13%	87%	+74%
都 dōu (all)	53%	87%	+34%
Make Sentences			
以前 yǐqián (a long time ago)	23%	90%	+67%
被 bèi (auxiliary)	23%	90%	+67%
什么 … 也 … shénme … yě (whatever… also)	40%	70%	+30%
每隔 měigé (every… period)	16%	70%	+54%
送给 sònggěi (give)	53%	93%	+40%

Errors in hand-writing words were dominated by the wrong arrangement and mistakes in choosing words in a sentence (Table 3).

Table 3. Word errors in handwriting.

Error\Number	1	2	3	4	5	6	7	8	9	10
Grammar	10	8	17	18	8	11	14	14	9	6
Characters	3	9	5	6	6	11	5	3	8	6
(No answer)	2	-	1	2	-	1	4	1	8	2
True	15	13	7	4	16	7	7	12	5	16
Total	30	30	30	30	30	30	30	30	30	30

Errors were found in grammar, word order and syntax, and sentence meaning. Meanwhile, in writing words, errors occurred in using correct words. For example, mistakes in writing the word 吗 become 马, and 评 became 枰. Students were unable to write the Chinese characters, for example, the letters "蔬菜", which were written as "shucai" (Figure 4).

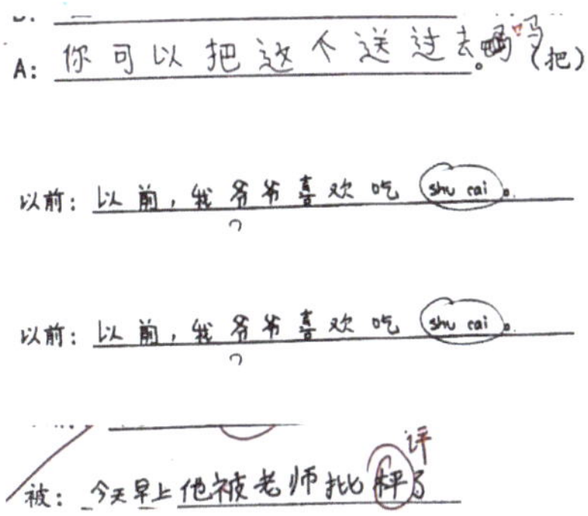

Figure 4. Errors in writing 吗 and 评.

There were other errors in that students could not order words correctly and use correct words in a sentence (Figure 5).

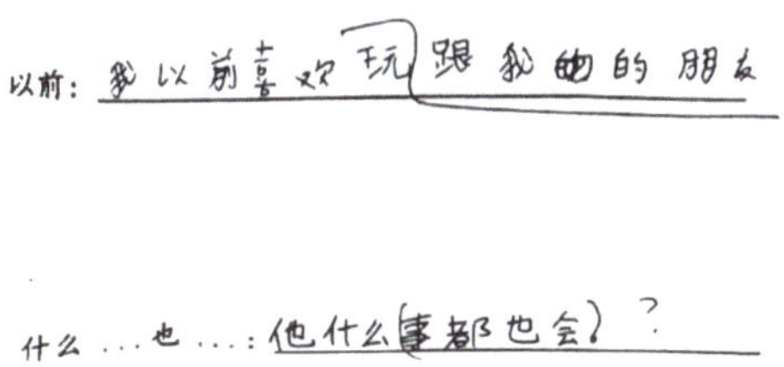

Figure 5. Students' errors in word order and meaning.

Most students made the mistakes of not filling in sentences/answers and of grammar in writing Chinese characters (Figure 6).

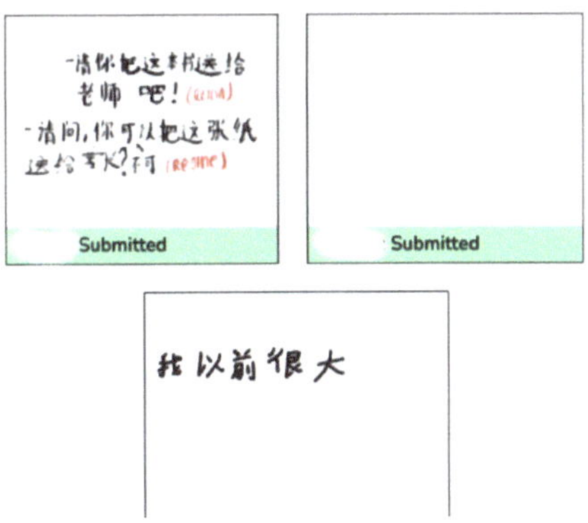

Figure 6. Students' errors in not filling sentence and grammar.

There is a significant difference in the use of Nearpod in vocabulary mastery, where students using Nearpod expressed more ideas. The error rate in grammar was higher than in handwriting. Most students used Nearpod when they did not know the correct answers. Figure 7 shows the number of errors before and after using Nearpod.

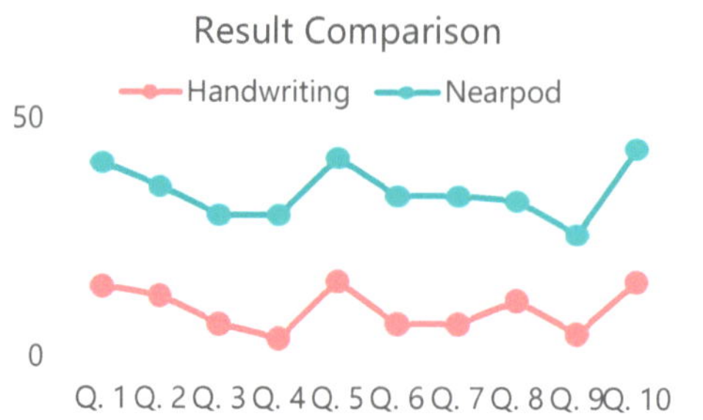

Figure 7. Difference in results of students before (in red) and after using Nearpod (in green).

4.2. *Student Interview*

The interview with students showed that Nearpod significantly influenced students' learning abilities (Table 4).

Table 4. Errors of students with Nearpod.

Error	1	2	3	4	5	6	7	8	9	10
Grammar	2	3	2	1	2	-	-	4	2	-
Characters	-	-	-	-	-	-	-	-	-	-
No answer	2	4	5	3	2	3	3	5	7	2
True	26	23	23	26	26	27	27	21	21	28
Total	30	30	30	30	30	30	30	30	30	30

Students using Nearpod were more active in learning vocabulary. However, there are still questions on the usage of Nearpod (Table 5).

Table 5. Questions and answers of students using Nearpod.

Questions	Answers			
	D*	C*	B*	A*
1. I am satisfied with the teaching system settings on Nearpod	1	7	14	8
2. I am satisfied with the way teachers explain on Nearpod	-	6	13	11
3. Nearpod teaching with the addition of multimedia makes me feel satisfied.	1	10	9	10
Questions	No	Unsure		Yes
4. Learning with Nearpod makes me able to remember longer.	3	15		12
5. Nearpod is easy to run.	7	7		16
6. Teaching with Nearpod can improve language skills.	1	15		14
7. Do you agree that all teachers should use Nearpod? Why?				
8. What are your suggestions for the Nearpod App?				

(A*: Very satisfied; B*: Satisfied; C*: Unsure; D*: Not Satisfied).

1. "Do you agree that all teachers should use Nearpod? Why?"
   21 students (70%) answered that it was necessary, but several disagreed with the following reasons.
   - No, when drawing Mandarin characters, the pen does not work well and often makes errors.
   - Not so, because it is complicated and lagging.
   - Yes, you must improve Internet constraints, and Nearpod is easier to run on specific devices, for example, laptops. If you want to use Nearpod for learning activities, it can be provided so students are okay with bringing things.

2. "What is your suggestion for Nearpod?"
    - It is good for learning activities, but I do not like how it works because it is hard to edit and run.
    - That loading is accelerated, and the draw feature is improved so that you can write more efficiently.
    - It needs to be more exciting with more tools.

5. Conclusions

Nearpod has a good effect in learning, especially in minimizing errors in the use of Mandarin vocabulary. However, Nearpod also gives students a challenge, especially for answering questions and feeling embarrassed if the teacher sees their answers. Students complained about Nearpod's memory use in devices causing lag. The results of this study showed that Nearpod affected learning Mandarin. As only 30 students participated in this study, further research is necessary to include more students and applications.

Author Contributions: Conceptualization, M.R.C.; methodology, M.R.C.; formal analysis, M.R.C. and Q.K.; writing—original draft preparation, M.R.C.; writing—review and editing, Q.K.; visualization, M.R.C.; supervision, M.R.C.; project administration, M.R.C.; funding acquisition, M.R.C. All authors have read and agreed to the published version of the manuscript.

Funding: This research was funded by Bina Nusantara University, grant number IDR001009.

Data Availability Statement: The further inquiries about the data can be directed to the corresponding author.

Acknowledgments: The authors gratefully acknowledge that the present research is supported by BINA NUSANTARA University.

Conflicts of Interest: The authors declare no conflict of interest.

References

1. Ying, Y.; Lin, X.; Yetty; Mursitama, T.N. Mobile Learning Based of Mandarin for College Students: A Case Study of International Department' Sophomores. In Proceedings of the 2017 11th International Conference on Information & Communication Technology and System (ICTS), Surabaya, Indonesia, 31 October 2017; IEEE: Piscataway, NJ, USA, 2017; pp. 281–286.
2. Wei, H.-C.; Chou, C. Online Learning Performance and Satisfaction: Do Perceptions and Readiness Matter? *Distance Educ.* **2020**, *41*, 48–69. [CrossRef]
3. Dumford, A.D.; Miller, A.L. Online Learning in Higher Education: Exploring Advantages and Disadvantages for Engagement. *J. Comput. High. Educ.* **2018**, *30*, 452–465. [CrossRef]
4. Palvia, S.; Aeron, P.; Gupta, P.; Mahapatra, D.; Parida, R.; Rosner, R.; Sindhi, S. Online Education: Worldwide Status, Challenges, Trends, and Implications. *J. Glob. Inf. Technol. Manag.* **2018**, *21*, 233–241. [CrossRef]
5. Rawendy, D.; Ying, Y.; Arifin, Y.; Rosalin, K. Design and Development Game Chinese Language Learning with Gamification and Using Mnemonic Method. *Procedia Comput. Sci.* **2017**, *116*, 61–67. [CrossRef]
6. Chua, N.A.; Tajuddin, A.J.B.A.; Soon, G.Y.; Zakaria, R.; Zaid, C.M.; Essa, M.A.E.F.I.; Ahmad, M. Mobile Applications in Mandarin Pedagogical Practice. *J. Phys. Conf. Ser.* **2020**, *1529*, 042055. [CrossRef]
7. Jureynolds; Ying, Y. Characteristics and Challenges of Chinese E-Learning Platforms in Indonesia. *J. Phys. Conf. Ser.* **2020**, *1477*, 042014. [CrossRef]
8. Mĕkota, T.; Marada, M. The Influence of Nearpod on Learning Social Geography in a Grammar School in Czecha. *Educ. Inf. Technol.* **2020**, *25*, 5167–5184. [CrossRef]
9. Chua, N.A.; Tajuddin, A.J.B.A.; Soon, G.Y.; Rashid, R.A.; Zakaria, R.; Zaid, C.M.; Ahmad, M. Classroom Research on Mandarin Foreign Language Learning Via Smartphone Applications. *J. Phys. Conf. Ser.* **2020**, *1529*, 042040. [CrossRef]
10. Liu, X. Improve Interactivity in Online Learning: Take Nearpod as an Example. *J. Educ. Humanit. Soc. Sci.* **2023**, *8*, 1954–1960. [CrossRef]
11. McClean, S.; Crowe, W. Making Room for Interactivity: Using the Cloud-Based Audience Response System Nearpod to Enhance Engagement in Lectures. *FEMS Microbiol. Lett.* **2017**, *364*, fnx052. [CrossRef] [PubMed]
12. Wang, J.; Chia, I. Engaging Students via Nearpod® in Synchronous Online Teaching. *Manag. Teach. Rev.* **2022**, *7*, 245–253. [CrossRef]
13. Hakami, M. Using Nearpod as a Tool to Promote Active Learning in Higher Education in a BYOD Learning Environment. *J. Educ. Learn.* **2020**, *9*, 119. [CrossRef]

14. Putra, A.P.; Arafik, M.; Pratiwi, I. Use of Nearpod to Enhance Student Engagement in Online Learning. In Proceedings of the 2021 7th International Conference on Education and Technology (ICET), Malang, Indonesia, 18 September 2021; IEEE: Piscataway, NJ, USA, 2021; pp. 298–303.
15. Ami, R.A. Optimalisasi pembelajaran bahasa indonesia menggunakan media pembelajaran berbasis aplikasi nearpod. *Bahtera Indones. J. Penelit. Bhs. Dan Sastra Indones.* **2021**, *6*, 135–148. [CrossRef]
16. Zhao, W. Applying Nearpod to the Teaching Chinese as a Second Language Class to Enhance Interactions and Collaborations in the Secondary Schools. In Proceedings of the 2021 4th International Conference on Humanities Education and Social Sciences (ICHESS 2021), Xishuangbanna, China, 29–31 October 2021.
17. Peng, H. Applying Nearpod to 10th-Grade History Courses to Improve Teaching Efficiency. In Proceedings of the 2021 4th International Conference on Humanities Education and Social Sciences (ICHESS 2021), Xishuangbanna, China, 29–31 October 2021.
18. Feri, A.; Zulherman, Z. Development of Nearpod-Based e Module on Science Material "Energy and Its Changes" to Improve Elementary School Student Learning Achievement. *Int. J. Educ. Learn.* **2021**, *3*, 165–174. [CrossRef]
19. Melinda Herwawan, N.; Balisar Panjaitan, N. The Influence of Using Nearpod to Improve Student's Vocabulary in Learning English as Foreign Language. *J. Pendidik. Dan Konseling* **2022**, *4*, 6076–6081.
20. Nadia Astarina, A.; Herlinda, R. Promoting active and interactive learning in a higher education online class. *Engl. J. Lit. UTama* **2022**, *6*, 534–543. [CrossRef]
21. Elizabeth Freire Espin, S.; Marcelo Rodriguez Cortez, D. Nearpod as a Gamification Resource for Teaching in Virtual Education: A Mathematical Case Study. In Proceedings of the 2022 International Conference on Inventive Computation Technologies (ICICT), Lalitpur, Nepal, 20 July 2022; IEEE: Piscataway, NJ, USA, 2022; pp. 177–183.
22. Qiao, Y.; Jia, X.; Wang, Y.; Wang, X. Research on the Influence of Competition Mechanism in Gamification Test on Learning Experiences and Learning Effects. In Proceedings of the 2022 IEEE 2nd International Conference on Educational Technology (ICET), Beijing, China, 25 June 2022; IEEE: Piscataway, NJ, USA, 2022; pp. 46–50.
23. Li, Q.; Yang, G.; Li, X.-L.; Han, M.; Zheng, X.-Q.; Li, J.-W. Integrating Problem Based Learning into Augmented Reality: The Effects on Learning Achievement in Chinese Writing Teaching. In Proceedings of the 2022 IEEE 2nd International Conference on Educational Technology (ICET), Beijing, China, 25 June 2022; IEEE: Piscataway, NJ, USA, 2022; pp. 115–119.
24. Leontyeva, I.A. Modern Distance Learning Technologies in Higher Education: Introduction Problems. *EURASIA J. Math. Sci. Technol. Educ.* **2018**, *14*, em1578. [CrossRef] [PubMed]
25. Hamidi, H.; Chavoshi, A. Analysis of the Essential Factors for the Adoption of Mobile Learning in Higher Education: A Case Study of Students of the University of Technology. *Telemat. Inform.* **2018**, *35*, 1053–1070. [CrossRef]
26. Cao, G.; Wang, M.; Xu, J. A Study on Game-Based Chinese Vocabulary Learning Tool Powered by Knowledge Graph. In Proceedings of the 2022 IEEE 2nd International Conference on Educational Technology (ICET), Beijing, China, 25 June 2022; IEEE: Piscataway, NJ, USA, 2022; pp. 41–45.

engineering proceedings

MDPI

Proceeding Paper

Using Digital Pictures to Enhance Students' Chinese Writing Skills †

Mei Rianto Chandra

Chinese Department, Bina Nusantara University, Jakarta 11480, Indonesia; mei.chandra@binus.edu

† Presented at the 2024 IEEE 4th International Conference on Electronic Communications, Internet of Things and Big Data, Taipei, Taiwan, 19–21 April 2024.

Abstract: In the past, it was not uncommon to take one image to represent an essay's contents. When writing an essay, an image is invariably formed in the mind. Using a qualitative descriptive method, a relationship between the number of digital images in the essay and the utilization of the essay was researched for 55 students. The results showed that the number of pictures was proportional to the number of words and the flow of the story in an essay but inversely proportional to the student's mastery of grammar skills. Such results provide a reference for teachers to pay attention to teaching grammar to use digital images in an essay.

Keywords: writing skill; narrative text; picture; Mandarin

1. Introduction

Composing is a process whereby ideas are put into text form; the text in an essay varies depending on the writer's content. Essays in the form of narrative are generally written about the author's experiences in the writer's style. Recently, the ways of writing narrative essays have changed. Online methods such as Gdoc (Google Documents) help writers do not type pinyin and insert digital images. Images help students write texts and impact writing abilities. Images help enhance their writing skills [1–3]. This means that images are a significant factor in developing students' writing skills and encourage them to come up with ideas for phrases in the target language [4]. Images replace writing instruction for students with diverse traits. However, previous related research lacks effort and idea development. Thus, teachers need to incorporate images to improve the writing skills of students [5–7].

2. Literature Review

Previous data showed that the application of images improved students' narrative text writing. Images can be used for concept development, sentence organization, vocabulary growth, convection, and the improvement of grammar usage [8]. Students who acquired writing proficiency through the utilization of visual aids demonstrated increased word output within the designated timeframe of 20 minutes, employed a greater number of cohesive devices, and exhibited a reduced frequency of grammatical errors in comparison to their counterparts who did not employ visual aids [9]. Images help students choose topics that suit their interests, make information easier to understand, inspire them to write more extended essays, and improve their writing abilities, especially regarding writing components and the creative use of images [10–12].

In teaching, images help students write descriptive texts. Using the Picture Learning Model (PLM), students can learn how to write narrative texts. Images can be used as a teaching tool as they provide background information and visualize scenarios. With images, students' writing exam scores significantly improved with fewer mistakes [2,6,13,14]. Using images may increase learning results in terms of students' writing abilities in English.

Citation: Chandra, M.R. Using Digital Pictures to Enhance Students' Chinese Writing Skills. *Eng. Proc.* **2024**, *74*, 64. https://doi.org/10.3390/engproc2024074064

Academic Editors: Shu-Han Liao, Teen-Hang Meen and Cheng-Fu Yang

Published: 19 September 2024

With image models, students can match their vocabulary to images and use them in the correct sequence. Students' understanding of narrative texts improves learning outcomes [1].

In the era of digitalization, teaching with images engages students to stimulate their enthusiasm for learning and lessen the issue of passive participation in class. Teachers must have the theoretical background to apply learning using digital images [13,15]. This implies that previous theories can be used to enrich the theoretical framework in the Image Strip Story.

3. Research Method

In this research, a qualitative research method was used for a case study. The outcome of students using images was analyzed. In total, 55 students were assigned for essay writing (Figure 1).

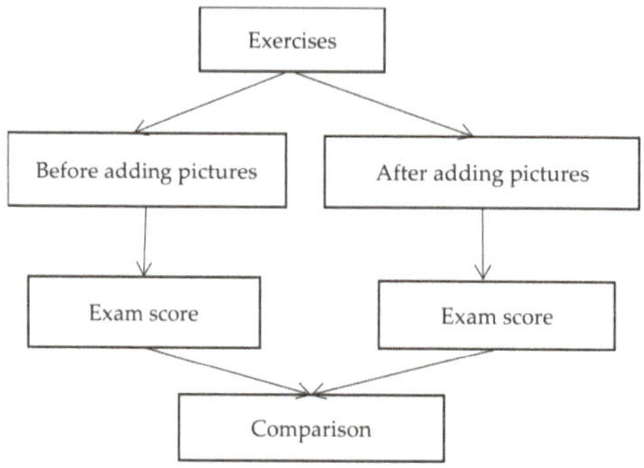

Figure 1. Research method.

4. Results and Discussion

This research was conducted in two stages of observation: before and after using digital images. In addition to assignments of narrative essays, images were inserted in recipes to assess students' writing abilities. Students were active in writing essays, and the resulting results improved (Figure 2).

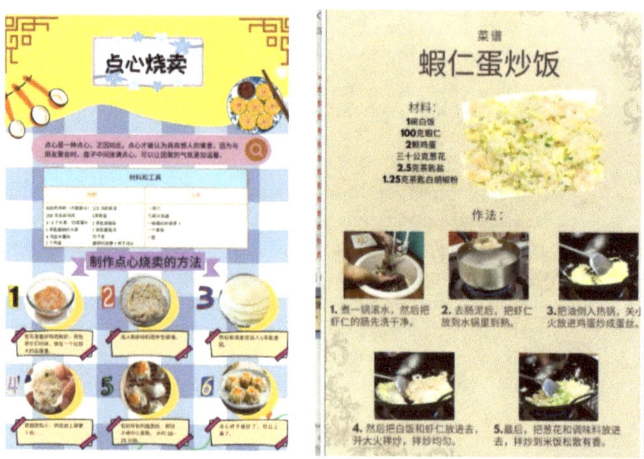

Figure 2. Student's projects.

Based on the pictures depicted above, the red lines delineate the areas where students can draw inspiration from the provided visuals for their writing. Consequently, the images can function as a navigational tool to direct their writing.

4.1. Analysis of Students' Essay

In composing narrative essays, most students used two or three digital images. With more images, the flow and the number of words were increased (Table 1). Based on the examples in Figure 3, students who insert images tend to write down the plot according to the images in their composition, which makes the use of images support students in writing narrative essays.

Table 1. Students' results in writing.

NO	A*	B*	C*	NO	A*	B*	C*
1	4	1	1	31	1	-	2
2	2	-	3	32	2	-	2
3	4	-	4	33	2	-	2
4	3	-	2	34	2	-	2
5	2	-	6	35	4	1	2
6	3	1	1	36	3	-	3
7	8	-	3	37	3	3	-
8	8	-	4	38	-	-	-
9	2	-	1	39	6	4	1
10	5	-	3	40	1	1	-
11	8	-	3	41	4	-	3
12	3	-	4	42	1	-	3
13	1	-	2	43	3	-	1
14	3	-	3	44	3	-	1
15	3	-	2	45	3	-	1
16	3	-	4	46	1	-	4
17	2	-	2	47	6	1	5
18	10	-	4	48	3	1	3
19	9	2	3	49	3	-	1
20	2	1	3	50	4	-	1
21	3	-	2	51	5	-	4
22	1	-	1	52	3	-	-
23	3	2	3	53	3	-	2
24	1	-	4	54	4	-	2
25	1	-	1	55	3	1	4
26	1	1	3				
27	1	-	5				
28	1	-	1				
29	3	-	4				
30	4	-	2				

Above the table, the description A* for article with total images inputed, B* for the total for wrong words and C* for total of grammatical errors.

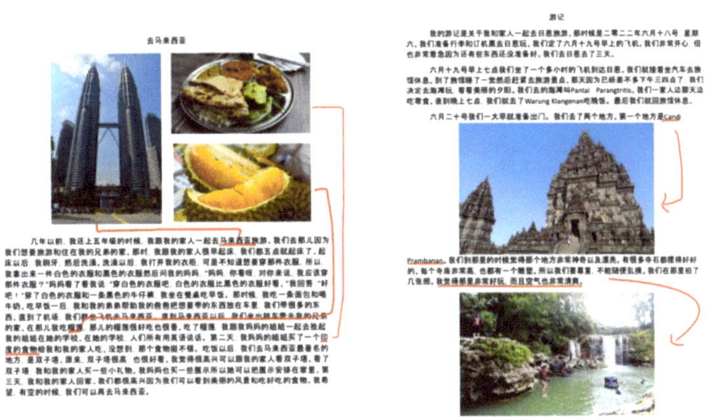

Figure 3. Student's projects.

4.2. Student's Mistakes

The most frequent mistakes in writing words were entering incorrect letters in the same pinyin, such's:

The word "小时 (xiǎoshí)" becomes "校师 (xiàoshī)"; the word "时候 (shíhou)" becomes "时后 (shíhòu)"; the word "自己 (zìjǐ)" becomes "自巳 (zìsì)"; The word "五 (wǔ)" becomes "无 (wú)"; the word "知道 (zhīdào)" becomes "这道 (zhè dào)".

From above the examples, this research finds out that grammatical mistakes were dominated by the order of the words:

3. 我们左右在巴厘岛六到七天。
(✓) 我们在巴厘岛六到七天左右。
= We're in Bali for about six to seven days.

4. 我们都五点就起床了。
(✓) 我们五点就起床了。
= We got up at five o'clock.

5. 因为我必须上大学从早上到下午。
(✓) 因为我必须从早上到下午上大学。
=Because I must go to college from morning to afternoon.

Most students did not pay attention to the context of the sentence, making the sentence's meaning and intent difficult to understand. Digital images can be used to enhance the student's cognitive progress. They also increased the skills of students. The scores ranged from 1 to 69%. Only four students did not show any improvement (Table 2).

Table 2. Students' exam results before and after inserting images.

NO	A *	B *	C *	NO	A *	B *	C *
1	92	92	=	31	85	98	↑ 13%
2	82	86	↑ 5%	32	90	98	↑ 8%
3	87	88	↑ 2%	33	90	98	↑ 8%
4	78	80	↑ 3%	34	80	98	↑ 18%
5	82	83	↑ 1%	35	90	97	↑ 7%
6	82	85	↑ 4%	36	60	97	↑ 38
7	89	91	↑ 2%	37	20	90	↑ 78%
8	85	85	=	38	40	100	↑ 60%
9	74	76	↑ 3%	39	90	90	=
10	75	77	↑ 3%	40	90	99	↑ 9%
11	87	92	↑ 6%	41	90	97	↑ 7%
12	71	74	↑ 4%	42	60	97	↑ 38
13	91	96	↑ 6%	43	90	99	↑ 9%
14	77	84	↑ 9%	44	85	99	↑ 14%
15	90	96	↑ 7%	45	15	99	↑ 85%
16	71	78	↑ 10%	46	80	96	↑ 17%
17	77	79	↑ 3%	47	90	94	↑ 4%
18	90	96	↑ 6%	48	95	98	↑ 3%
19	60	95	↑ 37	49	85	97	↑ 12%
20	90	96	↑ 6%	50	90	99	↑ 9%
21	90	98	↑ 8%	51	80	96	↑ 17%
22	60	99	↑ 39%	52	60	100	↑ 40
23	90	96	↑ 6%	53	90	98	↑ 8%
24	30	96	↑ 69%	54	85	98	↑ 13%
25	60	99	↑ 39	55	70	95	↑ 26%
26	40	95	↑ 58%				
27	50	95	↑ 47%				
28	90	99	↑ 9%				
29	95	95	=				
30	90	98	↑ 8%				

A*: score before using digital images; B*: score after using digital images; C*: progress in scores.

5. Conclusions

The use of digital images in student essays positively impacted students' learning abilities, where many students increased their ability to compose from zero to close to 10%. Students needed instructions in composing. Grammar plays an essential role in an essay. It is necessary to increase the number of students to generalize results.

Funding: This research was funded by Bina Nusantara University, grant number IDR001009.

Data Availability Statement: The further inquiries about the data can be directed to the corresponding author.

Acknowledgments: The author gratefully acknowledges that the present research is supported by BINA NUSANTARA University.

Conflicts of Interest: Chinese Linguistics, Chinese Teaching & Learning.

References

1. Hidayatullah, M.H. Improving Students' Writing Skill in Writing Narrative Text Through Image and Image Method. *JOEY J. Engl. Ibrahimy* **2022**, *1*, 35–41. [CrossRef]
2. Sarifah, N.T.; Apsari, Y. The use of image and image technique in improving student writing skill. *Proj. Prof. J. Engl. Educ.* **2020**, *3*, 664. [CrossRef]
3. Tri Endar Yogi Setiadi Saputra The Effectiveness of Image Series in Improving Students' Writing Skill at Mega Buana University. *DEIKTIS J. Pendidik. Bhs. Dan Sastra* **2023**, *3*, 111–124. [CrossRef]
4. Abdullah, Y.L.P.K.; Yunus, M.M. The use of pictures in improving students' writing. *Mod. J. Lang. Teach. Methods (MJLTM)* **2019**, 1–8.
5. Lidyawati, T.; Nirwanto, R. The effectiveness of image series toward the students' writing scores. In Proceedings of the Role of International Languages toward Global Education System, Palangka Raya, Indonesia, 25 June 2016.
6. Muchtar, A.A.; Rahmat, A.; Herlina, H. Improving Students' Narrative Text Writing Ability Through the Image and Image Learning Model. *Indones. Lang. Educ. Lit.* **2020**, *6*, 139. [CrossRef]
7. Naing, I.R.; Hamid, R. The Effectiveness of Image and Image Model in Improving the Students' Writing Skills at 8th Grade Students of SMPN 2 Pangkajene (An Experimental Research). Bachelor's Thesis, Universitas Galuh, Jawa Barat, Indonesia, 2021.
8. Ratminingsih, N.M. The Use of Personal Photographs in Writing in a Project-Based Language Learning: A Case Study. *New Engl. Teach.* **2015**, *9*, 102–118.
9. Navidinia, H.; Ozhan, A.R.; Younesi, A. Using Images in the English as Foreign Language (EFL) Classrooms: Exploring Its Potential Contribution for Developing Students' Writing Skill. *Asia Pac. J. Educ. Educ.* **2019**, *33*, 1–17. [CrossRef]
10. Ekarista, F. Improving Students' Writing Ability in Recount Text Using Image Series. *KnE Soc. Sci.* **2018**, *3*, 343. [CrossRef]
11. Kasih, A.; Gatot, S.Y.; Wardah, W. Improving students' process in writing procedure text by using image series. *J. Pendidik. Dan Pembelajaran Khatulistiwa* **2018**, 7. [CrossRef]
12. Sakkir, G. The effectiveness of images in enhance writing skill of senior high school students. *Interf. J. Lang. Lit. Linguist.* **2020**, *1*, 1–13.
13. Clarita, N.A.; Ashadi, A.; Amalia, U.; Juhansar, J. Utilizing Digital Image Series to Enhance Studentsâ€™ Performance in Writing Narrative Text. *EduLite J. Engl. Educ. Lit. Cult.* **2023**, *8*, 52. [CrossRef]
14. Erniwati, E.; Mertosono, S.R.; Rofiqoh, R.; Gente, R.A. Image Series in Teaching Writing Skills: A Literature Review. *Premise J. Engl. Educ.* **2022**, *11*, 679. [CrossRef]
15. Arik Kusuma Putra, I.G.N.; Supianti, G.A.P. The Implementation of E-Image Strip Story in English Writing. *J. Pendidik. Bhs. Ingg. Undiksha* **2023**, *10*, 285–290. [CrossRef]

engineering proceedings

Proceeding Paper

Role of Emotional Maturity and Social Support in Predicting Quarter-Life Crisis in Emerging Adulthood Using Multiple Linear Regression Analysis †

Muhamad Nanang Suprayogi * and Wira Bagus Santoso

Department of Psychology, Faculty of Humanities Bina Nusantara University, Jakarta 11480, Indonesia; wira.santoso@binus.ac.id
* Correspondence: msuprayogi@binus.edu

† Presented at the 2024 IEEE 4th International Conference on Electronic Communications, Internet of Things and Big Data, Taipei, Taiwan, 19–21 April 2024.

Abstract: This study aims to examine the role of emotional maturity and social support in predicting the level of quarter-life crisis in emerging adulthood. The employed research method was multiple linear regression analysis. The participants were individuals aged 18 to 29 years. Further, 122 participants were selected using convenience sampling. The data were collected using a questionnaire survey based on the Multidimensional Scale of Perceived Social Support to assess social support and the quarter-life crisis scale based on the theory by Robbins and Wilner. To assess emotional maturity, we used the emotional maturity scale based on the theory by Walgito. Emotional maturity and social support were important in predicting the level of quarter-life crisis in emerging adulthood. Higher levels of emotional maturity and social support were associated with lower levels of quarter-life crisis experiences in emerging adulthood.

Keywords: quarter-life crisis; emotional maturity; social support; emerging adulthood

Citation: Suprayogi, M.N.; Santoso, W.B. Role of Emotional Maturity and Social Support in Predicting Quarter-Life Crisis in Emerging Adulthood Using Multiple Linear Regression Analysis. *Eng. Proc.* **2024**, *74*, 65. https://doi.org/10.3390/engproc2024074065

Academic Editors: Shu-Han Liao, Teen-Hang Meen and Cheng-Fu Yang

Published: 20 September 2024

1. Introduction

Emerging adulthood or early adulthood is a transitional phase from adolescence to adulthood characterized by cognitive and psychological changes [1]. Every individual goes through this phase. The term emerging adulthood was introduced by Arnett [2] as a period or phase between adolescence and adulthood that occurs at around the ages of 18–29 years. According to Hurlock [3], the emerging adulthood period is a stage where individuals become more emotional, full of tension, encounter various issues, experience social isolation, and undergo changes in values and self-adjustment. During this time, individuals begin to explore their identity and the things they can do to prepare and plan for their future lives. In the emerging adulthood phase, individuals are required to become independent, solve their own life problems, determine their own path, and obtain suitable employment and career opportunities.

In a social world, the response of each individual to the demands from their surroundings inevitably varies. Several individuals may respond well to the demands and feel challenged to navigate through their upcoming life, while others may feel unprepared, excessively anxious, and pressured [4]. According to Arnett [5], when individuals are confronted with such situations, they respond seriously and enthusiastically with thorough preparation. However, they also lack sufficient preparation, leading to negative reactions such as feeling ambivalent, fearful, desperate, overwhelmed, powerless, and lacking confidence as they feel as if life is meaningless. These negative feelings cause an emotional crisis known as the quarter-life crisis [6]. Individuals in the emerging adulthood phase often face questions from their social environment that make them feel pressured. Various questions arise, including when to get married, when to graduate, when to have children, and others that seem to be never-ending [7].

According to Fischer [8], a quarter-life crisis occurs in the early- to mid-20s, caused by various pressures in life, especially concerning future prospects, encompassing issues of relationships, career, and social life. Nelson and Badger [9] stated that those who experience this crisis feel social symptoms such as anxiety about the future, loss of interest in previously enjoyed activities, physical changes such as decreased energy, and rapid emotional changes such as feeling sad without a clear reason. In this process, an individual goes through a phase of quarter-life crisis triggered by demands from family, friends, or oneself. The pressures easily lead to developing negative thoughts about their capabilities. According to Robbins and Wilner [10], the quarter-life crisis consists of seven aspects. Firstly, individuals experience indecision when faced with numerous life choices. This confusion arises due to the fear of making negative-impact mistakes. Next, individuals worry about interpersonal relationships, especially in the culture of Indonesia, where they are expected to marry and form relationships by their 30s. The problems and pressures in these relationships can disrupt their individual activities. Moreover, anxiety emerges because individuals in the emerging adulthood phase have aspirations and dreams that are difficult to attain, accompanied by feelings of worry and fear of failure. Depressive feelings can also arise when individuals face issues that disturb their minds and hinder their daily activities. Negative self-assessment leads individuals to doubt their abilities in facing life's challenges. Furthermore, such feelings while trapped in challenging situations cause individuals to feel stuck and contribute to them struggling to make the right decisions. Lastly, feelings of despair arise when an individual's hopes are unmet, leading to a sense of failure and self-disappointment.

Seventy percent of individuals in emerging adulthood experience a quarter-life crisis. A survey conducted by Gumtree.com found that 86% of 1000 young people admitted feeling pressured to achieve success in romance, finances, and their careers before the age of 30 years [11]. LinkedIn conducted a survey whose results indicated that 75% of those individuals aged 25–33 years experienced a quarter-life crisis [12]. Artiningsih and Savira [13] found that, among 63 adults in Surabaya, Indonesia, 55.6% had negative emotions related to their current condition, such as feeling empty when seeing photos of their friends with their partners, unworthy, and experiencing low self-esteem when they felt that they were not like their peers.

Two factors influence a quarter-life crisis, namely internal and external factors [14]. Internal factors are triggered from within oneself, one of which is related to emotional maturity. Hurlock [3] stated that individuals with emotional maturity carefully assess situations before taking action so that they do not act without prior thought. In this regard, individuals with emotional maturity do not feel confused when choosing future life paths because they consider the available options thoroughly beforehand. One of the external factors that influences the potential of a quarter-life crisis is social support.

Walgito [15] stated that emotional maturity comprises four important aspects. The first aspect is emotional control. Individuals with emotional maturity regulate their emotions and expressions effectively. They manage their emotions and determine when and how they express them even in situations of unstable emotions. For acceptance by oneself and others, emotionally mature individuals are capable of accepting their own and others' conditions based on reality. They understand their emotions and know the causes of those emotions. Individuals who take responsibility for their own self-control think objectively and have tolerance for various things when experiencing negative emotions. Lastly, individuals with emotional maturity make wiser decisions compared to those who do not possess it. This is because they think with careful consideration before making decisions.

Social support refers to the encouragement provided to others in the form of trust or attention with the intention of assisting them [16]. Social support evokes feelings of emotional closeness, being valued, feeling noticed, being safe, and feeling loved by one's environment [17]. Social support makes individuals feel cared for, loved, boosts their self-confidence, and improves their sense of competence. Zimet et al. [18] described social support as the assistance individuals receive from close individuals, including family, friends, and other significant individuals in their surroundings. Social support provides additional information and perspectives that help individuals to consider broader options and factors that may not have been considered before. Moreover, social support helps individuals to cope with the pressure and stress that might affect their ability to make rational decisions. Sarafino and Smith [19] proposed four important aspects of social support, including emotional support, instrumental support, informational support, and appraisal support.

2. Methods

2.1. Participants

One-hundred-eleven participants were recruited using a non-probability sampling method with a convenience sampling technique. The participants were in emerging adulthood and aged between 18 and 29 years (Table 1).

Table 1. Participants' demographic information.

Categories	n	%
Gender		
Male	33	27%
Female	89	73%
Age		
<20 years old	4	3.3%
20–25 years old	111	91%
>25 years old	7	5.7%
Educationlevel		
High School	65	53.3%
Bachelor's Degree	54	44.3%
Diploma	3	2.5%
Status		
Students/University Students	90	73.8%
Private/Public Employees	23	18.9%
Entrepreneur/Business Owner	2	1.6%
Unemployed	5	4.1%
Others	2	1.6%

2.2. Research Design

Using a predictive regression research design, we determined the role of independent variables in predicting the dependent variable. In this study, emotional maturity and social support variables were regarded as independent variables, while quarter-life crisis was the dependent variable. We employed multiple linear regression analysis with two dependent variables.

2.3. Measuring Tools

We used an adapted measurement tool [20] based on the aspects of quarter-life crisis [10]. The validity of this scale was assessed using content validity based on expert judgment. The reliability score of this scale was 0.856. The measured aspects of quarter-life crisis included decision-making anxiety, concerns about interpersonal relationships, feelings of anxiety, stress, negative self-assessment, feeling trapped in difficult situations, and feelings of hopelessness. The scale comprised 25 items with 13 favorable items and 12 unfavorable items. TA Likert scale with 4 responses was employed: 1 (Strongly Agree), 2 (Agree), 3 (Disagree), and 4 (Strongly Disagree).

An emotional maturity scale was developed by Walgito [15] and adapted by Eringtyas [21]. The emotional maturity scale was used to measure an individual's level of emotional maturity. The validity of this scale was assessed using content validity based on expert judgment. Additionally, the reliability score of this scale was 0.874. The measurement of individual emotional maturity included emotional control, self- and others' acceptance, responsibility, and decision-making. The scale comprises 23 items, with 12 favorable items and 11 unfavorable items. This variable will be measured using a Likert scale with 4 response alternatives: 1 (Strongly Agree), 2 (Agree), 3 (Disagree), and 4 (Strongly Disagree).

The Multidimensional Scale of Perceived Social Support (MSPSS) [18] was used to measure the variable of social support. The validity of this scale was assessed using content validity based on expert judgment. The reliability score of this scale was 0.871. The scale was used to gauge individuals' assessments of the adequacy of social support received from family, friends, and others. The questionnaire items for social support were adapted from the research of Juniastira [22]. With this scale, family support, friend support, and support from others were measured. The scale consisted of 12 items. For the assessment, a four-point Likert scale was used: 1 (Strongly Agree), 2 (Agree), 3 (Disagree), and 4 (Strongly Disagree).

3. Results

The coefficient of determination or adjusted R-square was 0.088 or equal to 8.8%. This Table indicates the contributions of social support and emotional maturity to a quarter-life crisis. Further, 91.2% of the quarter-life crisis was influenced by other variables that were not examined in this study (Table 2). The contributions of social support and emotional maturity to the quarter-life crisis are presented in Table 3.

Table 2. Results of R-square.

Model	R	R-Square	Adjusted R-Square	Standard Error of Estimate
1	0.322	0.104	0.088	4.257

Table 3. Results of multiple linear regression.

Model	Unstandardized Coefficients B	Unstandardized Coefficients *Std. Error*	Standardized Coefficients Beta	t	Significance
1 (*Constant*)	79.731	4.126		19.326	0.000
Social Support	−0.204	0.063	−0.285	−3.247	0.002
Emotional Maturity	−0.123	0.055	−0.196	−2.236	0.027

Each independent variable, namely emotional maturity and social support, plays a role in predicting a quarter-life crisis during emerging adulthood as the significance values of both variables were less than 0.05. Furthermore, the regression coefficient of social support is negative, indicating an inverse relationship between social support and a quarter-life crisis. The lower the received social support, the higher the likelihood of experiencing a quarter-life crisis and vice versa. The regression coefficient of the emotional maturity variable was also negative, indicating that lower levels of emotional maturity correlated with higher levels of quarter-life crises and vice versa.

4. Discussion

The results of this study revealed a significant role or influence of the emotional maturity variable in predicting a quarter-life crisis in emerging adulthood. These findings are supported by the research conducted by Johnson et al. [23], which demonstrated that emotional maturity played a crucial role in facing challenges and life conflicts in early adulthood. Individuals with higher levels of emotional maturity are inclined to experience lower levels of quarter-life crisis. Permatasari [24] examined the relationship between emotional maturity and a quarter-life crisis. They found a negative relationship, indicating that higher levels of emotional maturity correspond to lower levels of the experienced quarter-life crisis. These results align with the developmental theories that emphasize the importance of emotional maturity in achieving well-being and adaptation during early adulthood [2]. Individuals experiencing a quarter-life crisis often grapple with feelings of worry and anxiety, leading to insecurity due to uncertainty about the future [10]. However, individuals with emotional maturity can control and transform their emotions into a more positive outlook. An individual with strong emotional maturity is likely to navigate through crisis periods that encompass feelings of depression, worry, anxiety, and even frustration [4]. Therefore, emotional maturity serves as a protective factor for individuals in early adulthood, enabling them to better cope with the complexities of life's demands.

Social support plays a significant role in predicting a quarter-life crisis in emerging adulthood. Social support can be obtained from family, friends, the community, or someone considered special. The social support received by individuals during this transitional period provides emotional resources to cope with challenges and stresses. This is consistent with the research conducted by Misra and Castellanos [25], who found that social support is related to psychological adjustment and well-being during emerging adulthood. The four aspects of social support [19], namely emotional support, informational support, instrumental support, and appraisal support, are crucial for individuals in the transitional phase to independently face life's challenges. A lack of close interpersonal relationships and a sense of alienation from one's environment increase the likelihood of a quarter-life crisis in young adults [26].

The level of the quarter-life crisis experienced by individuals in emerging adulthood was moderate with 121 individuals (99.2%). This aligns with the majority of individuals' emotional maturity and social support being in the moderate range. Individuals need emotional maturity and sufficient social support to navigate through this crisis. A moderate level of quarter-life crisis indicates that individuals between the ages of 18 and 29 years are experiencing symptoms such as confusion about their life direction, dissatisfaction with their work or social relationships, and difficulty in finding meaning in life [10]. Therefore, it is important for individuals in emerging adulthood to effectively manage their quarter-life crisis. Emotional maturity and social support play a crucial role in addressing the quarter-life crisis. Emotional maturity helps individuals to manage complex and unstable emotions in this crisis [10]. Adequate social support, whether from friends, family, or the community, can provide individuals with the emotional and practical resources needed to overcome the pressures and challenges during the crisis period [27].

5. Conclusions

The results of this study revealed that social support and emotional maturity play a significant role in predicting the level of a quarter-life crisis. The negative regression coefficients in the multiple linear regression indicated that, the higher the levels of social support and emotional maturity an individual possesses, the lower the level of the quarter-life crisis. Conversely, lower levels of social support and emotional maturity correspond to higher levels regarding the quarter-life crisis. These findings highlight the importance of developing emotional maturity and enhancing social support for the psychological well-being of individuals in emerging adulthood. Such results are a basis for developing interventions and programs to strengthen emotional maturity and social support to help individuals cope effectively with quarter-life crises and achieve positive development in early adulthood.

Author Contributions: Conceptualization, M.N.S. and W.B.S.; methodology, M.N.S. and W.B.S.; software, M.N.S. and W.B.S.; validation, M.N.S.; formal analysis, M.N.S. and W.B.S.; data collection, W.B.S.; writing, M.N.S. and W.B.S. All authors have read and agreed to the published version of the manuscript.

Funding: This research received no external funding.

Institutional Review Board Statement: This study was conducted in accordance with the Declaration of Helsinki and all subjects gave their informed consent before they participated in this study.

Informed Consent Statement: Informed consent was obtained from all subjects involved in the study. The study has received the ethical approval from the ethical boards signed on 10 February 2023.

Data Availability Statement: Data are available in https://bit.ly/3MxPKNb. accessed on 15 April 2023.

Conflicts of Interest: The authors declare no conflicts of interest regarding the research and publication of this research article.

References

1. Shulman, S.; Feldman, B.; Blatt, S.J.; Cohen, O.; Mahler, A. Emerging adulthood: Age-related tasks and underlying self processes. *J. Adolesc. Res.* **2005**, *20*, 577–603. [CrossRef]
2. Arnett, J.J. Emerging adulthood: A theory of development from the late teens through the twenties. *Am. Psychol.* **2000**, *55*, 469. [CrossRef]
3. Hurlock, E.B. *Psikologi Perkembangan: Suatu Perkembangan Sepanjang Rentang Kehidupan*; Erlangga: Jakarta, Indonesia, 2009.
4. Nash, R.J.; Murray, M.C. *Helping College Students Find Purpose: The Campus Guide to Meaning-Making*; John Wiley & Sons: Hoboken, NJ, USA, 2009.
5. Arnett, J.J. Emerging adulthood: What is it, and what is it good for? *Child Dev. Perspect.* **2007**, *1*, 68–73. [CrossRef]
6. Atwood, J.D.; Scholtz, C. The quarter-life time period: An age of indulgence, crisis or both? *Contemp. Fam. Ther.* **2008**, *30*, 233–250. [CrossRef]
7. Herawati, I.; Hidayat, A. Quarterlife crisis pada masa dewasa awal di pekanbaru. *J. An-Nafs Kaji. Penelit. Psikol.* **2020**, *5*, 145–156. [CrossRef]
8. Fischer, K. *Ramen Noodles, Rent and Resumes: An after-College Guide to Life*; Supercollege, LLC: Belmont, CA, USA, 2008.
9. Nelson, L.J.; Badger, S. The quarter-life crisis: A developmental transition. In *Handbook of Adult Development and Learning*; Oxford University Press: Oxford, UK, 2010; pp. 247–265.
10. Robbins, A.; Wilner, A. *Quarterlife Crisis: The Unique Challenges of Life in Your Twenties*; Penguin: London, UK, 2001.
11. Hill, A. The Quarterlife Crisis: Young, Insecure and Depressed. 2011. Available online: https://www.theguardian.com/society/2011/may/05/quarterlife-crisis-young-insecure-depressed (accessed on 1 October 2023).
12. Ipelona, E. Quarter Life Crisis, Gejala Dan Cara Menghadapinya. *Kompas TV*, 2021. Available online: https://www.kompas.tv/article/233651/tgsl-quarter-life-crisis-gejala-dan-cara-menghadapinya (accessed on 13 October 2022).
13. Artiningsih, R.A.; Savira, S.I. hubungan Loneliness dan Quarter life crisis pada dewasa awal. *Character J. Penelit. Psikol.* **2021**, *8*, 1–11.
14. Rahajeng, A.L. *Hubungan Antara Dukungan Keluarga Dengan Quarter Life Crisis Pada Dewasa Awal Yang Bekerja*; Universitas Mercu Buana Yogyakarta: Depok, Indonesia, 2022.
15. Walgito, B. *Pengantar Psikologi Umum*; Andi: Yogyakarta, Indonesia, 2004.
16. Saronson. *Pengaruh Dukungan Sosial Terhadap Perilaku*; Penerbit Kencana: Jakarta, Indonesia, 2005.
17. Maziyah, F. *Hubungan Dukungan Sosial Dengan Tingkat Kecemasan Dalam Mengerjakan Skripsi Pada Mahasiswa Sekolah Tinggi Ilmu Kesehatan (STIKES) NU Tuban*; Universitas Islam Negeri Maulana Malik Ibrahim: Malang, Indonesia, 2015.
18. Zimet, G.D.; Dahlem, N.W.; Zimet, S.G.; Farley, G.K. The multidimensional scale of perceived social support. *J. Personal. Assess.* **1988**, *52*, 30–41. [CrossRef]
19. Sarafino, E.P.; Smith, T.W. *Health Psychology: Biopsychosocial Interactions*; John Wiley & Sons: Hoboken, NJ, USA, 2014.
20. Sumartha, A.R. *Pengaruh Trait Kepribadian Neuroticism Terhadap Quarter-Life Crisis Dimediasi Oleh Harapan Pada Mahasiswa Tingkat Akhir Universitas Islam Negeri Maulana Malik Ibrahim Malang*; Universitas Islam Negeri Maulana Malik Ibrahim: Malang, Indonesia, 2020.
21. Eriningtyas, R. *Hubungan Antara Kematangan Emosi Dan Kecenderungan Perilaku Berselingkuh Pada Individu Menikah*; Universitas Sanata Dharma Yogyakarta: Depok, Indonesia, 2018.
22. Juniastira, S. Hubungan Antara Dukungan Sosial Dan Kualitas Hidup Pada Pasien Stroke. 2018. Available online: https://dspace.uii.ac.id/handle/123456789/8391 (accessed on 1 October 2023).
23. Johnson, M.M.; Brown, E.S.; Davis, C.L. Emotional maturity and quarter life crisis in emerging adulthood: A longitudinal study. *J. Youth Adolesc.* **2021**, *50*, 518–533.
24. Permatasari, I. *Hubungan Kematangan Emosi Dengan Quarter Life Crisis Pada Dewasa Awal*; Universitas Muhammadiyah Malang: Malang, Indonesia, 2021.
25. Misra, R.; Castellanos, J. Identity and adjustment in emerging adulthood: Making a life without becoming your own worst enemy. *J. Adult Dev.* **2019**, *26*, 13–24.

26. Zhai, H.; Chen, L.; Zhang, X.; Liang, X. The Impact of Social Support on the Quarter-Life Crisis in Emerging Adults: A Moderated Mediation Model. *Front. Psychol.* **2020**, *11*, 1–10.
27. Luyckx, K.; Schwartz, S.J.; Berzonsky, M.D.; Soenens, B.; Vansteenkiste, M.; Smits, I.; Goossens, L. Capturing ruminative exploration: Extending the four-dimensional model of identity formation in late adolescence. *J. Res. Personal.* **2008**, *42*, 58–82. [CrossRef]

engineering proceedings

MDPI

Proceeding Paper

Technology Adaptation in Japan's Work Culture: Usage of Electronic Signatures (E-Signatures) in Post-COVID-19 Japan †

Diva Gabriela Prawiro, Fourmando Butar Butar, Jimmy Gotomo and Elisa Carolina Marion *

Japanese Department, Faculty of Humanities, Bina Nusantara University, Jakarta 11480, Indonesia; diva.prawiro@binus.ac.id (D.G.P.); fourmando.butar@binus.ac.id (F.B.B.); jimmy.gotomo@binus.ac.id (J.G.)

* Correspondence: emarion@binus.edu

† Presented at the 2024 IEEE 4th International Conference on Electronic Communications, Internet of Things and Big Data, Taipei, Taiwan, 19–21 April 2024.

Abstract: Hanko or signature seals are widely used by Japanese companies to sign business contracts. However, the COVID-19 pandemic has caused Hanko culture in Japan to become ineffective, especially in teleworking. The pandemic has also negatively affected the global economy, including Japan. To face this issue, the Japanese government has expanded the use of electronic signatures since 2020. Regardless of the government's efforts, many Japanese companies have not implemented the use of electronic signatures. Nevertheless, the prospects of utilizing electronic signatures in Japanese companies have increased due to post-COVID-19 socio-economic factors. We examined the problem of Hanko culture and how Hanko is replaced by electronic signatures in Japan's society through an inductive, descriptive, and qualitative method. By using those approaches, we discovered that, in the short run, Japanese companies will be forced to adapt to the use of electronic signatures to increase productivity post-economic crisis. In the long run, Japanese companies will be inclined to use electronic signatures to adapt to global trade conditions.

Keywords: Hanko; electronic signature; Japanese company; business manner

Citation: Prawiro, D.G.; Butar, F.B.; Gotomo, J.; Marion, E.C. Technology Adaptation in Japan's Work Culture: Usage of Electronic Signatures (E-Signatures) in Post-COVID-19 Japan. *Eng. Proc.* **2024**, *74*, 66. https://doi.org/10.3390/engproc2024074066

Academic Editors: Shu-Han Liao, Teen-Hang Meen and Cheng-Fu Yang

Published: 20 September 2024

1. Introduction

Hanko or better known internationally as "seals" is a strong Japanese business culture [1]. Despite that fact, as the COVID-19 pandemic catalyzed digitalization in all aspects of life, including businesses, Japanese Hanko culture is changing. The new culture of "teleworking", which promotes long distance working and interaction has made it difficult for companies to implement the use of Hanko. This is evident when activities outside one's home became restricted during the pandemic, while documents at companies still need to be signed by the employees [2]. Moreover, the effectiveness and efficiency of Hanko in modern times were questioned even before the pandemic. Personalized Hanko used to be a legitimate way to prove that someone is responsible for the approval of a certain contract or document. However, today, where Hanko can be mass-produced, two different people with the same names can use identical Hanko which increases the risk of the fraudulence in signing contracts [3]. Another weakness of Hanko culture is the fact that Japanese employees are at risk of being scapegoats if a document they have signed creates losses for their company. In other words, the use of Hanko can be a failsafe for companies to avoid losses at the expense of the reputation of their employees [4]. With technological advancement and the rise of electronic signatures, the use of Hanko can be replaced in the future by electronic signatures.

2. Method

We explore if and how electronic signatures replace *Hanko culture* in Japan. In this research, the following questions were answered.

1. What are electronic signatures?
2. What are the laws that dictate the use of electronic signatures in Japan?
3. How familiar are Japanese people with the use of electronic signatures?
4. What are the factors that drive the use of electronic signatures in post-pandemic Japan?

For the answers, hypotheses were proposed as follows.

1. In the short run, Japanese companies will be forced to use electronic signatures to boost the nation's economy in the post-COVID-19 era.
2. In the long run, Japanese companies will be dependent on the use of electronic signatures due to factors of economic and technological advancement.
3. Hanko culture will dissolve as the use of electronic signatures increases.

This research is a literature review that solely uses secondary data. The theories and data used were obtained from various resources including journals, news articles, and surveys made by both international and Japanese organizations. Relevant findings from those media were then analyzed through a descriptive and qualitative method. Moreover, an inductive approach was used in this research to establish links between theories from interdisciplinary subjects such as Japanese business manners, law, and economics to produce a general summary that answers the research question. This approach enabled the prediction of the long-term behavior of Japanese people regarding the use of electronic signatures.

3. Result and Discussion

An electronic signature is a digital seal on computer software. This type of seal is convenient because the legitimacy of the document is being checked directly by a non-sentient system, which decreases the possibilities for errors, inaccuracies, and fraud [5]. Unlike Hanko, which can be purchased or made by many other parties, the likelihood of an electronic signature being tampered with is low. In Japan, electronic signatures have been legalized by the "E-Signature Act" (Act No. 102 of 31 May 2000). This is an act that governs the legality of electronic signatures for certified business transactions [6]. Nonetheless, the implementation of electronic signatures is still limited, as shown in a survey conducted by Mizoguchi in 2022 regarding the use of electronic contracts in Japan [7]. In that research, Mizoguchi recruited 414 respondents, and their demographics are presented in Figure 1.

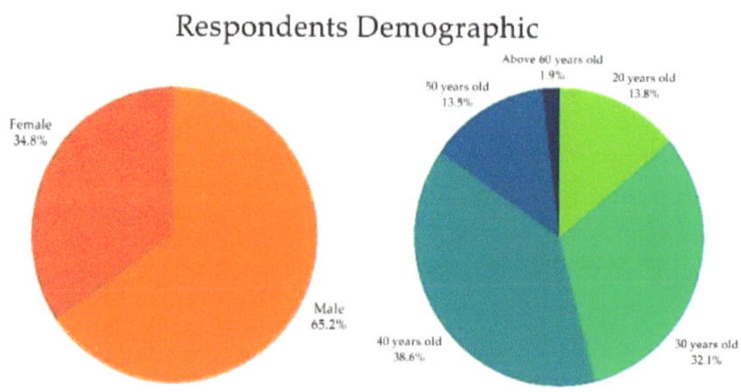

Figure 1. Chart of gender and age demographics of survey respondents (Mizoguchi, 2022).

In total, 65.2% of the respondents collected were males and 34.8% were females. The majority of the respondents were in their 40s (38.6%), 32.1% were in their 30s, 13.8% were in their 20s, 13.5% were in their 50s, and 1.9% were older than 60. The majority of the respondents belonged to Generation X (born around 1965–1980) and Millennials (born around 1991–1996). Figure 2 shows the respondents' professions. In total, 23% of the respondents were employed in the service industry, while less than 1% worked in the electricity and gas industry.

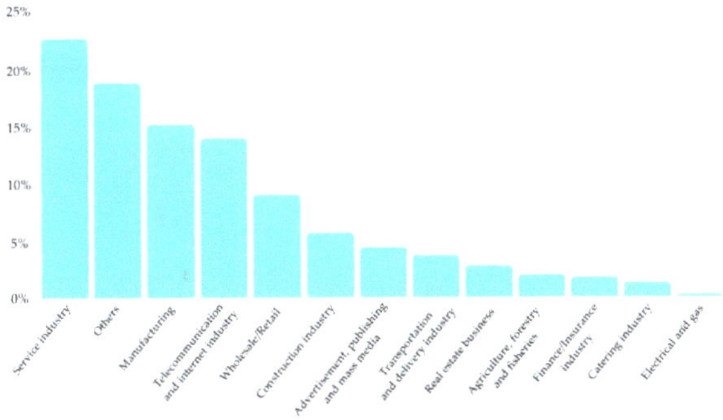

Figure 2. Professions of respondents.

Figure 3 shows that 76.1% of the respondents were aware of electronic contracts, while 23% were not. The majority of the respondents were aware of the existence of electronic contracts.

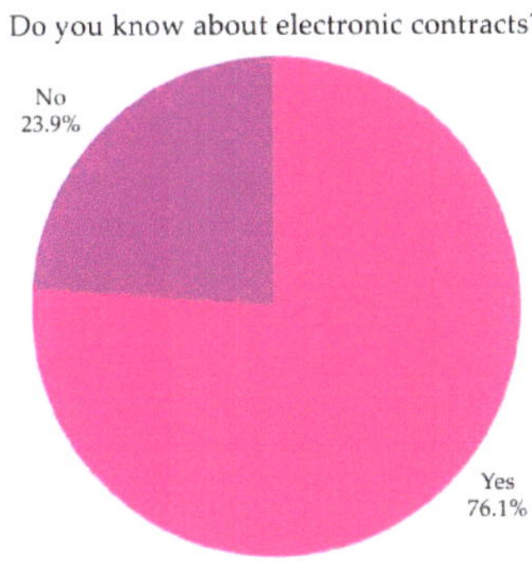

Figure 3. Awareness of electronic contracts (Mizoguchi, 2022).

Furthermore, Figure 4 shows that a total of 21.7% of the respondents thought that their companies were aware of electronic contracts, 60.9% of the respondents did not think so, and 17.4% did not know if their companies were aware. The majority of Japanese companies do not use electronic contracts. This implies that they do not use any electronic signatures in contracts.

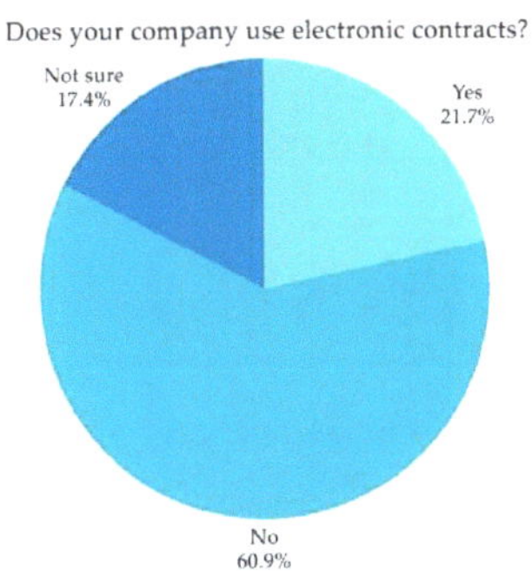

Figure 4. Company awareness of electronic contracts (Mizoguchi, 2022).

The use of electronic contracts varied depending on industry sector as shown in Figure 5.

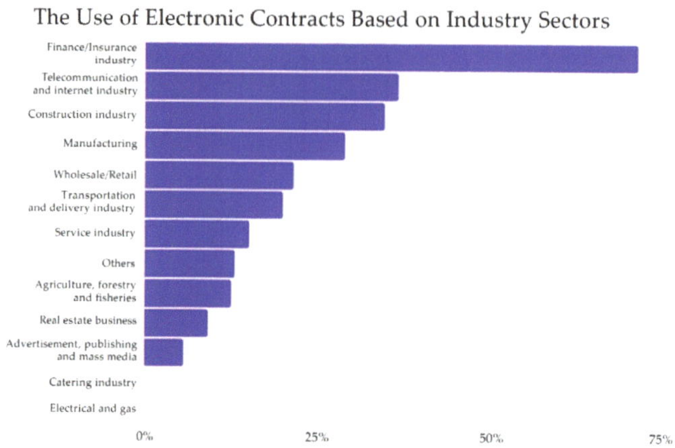

Figure 5. Use of electronic contracts by industry sector (Mizoguchi, 2022).

The leading industries for the use of electronic contracts were finance and insurance (71.4%), telecommunications and internet (36.8%), and construction (29%). They use digital contracts for error prevention and fraud deterrence. Finance and insurance benefit from document legitimacy and embezzlement prevention. The Japanese tax reform of 2021 requires companies to preserve transactions electronically starting from 2022. With the nature of the financial and insurance industry that correlates with many economic transactions, the tax reform boosts their need for electronic signatures and documents [8]. The construction industry handles numerous documents, while telecoms and internet are technology-oriented.

In total, 68.3% of the respondents supported electronic contracts, 2.7% were opposed, and 29% were unsure. Several respondents had never used electronic contracts. Supporters emphasized efficiency, cost savings, and convenience, while those who did not support them worried about the security, privacy, and the adversity of management (Figure 6).

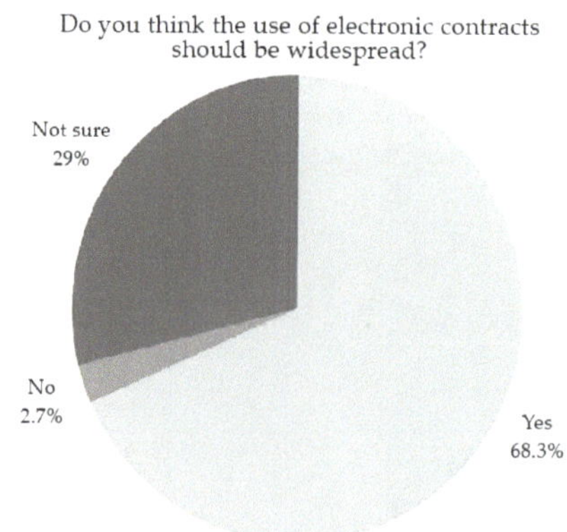

Figure 6. Use of electronic contracts (Mizoguchi, 2022).

Japanese employees, mostly Generation X and Millennials, are open to transitioning from Hanko to electronic signatures, which will lead Japanese companies to use them. Electronic signature adoption rates vary by industry involving many parties who are sensitive to errors in contracts or to the use of technological advancement.

The adoption of electronic signatures instead of Hanko is driven by social, technological, and economic changes in Japan. Since the 1990s, Japan has been facing economic stagnation [9]. This calls for an increase in economic growth. This condition is worsened by an aging population and a low birth rate. This affects the country's GDP since an aging population means slower economic growth [10]. This leads to Japan's dependency on foreigners to increase the country's economic circumstances, through tourism and goods that are exported to other countries. The COVID-19 pandemic has slowed global economic activity, including in Japan. The Japanese government has attempted to increase economic efficiency, including expanding the use of electronic contracts and signatures, as a response to the rise of teleworking. Currently, the pandemic has shown signs of being benign. However, Japanese companies implementing hybrid (online and on-site) offices have increased due to the efficiencies such as lowering the cost of transportation, lowering the cost of meeting venues, and networking with people from different places [11]. This results in the wider use of electronic signatures and contracts [12].

The Japanese yen has been depreciating in the past few years. The Japanese government can use this economic condition to increase its GDP by maximizing exports and establishing a trading policy with other countries [13]. The capability of electronic signatures to avoid duplication and inefficient bureaucracy can smoothen the process of international trade [14]. This strengthens the use of electronic signatures since other countries do not have Hanko culture.

4. Conclusions

The use of signature seals or Hanko has been a tradition of business in Japan. In recent years, the legitimacy, effectiveness, and efficiency of Hanko have been questioned. Advancement in technology has also led to the creation of electronic signatures, which is a digital type of seal that depends on computer software. The use of electronic contracts and signatures was recognized by the government in the "E-Signature Act" (Act No. 102 of 31 May 2000). Despite that, the majority of Japanese companies have not utilized electronic signatures in signing contracts. Social and technological advances have increased the interest of Japanese employees in implementing electronic signatures. Technology increases the effectiveness, efficiency, and convenience and reduces cost, time, and energy wasted. Furthermore, the use of electronic signatures is increasing under the teleworking and economic conditions in Japan for trading with other countries to increase Japan's GDP.

Several companies may be hesitant to adapt to the use of electronic signatures due to bureaucratic traditions and a poorer understanding of how to operate technology. In the short term, only big companies can adopt this technology due to their capital and manpower. Meanwhile, small companies may not use this technology due to limited capital and manpower. In the long term, as society embraces technological advancement, the capital and manpower needed to operate this technology will decrease. This means that slowly but surely Hanko culture will be replaced by electronic signatures. Further research is needed to compare bigger and smaller companies to determine different factors of using electronic signatures. The results can support or hinder the use of electronic signatures by Japanese companies.

Author Contributions: D.G.P., F.B.B. and J.G. provided the conceptualization, methodology, formal analysis, investigation, resources, data curation, writing—original draft preparation, writing—review and editing, and visualization. E.C.M. provided the validation, supervision, project administration, and funding acquisition. All authors have read and agreed to the published version of the manuscript.

Funding: This research and and its APC was funded by Bina Nusantara University's International Research Grant [029/VRRTT/III/2023].

Institutional Review Board Statement: Not applicable.

Informed Consent Statement: Not applicable.

Data Availability Statement: Most of the data that were used in this research were taken from a survey done by Mizoguchi in 2022. The data was taken from the resource below. Mizoguchi, H. [2022 Edition] Survey on Awareness and Usage of Electronic Contracting Services. [2022-Nenban] Denshi Keiyaku Saabisu no Ninchi-do to Riyou-ritsu ni Kansuru Ankeeto Chousa [Translated Title]. 2023. Available online: https://tng-marketing.com/freelance/questionnaire/post-1001/ (accessed on 15 July 2024). The authors of this research translated, paraphrased, and interpreted the data in English for the purpose in creating coherent answers to this research's question. Other secondary resources were also used to aid the synthesis of this research's conclusion. Please refer to the "References" of this research for further details regarding the data resources used in this research.

Conflicts of Interest: The authors declare no conflict of interest.

References

1. Widya, H.; Kirana, R.P. Hanko vs. sain: Kecenderungan minat mahasiswa universitas hiroshima terhadap pengesahan dokumen. *Japanology* **2016**, 5, 11–23.
2. Ryall, J. Coronavirus Hastens Japan's Shift away from Hanko Seals. *DW News*. 6 June 2020. Available online: https://www.dw.com/en/coronavirus-hastens-japans-shift-away-from-Hanko-seals/a-53783541 (accessed on 15 July 2024).
3. Aoki, Y. Japanese React to Trash Taste Complain about Japan. *That Japanese Man Yuta*. 20 December 2021. Available online: https://www.youtube.com/watch?v=MJkYBheHJKg&t=2s (accessed on 15 July 2024).
4. Beyer, V.L. The Japanese Hanko: Indispensable Signature Seals Or Idea Whose Time Has Gone? *Tokyo Weekender*. 29 June 2020. Available online: https://www.tokyoweekender.com/art_and_culture/japanese-culture/the-japanese-hanko-indispensable-signature-seals-or-idea-whose-time-has-gone/ (accessed on 15 July 2024).
5. Oka, K.; Sakamoto, Y. Legal Considerations for Electronic Contracts and Electronic Signatures. Deloitte. Available online: https://www2.deloitte.com/jp/en/pages/tax/articles/bt/japan-inbound-tax-legal-february-2022-no75.html# (accessed on 15 July 2024).
6. Electronic Signature Laws & Regulations-Japan. 2022. Available online: https://helpx.adobe.com/legal/esignatures/regulations/japan.html (accessed on 15 July 2024).
7. Mizoguchi, H. [2022 Edition] Survey on Awareness and Usage of Electronic Contracting Services. [2022-Nenban] Denshi Keiyaku Saabisu no Ninchi-do to Riyou-ritsu ni Kansuru Ankeeto Chousa [Translated Title]. 2023. Available online: https://tng-marketing.com/freelance/questionnaire/post-1001/ (accessed on 15 July 2024).
8. Arjunwadkar, P.; Yoshimoto, M. CFO Webinar 2021 December: Journey from Hankos to eSignatures. Deloitte. Nov. 2021. Available online: https://www2.deloitte.com/content/dam/Deloitte/jp/Documents/finance/cfop/jp-cfop-cfo-webinar-20211201.pdf (accessed on 15 July 2024).
9. Sheng, W. A Lesson Drawn from Japan-Style Economic Stagnation. Global Times. 2021. Available online: https://www.globaltimes.cn/page/202111/1239580.shtml (accessed on 15 July 2024).
10. Mühleisen, M.; Faruqee, H. Japan: Population Aging and the Fiscal Challenge. Finance & Development. 2001. Available online: https://www.imf.org/external/pubs/ft/fandd/2001/03/muhleise.htm (accessed on 15 July 2024).
11. Angle: Business Trips Has Changed Forever, without the Possibility of Returning to the State before COVID-19. Anguru: Kigyō no Shutchō ga Samagawari, Korona mae ni wa Modorazu [Translated Title]. Reuters. 2021. Available online: https://www.reuters.com/article/business-travel-covid-idJPKBN2G60DQ (accessed on 15 July 2024).
12. Sodsriwiboon, P.; Khera, P.; Rui, X. Japan's Digitalization Can Add Momentum for Economic Rebound. IMF News. 2022. Available online: https://www.imf.org/en/News/Articles/2022/05/31/CF-Japan-Digitalization-Can-Add-Momentum-for-Economic-Rebound (accessed on 15 July 2024).
13. Blink, J.; Dorton, I. *IB Economics Course Book 2nd Edition: Oxford IB Diploma Program*, 2nd ed.; Oxford University Press: Oxford, UK, 2012.
14. Hernandez, A.A. Adapting to Technological Change in the Workplace: An Assessment of the Effects of Information and Communication Technology on Older Workers. November 2014, pp. 30–31. Available online: http://hdl.handle.net/2345/bc-ir:104077 (accessed on 15 July 2024).

engineering proceedings

MDPI

Proceeding Paper

Application of Service-Based Learning to ASEAN Students in Taiwan: Teaching Air Quality †

I-Fei Luo [1,*], Darmamsyah Darmamsyah [2] and Sheng-Jie You [3]

1 Program of Learning Sciences, National Taiwan Normal University, Taipei 106, Taiwan
2 Chemical Engineering Department, Engineering Faculty, University of Lampung, Lampung 35141, Indonesia; darmansyah.1982@cycu.org.tw
3 Department of Environmental Engineering, Chung Yuan Christian University, Taoyuan 320, Taiwan; sjyou@cycu.edu.tw
* Correspondence: elisefeifei@gmail.com
† Presented at the 2024 IEEE 4th International Conference on Electronic Communications, Internet of Things and Big Data, Taipei, Taiwan, 19–21 April 2024.

Abstract: Service-based learning belongs to experiential education. It emphasizes experience in learning with services that benefit a provider and a recipient. Around 100,000 foreign students are coming to Taiwan to study every year. Most of them are from ASEAN countries. Taiwan provides an excellent experience in studying for foreign students. To strengthen their learning effect, we applied service-based learning through cooperation with professors from the Department of Environmental Engineering. Through the production, discussion, and revision of service-based learning and materials in-person or in online teaching, foreign students learn air quality-related knowledge effectively. Service-based learning was integrated into the competition method to enhance the learning memories of foreign students. As the ASEAN region is prone to climate change, service-based learning helps ASEAN countries cultivate governance leaders for a sustainable environment.

Keywords: service-based learning; Asean students; air quality

Citation: Luo, I.-F.; Darmamsyah, D.; You, S.-J. Application of Service-Based Learning to ASEAN Students in Taiwan: Teaching Air Quality. *Eng. Proc.* **2024**, *74*, 67. https://doi.org/10.3390/engproc2024074067

Academic Editors: Shu-Han Liao, Teen-Hang Meen and Cheng-Fu Yang

Published: 25 September 2024

1. Introduction

Service-based learning has the function of encouraging and assisting the self-learning of students. In service-based learning, students need to cooperate. Service-based learning can cultivate a spirit of teamwork, an understanding of the power of teams, and communication skills. In addition, contact with society (community) allows students to step out of their boundaries and encounter diverse people. In the process, students engage in conversations and interactions, understand different perspectives and needs, and interpret various matters from objective perspectives. This is beneficial for students to expand their worldviews and thoughts, encouraging their growth.

Service-based learning originated in the United States in the 1960s. John Dewey proposed that student learning must be the basis, and through planning courses and participating in service-based learning, students can develop themselves and learn how to communicate and cooperate. By participating in society (community), students can experience and engage in social (community) affairs. Through this participation, they discover social (community) problems and think about their causes to solve problems or help improve them. Society (community) activities make students aware of the community and assist in its development as citizens [1].

Taiwan has promoted service-based learning since 1980, beginning with various universities and colleges. In 2008, with the implementation of the nine-year integrated curriculum, service-based learning was incorporated into the educational activity. In the twelve-year national education system of 2014, service-based learning was included as a scoring item for admission without examination to encourage students to engage more in community service or participate in charitable activities and promote students' learning and civic literacy.

Battistoni (1997) [2] believed that service-based learning strengthens problem-solving skills, which are obtained through participating in community services. This involves many factors: searching for relevant information, taking action, and tracking results. Moreover, Jacoby (1996) [3] stated that service-based learning boosts the absorption and application of courses and improves students' interaction, participation, cooperation ability, and communication skills. Chen (2016) [4] thought that positive service-based learning experiences in self-growth, civic responsibility, and interpersonal relationships contribute to students' overall development. Indicators of psychological adjustment and self-identity are also positive, assisting students to amend their negative psychological status and explore and reassess their values or capabilities. Fertman et al. (1996) [5] proposed a four-stage model of service-based learning, which becomes a learning cycle. The four stages are preparation, service, reflection, and celebration. The preparation stage involves identifying the service target and direction; the service stage involves starting the service and contacting the service target; the reflection stage involves introspection after activities or contact, which can be carried out through group discussions or reports; the celebration stage involves affirming the students' previous service, such as through rewards, prizes, or certificates of recognition.

2. Method

Air quality-related knowledge is taught in English to ASEAN students in Taiwan. The topics include air pollution control equipment, air pollution policies, and solutions for air pollution. By imparting this knowledge, students are aware of the current status of air quality management and compare the situation with their countries. To motivate students' learning, the activity was provided in a service-based learning mechanism in this study. A total of 32 students participated in the activity in 14 groups. Each group designed a service-based activity for air quality knowledge. The participants served at least 10 students who were not the participants. Seven groups of the participants competed in the service-based learning activity, while the other group did not. The competition was evaluated based on the creativity and innovation of teaching materials (such as PPT design, pictures or video supplementary, Q&A game, etc.) by three judges. The participants completed a questionnaire (Table 1), which was designed to understand the effectiveness of service-based learning and the effect of competition. The questionnaire adopted a 5-point scale of the satisfaction degree. Service-based learning allowed students to transition from learners to instructors and strengthen their learning motivation.

Table 1. Questionnaire on a Likert 5-point scale.

	Questionnaire
1.	I understand how service-based learning operates.
2.	I like the design of the service-based learning course.
3.	Service-based learning courses help me to learn.
4.	I am interested in air pollution issues.
5.	Through service-based learning, I would like to expand my learning methods to learn air pollution-related knowledge.
6.	Because of the service-based learning design, I think my air pollution-related knowledge has improved.
7.	If there are competitions and bonuses (or prizes) at the end of the service-based learning, it will help improve my motivation to learn about air pollution issues.
8.	I understand the air pollution problem in my country.
9.	I hope I will have a contribution to the improvement of air pollution in my country.

Table 1. *Cont.*

Questionnaire
10. In teamwork, service-based learning may not be easy to operate efficiently due to the different backgrounds of the team members.
11. Through service-based learning, I will learn to communicate effectively.
12. I want to join community service work in the future.
13. If given the chance, I would like to volunteer to teach about air pollution.
14. If I have the opportunity in the future, I would like to introduce a service-based learning model to guide my students or the general public to learn.

3. Results

Most groups adopted webinars for service-based learning activities (Figure 1). The served students were from different countries, such as Taiwan, Indonesia, the Philippines, Vietnam, Pakistan, and Thailand. The language of communication was English. The shared topics included restaurant fume problems, the traditional Taiwanese culture of burning incense, indoor air quality issues, and others (Table 2). The fourteen groups in this study completed the service-based learning content. Each group conducted at least one webinar, with participants per session ranging from 14 to 108. A total of 589 participants joined the service-based learning activities. Coupled with interactions in the webinar, the service-based learning activities attracted participants' attention, deepened their impressions, and made the sharing more effective.

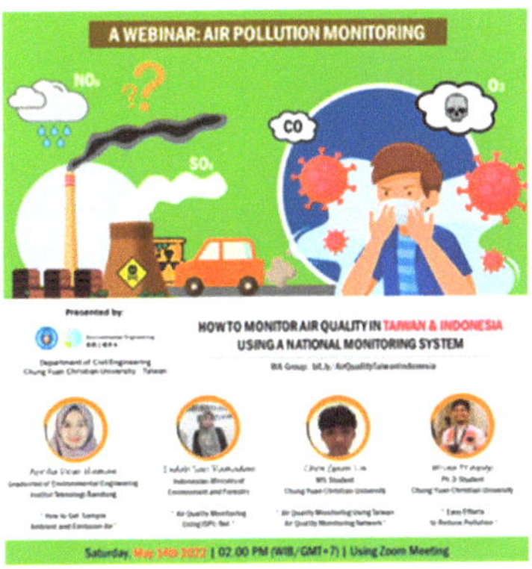

(**a**) Student's Webinar promotional flyer 1

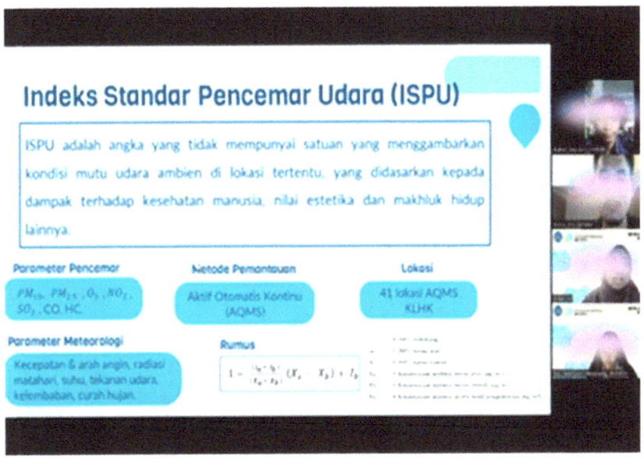

(**b**) Students' webinar

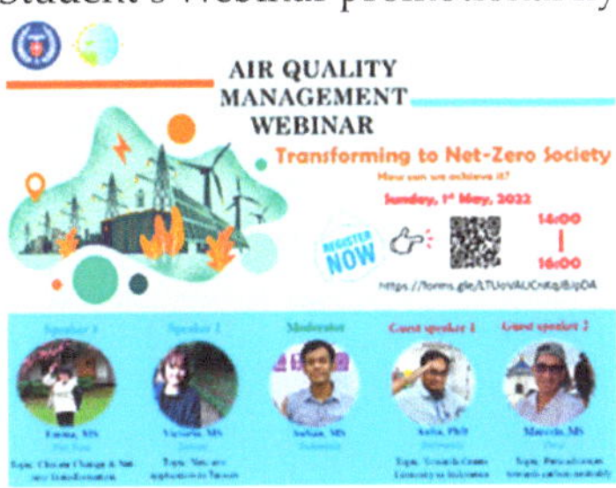

(**c**) Student's Webinar promotional flyer 2

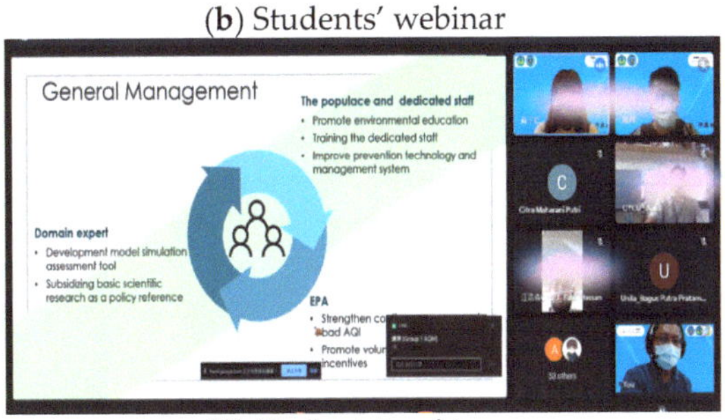

(**d**) Students' webinar

Figure 1. Examples of student service-based learning activities.

Table 2. Service-based learning activity for air quality management-related topics.

Group	Presentation Topic	Number of Participants	Activities
Group 1	Learn from R.O.C. (Taiwan): How can Taiwan be aware of its air pollution?	106	webinar and Q&A
Group 2	Indoor Air Pollutants in Various Settings	50	webinar and Slido
Group 3	Student's Awareness Of Environmental Air Pollution: A Study Case Of Yogyakarta City: Small Steps To Make Changes	40	webinar
Group 4	Earth Day: Addressing Air Pollution from Human Health	25	webinar
Group 5	Life Under the Smog of Forest and Wildfires (Case study: South Kalimantan)	43	webinar
Group 6	Greening Taiwanese Restaurants-Toward a sustainable culinary tourism	20	webinar
Group 7	Polluting in god's name	35	Physical activity
Group 9	Application Smart Cities as a Solution to Minimise Pollutants for Sustainable Development	42	webinar
Group 10	How to Get Sample Ambient and Emission Air	108	webinar and Video
Group 11	Air Quality Index: PM2.5	14	webinar and Quiz
Group 12	Breathe Better Air Campaign	30	webinar
Group 13	Fumigation Behavior as a Habit that Caused the Air Quality Degradation: Study Case: Reduce The Mosquito Population	26	webinar
Group 14	Towards Net-zero Society: An investigation of the public's willingness to change perceptions	50	webinar
Total		589	

The independent *t*-test results showed that the effect of competition on teaching material creativity was statistically significant at $p < 0.01$ (Table 3). The service-based learning activities of Q&A and interactive teaching (e.g., Slido) were beneficial for served students. They strengthened increased air quality-related knowledge ($p < 0.01$). Webinar teaching made education borderless, inspiring more students interested in the topic of air quality. It also allowed students to plan service-based learning activities and have opportunities to learn and practice. The questionnaire survey result (Figure 2) showed that competition enhanced the students' motivation for interactive service activities and made them search for more information on air quality or pollution. It also strengthened the knowledge of the air quality of the students who planned the service-based learning activities ($p < 0.01$). However, with competition, the participants had a limited impact on social contributions. It is necessary to explore how competition can be combined in cooperation for social benefits.

Table 3. Effect of competition on teaching material.

	Competition	No Competition
Mean	3.75	0.5
Variance	0.917	0.333
Observation	4	4
Pooled Variance	0.625	
Hypothesized Mean	0	
df	6	
t Stat	5.814	
$P(T \leq t)$ one-tail	0.001	
t Critical one-tail	1.943	
$P(T \leq t)$ two-tail	0.001	
t Critical two-tail	2.447	

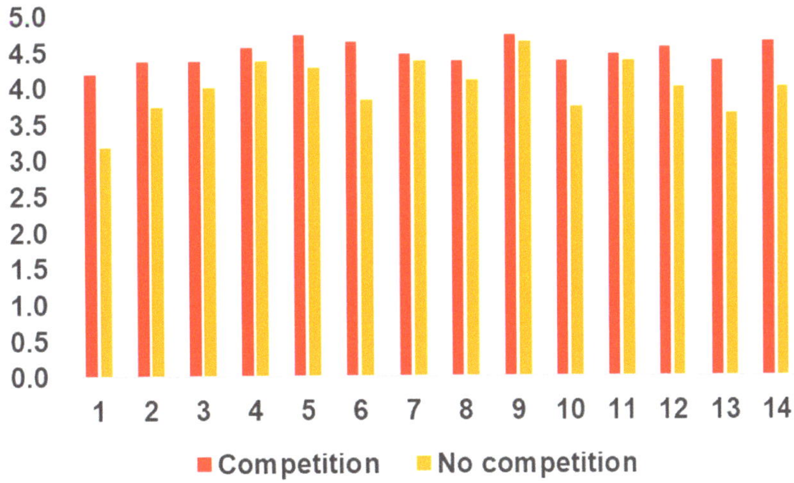

Figure 2. Questionnaire survey results.

4. Conclusions

Teamwork is valuable as it is used to coordinate diverse perspectives on problem-solving and enhance efficient and effective access to solutions. In air quality knowledge teaching, students were encouraged to think about related issues and actions. A competitive environment helps to absorb knowledge actively and increase extensive reading. Competition is a motivating factor for learning. Group activities help students cultivate teamwork and understand its importance. During teamwork, relationships and cohesion are formed, making tasks successful and complete. Students contributed their best performance and put in their efforts regardless of the result. The incentive-driven design of service-based learning activities strengthened teamwork, inspired participants' interest, and reinforced team members' learning about air quality-related knowledge.

Author Contributions: I.-F.L.: Writing—original draft, Writing—review and editing, Data curation, Formal analysis, Investigation, Methodology, Resources, Validation, Visualization. D.D.: Data curation, Validation, Investigation, Visualization. Methodology. S.-J.Y.: review and editing, Formal analysis, Resources, Investigation, Project administration, Funding acquisition. All authors have read and agreed to the published version of the manuscript.

Funding: This research received no external funding.

Institutional Review Board Statement: Not applicable.

Informed Consent Statement: Informed consent was obtained from all subjects involved in the study.

Data Availability Statement: No data were used for the research described in the article.

Acknowledgments: This research was supported by the Sustainable Environmental Education Center of Chung Yuan Christian University.

Conflicts of Interest: The authors declare no conflicts of interest.

References

1. Xu, M.; Lin, Z. *Service-Based Learning: Basic Concepts and Theoretical Foundations*; Hungyeh Publishing Co., Ltd.: Taipei, Taiwan, 2009.
2. Battistoni, R.M. Service-based learning and Democratic Citizenship. *Theory Into Pract.* **1997**, *36*, 150–156. [CrossRef]
3. Jacoby, B. *Associates, Service-Based Learning in Higher Education: Concepts and Practices*; Jossey-Bass: Hoboken, NJ, USA, 1996.

4. Chen, K.H. Preliminary Exploration of College Students' Service-based learning Experience and Growth Scale. *J. Holist. Educ.* **2016**, *14*, 63–103.
5. Fertman, C.I.; White, G.P.; White, L.J. *Service-Based Learning in the Middle School: Building a Culture of Service*; National Middle School Association: Westerville, OH, USA, 1996.

engineering proceedings

MDPI

Proceeding Paper

Analyzing Key Quality Attributes in Commercial Space Design Planning Using Impact Range Performance Analysis by Computer Software for Sustainable Development Goals †

Chun-Pin Huang [1], Chia-Hui Huang [1,*] and Chun-Chih Chen [2]

[1] Institute of Cultural and Creative Design, Tung-Fang Design University, Kaohsiung 829003, Taiwan; jimmyjimmy98886@gmail.com

[2] Department of Industrial Design, National Kaohsiung Normal University, Kaohsiung 824005, Taiwan; ccchen@nknu.edu.tw

* Correspondence: judy.tf.edu.tw@gmail.com

† Presented at the 2024 IEEE 4th International Conference on Electronic Communications, Internet of Things and Big Data, Taipei, Taiwan, 19–21 April 2024.

Abstract: For intensified global environmental and societal challenges, the Sustainable Development Goals (SDGs) have come to the forefront as a pivotal framework for corresponding action. For SDGs, the role of commercial spatial design and planning gains unique prominence. Using importance–performance analysis (IPA) with importance–performance–scope analysis (IPSA), we explore the SDGs' deployment and ramifications in commercial spatial planning in this study. By spotlighting pivotal SDG indicators, the study results underscore commercial spaces' performance in the environmental, social, and economic sectors. The combined analytical approaches were used to elucidate the present-day salience and efficacy of these attributes and highlight prospective trajectories for future evolution. The results offer a blueprint to empower designers and planners in the commercial realm to assimilate the SDGs effectively and design with environmental stewardship, social responsibility, and economic viability. The industry can have pragmatic strategic guidance aligned with global sustainable development imperatives.

Keywords: SDG indicators; commercial spatial planning and design; importance–performance analysis; importance–performance–scope analysis

Citation: Huang, C.-P.; Huang, C.-H.; Chen, C.-C. Analyzing Key Quality Attributes in Commercial Space Design Planning Using Impact Range Performance Analysis by Computer Software for Sustainable Development Goals. *Eng. Proc.* **2024**, *74*, 68. https://doi.org/10.3390/engproc2024074068

Academic Editors: Shu-Han Liao, Teen-Hang Meen and Cheng-Fu Yang

Published: 27 September 2024

1. Introduction

The global pandemic of COVID-19 profoundly impacted the perspectives of human life and reconfigured the structure of commerce. COVID-19 was not only a mere health crisis but revealed the inherent vulnerabilities and fluidity of the commercial milieu. From the rise of telecommuting to fundamental alterations in consumer behavior, the pandemic recalibrated the expectations of commercial environments. In this context, the design and planning of commercial activities for contemporary demands transcend design considerations. They directly implicate a business's sustainability and trajectory. In this overarching paradigm, consumer needs and expectations have been more multifaceted and nuanced, seeking a new method for shopping or consumption with an emphasis on health, safety, and environmental resilience. For businesses and consumers, the commerce industry necessitates prescient adjustments and innovations in both design and functionality.

Thus, this study, anchored in a consumer-centric paradigm, was conducted to explore the needs and anticipations of consumers in the post-pandemic epoch. Through analysis, orientations and strategies for commercial space design were proposed to guide companies to cultivate adaptable and enduring business frameworks.

2. Literature Review

2.1. Sustainable Development Goals (SDGs) and Commercial Design

In the aftermath of the pandemic, various sectors grapple with unparalleled challenges, ranging from the assimilation of cutting-edge technologies to radical transformations and reevaluating entrenched business models [1–5]. Thus, we researched business directions with an emphasis on the planning and design of commercial spaces. Architectural and strategic commercial spaces must be constructed according to the demands and epidemic prevention protocols. For example, shopping centers and retail stores need to amplify their sanitary provisions by adding more restrooms and disinfection points and establishing cleaning routines for touchscreens. Concurrently, astute spatial design and effective crowd regulation become indispensable to ensure social distancing measures. These measures help commercial spaces in the post-pandemic era to secure safety, comfort, and multifunctionality and aptly respond to the dynamic needs and anticipations of consumers.

2.2. Importance–Performance Analysis (IPA)

IPA is widely adopted in evaluating the operational efficiency of enterprises [6,7]. In IPA, questionnaires are formulated based on the attributes of products or services. Consumers are invited to appraise these attributes in terms of their 'importance' and 'performance'. These evaluations are plotted on a two-dimensional space with 'importance' on the Y-axis and 'performance' on the X-axis. Utilizing the mean values of both axes as a basis, the space is divided into four quadrants, each bearing its managerial implications. While IPA has been extensively used for various analytical purposes, it allows for decisions related to satisfaction and brand loyalty. However, it has limitations resulting in failing to effectively tackle the underlying issues. To address these shortcomings, the Impact Range Performance Analysis (IRPA) and impact-asymmetry analysis (IAA) theoretical frameworks, as well as the Penalty Reward Contrast Analysis (PRCA), were introduced to IPA [7]. In this approach, each attribute is represented by two distinct virtual variables: the Penalty Index (PI) and the Reward Index (RI). These indices are used to measure the influence of each attribute on overall customer satisfaction. PI assigns a value of 1 to the lowest scoring attribute with all other scores being 0. In contrast, the RI gives a score of 1 to the highest scoring attribute with other scores set to 0. The sum of the absolute values of the coefficients for the reward and penalty indices illustrates the magnitude of an attribute's influence on overall customer satisfaction as the Range of Impact on Overall Customer Satisfaction (RIOCS). The PRCA has two distinct functions. The first evaluates the RIOCS of each attribute, while the second determines the asymmetry of impact on customer satisfaction (Impact Asymmetry, IA). The computations are as follows.

$$\text{RIOCSi} = |\text{Ri}| + |\text{Pi}| \quad (1)$$

$$\text{SGPi} = \text{Ri}/\text{RIOCSi} \quad (2)$$

$$\text{DGPi} = |\text{Pi}|/\text{RIOCSi} \quad (3)$$

$$\text{IAi index} = |\text{SGPi}| - |\text{DGPi}| \quad (4)$$

$$|\text{SGPi}| + |\text{DGPi}| = 1 \quad (5)$$

where Ri represents the reward coefficient of attribute i, while Pi symbolizes its penalty coefficient, and RIOCS denotes the "Relative Importance of Customer Satisfaction". The RIOCS matrix delineates the influence of various quality attributes on overarching customer satisfaction. Satisfaction-Generation Potential (SGP) indicates the potential for a quality attribute to positively influence customer satisfaction. Conversely, Dissatisfaction-

Generation Potential (DGP) describes the potential of a quality attribute to adversely affect customer satisfaction. Lastly, Impact-Asymmetry (IA) quantifies the asymmetric influence on customer satisfaction when a particular quality attribute either improves or deteriorates.

3. Methodology

The Attractive Ergonomics Model (EGM) was used for in-depth interviews to discern factors of commercial space design and planning integrated with SDG indicators. For precise and targeted information during the in-depth interviews associated with attractive ergonomics, we bypassed traditional test samples. Instead, EGM interviews were conducted based on individual perceptions to avoid potential sample biases or undue influences and more accurately reflect the association of the SDG indicators and commercial space design. Twelve participants were selected for the interviews, including 6 interior designers, 3 commercial space operators, and 3 marketing planners with an average of over ten years of professional experience.

An IPA questionnaire survey was created based on the factors identified from the EGM interviews regarding the SDG indicators. An appropriate IPA questionnaire was curated after focus group discussions. This focus group consisted of 12 participants, including 6 interior designers, 3 commercial space operators, and 3 marketing planners, each with a professional tenure exceeding 10 years. We analyzed the attributes of SDGs in conjunction with commercial space design to understand participants' evaluations of each attribute and their satisfaction. We evaluated the attributes of commercial space designs integrated with the SDG indicators using metrics including RI, PI, RIOCS, SGP, DGP, and IA. These indicators were chosen to provide insights into various aspects of commercial space designs that incorporate the SDG indicators, ranging from satisfaction discrepancies to relative importance. The analysis results offer information with which concrete strategies and recommendations can be formulated in relevant fields.

4. Results and Discussion

4.1. EGM Interview

Utilizing the Attractive Ergonomics approach, 12 participants were interviewed in the Environment–Goal–Means (EGM) network diagram (Figure 1) to delve into the implications of the post-pandemic era on the planning and design of commercial spaces. Participant feedback was categorized into hygiene and safety, quality of life, spatial design, and sustainable development. The identified attractiveness factors were determined to exhibit substantial relevance from the consumer's vantage point as the primary attributes consumers value. These attributes impact satisfaction and purchasing intentions and reflect the evolving societal and economic trends and necessities.

A pronounced linkage was observed between waste management and green landscapes. After the pandemic, consumers tend to focus on environmental sustainability. Consequently, companies need to curtail waste and feature green spaces to enhance air quality and provide a relaxation zone. It is thus imperative to perform waste management and green landscaping to align with consumer expectations. Participation and sharing spaces encourage consumers to engage in and interact with commercial spaces. The shared space offers multifunctionality and choices resonating with consumers' inclination toward resource conservation. By integrating participation and shared spaces, diverse needs can be satisfied, leading to the creation of enticing environments.

In the post-pandemic era, the interrelation between hygiene, safety, and quality of life has been intensified. Consumers prioritize their health and safety in commercial spaces, seeking a potentially hazard-free environment. A clean, organized, and strictly hygienic space influences the consumer's quality of life. Such environments diminish stress by alleviating health concerns and enhance the overall experience. Moreover, a secure and hygienic space fortifies consumer trust. Such spaces reinforce the perception that companies prioritize the well-being of their customers and foster enduring trust and loyalty. They also generate positive word-of-mouth and social media endorsements, attracting potential patrons. Thus, hygiene, safety, and life quality are interwoven in commercial spaces.

The intricate interconnectedness of the attractive factors suggests that sustainable design in commercial space planning must be holistic, taking into account the diverse consumer preferences while balancing these elements. The efficacy of a commercial space relies on its adeptness in harmonizing these elements and ensuring a secure, eco-conscious, and gratifying customer experience. Understanding these interconnections from a consumer perspective is crucial for the optimal design and management of commercial spaces to meet consumer anticipations and have a lasting competitive edge for a sustainable and appealing future of commercial spaces.

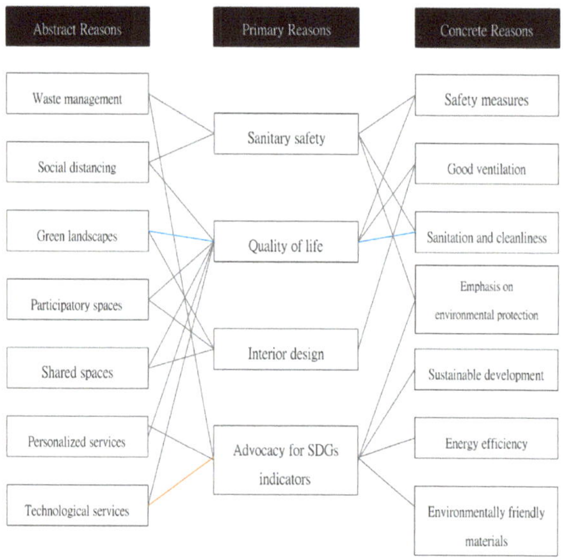

Figure 1. EGM interview.

4.2. IPA Results

In September 2023, we distributed a questionnaire for an online survey. The target participants included professionals such as commercial space operators, interior designers, and renovation specialists, as well as consumers acquainted with SDGs and those regularly using commercial spaces. Overall, 158 valid responses were obtained, and the reliability of the IPA questionnaire was assessed using Cronbach's α coefficient. The coefficient was 0.938, signifying the survey's reliability.

Table 1 shows safety protocols, efficient ventilation, and cleanliness in the "Maintain Strength" quadrant. These three quality attributes are regarded as supremely essential, reflecting exemplary standards, and highlighting their dominance and indispensability in commercial space design. Such results resonate with the contemporary societal emphasis on health and safety, especially in the ongoing context of pandemics and heightened environmental concerns. Thus, commercial space designers must prioritize these attributes to ensure their designs meet foundational necessities.

The "Priority for Improvement" quadrant identifies attributes such as environmental conservation, a focus on sustainability, energy efficiency, and efficient waste management. These elements are important, yet their performance is comparatively suboptimal. This indicates areas for improvement in commercial spaces, especially for sustainability. Within the SDGs framework, these attributes adhere to societal anticipations and mitigate negative environmental consequences. Hence, designers in the commercial space domain need to concentrate their efforts on developing and implementing more sustainable methodologies to enhance outcomes in these areas. Attributes such as eco-friendly material usage, social distancing design considerations, and personalized services were categorized under the "Secondary Improvement" quadrant. While these elements may not be as pivotal as other attributes, they need to be enhanced. Designers of commercial spaces must incorporate these aspects to enrich the holistic quality of their designs and ensure that they adapt to the constantly shifting consumer requirements and market dynamics. The "Excessive Emphasis" quadrant presents the provision of shared spaces but a lack of performance. This indicates that several commercial spaces focus overly on shared space configurations and neglect other integral quality aspects. Thus, designers must realign their priorities to balance their designs for diverse needs.

Table 1. IPA analysis results.

	Questionnaire Title	Importance (M = 4.42)	Satisfaction (M = 3.32)	IPA
1.	Diverse vegetarian options	4.93	3.51	I.
2.	Reducing food waste and providing recycling measures	4.83	3.38	I.
3.	Supporting local agriculture and farmers	4.92	3.76	I.
4.	Regulating energy conservation and resource efficiency	4.58	3.29	II.
5.	Sustainable fisheries and marine conservation	4.51	3.25	II.
6.	Eco-friendly tableware and reducing single-use plastic products	4.34	3.18	III.
7.	Supporting development in impoverished areas and increasing farmers' income	4.51	3.23	II.
8.	Promoting healthy eating choices and advocating a healthy lifestyle	4.28	3.27	III.
9.	Organic agricultural products and additive-free ingredients	4.29	3.39	IV.
10.	Water resource protection and conservation	4.23	3.25	III.
11.	Cultural exchange of ingredients and culinary fusion	4.20	3.28	III.
12.	Sustainable economic development and employment opportunities	4.09	3.25	III.
13.	Sustainable banquet venues and environmental design	4.34	3.24	III.
14.	Active promotion of local ingredients and agricultural products at banquets	3.82	3.20	III.

The IPA analysis results provide a reference for commercial space design and planning for SDGs. The results can guide designers to satisfy fundamental requirements and tackle the challenges of sustainability and societal accountability. This underscores the collaboration between researchers and practitioners and the continuous refinement of commercial space designs for evolving demands and societal values.

4.3. IRPA Results

RI in Table 2 indicates the respondents' evaluation of the importance of each quality attribute. Notably, attributes such as safety measures, optimal ventilation, hygiene and cleanliness, commitment to environmental conservation and sustainable development, and an emphasis on energy efficiency scored higher in RI. This underscores the respondents' perception that these attributes are crucial to the success of commercial space design. These findings resonate with the current societal emphasis on health, environmental consciousness, and sustainability, revealing their tangible impact on considerations in commercial space design. PI reflects the actual performance of each quality attribute. All attributes scored below zero. This suggests a potential for enhancement of these attributes in commercial space designs. Specifically, personalized services, the integration of technological solutions, the incorporation of green landscapes, and the provision of community engagement spaces scored low for PI, indicating their deficiency for deployment.

Table 2. IRPA analysis results.

	Items	RI	PI	RIOCS	SGP	DGP	IA
1.	SMEs' participation in social welfare activities	0.523	−0.496	1.019	0.513	0.487	0.026
2.	Gender equality employment opportunities	0.491	−0.557	1.048	0.469	0.531	−0.063
3.	Resource recycling implementation	0.555	−0.446	1.001	0.554	0.446	0.109
4.	Assistance to charitable organizations	0.585	−0.507	1.092	0.536	0.464	0.071
5.	Availability of SDGs-compliant products	0.533	−0.532	1.065	0.500	0.500	0.001
6.	Active promotion of SDGs	0.590	−0.499	1.089	0.542	0.458	0.084
7.	Price increases due to SDGs without affecting choices	0.577	−0.506	1.083	0.533	0.467	0.066
8.	Economic benefits from SDGs products/services	0.529	−0.506	1.035	0.511	0.489	0.022
9.	Uniqueness of SDG indicators	0.531	−0.525	1.056	0.503	0.497	0.006
10.	Provision of SDGs-related information	0.528	−0.566	1.094	0.483	0.517	−0.035
11.	Sense of security using SDGs products	0.532	−0.585	1.117	0.476	0.524	−0.047
12.	Creativity and innovation of SDGs products	0.573	−0.550	1.123	0.510	0.490	0.020
13.	Increased consumer awareness of SDGs	0.489	−0.571	1.060	0.461	0.539	−0.077
14.	Enhanced environmental knowledge from SDGs	0.546	−0.621	1.167	0.468	0.532	−0.064
	Mean (M)	0.542	−0.533	1.075	0.504	0.496	0.008

RIOCS captures the disparity between RI and PI, showing the areas of improvement for each quality attribute. RIOCS scores indicate required improvement: a positive value implies a need to elevate performance, whereas a negative value suggests that performance has already exceeded its perceived importance. In this context, commercial space designs need to be designed to enhance attributes such as personalized services, technological integration, green landscapes, and community engagement. SGP and DGP are used to decide the direction of improvements. SGP is related to attributes such as social distancing planning, the provision of shared spaces, and safety measures for enhancement. Conversely, DGP underscores the personalized services, technological integration, and the inclusion of green landscapes. IA is used for the assessment of the gap between RI and PI in commercial space design and its refinement. Commercial space design needs to be improved for quality attributes to meet the respondent's expectations and needs.

IRPA results provide a basis for assessing the quality attributes of commercial space design and planning. The results can be used to create a roadmap for designers and decision-makers and guide strategies for the sustainability and client satisfaction of commercial spaces. Moreover, they highlight the imperative for a holistic strategy, ensuring a balanced and superior performance for the attributes in commercial space design.

5. Conclusions

In an ever-evolving society and globalization, commercial space design stands at a crossroads with both opportunities and challenges. Originating from a consumer-centric perspective, we delved into commercial spaces for SDGs and integrated design strategies to meet the demands of sustainable development. Through multifaceted analyses, attributes that decisively influence consumer satisfaction were determined to understand the disparity between consumer expectations and experiences for the attributes. The results highlight that the commercial space has a value for 'safety measures', 'optimal ventilation', and 'hygiene and cleanliness'. Yet, performance related to 'environmental conservation and sustainability' needs to be improved. As environmental sustainability is gaining paramount attention, commercial spaces are more than just platforms for brand display and service. They manifest corporate culture and values. As such, innovation and sustainability emerge as the mission for commercial space design. The outcomes of this study offer strategic directions for commercial space design, prompting industry professionals to re-evaluate their designs and strategies from the consumer perspective. The present preliminary research needs to be expanded to investigate the expectations and needs of diverse consumer groups concerning commercial space design under the purview of the SDGs to offer comprehensive and actionable strategies.

Author Contributions: Conceptualization, C.-P.H. and C.-H.H.; methodology, C.-P.H.; software, C.-C.C.; validation, C.-P.H., C.-H.H. and C.-C.C.; formal analysis, C.-C.C.; investigation, C.-P.H.; resources, C.-P.H.; data curation, C.-P.H.; writing—original draft preparation, C.-P.H.; writing—review and editing, C.-P.H. and C.-H.H.; visualization, C.-C.C.; supervision, C.-H.H.; project administration, C.-H.H. All authors have read and agreed to the published version of the manuscript.

Funding: This research did not receive external funding.

Institutional Review Board Statement: Not applicable.

Informed Consent Statement: Not applicable.

Data Availability Statement: Data are contained within the article.

Conflicts of Interest: The authors declare no conflicts of interest.

References

1. Lai, J. An initial exploration of museum integration in virtual and physical realms in response to the metaverse during the post-pandemic era. *Mus. Cult.* **2022**, *24*, 77–104.
2. Wu, T.H.; Su, C.M.; Chen, X.T. A SWOT matrix analysis study on marketing strategies for unmanned intelligent hotels in the post-pandemic era. *J. Tour. Leis. Manag.* **2023**, *11*, 262–269.
3. Smith, S.W.; Shi, J.; Li, Z. Health communication and interdisciplinary research in the post-pandemic era. *J. Commun. Soc.* **2023**, *64*, 1–28.
4. Chang, Y.L.; Yeh, L.T.; Lee, Y.F. Analysis of consumer risk perception, restaurant safety trust, epidemic prevention measures, and consumption intentions in upscale restaurants during the post-pandemic era. *J. Sports Health Leis. Natl. Chia Yi Univ.* **2023**, *22*, 12–30.
5. Cheung, C.G. Investigation into the establishment and accessibility of museum collection interpretation data: A case study of the digital collections of artifacts at the National Palace Museum. *J. Technol. Mus.* **2022**, *26*, 25–47.
6. O'Sullivan, E.L. Improving performance with feedback. *Cornell Hotel. Restaur. Adm. Q.* **1991**, *32*, 31–40.
7. Hansen, E.; Bush, R.J. Understanding customer quality requirements: Model and application. *Ind. Mark. Manag.* **1999**, *28*, 119–130. [CrossRef]

engineering proceedings

MDPI

Proceeding Paper

Evaluation of Fabrication Process for Molybdenum Disulfide Quantum Dots in Organic Solvents Using Ultrasonic and Thermal Exfoliation †

Hon-Pan Yiu [1], Cheng-Jun Wu [1], Chuan Li [1,*] and Cho-Yin Lee [1,2,*]

1 Department of Biomedical Engineering, National Yang Ming Chiao Tung University, Taipei 112, Taiwan; yiuhonpan@gmail.com (H.-P.Y.); wuchengjunw@gmail.com (C.-J.W.)
2 Department of Radiation Oncology, Taoyuan General Hospital, Ministry of Health and Welfare, Taoyuan 330, Taiwan
* Correspondence: cli10@nycu.edu.tw (C.L.); choyin.lee@nycu.edu.tw (C.-Y.L.)

† Presented at the 2024 IEEE 4th International Conference on Electronic Communications, Internet of Things and Big Data, Taipei, Taiwan, 19–21 April 2024.

Abstract: When the size of the molybdenum disulfide (MoS_2) is reduced to a few nanometers, a distinctive photoluminescence is observed due to the strong effect of quantum confinement. In this study, we fabricated MoS_2 quantum dots (QDs) using a simple and green process. We dissolved the powder of MoS_2 in various solvents, including N-Methyl-2-pyrrolidone (NMP), ethanol (EtOH), and deionized water (DIW), and dispersed it by sonication or solvent-thermal exfoliation. The synthesized MoS_2 QDs were characterized for their optical properties. Transmission electron microscopy (TEM) was used to analyze the particle size and morphology; UV-visible spectrometer and photoluminescence tests were employed to measure optical absorption, bandgaps, and optical emission. The photothermal test was designed for the evaluation of the optothermal conversion. In vitro cultures of 3T3 fibroblast cells were evaluated for the biocompatibility of the MoS_2 QDs. Results from different experiments were cross-examined and analyzed to understand the relation among different syntheses, microstructures, and optical properties of MoS_2 QDs. A yield of 15% MoS_2 QDs was obtained when synthesized in ethanol by thermal exfoliation. They also showed satisfactory optothermal effects.

Keywords: molybdenum disulfide quantum dots (MoS_2 QDs); yield; photoluminescence; photothermal

Citation: Yiu, H.-P.; Wu, C.-J.; Li, C.; Lee, C.-Y. Evaluation of Fabrication Process for Molybdenum Disulfide Quantum Dots in Organic Solvents Using Ultrasonic and Thermal Exfoliation. *Eng. Proc.* **2024**, *74*, 69. https://doi.org/10.3390/engproc2024074069

Academic Editors: Shu-Han Liao, Teen-Hang Meen and Cheng-Fu Yang

Published: 29 September 2024

1. Introduction

Molybdenum disulfide (MoS_2) is an inorganic compound that belongs to the class of transition metal dichalcogenides. Its appendages are silvery black and are the main ore of molybdenite in nature [1]. Since bulk MoS_2 is a semiconductor with a narrow indirect band gap of approximately (~1.2 eV), it has been studied for photovoltaic and photocatalytic applications due to its strong absorption in the solar spectrum [2,3]. If the bulk size is reduced to a scale of dozens of nanometers, then the effects of quantum confinement dictate the electronic and optical properties of MoS_2. This phenomenon has been observed in MoS_2 films, nanoplates, and nanotubes [4,5].

Molybdenum disulfide (MoS_2) quantum dots (QDs) are biocompatible [6] and semiconductive with high photothermal conversion efficiency [7]. Li et al. have recently shown that MoS_2 flakes and ultra-small diameter MoS_2 QDs can be used in the renal pathway, thereby reducing long-term toxicity in kidneys. For the synthesis of MoS_2 QDs, top-down or bottom-up methods are used as available approaches. Chemical exfoliation, mechanical, electrochemical, emulsion, solvothermal, thermal ablation, and combined methods have been studied to produce MoS_2 QDs effectively. Each approach has advantages and shortcomings, but a common problem is the low yields of production. This is a challenge for up-scaling industrial production of MoS_2 QDs when compared to the production of carbon QDs [8].

The synthesis of MoS_2 QDs by the solvent–thermal process is relatively simple. The powder of MoS_2 is first dissolved in various solvents, including N-Methyl-2-pyrrolidone (NMP) and ethanol (EtOH), in deionized water (DIW). Then, either using sonication or solvent–thermal exfoliation, the MoS_2 QDs are produced. For the material characterization, transmission electron microscopy (TEM) is used to examine the particle size and morphology; UV-visible spectrometer and photoluminescence tests are used to measure the optical absorption, bandgaps, and optical emission. The in vitro cell culture of 3T3 fibroblast cells is assessed for the biocompatibility of MoS_2 QDs.

In this study, we used the sonification and solvent–thermal approach to investigate the synthesis of the MoS_2 QDs using different solvents. The results provide a reference for further research and the efficient manufacture of MoS_2 QDs.

2. Material and Method

2.1. Synthesis Method

Commercially available MoS_2 powders (~100–150 μm) were dispersed in ethanol (99.99%) by either ice-bath sonication (US) or solvent–thermal exfoliation (ST), as shown in Figure 1. Three solvents were used in this study: ethanol (EtOH), deionized water (DIW), and N-methyl-2-pyrrolidone (NMP). 20 mL of the solvents was used for the dispersion of MoS_2 powders. Following the dispersion, the solutions were centrifuged at 10,000 rpm for 15 min to remove the remaining bulk-size MoS_2. Then, the solutions were dialyzed by DIW through a dialysis membrane (molecular weight of 1 K Da) for three days to remove the excessive solvent. Finally, the dialyzed material was freeze-dried to increase its concentration.

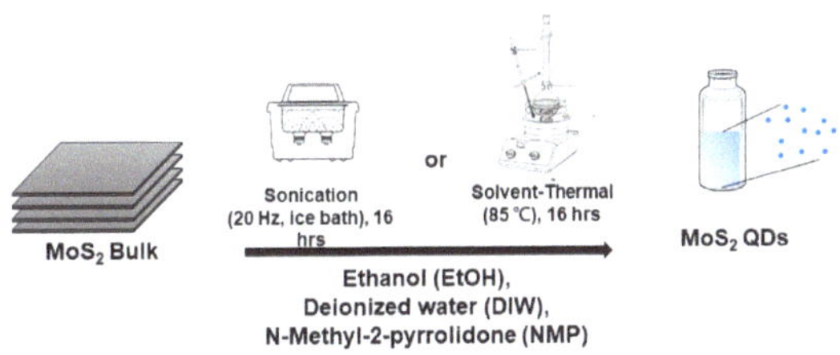

Figure 1. The synthesis of MoS_2 QDs.

2.2. Optical Characterization

The UV-VIS spectrum was measured using Biochrom Ultrospec 9000pc (Fisher Scientific Arendalsvägen Göteborg, Sweden). The range for optical absorption was between 300 and 800 nm. The Beer–Lambert law states that

$$I_T = I_0\, e^{-\varepsilon l c} \tag{1}$$

where I_T and I_0 are the intensity of transmitted and incident laser light, ε is the molar attenuation coefficient or absorptivity of the attenuating species, ℓ is the optical path length, and c is the concentration of the attenuating species. For simplicity, we combine the last three terms into one single absorbance A:

$$A \equiv \varepsilon l c = -\ln(I_T/I_0) \tag{2}$$

If the attenuation of an incident beam of light within a homogeneous solution is assumed to be absorption only. A conventional scale to represent the optical absorbance in solution is $\log_{10}$ instead of ln, so the optical absorbance of the sample is taken as:

$$A = -\log_{10}(I_T/I_0) = (1/\log_{10}(e))\ (I_T/I_0) \tag{3}$$

The photoluminance (PL) spectrum of MoS_2 QDs was measured with a multimode microplate reader (SPARK®, TECAN, Männedorf, Switzerland). The light source of the excitation laser ranges from 300 nm to 400 nm with a resolution of 10 nm. There was a shift of 45 nm for optical emission to avoid the overlapping between the excitation and emission. The image of MoS_2 QDs was examined with transmission electron microscopy (TEM) (JEM-2000EX II, JEOL, Tokyo, Japan) in magnified images obtained from ImageJ® 1.54j.

2.3. Ex-Vitro Photothermal Effect

The photothermal effect of MoS_2 QDs was assessed by direct irradiation using an 808 nm near-infrared (NIR) light-emitting diode (LED) laser at a distance of 20 mm. The specific near-infrared wavelength was selected considering its high transmission ratio into the human body and a range of therapeutic benefits such as reducing inflammation, pain, and increased blood flow [9,10]. The temperature variation was measured by a digital multimeter (600 V CAT III, Fluke Corporation, United States) every 15 s. The setup for the measurement is shown in Figure 2.

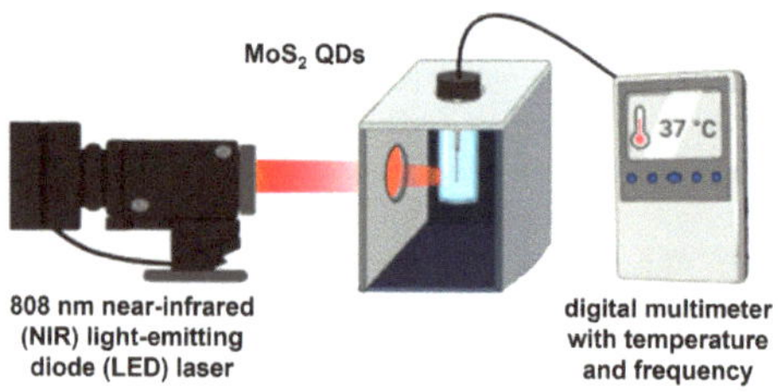

Figure 2. Illustration of ex vitro photothermal measure of MoS_2 QDs irradiated under 808 nm NIR LED laser.

2.4. In-Vitro Biocompatibility

To evaluate the biocompatibility of MoS_2 QDs, we used the 3-(4,5-dimethylthiazol-2-yl)-2,5-diphenyltetrazolium bromide (MTT) assay and analyzed the viability of 3T3 fibroblast cells cultured with MoS_2 QDs. 3T3 fibroblast cells were seeded in a 96-well tissue-culture plate at a density of 1×10^4 cells per well in a culture medium (Dulbecco's Modified Eagle Medium (DMEM), Gibco, New York, USA). The incubator (Thermo Forma 310, Thermo Fisher Scientific, Waltham, Massachusetts, USA) was controlled at 37 °C, a humidity of 95%, and a CO_2 flow of 5%. MoS_2 QDs of four different concentrations at 0.5, 0.25, 0.125, and 0.0625 mg/mL were mixed in the culture medium and tested for cell culture (testing group). The cell variability was assessed at 24 and 72 h after seeding. The MTT assay was measured by using a multimode microplate reader (SPARK®, TECAN, Männedorf, Switzerland) at the absorption peak of 560 nm. The biocompatibility was measured (n = 6) for the untreated (zero MoS_2 QDs, the control group) cells as follows:

$$\text{Relative Cell viability (\%)} = \text{(Average of Intensity of Testing Group)}/\text{(Average of Intensity of Control Group)} \times 100\% \quad (4)$$

3. Result

3.1. Yield of Synthesis

The yields of synthesis for MoS_2 QDs by different methods are presented in Table 1. Among the three solvents, ethanol (EtOH) resulted in a higher yield of 15%, especially in the solvent–thermal method. This is attributed to the high solubility of MoS_2 in ethanol (~0.1–5 mg/mL), by which a higher exfoliation rate resulted in [11,12].

Table 1. The yield of different synthesis methods and solvents for molybdenum disulfide QDs.

Synthesis	MoS_2 Weight (mg)	Solvent (mL)	Product Weight (MoS_2 QDs, mg)	Yield Ratio
Sonication Method (US)	200 mg	EtOH, 20 mL	14 mg	7.0%
		DIW, 20 mL	9 mg	4.5%
		NMP, 20 mL	6 mg	3.0%
Solvent-Thermal Method (ST)		EtOH, 20 mL	30 mg	15.0%
		DIW, 20 mL	4 mg	2.0%
		NMP, 20 mL	3 mg	1.5%

3.2. Characterization

3.2.1. Particle Size and Morphology

The particle size and morphology of MoS_2 QDs are shown in Figure 3, where the size of the particle was analyzed by ImageJ®. Except for NMP under the solvent–thermal process, all samples showed particles of less than 20 nm. Among all solvents, ethanol effectively exfoliated bulk MoS_2 to a few nanometers, whether by sonication or thermal treatment.

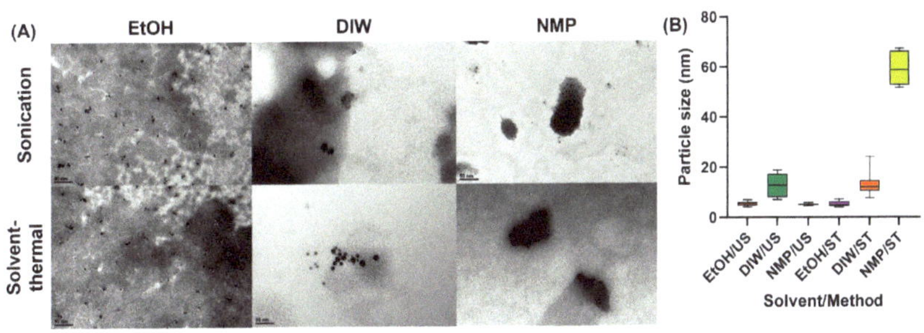

Figure 3. (**A**) TEM image and (**B**) particle size distribution of MoS_2 QDs synthesized using different methods and solvents.

3.2.2. UV-Visible Spectrum

Figure 4 shows the UV-Vis spectra of MoS_2 QDs. Broad absorption peaks in the UV range are common features of all samples, regardless of the method of synthesis. However, this broadband peak can be further broken down into two sub-band peaks. One shows a peak at 340 nm with the photon-induced excitons in MoS_2 QDs, and the other has a peak between 220 and 300 nm due to the quasi-continuous electronic band structures by quantum confinement [13]. For samples synthesized in ethanol, another broadband peak of around 795 nm was observed (Figure 4A,D). This peak is related to the optothermal excitation. Absorbed photons at this long wavelength provide a red-shift energy release in MoS_2 QDs.

3.2.3. Optical Absorbance

Given the UV-visible spectra, we estimated the absorbance of MoS_2 QDs using the Beer–Lambert law and Equation (3). Figure 5 shows the calculated absorbance of QDs. All samples exhibit high optical absorbance in the range of 200–400 nm for ultraviolet light. This is the signature of nanosized crystals where the quantum effects become noticeable. However, for QDs synthesized in EtOH, there is another broadband absorption in the range of 700–900 nm, which can be the conversion of near-infrared thermal energy.

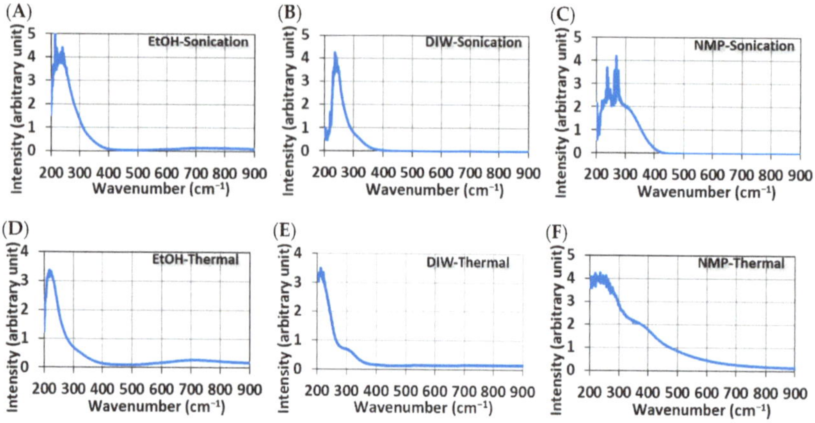

Figure 4. The UV-visible spectrum of MoS_2 QDs was synthesized using different methods and solvents. Ultrasonically in (**A**) EtOH, (**B**) DIW, and (**C**) NMP; Thermally in (**D**) EtOH, (**E**) DIW, and (**F**) NMP.

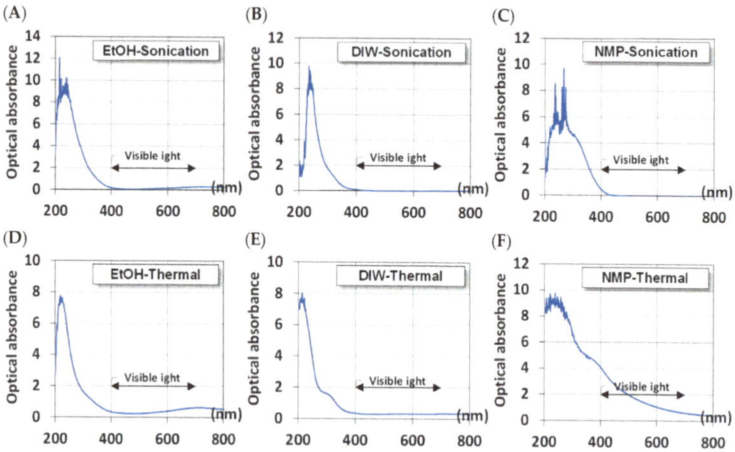

Figure 5. The optical absorbance of synthesized MoS_2 QDs using different methods and solvents. Ultrasonically in (**A**) EtOH, (**B**) DIW, and (**C**) NMP; Thermally in (**D**) EtOH, (**E**) DIW, and (**F**) NMP.

The NMP solvent presents a broad range of absorption due to the larger particle size of MoS_2, as shown in Figure 3 from the TEM image.

3.2.4. Photoluminescence

Figure 6 shows the photoluminescence of synthesized MoS_2 QDs. The highest intensity of optical emission from samples was found centered around 440–450 nm when the wavelength of the excitation laser was 340 nm. Interestingly, this result did not change by the method of synthesis or solvents. In other words, resonantly excited electrons in the synthesized QDs released energy by emitting photons almost along the same relaxation pathway or changes between the same energy levels [14]. According to the location of emission peaks, this fluorescence emission redshifted at the edge of blue light. However, the emission was broadband with a shoulder between 450 and 500 nm. This indicates the excited electrons have a two-stage energy release of photons. In the NMP solvent–thermal process, a broad photoluminescence peak was observed due to a larger deviation in the particle size distribution (Figure 3). The photoluminescence ebbed as the quantum confinement weakened when particles became larger [15].

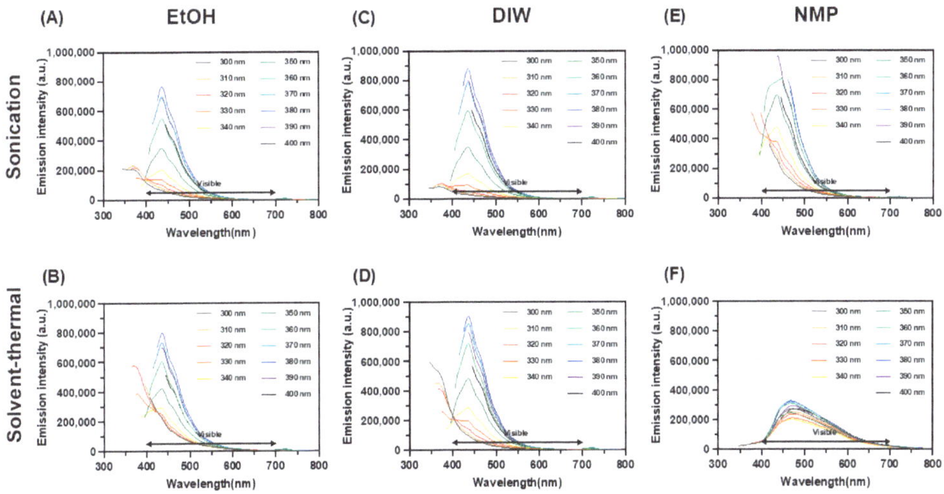

Figure 6. The photoluminescence spectrum of synthesized MoS_2 QDs using different methods and solvents as marked. Ultrasonically in (**A**) EtOH, (**B**) DIW, and (**C**) NMP; Thermally in (**D**) EtOH, (**E**) DIW, and (**F**) NMP.

The bangap of QDs can be estimated as $\Delta E = h(\Delta v) \approx h(C/\lambda_{emission})$. For the peaks at 440–450 nm, the corresponding bandgap is around 2.82–2.76 eV. The energy change between excitation and emission is around $\Delta E = h(\Delta v) \approx h(C/\lambda_{incident} - C/\lambda_{emission}) = 0.8288 - 0.8914$ eV. A freestanding monolayer MoS_2 is predicted to have direct bandgaps around 1.8–2.8 eV, and the bulk MoS_2 (hexagonal and rhombohedral symmetry) showed narrower indirect bandgaps around 1.2 eV [16–21]. Based on the nature of multiple bandgaps of polycrystallinity in QDs, the estimated bandgap from the photoluminescence spectra was roughly within the upper bound of the findings in the other studies.

3.3. Photothermal Effect

The UV-VIS absorption spectra showed the presence of a broadband peak around 795 nm. This absorption is useful for clinical treatment if properly utilized [22]. Figure 7 shows the variation of temperature when samples of MoS_2 QDs were exposed to an 808 nm LED laser. MoS_2 QDs synthesized in EtOH showed the temperature rise to 50 °C in 300 s. Other samples had a smaller temperature rise of around 25–30 °C in 300 s. The photothermal effect occurred due to the absorption of photons in the whole spectra, though the broadband peak had a major contribution to the effect because of the vicinity of 808 and 795 nm. At the wavelengths, the photon energy becomes more readily absorbed. MoS_2 QDs synthesized in EtOH convert the energy efficiently because of their smaller size. The solvent–thermal synthesized NMP MoS_2 QDs were noticed for their higher photothermal effect (temperature rise to 45 °C in 300 s). Figure 6F shows the broadband absorption that explains the enhanced photothermal conversion [23].

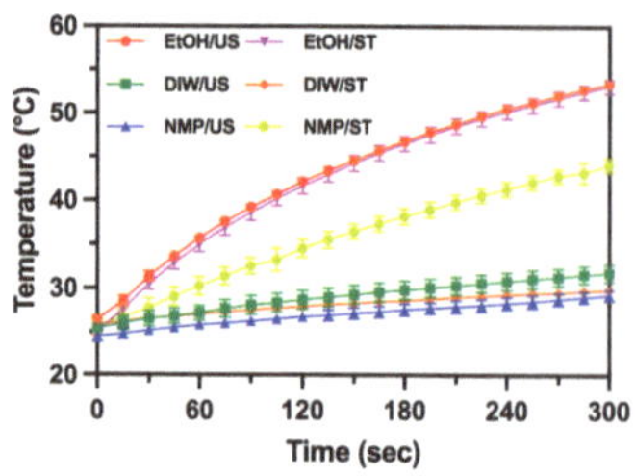

Figure 7. The temperature variation of synthesized MoS_2 QDs using different methods and solvents is marked. Samples were exposed to an 808 nm LED laser continuously.

3.4. Biocompatibility Evaluation

Figure 8 shows the relative cell viability for in vitro culture of 3T3 fibroblast cells. Only MoS_2 QDs synthesized in the EtOH solvent–thermal process were tested in the in vitro cell culture because of their high optothermal effect. For medium mixed with MoS_2 QDs, the viability was reduced as the concentration of MoS_2 increased. However, the low concentration of 00625 and 0.125 mg/mL was appropriate for the treatment of cells, particularly after 72 h when cells were stabilized and started to proliferate. The relative cell viability of these two concentrations was maintained at a level above 90% in 72 h after seeding.

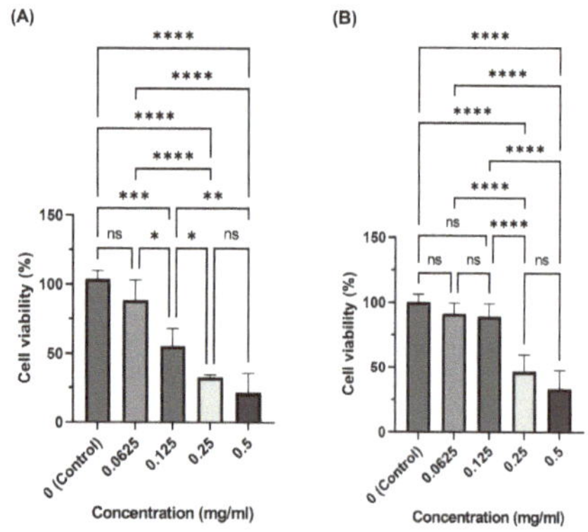

Figure 8. The biocompatibility of EtOH/ST MoS_2 QDs at (**A**) 24 hr and (**B**) 72 hr. (p-value: ****: 0.0001%, ***: 0.001%, **: 0.01%, *: 0.05%, ns: not significant).

4. Conclusions

The experimental results of this study showed the following findings: MoS_2 QDs were successfully synthesized using ultrasonic and thermal exfoliation in various solvents, including EtOH, DIW, and NMP. The most effective solvent to yield MoS_2 QDs was EtOH because of the high solubility of MoS_2 in EtOH (~0.1–5 mg/mL), which leads to a higher exfoliation rate. The UV-visible spectra of MoS_2 QDs showed a broadband absorption peak around 340 nm due to the photon-induced excitons. A smaller broadband peak around 795 nm was observed in the UV-visible spectra, related to the optothermal excitation. The photoluminescence of MoS_2 QDs showed the highest emission intensity at 440–450 nm with the excitation laser of 340 nm. This fluorescence emission was redshifted and broadband at the edge of blue light. Temperature variation in the photothermal test under an 808 nm LED laser showed that MoS_2 QDs synthesized in EtOH had the temperature rise to 50 °C in 300 s. Other samples had a smaller temperature rise of around 25–30 °C in 300 s. The result of in vitro 3T3 fibroblast cell culture indicated that low concentrations (0.0625 and

0.125 mg/mL) of MoS_2 QDs in the EtOH solvent–thermal process were appropriate for maintaining cell viability.

Author Contributions: Conceptualization, H.-P.Y. and C.-J.W.; methodology, H.-P.Y., C.-J.W. and C.-Y.L.; validation, H.-P.Y.; formal analysis, H.-P.Y.; investigation, C.-J.W.; resources, H.-P.Y.; data curation, C.L. and C.-Y.L.; writing—original draft preparation, review, and editing, H.-P.Y., C.L. and C.-Y.L.; visualization, H.-P.Y.; supervision, C.L. and C.-Y.L.; project administration, C.-Y.L. and C.L.; funding acquisition, C.-Y.L. and C.L. All authors have read and agreed to the published version of the manuscript.

Funding: The funding was funded by Taoyuan General Hospital, the Ministry of Health and Welfare (PTH113060), the Nation Science and Technology Council (NSTC 112-2622-E-A49-017), and the Joint Developed Project of Taiwan Semiconductor Research Institute (JDP113-Y1-093).

Institutional Review Board Statement: Not applicable.

Informed Consent Statement: Not applicable.

Data Availability Statement: The raw data supporting the conclusions of this article will be made available by the authors upon request.

Acknowledgments: This work was supported by the Electron Microscopy Facility at National Yang Ming Chiao Tung University and the Center for Plasma and Thin Film Technologies at the Ming Chi University of Technology.

Conflicts of Interest: Author C. Y. Lee is an adjunct professor in the Department of Biomedical Engineering and also an M.D. of Radiology at Taoyuan General Hospital. There are no conflicts of interest for his role in this study. The remaining authors declare that the research was conducted in the absence of any commercial or financial relationships that could be construed as a potential conflict of interest.

References

1. Mitchell, P.C.H.; Outteridge, T.; Kloska, K.; McMahon, S.; Epshteyn, Y.; Roger, F.S.; Burkin, A.R.; Dorfler, R.R.; Laferty, J.M.; Leichtfried, G.; et al. Molybdenum and Molybdenum Compounds. *Ullmann's Encycl. Ind. Chem.* **2020**, 1–63. [CrossRef]
2. Splendiani, A.; Sun, L.; Zhang, Y.; Li, T.; Kim, J.; Chim, C.Y.; Galli, G.; Wang, F. Emerging Photoluminescence in Monolayer MoS_2. *Nano Lett.* **2010**, *10*, 1271–1275. [CrossRef] [PubMed]
3. Wu, F.Y.; Cheng, Y.S.; Wang, D.M.; Li, M.L.; Lu, W.S.; Xu, X.Y.; Zhou, X.H.; Wei, X.W. Nitrogen-Doped MoS_2 QDs: Facile Synthesis and Application for the Assay of Hematin in Human Blood. *Mater. Sci. Eng. C* **2020**, *112*, 110898. [CrossRef]
4. Jiang, J.; Chen, Z.; Hu, Y.; Xiang, Y.; Zhang, L.; Wang, Y.; Wang, G.C.; Shi, J. Flexo-Photovoltaic Effect in MoS_2. *Nat Nanotechnol* **2021**, *16*, 894–901. [CrossRef] [PubMed]
5. Guo, Y.; Li, J. MoS_2 QDs: Synthesis, Properties and Biological Applications. *Mater. Sci. Eng. C* **2020**, *109*, 110511. [CrossRef]
6. Chen, X.; Park, Y.J.; Kang, M.; Kang, S.K.; Koo, J.; Shinde, S.M.; Shin, J.; Jeon, S.; Park, G.; Yan, Y.; et al. CVD-Grown Monolayer MoS_2 in Bioabsorbable Electronics and Biosensors. *Nat. Commun.* **2018**, *9*, 1690. [CrossRef]
7. Gan, X.; Zhao, H.; Quan, X. Two-Dimensional MoS_2: A Promising Building Block for Biosensors. *Biosens. Bioelectron.* **2017**, *89*, 56–71. [CrossRef]
8. Guo, Y.; Zhang, L.; Zhang, S.; Yang, Y.; Chen, X.; Zhang, M. Fluorescent Carbon Nanoparticles for the Fluorescent Detection of Metal Ions. *Biosens. Bioelectron.* **2015**, *63*, 61–71. [CrossRef]
9. Museux, N.; Perez, L.; Autrique, L.; Agay, D. Skin Burns after Laser Exposure: Histological Analysis and Predictive Simulation. *Burns* **2012**, *38*, 658–667. [CrossRef]
10. Svobodova, B.; Kloudova, A.; Ruzicka, J.; Kajtmanova, L.; Navratil, L.; Sedlacek, R.; Suchy, T.; Jhanwar-Uniyal, M.; Jendelova, P.; Machova Urdzikova, L. The Effect of 808 nm and 905 nm Wavelength Light on Recovery after Spinal Cord Injury. *Sci. Rep.* **2019**, *9*, 7660. [CrossRef]
11. Huang, H.; Liu, N.; Wang, X.; Zhong, M.; Huang, X. Application of Hydrothermal and Solvothermal Method in Synthesis of MoS_2. *Mater. Plast.* **2022**, *59*, 26–35. [CrossRef]
12. Li, Z.; Fan, R.; Hu, Z.; Li, W.; Zhou, H.; Kang, S.; Zhang, Y.; Zhang, H.; Wang, G. Ethanol introduced synthesis of ultrastable 1T-MoS_2 for removal of Cr (VI). *J. Hazard. Mater.* **2020**, *394*, 122525. [CrossRef]
13. Chikan, V.; Kelley, D.F. Size-Dependent Spectroscopy of MoS_2 Nanoclusters. *J. Phys. Chem. B* **2002**, *106*, 3794–3804. [CrossRef]
14. Kira, M.; Jahnke, F.; Koch, S.W. Quantum Theory of Secondary Emission in Optically Excited Semiconductor Quantum Wells. *Phys. Rev. Lett.* **1999**, *82*, 3544–3547. [CrossRef]
15. Hari Krishna, P.; Ramrakhiani, M. Nano Particle Size Effect on Photo-Luminescence. *Int. J. Nanotechnol. Appl.* **2010**, *4*, 13–19. [CrossRef]

16. Cao, H.; Wang, H.; Huang, Y.; Sun, Y.; Shi, S.; Tang, M. Quantification of Gold(III) in Solution and with a Test Stripe via the Quenching of the Fluorescence of Molybdenum Disulfide QDs. *Microchim. Acta* **2017**, *184*, 91–100. [CrossRef]
17. Ryou, J.; Kim, Y.S.; Kc, S.; Cho, K. Monolayer MoS_2 Bandgap Modulation by Dielectric Environments and Tunable Bandgap Transistors. *Sci. Rep.* **2016**, *6*, 29184. [CrossRef]
18. Kobayashi, K.; Yamauchi, J. Electronic structure and scanning-tunneling-microscopy image of molybdenum dichalcogenide surfaces. *Phys. Rev. B* **1995**, *51*, 17085–17095. [CrossRef] [PubMed]
19. Yun, W.S.; Han, S.W.; Hong, S.C.; Kim, I.G.; Lee, J.D. Thickness and strain effects on electronic structures of transition metal dichalcogenides: 2H-MX2 semiconductors (M = Mo, W; X = S, Se, Te). *Phys. Rev. B* **2012**, *85*, 033305. [CrossRef]
20. Cheiwchanchamnangij, T.; Lambrecht, W.R.L. Quasiparticle band structure calculation of monolayer, bilayer, and bulk MoS_2. *Phys. Rev. B* **2012**, *85*, 205302. [CrossRef]
21. Qiu, D.Y.; da Jornada, F.H.; Louie, S.G. Optical spectrum of MoS_2: Many-body effects and diversity of exciton states. *Phys. Rev. Lett.* **2013**, *111*, 216805. [CrossRef] [PubMed]
22. Wu, X.; Suo, Y.; Shi, H.; Liu, R.; Wu, F.; Wang, T.; Ma, L.; Liu, H.; Cheng, Z. Deep-Tissue Photothermal Therapy Using Laser Illumination at NIR-IIa Window. *Nanomicro Lett.* **2020**, *12*, 38. [CrossRef] [PubMed]
23. Jiang, Q.; Zeng, W.; Zhang, C.; Meng, Z.; Wu, J.; Zhu, Q.; Wu, D.; Zhu, H. Broadband Absorption and Enhanced Photothermal Conversion Property of Octopod-like Ag@Ag2S Core@shell Structures with Gradually Varying Shell Thickness. *Sci. Rep.* **2017**, *7*, 17782. [CrossRef] [PubMed]

engineering proceedings

MDPI

Proceeding Paper

Charm Factors of Clay and Composite Materials in Aesthetic Education Curriculum †

Qiu-Ying Lu [1] and Chia-Hui Huang [2,*]

1 Institute of Arts and Crafts, Tung-fang Design University, Kaohsiung 82941, Taiwan; luqiuying1976@gmail.com
2 Institute of Cultural and Creative Design, Tung-fang Design University, Kaohsiung 82941, Taiwan
* Correspondence: judy.tf.edu.tw@gmail.com
† Presented at the 2024 IEEE 4th International Conference on Electronic Communications, Internet of Things and Big Data, Taipei, Taiwan, 19–21 April 2024.

Abstract: The significance of aesthetic education is increasingly acknowledged for its role in enhancing students' motivation for creativity, aesthetic sensibility, critical thinking, and imagination. This enhancement enriches the practice of art education, providing students with expansive learning experiences. Focusing on the use of clay and composite materials in aesthetic education, we analyzed how the curriculum and creative courses can increase the attractiveness of learning. The incorporation of clay and composite materials into the presentation of athletic figures affected students' artistic endeavors. The diversity of the course content and artistic skills are important factors in augmenting creative activities. Hence, educators need to consider such attributes in the development and execution of curricula in aesthetic education and stimulate students' artistic innovation and potential. The results of this study suggest a way to improve aesthetic education and composite material creation courses to elevate students' creativity and artistic competencies.

Keywords: aesthetic education; curriculum design; charm factors; Kano model

Citation: Lu, Q.-Y.; Huang, C.-H. Charm Factors of Clay and Composite Materials in Aesthetic Education Curriculum. *Eng. Proc.* **2024**, *74*, 70. https://doi.org/10.3390/engproc2024074070

Academic Editors: Shu-Han Liao, Teen-Hang Meen and Cheng-Fu Yang

Published: 7 October 2024

1. Introduction

We examined Taiwan's aesthetic education development plan to enhance children's artistic literacy and creativity by teaching the courses "Aesthetic Education from Early Childhood to Lifelong Learning" and "Aesthetics as a Lifestyle." With limited school resources, extracurricular art classes using clay and composite materials have fostered artistic skills and the emotional expression of students. Focusing on consumers' needs and satisfaction with clay and composite materials, material selection and course quality were examined in aesthetic education. The importance of course design to CS and preferences was explored using the Kano model. The intricate relationship between motivations and satisfaction levels was also explored to address the complexities of aesthetic education. Through the analysis, we identified a way to boost CS. The results helped to offer recommendations for clay-based aesthetic education courses in terms of goal setting and decision making. The results also contribute to enhancing educational practices in aesthetic education using clay and composite materials to align with changing consumer expectations. Educators and curriculum designers need to adapt the results to evolve with demands in aesthetic education, highlighting the importance of a responsive approach.

2. Literature Review

2.1. Aesthetic Education Curriculum

The increasing emphasis on aesthetic education is evident. Research at Donghai Elementary School on sixth graders showed the success of interdisciplinary approaches in aesthetic education, utilizing scaffolding theory, cooperative learning, and creative thinking, enhanced by technology and color exploration [1]. Another study demonstrated how physical education integrated athletics and aesthetics to increase confidence and aesthetic appreciation [2]. Advancements in early childhood teaching include teaching aesthetic principles to enrich art comprehension and appreciation in young children [3].

The application of aesthetic education principles was researched for creating engaging and creative courses [4]. The use of clay and composite materials in aesthetic education increased adaptability, sensory experiences, and aesthetic appreciation in children [5]. Children used composite materials for creative expression [6]. The significance of composite materials in children's visual arts was also proved in Ref. [7]. For upper elementary students' aesthetic perception and art appreciation skills, the importance of aesthetic education was highlighted [8]. By integrating aesthetic concepts into curriculum design, children's awareness and appreciation of the aesthetics of clay and composite materials can be added to aesthetic education.

2.2. Kansei Engineering

Kansei Engineering, initiated in 1991 by Masato Ujigawa and later integrated into the Japan Society of Kansei Engineering in 1998, focuses on creating products and spaces with attractive qualities. To study consumer senses and perceptions and to identify unique product characteristics, the Evaluation Grid Method (EGM) is used for user interviews and comparative analyses [9]. Recent advancements in Kansei Engineering have led to various designs that transform and quantify human perceptions and feelings towards objects, making product design more attuned to consumer emotional expectations [10]. The need for market-oriented design is emphasized in new product development by integrating consumers' aesthetics and individual needs to create appealing products [11]. In aesthetic education, clay and composite materials are not just creative mediums, but connectors between aesthetic literacy and emotional expression. This study suggests that by integrating the creative process with consumer psychology and principles of aesthetic education, its value and future development potential can be better understood within the context of aesthetic education.

2.3. Research Methodology: Application of the Kano Model

The Kano model plays a pivotal role in how consumers evaluate product quality, focusing on identifying product standards or features that significantly enhance satisfaction [12]. A bidirectional model was proposed, elucidating the multifaceted relationships between customer satisfaction (CS) and product feature performance [13]. This model classifies product features into five distinct categories, with each category exhibiting unique dynamics in affecting CS, as illustrated in Figure 1.

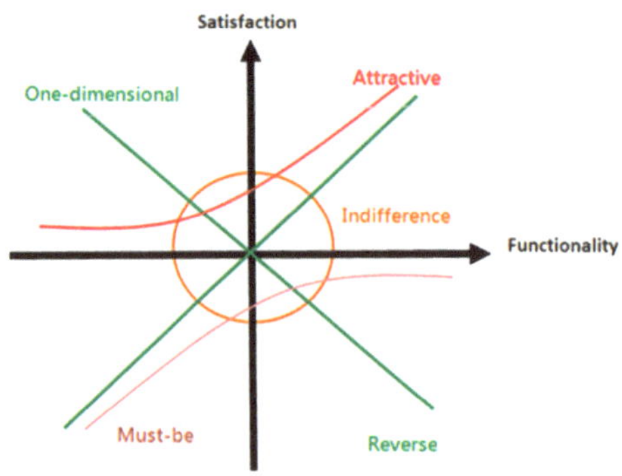

Figure 1. Kano model of CS.

The Kano model is used to classify customer requirements to understand its effectiveness in product needs [14]. It enables designers to make informed strategic decisions in product development. Investing in basic quality aspects may not be as beneficial as enhancing attributes or features, which influence CS and quality perception. The model proves useful in scenarios with limited resources, where all product features cannot be improved. It helps identify features that impact CS and importance, guiding optimal product development strategies. In this study, the Kano model was applied to aesthetic education in a curriculum design involving clay and composite materials. The research framework was identified and categorized according to the learner's needs, helping educators understand which aspects effectively enhance learner satisfaction and engagement. The Kano model distinguishes essential elements (basic needs), appealing aspects (motivators), and elements that, while not crucial, significantly improve the learning experience (performance needs). The use of clay and composite materials in aesthetic courses, for instance, is a motivator, offering unique sensory and creative experiences that increase learner satisfaction and course engagement. The Kano model in aesthetic education curricula with clay and composite materials allows for aligning closely with learner expectations, enhancing educational effectiveness. This approach helps educators design courses that are educationally sound, engaging, and stimulating for creative thinking.

3. Methodology

To elucidate the charm factors in aesthetic education curriculum design using clay and composite materials, we adopted the EGM and the Kano Model.

3.1. *Evaluation Grid Method*

EGM is a profound qualitative tool. It was deployed to dissect the nuanced perceptions and evaluative criteria of educators and learners in aesthetic education involving clay and composite materials in this study. A panel was formed with educators who were experienced in aesthetic education, experts in curriculum design, and psychologists. They reviewed the model through interviews focusing on creative learning. The interviews were conducted to unearth the underlying needs, interactive dynamics, and detailed assessments regarding the implementation and impact of clay and composite materials in aesthetic education.

3.2. *Application of the Kano Model*

The Kano Model was utilized to construct a dual-focused questionnaire and determine the satisfaction and dissatisfaction factors of educators and learners for the use of clay and composite materials in aesthetic education. This model was used to identify the attributes that significantly enhance educational experiences and distinguish between critical "basic" factors that cause dissatisfaction if unmet and "motivator" factors that elevate the learning experience. The questionnaire was created, encompassing elements relevant to the use of these materials in aesthetic education to scrutinize the importance and expectations. The results provide an understanding of their influence on educational satisfaction and outcomes. By integrating these methods, the effective use of clay and composite materials in aesthetic education curriculum design was assessed. Based on the results, we proposed recommendations for curriculum developers, educators, and professionals in aesthetic education for enhancing the engagement, creativity, and overall learning experience of students.

4. Results and Discussion

4.1. *EGM Findings*

Factors influencing students' decision making in aesthetic education were determined, focusing on a curriculum design with clay and composite materials. Three main factors were determined to affect aesthetic literacy, formative design skills, and creativity. These factors were crucial in evaluating the appeal of aesthetic education curricula (Figure 2). Assessments within aesthetic education curricula are crucial for evaluating students' understanding and expression of beaut, as it is important to enhance artistic literacy, expand aesthetic knowledge, and increase perceptual awareness and appreciation abilities. Students were engaged in the detailed analysis of visual elements and used artistic techniques and color theory, nurturing their unique artistic styles and innovative thinking. Curriculum design with clay figures in aesthetic education encourages the creation of personalized sculptural creations, stimulating students' creative thinking. The creation of clay figures blends clay's tactile properties with diverse materials and techniques to achieve dynamics and intricate forms. Accessories and color coordination can be used to enhance visual impact, ignite imagination, and improve observational, reflective, and expressive abilities, leading to distinctive artistic styles.

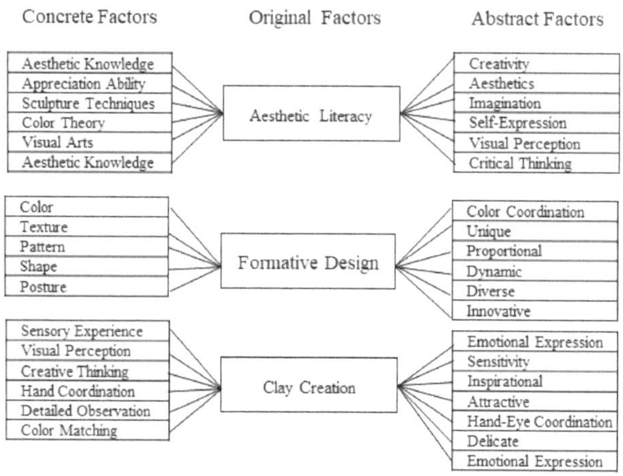

Figure 2. EGM results.

Hands-on clay activities in aesthetic education enrich sensory experiences and creativity. They improve hand–eye coordination and three-dimensional visual perception, and deepen students' understanding of color, shape, and proportion. This process boosts aesthetic literacy and critical art appreciation, with creation serving as a medium for emotional expression and psychological relief. Thus, creation using clay needs to become a part of aesthetic education, advancing technical skills, sensory experiences, creativity, aesthetic comprehension, and emotional expressiveness.

4.2. *Results of the Kano Model*

4.2.1. Kano Quality Attributes

Utilizing the Kano model's bidirectional questionnaire, we identified factors for students in aesthetic education with clay and composite materials. The frequency analysis results revealed that students focused on fundamental attributes such as creativity development, hand–eye coordination, and artistic skills, which collectively formed the 12 charm qualities listed in Table 1, resonating with diverse student interests and needs. Students enjoyed the creative process involving clay and composite materials, drawing from their life experiences. Clay-based athletic figure creation in the curriculum appealed to students, who wanted to present their favorite sports in clay. Creativity development in aesthetic education enhances creative skills and bolsters innovative thinking, problem-solving, confidence, and expressiveness, contributing to students' emotional and psychological growth. Skills such as hand–eye coordination and artistic techniques are crucial for refining artistic precision and quality for perceptual, observational, and creative growth, and confident artistic expression. Aesthetic education, thus, becomes an integral part of daily life. Teaching "artistic style" allows students to diversify their creative expressions, while "aesthetic cultivation" and "aesthetic appreciation" expand their understanding and sensitivity towards beauty, stimulating creativity. The clay creation activities enhance "spatial imagination" and "visual art" skills, offering students a rich experiential value and heightening their course engagement. These charm qualities play a significant role in enhancing student involvement and the overall value of aesthetic education.

Table 1. Classification in Kano Model.

Factor Items	Weighted Classification of Kano Quality Attributes (%)						Kano Quality Classification
	M	O	I	A	Q	R	
1.Development of Creativity	6	34.5	13.1	44	2.4	0	A
2.Hand–Eye Coordination Skills	7.1	51.2	11.9	27.4	1.2	1.2	A
3.Artistic Creation Techniques	6	39.3	8.3	44	1.2	1.2	A
4.Cultivation of Aesthetic Sensibility	3.6	41.7	11.9	41.7	0	1.2	A
5.Aesthetic Appreciation Skills	3.6	36.9	8.3	48.8	1.2	1.2	A
6.Artistic Style	4.8	28.6	16.7	50	0	0	A
7.Emotional Expression	6	44	11.9	35.7	1.2	1.2	O
8.Stress Relief	6	44	11.9	35.7	1.2	1.2	O
9.Relaxation and Emotional Stability	3.6	50	9.5	34.5	1.2	1.2	O
10.Spatial Imagination	8.3	36.9	7.1	46.4	0	1.2	A
11.Problem-Solving Skills	7.1	40.5	13.1	36.9	1.2	1.2	A
12.Visual Arts	3.6	28.6	9.5	50	3.6	4.8	A

4.2.2. Kano Quality Improvement Indicators

The "CS Coefficient" in the Kano model analysis elucidates the degree to which the adequacy or inadequacy of a product's quality influences CS or dissatisfaction by using the "Satisfaction Improvement Coefficient" and the "Dissatisfaction Resolution Coefficient" [15]. The formula for the "extent of satisfaction" is given as (A + O)/(A + O + M + I) (1), and for "dissatisfaction resolution," it is -(M + O)/(A + O + M + I) (2), where A denotes Attractive qualities, O represents One-dimensional, M stands for Must-be, and I signifies Indifferent (frequency) (Figure 3).

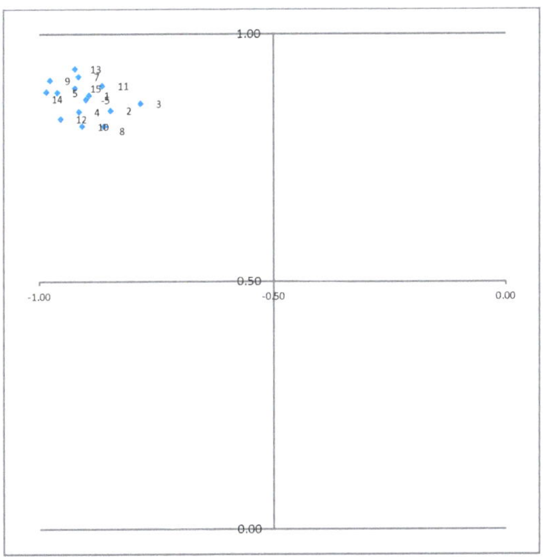

Figure 3. Matrix of Kano quality improvement indicators.

Applying CS-customer dissatisfaction (DS) values to ascertain the Kano model's quality attributes, the attributes in the upper right quadrant were categorized as Attractive qualities. These attributes surpassed basic consumer expectations, thereby providing additional satisfaction. Following a clockwise sequence, the quality attributes were classified as Indifferent, Must-be, and One-dimensional, respectively. The Attractive qualities are closely linked to consumer satisfaction, with their enhanced performance correlating with increased consumer contentment. Among the 12 evaluated factors, 9 were identified as Attractive qualities, which coincided with the Kano model's mode statistical outcomes. These particular items mirror consumer expectations, and their performance levels impact CS. In strategic planning, it is crucial to prioritize these Attractive quality items due to their significant influence within services or products.

4.2.3. Kano Weighting Method

The Kano Weighting Method is used for increasing satisfaction and mitigating dissatisfaction in determining CS. By comparing the "CS Increase Coefficient" and the "DS Reduction Coefficient" (Equation (1), the method identifies the attribute with the greatest impact (the coefficient with the larger absolute value). Initially, qualities lacking differentiation were omitted from consideration using (Equation (2).

$$C_i = \mathrm{Max}\left[\frac{CS_i}{\sum_i^m CS_i}, \frac{CD_i}{\sum_i^m CD_i}\right] \quad (1)$$

$$W_i = \frac{C_i}{\sum_i^m C_i} \quad (2)$$

According to the weight analysis results from the Kano model (Table 2), the two factors with the highest significance were found: "Artistic Creation Techniques" (0.101) and "Spatial Imagination"(0.093). These factors were associated with consumer expectations and satisfaction. In clay and composite material creation contexts, students had explicit expectations regarding the output, seeking acknowledgment and comprehension of their artistic skills and imaginative prowess. Therefore, the considerable weights attributed to "Artistic Creation Techniques" and "Spatial Imagination" reflected a strong desire for their input and perspectives to be thoroughly respected and recognized within the clay creation course.

Table 2. Satisfaction and dissatisfaction degree and coefficient weights of quality attributes.

Quality Elements	CS/SUM	DS/SUM	MAX	Weights
1. Development of Creativity	0.805	−0.415	0.081	0.075
2. Hand–Eye Coordination Skills	0.805	−0.598	0.081	0.108
3. Artistic Creation Techniques	0.854	−0.463	0.086	0.083
4. Cultivation of Aesthetic Sensibility	0.843	−0.458	0.085	0.082
5. Aesthetic Appreciation Skills	0.878	−0.415	0.088	0.075
6. Artistic Style	0.786	−0.333	0.079	0.06
7. Emotional Expression	0.817	−0.512	0.082	0.092
8. Stress Relief	0.817	−0.512	0.082	0.092
9. Relaxation and Emotional Stability	0.866	−0.549	0.087	0.099
10. Spatial Imagination	0.843	−0.458	0.085	0.082
11. Problem-Solving Skills	0.793	−0.488	0.08	0.088
12. Visual Arts	0.857	−0.351	0.086	0.063

Regarding the Kano model, the factors with the lowest weights were identified as "Emotional Expression" (0.074) and "Hand–Eye Coordination Skills" (0.076). Although these factors had relatively lower weights, this did not diminish their importance. Compared to other factors, these were perceived by consumers as basic or fundamental, being expected elements within the course design. For instance, emotional expression and hand–eye coordination were regarded as essential components in aesthetic education involving clay creation. Hence, the reduced weights of these foundational factors reflected their perceived elementary nature within the curriculum, particularly in comparison to factors that more directly address and fulfill specific consumer needs.

5. Conclusions

We explored the attributes influencing decision making in creating athletic figures with clay and composite materials. Through qualitative and quantitative analyses, various key factors were revealed. The results of the Kano model indicated that nine attributes were classified as Attractive qualities, which were especially valued by students and teachers in the decision-making process for clay athletic figure creation. These attributes met basic expectations and impacted CS in "Artistic Creation Techniques" and "Spatial Imagination" as the most influential factors. The results underscore the role of technical skill, imaginative capacity, and creativity in the creative process as being pivotal to enhancing CS. Recognizing the significance of the Attractive factors improves teaching quality and strengthens customer relationships. To optimize the outcomes in clay athletic figure creation and increase CS, course designers need to consider these decision-influencing attributes. The continuous refinement of course design and the fostering of long-term trust with consumers is recommended, too. Despite the Attractive qualities, consumer expectations and needs are changing. More research is necessary to develop a creative process model for course designers and educators to further investigate.

Author Contributions: The contribution of the authors to the paper include the provision of study materials or patients by Q.-Y.L. and the critical revision of the article for important intellectual content and the final approval of the article by C.-H.H. C.-H.H. also provided administrative, technical, or logistical support. All authors have read and agreed to the published version of the manuscript.

Funding: This research did not receive external funding.

Institutional Review Board Statement: Not applicable.

Informed Consent Statement: Not applicable.

Data Availability Statement: Data are contained within the article.

Conflicts of Interest: The authors declare no conflicts of interest.

References

1. Chen, S.-Y. A Study on the Implementation of Cross-Disciplinary Aesthetic Education at a Primary School: A Case Study of Sixth-Grade Students at Donghai Elementary School. Master's Thesis, National Taitung University, Taitung, Taiwan, 2022.
2. Zhuang, W.-X. Research on the Implementation of Aesthetic Education in the Field of Physical Education. Master's Thesis, National Taipei University of Education, Taipei, Taiwan, 2022.
3. Yin, Y.-M. An Action Research on Aesthetic Education: A Case Study of Children's Rhythmic Teaching. Master's Thesis, National Taipei University of Education, Taipei, Taiwan, 2020.
4. Chen, C.-Y. A Case Study on Curriculum Design and Practice of Aesthetic Education. Master's Thesis, Department of Fine Arts, National Taiwan Normal University, Taipei, Taiwan, 2021.
5. Chen, G.-Y. The Impact of Clay Sculpting Activities on Preschool Children's Aesthetic Education. Master's Thesis, Asia-Pacific Institute of Creativity, Toufen, Taiwan, 2016.
6. Qiu, Y.-R. A Study on Multifaceted Media Art in Creative Curriculum for Indigenous Children. Master's Thesis, National Taichung University of Science and Technology, Taichung, Taiwan, 2021.
7. Chen, W.-Y. An Action Research on Integrating Mixed Media Design in Visual Arts Teaching for Upper Primary Students. Master's Thesis, National Taichung University of Education, Taichung, Taiwan, 2016.
8. Zheng, J.-Q. An Action Research on Integrating Aesthetic Perception, Appreciation, and Creation into Visual Arts Curriculum for Upper Primary Students. Master's Thesis, National Taichung University of Education, Taichung, Taiwan, 2012.

9. Sanui, J. Visualization of users' requirements: Introduction of the Evaluation Grid Method. In Proceedings of the 3rd Design & Decision Support Systems in Architecture & Urban Planning Conference, Spa, Belgium, 18–21 August 1996; Volume 1, pp. 365–374.
10. Wang, Z.-Y. Affective Engineering-Based Artificial Expression Analysis. Master's Thesis, Graduate Institute of Optomechatronic Engineering, National Central University, Taoyuan, Taiwan, 2008.
11. Asano, H. *Practice of Miryoku Engineering: The Steps to Create Popular Products*; Kaibundo; Haiwen Hall: Tokyo, Japan, 2001.
12. Kano, N.; Rakugi, S.; Takahashi, F.; To, S. Attractive Quality and Must-Be Quality. *Qual. Control J.* **1984**, *21*, 33–41.
13. Matzler, K.; Hinterhuber, H.H. How to Make Product Development Projects More Successful by Integrating Kano's Model of CS into Quality Function Deployment. *Technovation* **1998**, *18*, 25–38. [CrossRef]
14. Berger, C.; Blauth, R.; Boger, D. Kano's Methods for Understanding Customer-defined Quality. *Cent. Qual. Manag. J. Fall* **1993**, 3–35.
15. Sireli, Y.; Kauffmann, P.; Ozan, E. Integration of Kano's Model into QFD for Multiple Product Design. *IEEE Trans. Eng. Manag.* **2007**, *54*, 380–390. [CrossRef]

engineering proceedings

Proceeding Paper

Digital Ghost: Application of Holographic Projection on Protection of Guangdong Puppet Show †

Song Xu [1], Chen Li [1,*], Peng-Wei Hsiao [2] and Huan Hu [1]

[1] School of Design and Art, Beijing Institute of Technology, Zhuhai 519088, China; xusong@bitzh.edu.cn (S.X.); 181111100241@bitzh.edu.cn (H.H.)
[2] Department of Visual Arts, Macao Polytechnic University, Macau 999078, China; pwhsiao@ipm.edu.mo
* Correspondence: lichen@bitzh.edu.cn

† Presented at the 2024 IEEE 4th International Conference on Electronic Communications, Internet of Things and Big Data, Taipei, Taiwan, 19–21 April 2024.

Abstract: Guangdong puppetry, a 700-year-old intangible cultural heritage, faces declining popularity due to economic influences and evolving youth interests. The shrinking audience and a lack of successors to inherit this tradition further compound the issue. This research aims to revitalize the puppet show by preserving its traditional roots, exploring new possibilities, and engaging the younger generation. Divided into three stages—preliminary investigation, role modeling, and holographic projection device design—the study utilizes field research, literature review, questionnaires, and experiments. Information is gathered through venue visits, which is followed by questionnaire distribution and 3D model creation based on survey results. The final stage involves designing and testing a holographic projection booth.

Keywords: Guangdong puppet show; holographic projection; interaction design; intangible cultural heritage

Citation: Xu, S.; Li, C.; Hsiao, P.-W.; Hu, H. Digital Ghost: Application of Holographic Projection on Protection of Guangdong Puppet Show. *Eng. Proc.* **2024**, *74*, 71. https://doi.org/10.3390/engproc2024074071

Academic Editors: Shu-Han Liao, Teen-Hang Meen and Cheng-Fu Yang

Published: 14 October 2024

1. Introduction

The Guangdong puppet show is an essential aspect of Cantonese culture. Cantonese culture is a regional culture that is primarily found in southern China. It is currently available in Cantonese-speaking locations such as the Greater Bay Area of Guangdong, Hong Kong, and Macao (Figure 1). Due to societal progress and generational shifts, the Guangdong puppet performance is now an intangible cultural heritage rather than part of the mainstream culture of young people in Guangdong. The show is protected as an intangible cultural heritage by the government. Ordinary young people in the Guangdong–Hong Kong–Macao Greater Bay Area nowadays find it difficult to attend the Guangdong puppet show, let alone experience the cultural genes in this intangible cultural asset. The rapid advancement of information technology has created new opportunities for Guangdong Puppet show researchers and practitioners. Holographic projection is a very new type of media technology. Holographic projection technology in the digital age bridges the gap between reality and virtual reality by presenting floating pictures in actual space, resulting in a novel visual viewing experience, and this suspension is similar to the techniques employed in Guangdong puppet shows.

The recent findings from a study highlight a sustained interest among local administrations in providing ongoing support and guidance for significant intangible cultural heritage projects [1]. Furthermore, a separate study has delved into establishing a quantitative dimension for the preservation of Chinese cultural heritage [2]. Another research initiative aims to enhance the 3D design workflow by employing wearable motion capture (Mocap) systems for virtual humans [3]. In addition, a study has explored the application of true-color holograms for the conservation of museums and ancient Greek artifacts [4]. Lastly, there is a research endeavor focused on experimenting with both immersive and non-immersive virtual reality to craft a distinctive fusion of sound and sensory experiences for cultural heritage [5]. Consequently, the objective of this research is to examine the possibilities in design and production, along with the technological approach, for combining holographic projection technology with the essential qualities of Guangdong puppet performances.

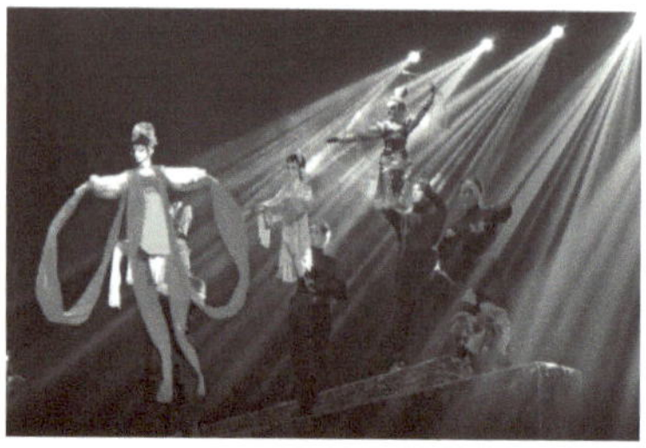

Figure 1. Guangdong puppet show scene.

2. Materials and Methods

Three key technologies have been employed in this study: 3D modeling, non-realistic modeling, and holographic projection. Among these, 3D modeling is the most commonly used to design and digitize the characters in the Guangdong puppet show. Non-realistic modeling technology is used to boost job productivity. Rather than pursuing the most realistic picture possible, we require rapid prototyping and iteration in early prototype design. Holographic projection is the principal technology used in this investigation. It depicts non-realistic 3D models that are used to examine the interaction of actual and virtual space. A study studied the impact of tourist satisfaction and brand loyalty on brand equity by introducing mixed reality technology to cultural heritage protection to improve tourist user experience [6]. A similar study is being conducted in which they evaluate the use of new interactive technologies to improve customer experience and client loyalty [7].

2.1. Three-Dimensional (3D) Modeling

Three-dimensional (3D) modeling is an essential element of digital modeling technology, and Autodesk's 3D software is the go-to option for producers. The bundle includes two notable programs, 3DMax and MAYA, which are widely used for creating models. 3DMax is the preferred choice for architectural and landscape modeling and boasts sophisticated tools that cater specifically to those fields. On the other hand, MAYA is a top-rated platform for character modeling, leveraging powerful features to bring virtual characters to life with precision and detail (Figure 2). This versatile suite of software supports producers across diverse industries, allowing them to create sophisticated digital models for architecture, landscapes, and character design with ease and confidence.

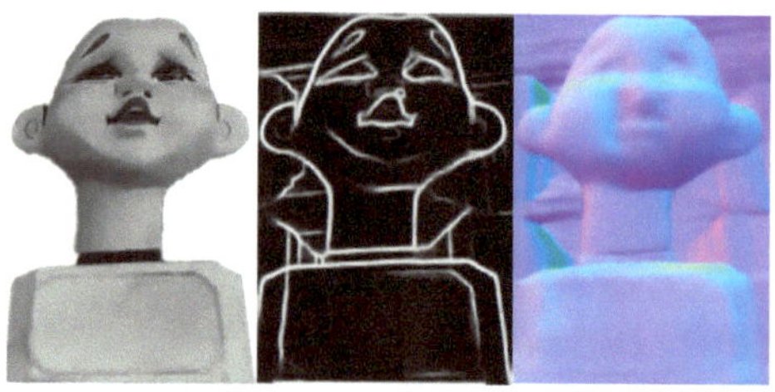

Figure 2. Traditional puppet head (left to right: model, line draft, normal map).

Scholars have increasingly embraced 3D modeling tools for cultural conservation studies in recent years. With the aid of AR and LiDAR technology, a team of researchers successfully created a highly detailed 3D model of the Lantern Festival using nothing but a smartphone [8]. In a separate study, the literature surrounding the preservation of intangible cultural assets through 3D technologies was categorized into 12 distinct groups, allowing for a more comprehensive analysis of the topic [9]. Furthermore, another group of researchers utilized cutting-edge UAV imagery and 3D laser scanning technology to digitally preserve the cultural landscape heritage of Mount Lushan with remarkable precision and accuracy [10].

The advantages of 3D modeling over traditional manual modeling are indisputable. Being carried out digitally, 3D modeling is strongly associated with the digital environment, and the mathematical model can be displayed on various devices using computer vision technology. As a result, 3D modeling is one of the primary technologies that connect reality and virtuality, offering immense possibilities. The digital world transcends time and location, which makes Guangdong's puppet performance in the digital environment more comprehensive than the conventional form. This work uses three-dimensional modeling technology to bridge virtuality and reality, portraying the Guangdong puppet performance model in virtual space in the most sci-fi way.

2.2. Non-Realistic Modeling

With the help of non-realistic 3D modeling, designers can produce unique and inventive objects without being constrained by the constraints of realistic modeling techniques. Unlike traditional 3D modeling techniques that strive to produce an accurate portrayal of real-world objects, non-realistic modeling methods apply artistic freedom to create unique and remarkable designs. A study conducted over a decade ago presented an algorithm for 3D collage generation using non-realistic modeling technology. This algorithm was found to be exceptionally useful in handling complex 3D processing tasks [11]. Another study used this technology to create interactive exhibition pieces that showcase the splendor of a monastery [12]. These examples demonstrate the immense potential of non-realistic 3D modeling to push the boundaries of creativity and innovation.

Non-realistic modeling is an approach that offers three significant advantages over realistic modeling methods: high efficiency, small model size, and rapid speed. With non-realistic modeling, designers can achieve greater work efficiency than with realistic modeling methods. Unlike realistic modeling, which requires designers to spend a lot of time on modeling tasks to achieve expressive model details, non-realistic modeling provides block modeling or facet modeling technology, making it easier for designers to finish the prototype design of the model or even the subsequent enhanced design. Even if the existing common non-realistic modeling methods, such as low-surface modeling, are not suitable, designers can use other techniques to complete the task. Additionally, non-realistic models have the advantage of being smaller in volume than realistic models. With these benefits, non-realistic modeling is a highly efficient and effective approach for designers to complete their tasks. Non-realistic 3D models unquestionably have several advantages over realistic ones. They have a lower mesh count, which means they have fewer materials and shading. As a result, they require less bandwidth, making them far easier to transport and display in the virtual world. The second advantage of non-realistic models is their production speed. They can be designed much more quickly in digital space. Traditional 3D modeling often produces two sets of models: a high model and a low model. By applying the low-details model to the texture produced by the high-details model, a faster visual representation is produced. A designer can omit this step and complete the model considerably more quickly, though, by beginning with a low-plane model. Moreover, most low-detail models are as good as high-detail models in future interface design, which makes them the best option for prototyping.

2.3. Holographic Projection

In contrast to Pepper's ghost illusion technology, holographic projection technology stands as a well-established and advanced industry technology, boasting distinct advantages in this research. This technology encompasses three main categories: gas projection, air projection, and reflection projection. In the specific context of this study, holographic film served as the imaging medium, and glass acted as the projection surface. Three crucial characteristics distinguish holographic projection technology: its ability to offer a 360° vision, adjust the size of the projection, and interchange content seamlessly. The utilization of holographic projection technology introduces unprecedented flexibility in stage placement compared to traditional Cantonese puppet shows. Remarkably, this flexibility is achieved without the necessity for a separate performance and display stage, highlighting the efficiency and innovation inherent in holographic projection techniques (Figure 3).

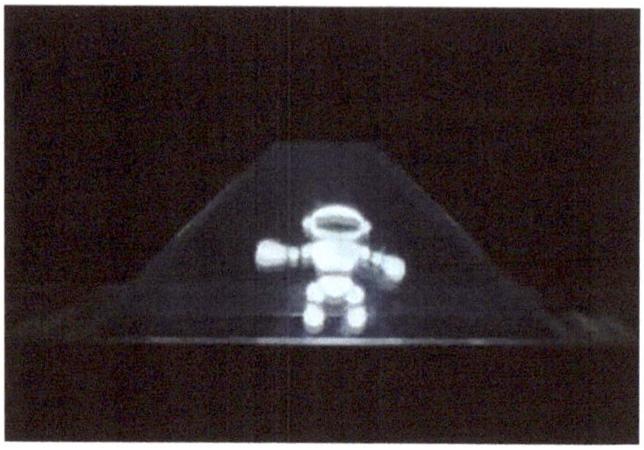

Figure 3. Hologram projection real scene.

Comparing holographic projection booths to conventional stages reveals several benefits. First of all, they offer better efficiency, more storage capacity, and simple display content switching. Conventional stages, on the other hand, offer little room for performers. Second, holographic projection technology is more adaptable than traditional stages, which are limited by the size of the performance area. This makes it a better option. Lastly, if a power source is available, 360-degree performances can be hosted by holographic projection booths. All things suggested, holographic projection technology offers a better and more adaptable stage for putting on shows. Holographic projection technology boasts the unique advantage of a 360-degree display ability, which is a significant departure from traditional Cantonese puppet shows. Unlike the conventional setup, where one side of the stand remains hidden, our holographic projection booth empowers the audience to relish the show from multiple perspectives. As a critical element of digital media, holographic projection technology seamlessly bridges the gap between the real world and virtual space. This breakthrough has the potential to revolutionize Guangdong puppet performances and even pave the way for them to enter the metaverse.

Over the past couple of years, the use of holographic projection technology has increased significantly especially in the museum industry. For instance, a study found that museums using X-reality technologies, such as ARVRXR, create an immersive experience where visitors can interact with virtual agents as if they were real [13]. Similarly, a research team explored how to preserve Kunqu Opera in China through the mediating role of authenticity on experience quality and satisfaction [14]. Another team designed an IntARSI system for the New Museum of Civilization in Rome (MuCIV), offering visitors a multisensory and enhanced experience [15]. Moreover, a study found that improving perceived authenticity and tourist interaction could enhance the nostalgic experience of vintage hotels. Self-congruity acted as a mediator for this interaction, while digital technology acted as a moderator, reducing it [7].

3. Results

This research is organized into three stages: preliminary investigation, role modeling, and holographic projection device design. We utilized various research methods, including field investigation, literature research, questionnaire surveys, experiments, and others, to ensure comprehensive results. Our research team visited the existing puppetry venues in Guangdong to collect first-hand information, providing a strong foundation for our study. Based on the preliminary results, we designed and distributed questionnaires to gather more data. We then used the results of the questionnaire survey to design a 3D model, taking into account various factors. Finally, we designed the holographic projection booth, and the 3D model was imported for testing. We are confident that the methodology used in this research will provide valuable insights into the design and development of holographic projection devices.

3.1. Questionnaire

This study's preliminary investigation consisted mostly of three tasks: field investigation, literature research, and a questionnaire survey. The goal is to collect data from many sources and then compare it to obtain results for design studies. On 6 November 2021, the research team traveled to the Guangzhou Province Puppet Aat Theater to conduct field research and gather first-hand knowledge by attending Guangdong puppet shows. After returning to the lab, we looked through numerous books to learn more about Guangdong puppet shows. Based on the main data from the field survey and the secondary data from the literature study, we created a questionnaire for a general young population and distributed it via the Internet. A total of 161 questionnaires were gathered, of which 161 were legitimate. According to the results of the questionnaire survey, 38.51% of people were very willing to "learn about the intangible cultural heritage of puppet shows", and their readiness to "try a new way of puppet show experience" was comparable, except for 6 people who selected "very unwilling". The percentage of people who selected "willing, general, unwilling" was around 25%. When asked, "What do you think are the limitations of puppetry?" 87.58% chose "single form of expression", and when asked, "Should traditional elements be retained in the shape of a puppet show?" (47.2%), the most common answer was "keep a little". When asked if they agreed to the combination of puppet performance and holographic projection, 36.65% responded "very willing".

3.2. The 3D Modeling

The 3D design segment encompasses three primary facets: 3D model appearance design, 3D model function design, and 3D model animation design. Initially, researchers embarked on crafting 3D models of puppet characters, primarily humanoid in form, drawing upon preliminary research findings. The model's skin is intricately designed following the completion of the mesh design for the model surface. The skin drawing phase focuses on creating the material sphere and mapping the UV topology. Employing a technique known as non-realistic modeling, three-dimensional models were generated in this study, significantly simplifying the mesh complexity and expediting the modeling process (Figure 4).

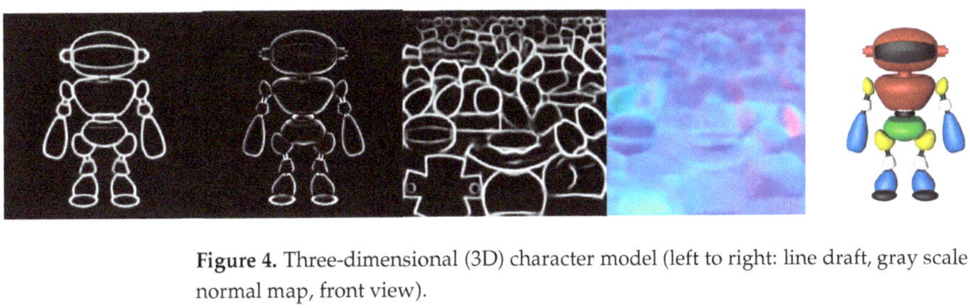

Figure 4. Three-dimensional (3D) character model (left to right: line draft, gray scale draft, UV map, normal map, front view).

Considering the puppet-like motion integral to the character, this aspect was factored in from the model's inception. The decision to model the characters after imitation robots was deliberate, incorporating joints akin to puppets into the humanoid form. To streamline the design process, the head area of the 3D character was specially treated, with facial features covered by large VR glasses, facilitating a more efficient design process.

Upon completing the visual design, the animation design phase commenced, involving three key pieces of work. Initially, the researchers designed the skeleton for the 3D character model using a full-body inverse kinematics (IK) solver, encompassing primary skeletons such as the spine, left arm, left hand, right arm, right hand, left leg, left toe, right leg, and right toe. Subsequently, components and controllers of the 3D character model's skeleton were adjusted accordingly, aligning joints and mesh and configuring the controller for seamless integration with subsequent animations. The 3D model skeleton was then bound by the 3D model, allowing the team to animate the puppet show in accordance with its specific requirements.

This comprehensive approach to 3D design not only involved a meticulous consideration of appearance but also extended to the functional and animated aspects, ensuring a holistic and integrated process. Through the strategic incorporation of non-realistic modeling and the deliberate choice of puppet-like features, the researchers aimed to optimize the efficiency and flexibility of their 3D design workflow, ultimately tailoring the puppet show to their unique creative and technical specifications.

3.3. Hologram Pyramid Booth

The design of a hologram projection booth involves two crucial components: the design of the holographic projection booth itself and the production and integration of holographic projection materials (Figure 5). The process commenced with the transformation of a pre-made miniature into a pyramid, utilizing PVC transparent film as the display light source and an Android phone as the image source. The creation of a holographic projection sample involved the application of Adobe After Effects 2020 non-linear audio and video editing tools. To construct a holographic projection test prototype, a holographic projection video, an Android phone, and the actual holographic projection booth were employed. Through a series of rigorous tests, the research team meticulously identified the dimensions, proportions, and other essential parameters of the 3D model. Additionally, we determined the animation time required for an initial performance of the Guangdong puppet show, amounting to approximately 60 to 300 s (Figure 6).

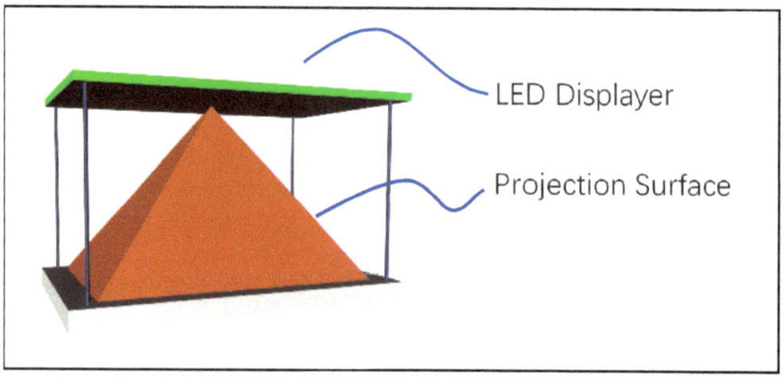

Figure 5. Hologram pyramid booth blueprint.

The subsequent step involved the construction of a life-sized (1:1) holographic projection booth, utilizing materials procured from the Internet. This booth comprised three primary components: a truss, a bracket, and a projection pyramid. The truss, crucial for stability, portability, display convenience, and adaptability, was crafted from a lightweight yet durable aluminum alloy. Four straight-angle iron bars constituted the stand, ensuring robust support for the structure. The projection pyramid, consisting of four glass pieces, each affixed with a holographic projection film, housed a 24-inch LED display. During the projection direction selection process, the team opted for top projection, effectively concealing the projection surface and facilitating seamless projection.

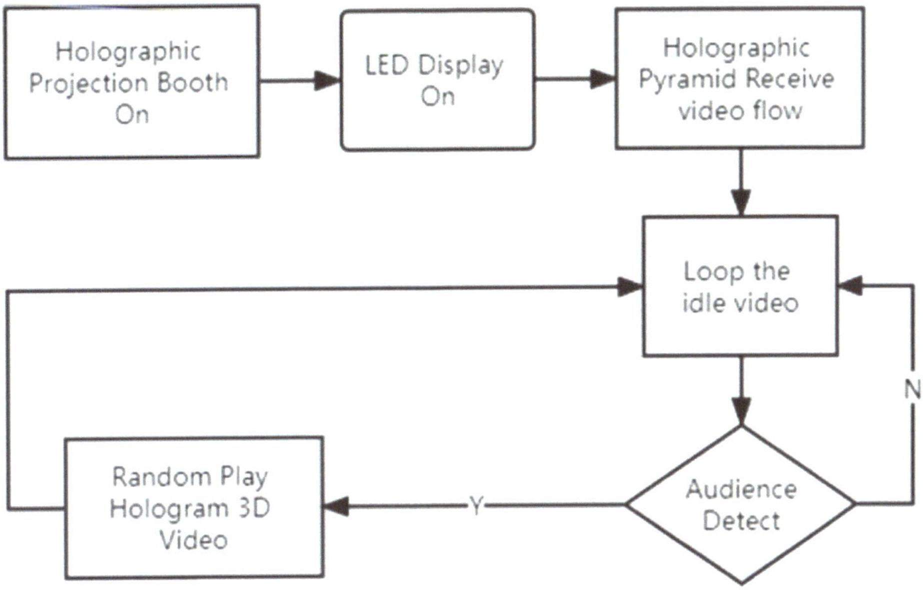

Figure 6. Hologram pyramid booth interaction flow.

The meticulous engineering and selection of materials ensured that the holographic projection booth met the specific requirements for stability, portability, and display quality. The truss's aluminum alloy construction enhanced its portability while maintaining structural integrity. The strategic use of holographic projection film on the glass pieces of the pyramid contributed to an optimal display, aligning with the project's objectives. The research team's detailed examination of dimensions, proportions, and animation time underscored a commitment to precision in crafting a holographic projection booth tailored to the unique demands of the Guangdong puppet show. Ultimately, this multifaceted approach resulted in a functional and purpose-built hologram projection booth that was ready to showcase the immersive fusion of technology and traditional puppetry (Figure 7).

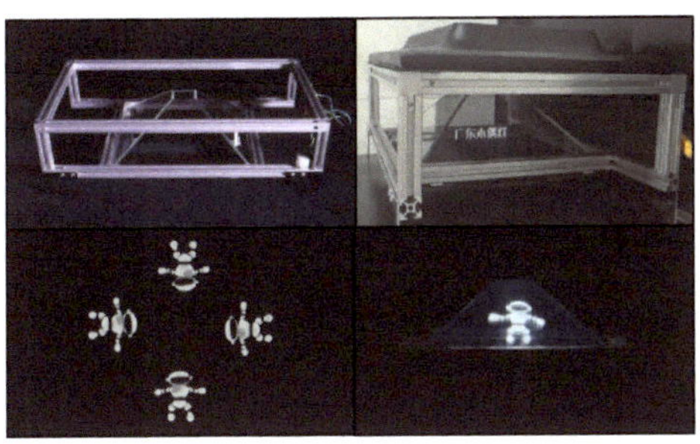

Figure 7. Hologram pyramid booth physical structure.

4. Discussion

4.1. Holographic Projection Technology to Protect Intangible Cultural Heritage

Holographic projection technology, a well-established innovation, has found a novel application in the preservation of intangible cultural assets, which are exemplified by its integration into the realm of the Guangdong puppet show. The evolution of this technology has brought about three significant advancements that are reshaping the traditional puppet show experience. Firstly, the holographic pyramid booth emerges as a transformative force capable of catapulting the traditional Guangdong puppet show into the digital era, especially within the evolving landscape of the metaverse. This transition represents a seamless blend of heritage and modernity, offering audiences a dynamic and engaging spectacle. Secondly, holographic projection transcends the temporal constraints associated with traditional puppet theater. Audiences can now relish the Guangdong puppet performance from the comfort of their homes, breaking free from the limitations of fixed showtimes. For those seeking an immersive encounter, the option to attend live performances in theaters remains open, providing a flexible and inclusive experience. Lastly, the holographic projection booth introduces a remarkable aspect of 360° transparency, presenting a visually diverse and distinctive form compared to the conventional Guangdong puppet show. This transparency poses new challenges, necessitating the creation of innovative 360-degree scene performance scripts and the incorporation of transparent visual content to convey intricate plot details. Consequently, practitioners and enthusiasts of the Guangdong puppet show are presented with a wealth of new content to explore and innovative challenges to overcome, aligning with the evolving landscape of the metaverse. In essence, holographic projection technology not only preserves cultural heritage but also propels it into the future, offering an array of possibilities for both creators and audiences. The marriage of tradition and cutting-edge technology not only ensures the longevity of the Guangdong puppet show but also opens up new avenues for creativity, interaction, and engagement in the ever-evolving metaverse era.

4.2. Research Deficiencies and Future Improvement

This study exhibits three notable limitations that warrant attention for future improvements. The first limitation pertains to character creation, where the conservative 3D modeling method was employed when conclusive research results were unavailable. This conservative approach led to a role model that deviated from the conventional modeling of Guangdong puppet shows. Addressing this flaw could involve leveraging advanced technologies like 3D scanning and motion capture in future studies to enhance the fidelity and authenticity of character creation. The second limitation revolves around the size of the stage within the holographic projection booth. The current dimensions constrain the inclusion of multiple roles or intricate tale performances, which is primarily due to the utilization of a 24-inch LED display as imaging equipment. A potential remedy involves expanding the image size, perhaps by incorporating an ultra-short focal projector, accommodating more complex and nuanced performances. The third limitation concerns the impact of lighting on the holographic projection booth's performance. The mainstream LED or LCD screens used in the current setup exhibit a relatively low brightness count, approximately 300 nits. This limitation hampers the booth's visibility during daylight hours, potentially rendering it invisible in bright environments. To overcome this challenge, adopting a laser projector with a brightness exceeding 3000 Lm could significantly enhance visibility in various lighting conditions. Moreover, the study suggests that integrating interactive technology has the potential to elevate user engagement within the holographic projection booth. This recommendation implies that future research could explore interactive features to enhance the overall user experience, fostering greater interaction and immersion. In conclusion, while the current study contributes valuable insights, addressing these identified limitations in character creation, stage size, and lighting conditions could substantially enhance the holographic projection booth's effectiveness, realism, and adaptability for diverse settings and performances. Embracing cutting-edge technologies and refining technical specifications are key steps toward overcoming these challenges and advancing the field of holographic puppetry.

Author Contributions: Conceptualization, S.X., C.L., P.-W.H. and H.H.; methodology, S.X., P.-W.H. and C.L.; software, S.X.; hardware, H.H.; validation, S.X. and C.L.; formal analysis, S.X.; investigation, S.X. and H.H.; resources, S.X., and P.-W.H.; data curation, S.X. and C.L.; writing—original draft preparation, S.X. and H.H.; writing—review and editing, S.X. and C.L.; visualization, S.X. and H.H.;

supervision, C.L.; project administration, C.L. and P.-W.H.; funding acquisition, C.L. and P.-W.H. All authors have read and agreed to the published version of the manuscript.

Funding: This study was supported by the School of Design and Art, Beijing Institute of Technology, Zhuhai (ZX-2020-031) and the Department of Visual Arts, Macao Polytechnic University (RP/FAD-02/2022).

Institutional Review Board Statement: Not applicable.

Informed Consent Statement: Not applicable.

Data Availability Statement: Not available due to privacy restrictions.

Acknowledgments: We would like to express our heartfelt appreciation to the School of Design and Art for generously lending us the experimental venue, which played a critical role in the successful completion of our research.

Conflicts of Interest: The authors declare no conflicts of interest.

References

1. Shih, N.-J.; Chen, T.-Y. Assessment of Lantern Festivals by Government Procurements. *Sustainability* **2022**, *14*, 5147. [CrossRef]
2. Li, M.; Wang, Y.; Xu, Y.Q. Computing for Chinese cultural heritage. *Vis. Inform.* **2022**, *6*, 1–13. [CrossRef]
3. Karuzaki, E.; Partarakis, N.; Patsiouras, N.; Zidianakis, E.; Katzourakis, A.; Pattakos, A.; Kaplanidi, D.; Baka, E.; Cadi, N.; Magnenat-Thalmann, N.; et al. Realistic Virtual Humans for Cultural Heritage Applications. *Heritage* **2021**, *4*, 4148–4171. [CrossRef]
4. Sarakinos, A.; Lembessis, A. Color Holography for the Documentation and Dissemination of Cultural Heritage: OptoClonesTM from Four Museums in Two Countries. *J. Imaging* **2019**, *5*, 59. [CrossRef] [PubMed]
5. Pietroni, E. Mapping the Soundscape in Communicative Forms for Cultural Heritage: Between Realism and Symbolism. *Heritage* **2021**, *4*, 4495–4523. [CrossRef]
6. Bae, S.; Jung, T.H.; Moorhouse, N.; Suh, M.; Kwon, O. The Influence of Mixed Reality on Satisfaction and Brand Loyalty in Cultural Heritage Attractions: A Brand Equity Perspective. *Sustainability* **2020**, *12*, 2956. [CrossRef]
7. Elshaer, I.A.; Azazz, A.M.S.; Fayyad, S. Authenticity, Involvement, and Nostalgia in Heritage Hotels in the Era of Digital Technology: A Moderated Meditation Model. *Int. J. Environ. Res. Public Health* **2022**, *19*, 5784. [CrossRef] [PubMed]
8. Shih, N.J.; Diao, P.H.; Qiu, Y.T.; Chen, T.Y. Situated ar simulations of a lantern festival using a smartphone and lidar-based 3d models. *Appl. Sci.* **2020**, *11*, 12. [CrossRef]
9. Skublewska-Paszkowska, M.; Milosz, M.; Powroznik, P.; Lukasik, E. 3D technologies for intangible cultural heritage preservation—Literature review for selected databases. *Herit. Sci.* **2022**, *10*, 3. [CrossRef] [PubMed]
10. Cai, Z.; Fang, C.; Zhang, Q.; Chen, F. Joint development of cultural heritage protection and tourism: The case of Mount Lushan cultural landscape heritage site. *Herit. Sci.* **2021**, *9*, 86. [CrossRef]
11. Gal, R.; Sorkine, O.; Popa, T.; Sheffer, A.; Cohen-Or, D. 3D collage: Expressive non-realistic modeling. In Proceedings of the 5th International Symposium on Non-Photorealistic Animation and Rendering, San Diego, CA, USA, 4–5 August 2007.
12. Rodríguez-Miranda, Á.; Valle Melón, J.M.; Korro Bañuelos, J.; Elorriaga Aguirre, G. Interactive virtual representation of the disappeared convent of El Carmen (Logroño) generated from a paper craft model. *Virtual Archaeol. Rev.* **2021**, *12*, 77–89. [CrossRef]
13. Margetis, G.; Apostolakis, K.C.; Ntoa, S.; Papagiannakis, G.; Stephanidis, C. X-Reality Museums: Unifying the Virtual and Real World Towards Realistic Virtual Museums. *Appl. Sci.* **2021**, *11*, 338. [CrossRef]
14. Lu, W.; Su, Y.; Su, S.; Zhao, J.; Zhang, L. Perceived Authenticity and Experience Quality in Intangible Cultural Heritage Tourism: The Case of Kunqu Opera in China. *Sustainability* **2022**, *14*, 2940. [CrossRef]
15. Pietroni, E.; Pagano, A.; Biocca, L.; Frassineti, G. Accessibility, Natural User Interfaces and Interactions in Museums: The IntARSI Project. *Heritage* **2021**, *4*, 567–584. [CrossRef]

engineering proceedings

MDPI

Proceeding Paper

A Study on Eyewear Design Quality Using the Kano Two-Dimensional Quality Model †

Hsiao-Ni Su

Department of Optometry, College of Health Sciences, Hsin Sheng Junior College of Medical Care and Management, Taoyuan 32544, Taiwan; keisutokyo@hsc.edu.tw

† Presented at the 2024 IEEE 4th International Conference on Electronic Communications, Internet of Things and Big Data, Taipei, Taiwan, 19–21 April 2024.

Abstract: In the recent consumer market, eyewear has gone beyond the improvement of visual function and is used for the individual style and the symbolization of social standing. Consequently, the aesthetic design of eyewear influences consumer purchasing decisions. Thus, it is necessary to investigate how eyewear design incorporating elements with aesthetic appeal can enhance the sensory experiences of consumers, thereby intensifying their preference for products and fostering their intent to purchase. Utilizing the Evaluation Grid Method (EGM), the design characteristics of eyewear products in the market were explored to assess how these characteristics affect consumer selections. A quantitative analysis of the key quality attributes in eyewear design was conducted using the Kano Model. The results demonstrated a nonlinear relationship between design attributes and consumer satisfaction, confirming the relevance of the Kano Model's classification. By providing a multi-dimensional quality, the Kano Model elucidated variations in consumer quality requirements for eyewear design, allowing designers and manufacturers to strategically enhance key product design elements, thus creating items with greater market appeal. The results provide recommendations for the improvement of product design aesthetics to increase visual allure for consumers and strengthen market competitiveness.

Keywords: eyewear design; design quality; Kansei engineering; Kano mode

Citation: Su, H.-N. A Study on Eyewear Design Quality Using the Kano Two-Dimensional Quality Model. *Eng. Proc.* **2024**, *74*, 72. https://doi.org/10.3390/engproc2024074072

Academic Editors: Shu-Han Liao, Teen-Hang Meen and Cheng-Fu Yang

Published: 16 October 2024

1. Introduction

In the consumer-driven market, practitioners must understand and assess the integral role of the quality attributes of eyewear design in cultivating and sustaining brand competitiveness. The complexity of product design quality demands that companies satisfy the consumers' fundamental functional requirements and identify and leverage the latent elements of allure for consumer satisfaction. Kansei Engineering and the Kano Model furnish a research framework to decode the nonlinear dynamics of consumer satisfaction and appraise the contributions of various quality attributes. This study, through its empirical application, aims to investigate the particular quality facets of eyewear design that significantly influence consumer satisfaction. The findings can be used to direct the orientation for design innovation and encourage focused product enhancements for consumer experience and product market viability.

2. Literature Review

2.1. Research in Eyeglass Design

In the consumer-oriented market, stakeholders must recognize and evaluate the quality attributes of eyeglass design to establish and maintain brand competitiveness. The multifaceted nature of product design quality demands that companies fulfill the fundamental functional requirements of consumers and grasp implicit and charming elements capable of eliciting profound customer satisfaction. Ergonomic charm and the Kano Model provide a framework for understanding the nonlinear characteristics of consumer satisfaction, as well as the differential contributions of various quality attributes to satisfaction. Therefore, it is necessary to unveil which elements in eyeglass style design have a decisive impact on consumer satisfaction and guide the strategic positioning of design. The result promotes targeted product improvements for optimizing consumer experience and enhancing market performance.

Contemporary eyeglass design has been studied to assess aesthetic and functional elements and their impact on consumer preferences. The evolution of professional image and personalized demands propels design innovation. Research on eyeglass frames for different professions emphasized the significance of professional image in choosing frames, suggesting positive attributes such as expertise and youthful appearance [1]. This guides optometrists to broaden the spectrum of choices in the retail industry.

As a fashion accessory, eyeglasses serve a crucial function in the dynamic between design and fashion trends in the 21st century. Design trends shift with cultural and popular changes, where the synergy of color and image assumes critical importance in fashion design [2]. Furthermore, eyewear research has expanded to consider the bifunctional role of eyeglasses in both fashion and health, with [3] offering a fresh perspective on how design practices can satisfy both contemporary fashion trends and health needs, proposing the creation of eyewear that conforms to health standards while retaining a fashionable allure. In the exploration of eyeglass design for fit, Peng [4] identified the challenges faced when Taiwanese design data depend on foreign standards, advocating for the application of scientific data to enhance eyeglass design for improved wearing comfort and ocular health. Additionally, the commercial design and evaluation of eyeglasses, through computer-aided design and product flaw analysis, have increased the development efficiency from conceptualization to mass production, enriching the consumer experience with glasses utilizing 3D display technologies [5]. Within the scope of individualized eyeglass design, consumer preference-based design approaches have introduced interactive design interfaces that promote consumer involvement in the design process, facilitating personalized adjustments to eyeglasses [6]. In the research on eyeglass design, it is necessary to integrate style and functionality, the personal needs of consumers, professional imagery, and product comfort. The results provide a basis for the development of eyeglass design, thereby crafting fashionable and functional products.

2.2. Kano Model

Amidst the swift shifts within the global marketplace, companies must comprehend the needs of consumers and probe how these needs influence customer satisfaction [7]. The Kano Model has been widely implemented in recent years [8]. Stemming from the research of Kano et al. [9], this model amends the perceptions of quality management [10]. The 'unidimensional' notion of quality introduces a nuanced classification of quality [11]. The Kano Model delineates quality into five principal categories, suggesting that each category affects consumer satisfaction distinctly [12]. The Kano model of customer satisfaction categorizes product attributes into five distinct categories, providing insights into how different attributes impact customer satisfaction (Figure 1).

- The Must-be Quality constitutes the essential requirements anticipated by consumers [13]. A failure to meet the quality results in dissatisfaction, whereas satisfaction does not increase proportionally once these requirements are adequately met [14].
- The One-dimensional Quality is related to the demands that consumers have for the product [15]. The relationship between meeting the one-dimensional quality and consumer satisfaction is linear, indicating that as these demands are more effectively satisfied, consumer satisfaction also increases accordingly [16].
- The Attractive Quality includes the needs not indicated by consumers but which, if met, enhance their satisfaction [10].

The Kano Model enables companies to ascertain important consumer needs and distinguish and innovate their offerings to secure differentiation from their competitors [17].

This model equips companies with an encompassing instrument to understand consumer needs, thereby promoting heightened customer satisfaction [18].

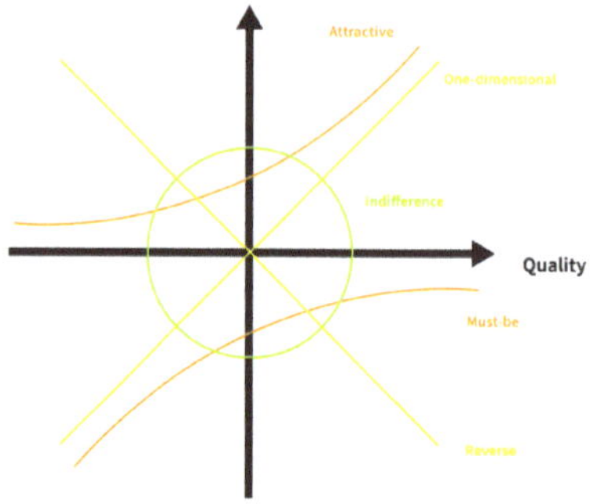

Figure 1. Kano model of customer satisfaction.

3. Methodology

In this research, the attributes of eyeglass design and their impact on consumer satisfaction were explored. The Expressed Goal Method (EGM) was utilized for in-depth interviews, coupled with the Kano model for a dual-structured questionnaire. After the EGM interviews, the features of the eyeglass design were decoded. Seven respondents with rich experience in eyeglass design and diverse backgrounds (four males and three females from product design, fashion analytics, and marketing strategy sectors) were interviewed to construct an attractiveness factor diagram. Subsequently, a bidirectional questionnaire using the Kano model was employed to understand respondents' perceptions and requirements for eyewear design. A total of 127 valid responses were gathered from young respondents. The questionnaire items included the following.

- Positive dimension: what are your feelings when the eyeglasses you intend to purchase feature modern design elements?
- Negative dimension: what are your feelings when the eyeglasses you intend to purchase do not incorporate modern design elements?

To verify the survey's reliability, Cronbach's Alpha analysis was performed. The Cronbach's Alpha for the survey was 0.930, with the positive dimension scoring 0.923 and the negative dimension scoring 0.973. These high coefficients indicated a high degree of reliability in assessing respondents' reactions to eyeglass design attributes.

4. Results and Discussion

4.1. Analysis of EGM Interviews

Figure 2 summarizes the results of the interview. The design attributes of eyewear were presented into Concrete, Original, and Abstract Factors. Original Factors were identified as Comfort, Design Style, Durability, and Value for Money, with each category further explicating related characteristics. Concrete Factors for Comfort included nose pads, temple arms, materials, weight, design shape, and the frame. These attributes are directly experienced by the customer and influence product satisfaction. Abstract Factors, in contrast, are perceptions derived from customer experience, encompassing qualities such as softness, fit, lightness, sturdiness, breathability, a pressure-free experience, and security, which customers typically come to appreciate and evaluate over time.

In Design Style, Concrete Factors comprised visually distinguishable attributes such as color, shape, texture, decorations, and branding. Conversely, Abstract Factors such as modernity, classic appeal, innovation, uniqueness, multifunctionality, and fashion sense were subjective evaluations shaped by individual preferences and cultural contexts.

Durability's Concrete Factors pertain to measurable and testable attributes, including material strength, structural design, joints, lenses, and coatings. Abstract Factors such as robustness, scratch resistance, longevity, impact resistance, resistance to deformation, and thermal tolerance reflect customers' expectations and perceptions regarding product longevity. The Concrete Factors are related to Value for Money, including material costs, design fees, manufacturing expenditures, brand influence, and market positioning. Companies must consider these critical tangible attributes for pricing and market strategies. At the abstract level, Value for Money includes subjective evaluations by customers, such as competitive pricing, perception of luxury, affordability, premium quality, perceived worth, assurance, and market competitiveness.

The attractive attributes of eyewear design consist of an analytical framework for assessing eyewear design quality and addressing the tangible technical requirements of product design and production and the emotive needs and anticipations of consumers. Using this model, designers and manufacturers can enhance their comprehension of, and alignment with, market needs and product offerings, thus creating products that not only satisfy practical use requirements but also meet the expectations of consumers.

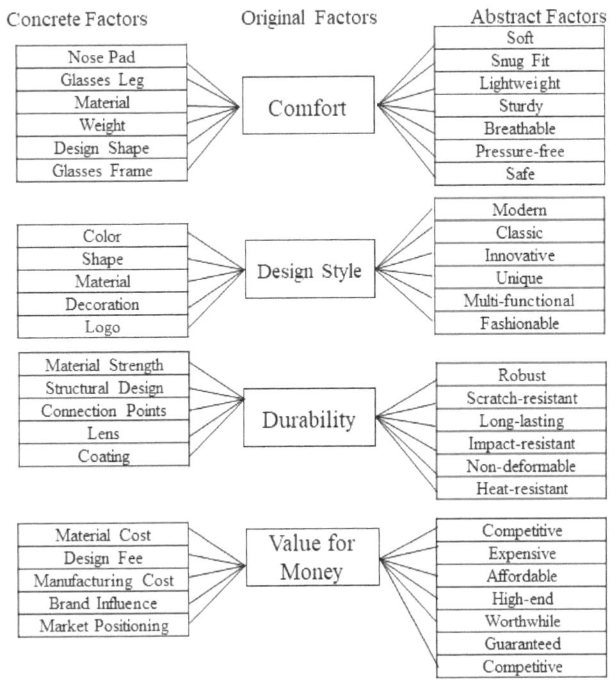

Figure 2. Analysis framework of EGM Interviews.

4.2. Analysis of Kano Model Results

4.2.1. Classification of Quality Attributes

Using the bidirectional questionnaire of the Kano Model, the quality attributes were identified by the respondents using the predominant quality attribute. Table 1 shows the four Attractive Quality factors, six Must-be Quality factors, one One-dimensional Quality factor, and one Indifferent Quality factor. In contemporary consumer culture, eyeglasses serve as emblems of fashion trends and personal style beyond the function of vision correction. The Kano Model dissects multi-faceted quality characteristics and delineates consumer expectations and predilections for various design quality features and their impact on consumer satisfaction. As shown in Table 1, Must-be Quality (M) attributes such as innovation and multifunctionality were epitomized by innovative designs, versatile functionality, unprecedented characteristics, and novel materials. Such attributes are anticipated by consumers, and their absence causes marked dissatisfaction. Therefore, companies need to pursue technological innovation and multifunctional solutions to satisfy the requirements of consumers' usage. Additionally, design elements need to be identified as Attractive Quality (A) attributes of modern aesthetics, distinctiveness, and alignment with prevailing trends. These traits elevate consumer satisfaction, whereas their absence does not engender dissatisfaction. Designers MUST exploit these elements to engender a 'wow' factor, enhancing the allure of the product.

Designs being characterized as timeless and incorporating fashion elements and are considered as One-dimensional Quality (O) attributes, which suggests a direct relationship between these features and consumer satisfaction. The explicit portrayal of branding and minimalist design (I) affect satisfaction levels, as they attract niche customers. With these qualities, eyewear must be designed to satisfy functional requirements while also catering to consumer desires for aesthetic appeal and individualistic expression. In a competitive environment, this approach allows for design strategies that augment the consumer experience with additional value while preserving essential functionality.

The Kano Model was used to explore the relationship between eyewear design quality attributes and consumer satisfaction, and provide user-centric data for strategic design and marketing decisions. Understanding the influence of these attributes on consumer perceptions, companies need to craft eyewear designs to fulfill fundamental requirements and add value.

Table 1. Factors of Kano Model.

Factor Items	Weighted Classification of Kano Quality Attributes (%)						Kano Quality Classification
	M	O	I	A	Q	R	
1. Embodying contemporary attributes	4.9	15.8	13.8	65.5	0.0	0.0	A
2. Timeless design	36.9	46.8	6.4	8.4	1.5	0.0	O
3. Cutting-edge design	56.7	38.9	2.5	2.0	0.0	0.0	M
4. Distinctive characteristics	3.9	25.6	7.4	62.6	0.5	0.0	A
5. Versatile design	67.0	18.2	4.4	2.5	6.4	1.5	M
6. Fashion-forward elements	66.0	18.2	1.5	0.5	12.3	1.5	M
7. Trend-conscious design	4.9	24.6	10.3	57.6	2.0	0.5	A
8. Novel features	70.4	19.7	4.4	0.5	4.9	0.0	M
9. Innovative material use	69.5	18.7	3.4	1.0	7.4	0.0	M
10. Specialized decorative accents or details	75.4	15.8	3.0	0.5	4.9	0.5	M
11. Prominent logo or brand display	16.7	14.3	35.5	28.6	3.0	2.0	I
12. Minimalistic approach	1.5	33.0	6.4	59.1	0.0	0.0	A

4.2.2. Kano Weighting Method

The Kano Weighting Method operates to increase satisfaction and mitigate dissatisfaction gain in determining consumer satisfaction. By comparing the "Customer Satisfaction (CS) Increase Coefficient" and the "Customer Dissatisfaction (CD) Reduction Coefficient", the method is used to identify the attribute with the greatest impact (the coefficient with the larger absolute value) (Equation (1)). Initially, qualities lacking differentiation are omitted from consideration and determined by using Equation (2).

$$C_i = \mathrm{Max}\left[\frac{CS_i}{\sum_i^m CS_i}, \frac{CD_i}{\sum_i^m CD_i}\right] \tag{1}$$

$$W_i = \frac{C_i}{\sum_i^m C_i} \tag{2}$$

Table 2 presents the relative weights within the Kano model and a discernible pattern in consumer satisfaction and dissatisfaction with a product or design. The weights derived from the Kano analysis present consumer anticipations towards brands and products and show trends within the contemporary marketplace. A weight associated with the attribute of "brand or logo" underscores the salience of brand identity. A brand transcends its emblematic logo or nomenclature and embodies a testament to quality, dependability, and societal identity. Consumers' purchasing decisions extend beyond the product's functional or aesthetic attributes, encompassing an alignment with the ethos and values emblematic of the brand. Similarly, the considerable weight of "innovative special materials" suggests a consumer inclination towards novel and distinctive experiences. The weight was used to distinguish cutting-edge technologies for enhanced performance. Such products have advantages over the competing ones. The weights of "fashion trends" and "fashion elements" underscore consumer predilections for functional utility or efficacy. Emotional aspiration exists to identify the personal and sartorial acumen of the eyewear. The weights attributed to "classic design" and "simplicity" suggest that in the vanguard of innovation and style, traditional or simple designs may not align with the preferences of the consumer.

The data derived from the Kano model's weighting system offer information on consumer predilections and trends in the market. For brand designers, this underscores imperative innovation with the emotional rapport with consumers, as a strategy to obtain differentiation in a competitive market.

Table 2. Discrimination of quality attributes and weights of satisfaction coefficients.

Quality Elements	CS	DS	CS/SUM	DS/SUM	MAX	Weights
1. Embodying contemporary attributes	0.69	−0.34	0.083	0.037	0.087	0.080
2. Timeless design	0.65	−0.42	0.077	0.046	0.065	0.060
3. Cutting-edge design	0.62	−0.48	0.074	0.053	0.078	0.071
4. Distinctive characteristics	0.58	−0.55	0.069	0.061	0.076	0.070
5. Versatile design	0.57	−0.55	0.068	0.061	0.077	0.070
6. Fashion-forward elements	0.66	−0.50	0.079	0.056	0.080	0.073
7. Trend-conscious design	0.58	−0.52	0.069	0.058	0.085	0.078
8. Novel features	0.53	−0.50	0.063	0.055	0.079	0.072
9. Innovative material use	0.55	−0.44	0.066	0.049	0.088	0.081
10. Specialized decorative accents or details	0.60	−0.39	0.072	0.043	0.072	0.066
11. Prominent logo or brand display	0.46	−0.46	0.055	0.050	0.100	0.091
12. Minimalistic approach	0.57	−0.48	0.068	0.053	0.068	0.062

5. Conclusions

Using the EGM interview method and the Kano Model, the consumer quality attributes were determined to elucidate the relationship between the attractive factors of eyewear design and consumer satisfaction. The Kano Model's results indicated that innovative materials, multifunctionality, and fashionable elements were the determinants of consumer satisfaction in the 'Must-be Quality' and 'One-dimensional Quality' categories. The existence or improvement of these attributes increased consumer satisfaction. Herein, innovation and multifunctionality were identified as basic requirements and essential elements to enhance consumer satisfaction in eyewear design. Contemporary aesthetics, personalized elements, and alignment with fashion trends forged strong brand associations with the consumer, thereby bolstering their intent to purchase. The result of the interview validated charm factors such as distinctive ornamentation or details and the incorporation of innovative materials, which affected consumer evaluation. In designing new eyeglass models, designers pay particular attention to the incorporation of these elements. Although a logo or brand is not an important factor, differentiated brand presentation is imperative to raise recognition in the marketplace. Such results can be used to transform consumer needs and preferences into tangible design references. It is necessary to integrate innovative materials and technologies to craft products with enhanced functionality to satisfy the fundamental needs of consumers. It is also necessary to use the results of the Kano Model for products to meet the demands of various consumers and prioritize functionality or unique designs.

Funding: This research did not receive external funding.

Institutional Review Board Statement: This study did not involve humans or animals, and therefore, ethical review and approval were not required.

Informed Consent Statement: Not applicable, as the study did not involve humans.

Data Availability Statement: Data sharing is not applicable to this article as no datasets were generated or analyzed during the current study.

Conflicts of Interest: The author declares no conflicts of interest.

References

1. Huarng, K.; Lin, Y.-C. A Study on Filling a Prescription According to Different Professional Images and Face Shapes. *J. Bus. Des.* **2020**, *24*, 1–20.
2. Jung, H.-H. A Study on the Conditions of 21st Century Eyewear Design and Total Fashion Trends—Focused on Clothing, Hair, and Makeup. *J. Korean Ophthalmic Opt. Soc.* **2005**, *10*, 17–25.
3. DeLong, M.; Daly, C. Eyewear, Fashion, Design, and Health. *Fash. Pract. J. Des. Creat. Process Fash. Ind.* **2015**, *5*, 117–127. [CrossRef]
4. Peng, G.-Y. Human Facial Measurement Survey for Eyewear Design. *J. Des.* **2009**, *6*, 17–31.
5. Liu, I.-M. Study on the Design of Shutter Glasses. Master's Thesis, Precision and Automation Engineering Program, College of Engineering, National Chiao Tung University, Taipei City, Taiwan, 2013.
6. Huang, Y.-X.; Li, Y.-R. Generative Product Design by Form Preferences with Kansei Evaluations—A Case Study of Eyeglasses Design. *J. Kansei* **2017**, *5*, 60–82.
7. Chen, J.K.; Chen, I.S. Kano's Model and Customer Satisfaction. *Int. J. Commer. Strategy* **2010**, *2*, 45–50.
8. Matzler, K.; Hinterhuber, H.H. How to Make Product Development Projects More Successful by Integrating Kano's Model of Customer Satisfaction into Quality Function Deployment. *Technovation* **1998**, *18*, 25–38. [CrossRef]
9. Kano, N.; Seraku, N.; Takahashi, F.; Tsuji, S. Attractive Quality and Must-Be Quality. *J. Jpn. Soc. Qual. Control* **1984**, *14*, 39–48.
10. Berger, C.; Blauth, R.; Boger, D. Kano's Methods for Understanding Customer-Defined Quality. *Cent. Qual. Manag. J.* **1993**, *2*, 3–36.
11. Tan, K.C.; Shen, X.X. Integrating Kano's Model into Internal/External Customer Satisfaction. *Total Qual. Manag.* **2000**, *11*, 813–819.
12. Sireli, Y.; Kauffmann, P.; Ozan, E. Integrated Application of Kano's Model and AHP to R&D Projects. *J. Eng. Des.* **2007**, *18*, 167–183.
13. Anderson, E.W.; Sullivan, M.W. The Antecedents and Consequences of Customer Satisfaction for Firms. *Mark. Sci.* **1993**, *12*, 125–143. [CrossRef]
14. Oliver, R.L. *Satisfaction: A Behavioral Perspective on the Consumer*; Irwin/McGraw-Hill: New York, NY, USA, 1997.
15. Kotler, P.; Armstrong, G. *Principles of Marketing*; Pearson Education: London, UK, 2010.
16. Shahin, A. Integration of Fuzzy Logic and Kano's Model in Quality Function Deployment. *Int. J. Qual. Reliab. Manag.* **2004**, *21*, 731–746. [CrossRef]
17. Tan, K.C.; Pawitra, T.A. Integrating SERVQUAL and Kano's Model into QFD for Service Excellence Development. *Manag. Serv. Qual. Int. J.* **2001**, *11*, 418–430. [CrossRef]
18. Wittink, D.R.; Bayer, L.R. Measuring Product Perceptions: A Structural Analysis of the Relationship Between Attribute Judgments and Overall Evaluations. *J. Consum. Mark.* **1994**, *6*, 14–23.

engineering proceedings

Proceeding Paper

Key Advantages of Digital Learning in Group Decision Support System: Benefit Evaluation and Its Perspective †

Shu-Chin Huang [1], Hung-Yu Lin [1], Yi-Chang Chen [1,*] and Chih-Wen Hsiao [2]

[1] Department of Business Administration, Chaoyang University of Technology, Taichung 413310, Taiwan; schuang2@gm.cyut.edu.tw (S.-C.H.); s10117083@gmail.com (H.-Y.L.)
[2] Ph.D. Program of Business Administration in Industrial Development, Chaoyang University of Technology, Taichung 413310, Taiwan; chih1124@ms21.hinet.net
* Correspondence: t2003151@cyut.edu.tw
† Presented at the 2024 IEEE 4th International Conference on Electronic Communications, Internet of Things and Big Data, Taipei, Taiwan, 19–21 April 2024.

Abstract: In today's dynamic business landscape, companies need to enhance problem-solving efficiency to produce products or services to meet evolving customer needs. Fostering creative talent and utilizing Group Decision Support Systems (GDSS) have become crucial in the management of human resources and marketing. While empirical studies demonstrate the positive impact of GDSS on learning, a gap exists in understanding its correlation with outcomes like enhanced creativity. Thus, qualitative research is needed to uncover the cognitive processes for favorable results with the adoption of GDSS. We explored the relationship between Project-Based Learning (PBL), GDSS deployment, and outcomes in a cross-organizational study. Results highlighted PBL activities facilitated by GDSS and the key benefits of digital learning, and managerial and academic considerations were proposed.

Keywords: group decision supporting systems (GDSS); benefit evaluation; e-learning

Citation: Huang, S.-C.; Lin, H.-Y.; Chen, Y.-C.; Hsiao, C.-W. Key Advantages of Digital Learning in Group Decision Support System: Benefit Evaluation and Its Perspective. *Eng. Proc.* **2024**, *74*, 73. https://doi.org/10.3390/engproc2024074073

Academic Editors: Shu-Han Liao, Teen-Hang Meen and Cheng-Fu Yang

Published: 23 October 2024

1. Introduction

To improve learners' learning effectiveness, it is necessary to use information technology effectively. Though the COVID-19 pandemic is over, it still affects our lives and work behaviors as it creates different experiences in learning activities. The Means–End Chain method provides three-level element connections at the attribute, result, and value levels to form a hierarchical relationship [1–4]. This hierarchical relationship presents the number of source links of elements and the number of times the element links are extended. The former is the In-Degrees (IDs) frequency and the latter is the Out-Degrees (ODs) frequency.

Benefit evaluation is used to judge the relative importance and specificity of various elements in the benefit structure. The three indicators of abstractness, centrality, and prestige are widely used in the evaluation and their values range between 0 and 1 [5]. The degree of abstraction is used to understand the degree of the benefit element in achieving the goal. The higher the value, the more abstract the benefit element is. The ratio is used to measure the ratio of IDs to ODs. The higher the centrality, the higher the proportion of IDs and ODs of the benefit element to total IDs and ODs. This means the benefit element plays an important role in the relationship between IDs and ODs. The ratio of the sum of IDs and ODs to the 'total number of links' is used for the measurement of benefit factors. The more the benefit, the higher the proportion of IDs to the total number of links. The ratio of the number of IDs to the number of total links is used to evaluate the importance of the benefit element in achieving the goal also using centrality and benefits.

In this study, we analyzed the characteristics of digital learning using a Group Decision Support System and explored the benefit elements that participants value when learning in a Group Decision Support System. Benefits were evaluated to select important benefit factors.

2. Research Method

2.1. Research Design

To understand the connection between the implementation of topic-based learning and the Group Decision Support System, we conducted cross-organizational research for four months, in which the participants implemented innovative products in a Group Decision Support System. Naming and designing advertising slogans were used in project-based learning (PBL). The participants were students from various departments of three different colleges. A total of 168 participants were split into 42 groups, with each group comprising 4 participants. Each group included members of different genders, different colleges, different majors, and different regions. Thus, face-to-face discussions were difficult, and virtual group discussions were adopted.

2.2. Data Collection

We randomly selected 66 participants for interviews to obtain data for PBL in a Group Decision Support System and explored the key benefits of digital learning. The soft laddering method, one-to-one in-depth interviews, and a semi-structured questionnaire were used. On average, each person provided 2 to 3 items of learning experiences with an average of 2.55. The data obtained from the interviews were analyzed by three experts to extract the characteristic PBL activities. Using the benefit evaluation analysis, the key benefits of digital learning were identified.

2.3. Definitions

The variables of this study included digital learning attributes and digital learning benefits (Table 1).

Table 1. Operationalizing definitions of research concepts.

Code	Benefit Element	Definition	Description
	Attribute element		
A01	Information integration and classification	Ability to integrate and classify information	Thematic classification, columnar data display, data integration, and publication
A02	Immediacy	Not limited by time and space, providing the function to express opinions at any time	No time limit, not affected by time and space, can leave messages at any time
A03	Easy to operate	System is simple to operate and easy to learn	Easy to use, convenient and simple to operate
A04	Competition format	Implement project-based learning in a competitive format	Presented as a group competition
A05	Matchmaking group	Form a group of unfamiliar participants	Group up and cooperate with people you don't know
A06	Account and password protection	Protect participants' personal information with account and password	Account and password protection
A07	Anonymity	System operates anonymously	Anonymous
A08	Recordable information	System provides data storage	Computer record information
A09	Open platform	Platform for participants to discuss and share information	Platform where you can post URLs, post different messages, search and post different messages, and express your creativity
A10	Gamified learning	Provide participants with lively and stress-free interactive activities	More interactive among peers, presented in a lively, interesting, and less stressful way

Table 1. *Cont.*

Code	Benefit Element	Definition	Description
	Benefit element		
C01	Improving work efficiency	Operating time is flexible, increasing the time individuals can participate in activities	Save time, let the game go smoothly, have more time to discuss, do more things, enrich ourselves, facilitate discussion, have more time to think
C02	More chance of victory	Increase the likelihood of winning	Not to admit defeat, for honor, to gain fame, and to gain recognition from others
C03	Stimulating ideas	Generating or adding ideas through others or oneself	Inspire more ideas, you can throw ideas on it at any time, inspire your own ideas through other people's ideas, and a pile of ideas makes it easier to think.
C05	Increasing enthusiasm for participation	Promote participants to be more enthusiastic about using the system	More enthusiastic participation, convenient for discussion, easy to reach consensus, interesting, novel, and more want to use, stimulate curiosity
C06	Changing mindset	Change personal thinking patterns without being limited by existing thinking frameworks	Activate brain cells, break through existing ideas, improve creative quality, improve thinking, and integrate thinking
C07	Developing group spirit	Sense of the overall situation and a spirit of mutual assistance for collaboration and cooperation	Cultivate group chemistry and learn from each other's different strengths
C09	Meeting new friends	Make new friends and expand your network	Expand your circle of friends and expand your network
C10	Privacy	Ideas are protected	Attention to personal privacy and the protection of your ideas or data
C11	Improving competitiveness	Improve capabilities that can be demonstrated in competition	Improve competitive advantage, show ambition, and enhance competitiveness through group competition, future considerations, and future planning
C13	Expressing ideas freely	Express ideas freely without restraint	Easy to express ideas, express ideas without pressure, throw away whatever comes to mind, and think randomly
C14	Improving learning effectiveness	Opportunities to learn more and improve learning outcomes	Learn more, gain new knowledge easily, gain something, accumulate knowledge and experience

2.4. Analysis Method

We used the content analysis method to analyze the interview content of interviewees. The content analysis method is used to extract and analyze the central tendency of important concepts [6]. We conducted a literature review to determine the research scope and subject areas. For research samples, we established category rules to code the data and obtain the data statistics. The important concepts and occurrence of elements at each level were analyzed. To understand the importance of the attribute level and the interest level, abstraction, concentration, and prestige were used for analysis using the following.

1. Abstraction degree calculation method

$$\text{Degree of abstraction} = \text{number of IDs}/(\text{number of IDs} + \text{number of ODs}) \quad (1)$$

2. Concentration calculation method

$$\text{Centrality} = (\text{number of IDs} + \text{number of ODs})/\text{total number of links} \quad (2)$$

3. Prestige calculation method

$$\text{Prestige} = \text{number of IDs}/\text{total number of links} \quad (3)$$

2.5. Reliability and Validity Analysis

Intercoder reliability was used to test reliability, and the jury method was employed to ensure research validity. Three coders were classified to code the data and compare the analysis results. The average agreement of the three evaluators was 0.82. The reliability was calculated as follows.

$$\text{Reliability} = (\text{number of evaluators} \times \text{average mutual agreement})/[1 + (\text{number of evaluators} - 1) \times \text{average mutual agreement}] = (30.82)/(1 + 20.82) = 0.93 \quad (4)$$

The reliability was 0.93, which met the standard threshold (0.85) recommended by Kassarjain [7]. In the jury method, one professor and three graduate students familiar with the Means–End chain and the Group Decision Support System were invited.

3. Results

3.1. Group Decision Support System-Oriented Digital Learning Activities

The characteristics of digital learning were presented as 10 attribute elements. "Immediacy" was mentioned most frequently by 56.06% of the participants. More than half of the participants were not affected by time and space restrictions, and they thought the ability to express their opinions at any time was the most important in this learning model. "Recordable data (39.39%)", "anonymity (33.33%)", "open platform (31.82%)", and "competition format (30.30%)" were mentioned as the elements (Table 2). The functions and characteristics of the Group Decision Support System (immediacy, recordable data, anonymity, open platform) were found to be important. (see Table 2)

Table 2. Attribute occurrences.

Code	Attribute	Frequency	No. of Freq. Ratio	No. of People Ratio
A02	Immediacy	37	26.06%	56.06%
A08	Recordable information	26	18.31%	39.39%
A07	Anonymous	22	15.49%	33.33%
A09	Open platform	21	14.79%	31.82%
A04	Competition format	20	14.08%	30.30%
A10	Like a game	19	13.38%	28.79%
A05	Match strangers to group up	17	11.97%	25.76%
A01	Information integration and classification	9	6.34%	13.64%
A03	Easy to operate	7	4.93%	10.61%
A06	Account and password protection	1	0.70%	1.52%
	Total (66 participants)	142	100.00%	271.21%

3.2. Key Benefits of Digital Learning

We interviewed the participants to explore the benefits of digital learning. Among the 11 digital learning benefits, stimulating ideas was mentioned the most by the respondents, with 47 mentions, accounting for 71.21% of the 66 participants. More than 70% of the participants believed that such a learning design helped them have "stimulating ideas". The other mentioned benefits included "Improving work efficiency (45.45%)", "Freely expressing ideas (50.00%)", "Changing mindset (44.78%)", "Increasing enthusiasm for participation (40.91%)", and "Improving learning effectiveness (40.91%)" (Table 3).

Table 3. Key benefits of digital learning.

Code	Attribute	Frequency	No. of Freq. Ratio	No. of People Ratio
C03	Stimulating ideas	47	17.60%	71.21%
C01	Improving work efficiency	37	13.86%	56.06%
C13	Expressing ideas freely	33	12.36%	50.00%
C06	Changing mindset	30	11.24%	45.45%
C05	Increasing enthusiasm for participation	27	10.11%	40.91%
C14	Improving learning effectiveness	27	5.24%	40.91%
C11	Improving competitiveness	19	7.12%	28.79%
C07	Developing group spirit	17	6.37%	25.76%
C09	Meeting new friends	16	5.99%	24.24%
C02	More chance of victory	12	4.49%	18.18%
C10	Privacy	2	0.75%	3.03%
	Total (66 participants)	267	100.00%	404.55%

3.3. Benefit Evaluation of Digital Learning

We evaluated 11 learning benefit elements of digital learning in terms of abstractness, centrality, and prestige. Abstractness was mentioned most frequently by participants as "Privacy", followed by "Meeting new friends", and "Changing thinking". For centrality and prestige, "Stimulating ideas" was the most mentioned followed by "Improving work efficiency" and "Expressing ideas freely". In digital learning, "Stimulating ideas", "Improving work efficiency", and "Expressing ideas freely" were important benefit elements (see Table 4).

Table 4. Benefit evaluation results of digital learning.

Code	Benefit Element	In	Out	I+O	Abstractness	Centrality	Prestige
C01	Improving work efficiency	37	37	74	0.500	0.166	0.083
C02	More chance of victory	12	12	24	0.500	0.054	0.027
C03	Stimulating ideas	47	48	95	0.495	0.213	0.106
C05	Increasing enthusiasm for participation	27	27	54	0.500	0.121	0.061
C06	Changing mindset	31	30	61	0.508	0.137	0.070
C07	Developing group spirit	17	17	34	0.500	0.076	0.038
C09	Meeting new friends	16	15	31	0.516	0.070	0.036
C10	Privacy	2	1	3	0.667	0.007	0.004
C11	Improving competitiveness	19	19	38	0.500	0.085	0.043
C13	Expressing ideas freely	33	33	66	0.500	0.148	0.074
C14	Improving learning effectiveness	27	27	54	0.500	0.121	0.061

4. Conclusions

The digital PBL in the Group Decision Support System showed "Immediacy", "recordable data", "anonymity", "open platform", and "competition format". On the asynchronous system platform, the digital PBL allowed learners to be multifunctional (without time and space restrictions, store and share learner opinions, everyone has a fair right to express their opinions, participate anonymously without pressure, and use competitions to enhance participation and stimulate engagement). It provided learners with a rich learning experience. A total of 11 benefits in the digital PBL were determined, among which "stimulating ideas", "improving work efficiency", "expressing ideas freely", "changing mindset", "increasing enthusiasm for participation", and "enhancing learning effectiveness" were important. The Group Decision-making Support System directly impacted learners' way of thinking (stimulating ideas and changing mindset) and allowed for benefits in learners' learning process such as improving participation enthusiasm, work efficiency, learning effectiveness, involving attitude, learning process, and learning results. The important key factors in digital learning included "stimulating ideas", "improving work efficiency", and "expressing ideas freely". By sharing information in the Group Decision Support System, learners can generate more diverse ideas in a stress-free digital learning environment and express their ideas freely without inhibition. In the asynchronous system, the group members participated in learning to learn flexibly without being restricted by time and space. Such benefits meet the needs of college students whose lives and schedules are very tight.

The Group Decision-making Support System combined with digital PBL allows for the functions of the platform and benefits such as "stimulating ideas", "improving work efficiency", and "freely expressing ideas". PBL with competition strengthens the learning behavior of participants. It is recommended for teachers to combine group decision-making platforms and PBL to diversify learning activities and designs. Then, learning participation and activities can be used to bring benefits. The Group Decision Support System enables group interaction and cooperation in a virtual environment. Although it brings diverse benefits, it may have negative effects. The benefits are also limited to the system. Therefore, more learning activities are demanded in the learning activities for students to have diverse learning experiences.

Author Contributions: Conceptualization, S.-C.H., H.-Y.L. and Y.-C.C.; methodology, S.-C.H.; writing—original draft preparation, H.-Y.L. and C.-W.H.; writing—review and editing, Y.-C.C. and C.-W.H. All authors have read and agreed to the published version of the manuscript.

Funding: This research received no external funding.

Institutional Review Board Statement: Not applicable.

Informed Consent Statement: Not applicable.

Data Availability Statement: Data sharing is not applicable to this article.

Acknowledgments: All subjects' enthusiastic participation is greatly appreciated.

Conflicts of Interest: The authors declare no conflicts of interest.

References

1. Gutman, J. A means-end chain model based on consumer categorization processes. *J. Mark.* **1982**, *46*, 60–72. [CrossRef]
2. Gutman, J. Means–end chains as goal hierarchies. *Psychol. Mark.* **1997**, *14*, 545–560. [CrossRef]
3. Zanoli, R.; Naspetti, S. Consumer motivations in the purchase of organic food: A means-end approach. *Br. Food J.* **2002**, *104*, 643–653. [CrossRef]
4. Zhao, Y.; Agyeiwaah, E. Exploring value-based motivations for culture and heritage tourism using the means-end chain and laddering approach. *J. Herit. Tour.* **2023**, *18*, 594–616. [CrossRef]
5. Pieters, R.; Baumgartner, H.; Allen, D. A means-end chain approach to consumer goal structures. *Int. J. Res. Mark.* **1995**, *12*, 227–244. [CrossRef]
6. Krippendorff, K. Content analysis. *Int. Encycl. Commun.* **1989**, *1*, 403–407.
7. Kassarjian, H.H. Content analysis in consumer research. *J. Cons. Res.* **1977**, *4*, 8–18. [CrossRef]

engineering proceedings

Proceeding Paper

Satisfaction with Research-Based Learning and Academic Performance by Big Data Analysis †

Gabriela Torres-Delgado [1], Sofía Ramos-Pulido [2,*] and Neil Hernández-Gress [2]

1 School of Humanities and Education, Tecnologico de Monterrey, Monterrey 64849, Mexico; gtorresd@tec.mx
2 School of Engineering and Science, Tecnologico de Monterrey, Monterrey 64849, Mexico; ngress@tec.mx
* Correspondence: a00834077@tec.mx

† Presented at the 2024 IEEE 4th International Conference on Electronic Communications, Internet of Things and Big Data, Taipei, Taiwan, 19–21 April 2024.

Abstract: Data science analysis was used to investigate the association between Research-Based Learning (RBL) and student's academic performance. The research professors certified in RBL participated in this research. The participants used an advanced platform with over 500 resources. Tutors guided students in designing, implementing, and evaluating the RBL. We employed a quantitative and quasi-experimental design without a control group, correlational analysis, and ex post facto elements. A satisfaction survey was administered after the capacitation. In total, 342 teachers were trained and received accreditation. The analyses incorporated non-conventional data science methods such as correlation analysis, principal component analysis, and unsupervised learning utilizing the Density-Based Spatial Clustering Application with Noise algorithm. The professors' satisfaction with RBL was related to student's academic performance, which was found in clustering analysis.

Keywords: Research-Based Learning; academic performance; teacher training; higher education; educational innovation; unsupervised learning; algorithm; professional education

Citation: Torres-Delgado, G.; Ramos-Pulido, S.; Hernández-Gress, N. Satisfaction with Research-Based Learning and Academic Performance by Big Data Analysis. *Eng. Proc.* **2024**, *74*, 74. https://doi.org/10.3390/engproc2024074074

Academic Editors: Shu-Han Liao, Teen-Hang Meen and Cheng-Fu Yang

Published: 24 October 2024

1. Introduction

The COVID-19 pandemic significantly changed university teaching and learning approaches. Videoconferences became the norm, the demand for information and communication technology (ICT) surged, and evaluation systems were redesigned. This transformation also increased the workload for teachers and students, highlighting deficiencies in ICT proficiency and resulting in feelings of isolation and disorientation [1]. The pandemic has exposed a substantial gap in educational institutions regarding infrastructure and teaching and research staff training. However, institutions have responded swiftly and creatively to these challenges. Educators have enhanced their training and shown greater interest in resources and strategies to improve teaching [2].

Inquiry-based learning emerges as a powerful teaching strategy, adaptable to various disciplines and educational objectives. College instructors employ a range of classifications or vocabularies to delineate investigative learning assignments from basic to advanced levels of achievement. This versatility underscores the effectiveness and adaptability of inquiry-based learning, instilling confidence in its application across diverse educational settings [3].

At the educational institution where this research was conducted, Challenge-Based Research [4,5] was promoted to accelerate solutions to societal issues. This methodology combines innovation with pedagogical practices. Additionally, faculty members integrate their teaching with research via Research-Based Learning (RBL), addressing the need for meaningful learning experiences and providing engaging teaching formats that captivate students' interest [6]. This professional development initiative is implemented through a completely digital and utterly online model featuring a portal rich with over 500 high-quality instructional materials.

The courses or topics considered for RBL are taught in the different schools of the institution, including the School of Humanities and Education, School of Engineering and Sciences, School of Medicine and Health Sciences, School of Business, School of Architecture and Design, and School of Social Sciences and Government at a university in Mexico. The university's high school system is integrated into this framework. Moreover, faculty members of different undergraduate and high school programs actively engage in RBL initiatives and are trained through an accredited RBL workshop.

In this study, we observed the satisfaction of professors who have undergone RBL accreditation. Taking the initiative to assess this process, we calculated and analyzed the correlation between the contentment levels of RBL-accredited educators and student's academic progress. Then, the impact of RBL on teacher satisfaction and student learning outcomes was investigated with unsupervised learning.

2. Inquiry-Based Learning and Academic Achievement

It has been observed that researchers and professionals do not collaborate and lack synchronization [7]. This disconnect might dissipate student's engagement in experiential learning through research. RBL approaches can potentially foster a favorable transformation. Educators undergo professional growth by participating in research and developmental endeavors. Research initiatives directly impact teaching quality, bolster student motivation and engagement, and shape the academic atmosphere concerning faculty research endeavors. Furthermore, when educational institutions prioritize research, students actively participate and cultivate interactions, perseverance, intellectual curiosity, critical thinking abilities, and other skills [8].

The study of learning through student accomplishment is becoming increasingly indispensable. Students actively engage in learning, employ meaningful tactics, attain enhanced academic outcomes, and showcase competencies and engagement in their assignments and academic endeavors. Several universities recognize the benefits and have integrated RBL into their educational programs and embedded it within the syllabus [9]. This approach offers an opportunity for myriad students to engage in research endeavors, especially in technology, science, engineering, and mathematics (CTIM), leading to a rich learning experience [10]. Moreover, the RBL methodology fosters cognitive and affective-emotional growth for research in alternative fields, like the social sciences [6].

In RBL, four distinct modes of student involvement in inquiry are distinguished. Students express enthusiasm for the research results or process, while others adopt active or passive roles. These modes are combined in four modalities to establish the link between teaching and research [9].

- Research-Guided Learning: **students** acquire knowledge from the findings of investigations.
- Research-led: students learn about research outcomes with the teacher determining the communication strategy.
- Research-oriented: students derive learning from the research process in this mode.
- Research-based: students assume the role of researchers, engaging directly in the research process.

Reference [11] defines RBL as a procedure where students regulate themselves, assisted by their research inquiries. Through the progression of research projects, students engage in cognitive, behavioral, and affective activities that demonstrate the advantages of conducting RBL [12]. In RBL [3], (1) scientific investigation is utilized in the teaching–learning process, (2) teaching centers on the learner, (3) learning is stimulated by raised inquiries and questions, (4) an instructor assumes the role of the facilitator, learning results from the construction of knowledge that promotes cognition and metacognition, and (5) self-direction is encouraged. Students who engage in RBL report enhanced learning experiences and increased academic attainments. Once students become enthralled with a research project that they can conduct independently, they never revert to their previous methods [12], but transform.

An understanding of learning through the RBL approach is enabled in an interpretative process that leads to understanding reality [13]. Learning is manifested through the capacity to debate and even bolster practical experiences. Practical learning entails solving problems, honing skills through encounters with real-world issues, and suggesting viable solutions that can be implemented with expert guidance. Learning comprehension is observed when the student assumes an active role. Engaging in a science project transcends the mere completion of another assignment for the student [12]. It represents an encounter involving self-discovery, wherein they take on, often for the first time, the responsibility for their self-learning. This demands intellectual maturity in conducting research and assuming accountability for the process. Moreover, as previously discussed, integrating teaching with research entails advantages for the institution.

Several studies notice the significance of RBL in influencing students' academic achievements and enhancing their learning outcomes (Table 1). It is crucial to carry out further research to identify the factors that enhance the learning patterns and research activities of both teachers and students. This increases their performance, skill development, and overall learning. It is beneficial to receive feedback from some of their teachers [8].

Table 1. Similar studies to this research.

Reference	Description	Method	Data Analysis	Findings
[14]	Assess the influence of research-oriented learning on students' academic outcomes and evaluate their contentment with the experience.	The study utilized longitudinal data to determine if RBL improved learning, academic performance, and overall satisfaction.	Linear and logistic regression analysis	A positive correlation exists between academic performance and RBL. The authors concluded that research-based learning can enhance students' engagement and knowledge acquisition.
[15]	It is a method for designing a research-oriented course. It enables faculty across various fields to involve students in innovative manners.	Qualitative	Qualitative	Research-based learning is a potent pedagogical approach for developing self-directed students. Successful completion of Inquiry 1SS3 correlates with learners achieving passing grades, maintaining positions on the dean's honor roll, and persisting in their university studies.
[16]	To assess the impact of training digital stories through RBL on the inclination of prospective educators to embrace technology instruction	Experimental study utilizing a convergent parallel design.	Shapiro–Wilk test and *t*-test.	The study suggests that preparing digital stories through an inquiry-based learning approach significantly reduces forthcoming teachers' resistance toward technology-based teaching and performing research.
[17]	The paper summarizes the creation and implementation of four integrated laboratory sessions at the School of Medicine, King Saud University.	It is based on promoting inquiry-based learning and motivating students to engage in collaborative tasks within small groups.	The chi-squared test, Mann–Whitney U, and Cronbach's alpha.	The research also demonstrated that the revised design promoted self-guided learning, knowledge integration, and apprenticeship among students.

3. Method

After completing the training program, a satisfaction survey was administered to a non-random convenience sample of professors to evaluate their contentment level. A focus group examined the survey to ensure its quality, assessing the content and structure of each question. We employed a quantitative, quasi-experimental design without a control group and ex post facto aspects. Correlational analysis, principal components, and the Density-Based Spatial Clustering Application with Noise (DBSCAN) algorithm for clustering were utilized for analysis.

3.1. Intervention

Educators were certified through the RBL workshop using the digital plus model (100% online format) in response to the confinement restrictions imposed by the COVID-19 pandemic. The state-of-the-art platform provided instructors with more than 500 resources, including complimentary courses, library tutorials, templates, readings, websites, and research hubs. The professors devised an RBL strategy based on the approaches outlined in Ref. [9]. Mentors provided feedback to teachers who utilized the platform featuring RBL resources as a tool. They conceived, formulated, executed, and evaluated an RBL strategy for their designated classes within one semester. The educators were assessed using rubrics and student evidence. The students acquired and honed competencies through research and presentation of their findings. At the culmination of the intervention, a participant satisfaction survey was administered, and the educators received acknowledgment in their profiles. The trained educators facilitated their students' learning through research endeavors.

3.2. Sample

The sample consisted of 342 educators, with 41% being female and 59% male. Of the instructors, 18% are affiliated with SNI, the national research system in Mexico. In terms of age, 32% were aged between 25 and 40, 31% between 41 and 50, 28% between 51 and 60, and 8% were over 60. Further, 42% taught in the School of Engineering and Sciences, followed by the Business School at 18%; the School of Social Sciences and Government at 10%; the School of Humanities and Education at 9%; the School of Architecture and Design at 7%; and the remainder included preparatory schools (high schools), the School of Medicine, and administrative sectors.

3.3. Data Analysis

The responses were coded for descriptive analysis, and dummy variables were created for the categorical variables for the school and campus. Subsequently, correlation analysis was conducted to explore the relationships between these variables. To delve into the structure of the dataset, dimensionality reduction was conducted using principal component analysis (PCA) [18]. This statistical technique was used to extract essential information from the dataset by creating new features named principal components, a new collection of orthogonal variables [19]. Dimensionality is successfully reduced when a small number of components explain a significant portion of the total variance, enabling the identification of patterns, trends, and outliers [20].

The Python library sklearn was used in PCA. Notably, the two main components elucidated 74% of the data's variability, with the first accounting for 61% and the second for 13%. Consequently, these components were plotted to visualize potential patterns or clusters. Irregular clustering patterns were observed, prompting further investigation through unsupervised analysis of a non-convex clustering structure. The DBSCAN algorithm was employed to identify clusters as high-density regions separated by low-density areas [21].

The DBSCAN procedure was introduced in Ref. [22]. This method operates with just two parameters: the neighborhood size (eps) and the minimum number of points required to constitute a cluster (minPts). DBSCAN identifies clusters by seeking regions where points are densely packed, with sparse spaces between them [23]. While the algorithm employs a Euclidean algorithm to compute similarity, alternative metrics can also be utilized. DBSCAN offers benefits, including the ability to detect groups of any shape, straightforward parameter interpretation, and efficient performance even with large datasets [22].

4. Results and Discussions

4.1. Descriptive Analysis

In total, 95% of the respondents expressed satisfaction with implementing and utilizing RBL, rating themselves as either satisfied or extremely satisfied. Additionally, 5% scored themselves as somewhat satisfied, indicating the significance of using RBL. When RBL was implemented, teachers trained in RBL under the institution's educational model reported that the following six activities were frequently employed by students. First, efficient search strategies, planning, and specialized database management accounted for 41%. Second, the analysis of scientific articles represented 37%. Theoretical framework elaboration, elaboration/execution of projects, teamwork, and bibliographical analysis accounted for 22–24%.

In total, 98% of the teachers believed that the Challenge-Based Learning (CBL Model) must be linked with RBL to achieve greater rigor, quality, performance in learning, and student aptitude development. Further, 92% believed that the RBL strategy is necessary for the educational model of the institution where the research was developed, particularly within the CBL strategy. Teachers also recommended that the learning units designed for the educational model must integrate CBL-RBL.

The professors used RBL in classes of varying sizes, from 2 to 245 students, with 30 students being the most common (8%). Regarding academic performance, 56% of the respondents stated that their grades improved when RBL was used, 34% reported that an increase did not apply because of how the courses are usually evaluated, and 10% reported no improvement. Table 2 summarizes the percentage increase distribution in academic performance when RBL was implemented. Scopus was the most used database among teachers, with 43.7% implementing it in RBL. Web of Science and Elsevier followed, with 28 and 27.6% usage.

Table 2. Percentage growth with RBL implementation.

Increase in Academic Performance		Percentage
Yes	1–5%	12%
	6–10%	17%
	11–20%	14%
	>20%	13%
NA		34%
No		10%

4.2. Correlation Analysis

The assessment of the RBL certification course and instructors' contentment in executing and employing the RBL framework showed a correlation coefficient of 0.38. The rise in academic performance percentage associated with RBL utilization and the satisfaction level in implementing and utilizing the RBL framework showed a correlation coefficient of 0.35. Instructors' satisfaction with the RBL model was positively correlated with evaluating the RBL certification and students' academic achievement. Therefore, prioritizing instructor contentment with pedagogical approaches is crucial, as it directly impacts student outcomes.

4.3. Unsupervised Learning

In the PCA, the clustering of the two principal components was irregular. Consequently, the DBSCAN algorithm was employed, utilizing the Scikit-Cluster function, with Euclidean distance utilized for the distance matrix. The determination of the neighborhood size and cluster count was based on the plot of the two principal components, with eps established at 0.0003 and minPts set at five. Figure 1 illustrates the outcomes of the clustering analysis.

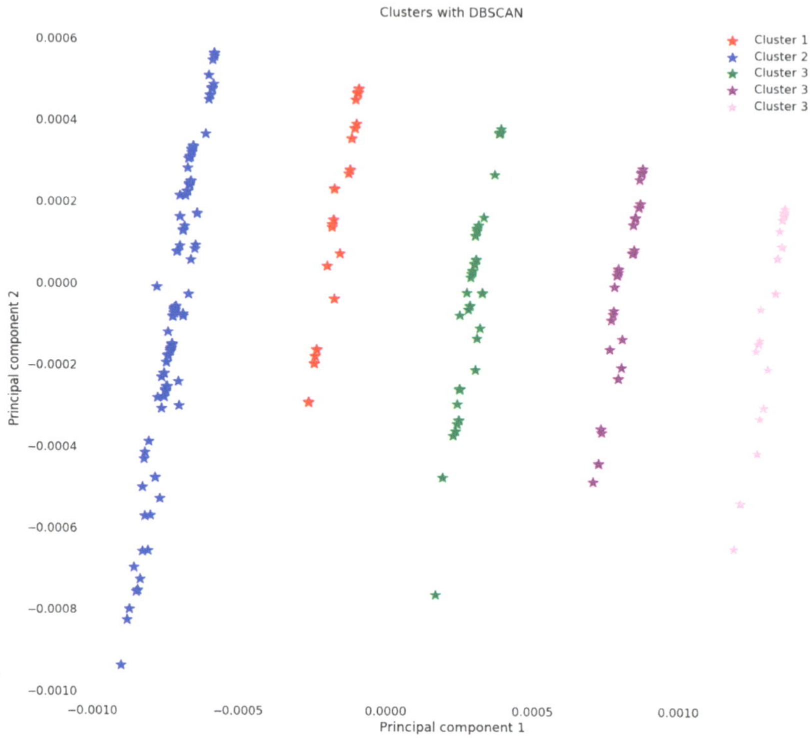

Figure 1. Results of unsupervised DBSCAN algorithm.

The DBSCAN algorithm was used to effectively group the irregular clusters. Table 3 presents several noteworthy details for each group. In Figure 1, the red cluster (Cluster 1) represents teachers who have witnessed a 1–5% increase in their students' academic performance. The largest group, identified as the blue cluster (Cluster 2), exhibits no notable increase in academic performance. Cluster 3 (green) pertains to teachers who have observed a performance increase between 6 and 10%, while Cluster 4 (purple) denotes an increase between 11 and 20%. Lastly, Cluster 5 (pink) comprises cases where the increase exceeded 20%.

Table 3. Clustering statistics.

Group		1	2	3	4	5
Cluster Size		11%	45%	17%	14%	13%
Female (1)		42%	43%	32%	30%	46%
How satisfied are you with implementing and using the RBL model?	Very good	60%	50%	70%	77%	72%
	Good	37%	38%	28%	23%	26%
	Regular	3%	11%	2%		2%
Would you consider it essential to integrate the CBL framework with the RBL approach to enhance the rigor, quality, and effectiveness of learning, as well as the development of student competencies?	Extremely satisfied	47%	21%	36%	64%	70%
	Very satisfied	53%	72%	64%	36%	30%
	Somewhat satisfied		7%			

Table 3. *Cont.*

Group		1	2	3	4	5
Did the academic performance increase with the RBL accreditation?	Yes	100%	5%	100%	100%	100%
	No		23%			
	NA		72%			
How much was the percentage increase?	NA	0%	100%	0%	0%	0%
	(1–5%)	100%	0%	0%	0%	0%
	(6–10%)	0%	0%	100%	0%	0%
	(11–20%)	0%	0%	0%	100%	0%
	>20%	0%	0%	0%	0%	100%

No significant distinctions were detected among the clusters based on age groups, gender, SNI membership, campus, or school. Clusters 4 and 5 exhibited the most notable enhancements in academic performance, which indicated higher levels of satisfaction with the implementation of the RBL model with rates of 77 and 72%, compared to Cluster 2, which reported only 50% being extremely satisfied with RBL implementation. Conversely, Cluster 5 demonstrated the most substantial increase in academic performance and displayed predominant utilization of databases for RBL implementation (80%).

5. Conclusions

In this research, the positive impact of implementing RBL on academic performance was determined. It reaffirmed the effectiveness of the unsupervised learning algorithm DBSCAN in identifying irregular clustering patterns within educational contexts, underscored by its reliability and applicability in educational research. The results highlighted the role of teacher satisfaction in RBL implementation, which directly influenced students' academic outcomes. RBL enabled a wide range of successful activities, including strategic planning, efficient database management, article analysis, theoretical framework development, research project execution, bibliographic analysis, and collaborative teamwork. This versatility of RBL underscores its potential to enhance various aspects of education. Thus, fostering teacher satisfaction with RBL implementation is essential in fostering students' academic success.

Author Contributions: Conceptualization, G.T.-D. and S.R.-P.; methodology, G.T.-D., S.R.-P. and N.H.-G.; validation, G.T.-D., S.R.-P. and N.H.-G.; formal analysis, S.R.-P.; investigation, G.T.-D. and S.R.-P.; resources, G.T.-D.; data curation, G.T.-D.; writing—original draft preparation, G.T.-D. and S.R.-P.; writing—review and editing, G.T.-D., S.R.-P. and N.H.-G.; visualization, S.R.-P.; supervision, G.T.-D., S.R.-P. and N.H.-G.; project administration, G.T.-D. and N.H.-G.; funding acquisition, G.T.-D. All authors have read and agreed to the published version of the manuscript.

Funding: This research received no external funding.

Informed Consent Statement: Informed consent was obtained from all subjects involved in the study.

Data Availability Statement: The data can be shared upon formal request to the corresponding author.

Acknowledgments: The authors thank the Writing Lab at the Institute for the Future of Education, ITESM for their invaluable technical assistance in developing this work.

Conflicts of Interest: The authors declare no conflict of interest.

References

1. Gómez-Hurtado, I.; García-Rodríguez, M.D.P.; Falcón, I.G.; Coronel-Llamas, J.M. Adaptación de las Metodologías Activas en la Educación Universitaria en Tiempos de Pandemia. *Rev. Int. Educ. Para Justicia Soc.* **2020**, *9*, 415–433. [CrossRef]
2. García-Peñalvo, F.-J. El Sistema Universitario Ante la COVID-19: Corto, Medio y Largo Plazo. 12 May 2020. Available online: https://www.universidadsi.es/sistema-universitario-covid-19/ (accessed on 1 January 2023).
3. Aditomo, A.; Goodyear, P.; Bliuc, A.-M.; Ellis, R.A. Inquiry-based learning in higher education: Principal forms, educational objectives, and disciplinary variations. *Stud. High. Educ.* **2011**, *38*, 1239–1258. [CrossRef]

4. ITESM. Challenge Based Research. 2021. Available online: https://tec.mx/en/challenge-based-learning/ (accessed on 1 January 2024).
5. Bogers, M.; Chesbrough, H.; Moedas, C. Open Innovation: Research, Practices, and Policies. *Calif. Manag. Rev.* **2018**, *60*, 5–16. [CrossRef]
6. Wessels, I.; Rue, J.; Gess, C.; Deicke, W.; Ziegler, M. Is research-based learning effective? Evidence from a pre–post analysis in the social sciences. *Stud. High. Educ.* **2021**, *46*, 2595–2609. [CrossRef]
7. Nardello, C.M.J.G.M. Understanding Enterprise Architecture with Topic Modeling. In Proceedings of the 20th International Conference on Enterprise Information Systems, Madeira, Portugal, 21–24 March 2018; pp. 640–648.
8. Debarun, C.; Biswas, W. Motivating factors in a teacher's research and developmental activities and their impact on effective quality teaching in higher education institutions. *J. Appl. Res. High. Educ.* **2019**, *12*, 609–632.
9. Healey, M.; Jenkins, A. Developing Undergraduate Research and Inquiry. Innovations in Education and York. *High. Educ. Acad.* **2009**, 1–156.
10. Linn, M.; Palmer, E.; Baranger, A.; Gerard, E.; Stone, E. Education. Undergraduate research experiences: Impacts and opportunities. *Am. Assoc. Adv. Sci.* **2015**, *347*, 1261757.
11. Huber, L. Forschungsbasiertes, Forschungsorientiertes, Forschendes Lernen: Alles dasselbe? *Hochschulforschung* **2014**, *62*, 22–29.
12. Lopatto, D. Science in Solution: The Impact of Undergraduate Research on Student Learning. *Res. Corp.* **2009**.
13. Cabanach, R. Concepciones y enfoques de aprendizaje. *Rev. Psicodidáctica* **1997**, *4*, 5–39.
14. Zafra-Gómez, J.L.; Román-Martínez, I.; Miranda, M.E.G. Measuring the impact of inquiry-based learning on outcomes and student satisfaction. *Assess. Eval. High. Educ.* **2015**, *40*, 1050–1069. [CrossRef]
15. Justice, C.; Rice, J.; Warry, W.; Inglis, S.; Miller, S.; Sammon, S. Inquiry in higher education: Reflections and directions on course design and teaching methods. *Innov. High. Educ.* **2007**, *31*, 201–214. [CrossRef]
16. Konokman, G.Y.; Yelken, T.Y. Preparing Digital Stories through the Inquiry-Based Learning Approach: Its Effect on Prospective Teachers' Resistive Behaviors toward Research and Technology-Based Instruction. *Educ. Sci. Theory Pract.* **2016**, *16*, 2141–2165.
17. Azer, S.A.; Hasanato, R.; Al-Nassar, S.; Somily, A.; AlSaadi, M.M. Introducing integrated laboratory classes in a PBL curriculum: Impact on student's learning and satisfaction. *BMC Med. Educ.* **2013**, *13*, 71. [CrossRef] [PubMed]
18. Wold, S.; Esbensen, K.; Geladi, P. Principal component analysis. *Chemom. Intell. Lab. Syst.* **1987**, *2*, 37–52. [CrossRef]
19. Abdi, H.; Williams, L.J. Principal component analysis. *Wiley Interdiscip. Rev. Comput. Stat.* **2010**, *2*, 433–459. [CrossRef]
20. Richardson, M. Principal Component Analysis. 2009. Available online: http://aurora.troja.mff.cuni.cz/nemec/idl/09bonus/pca.pdf (accessed on 18 July 2022).
21. Scikit-Learn Developers, "Clustering", 2007–2022. Available online: https://scikit-learn.org/stable/modules/clustering.html# (accessed on 4 April 2022).
22. Ester, M.; Kriegel, H.P.; Sander, J.; Xu, X. A density-based algorithm for discovering clusters in large spatial databases with noise. In Proceedings of the 2nd International Conference on Knowledge Discovery and Data Mining, Portland, OR, USA, 2–4 August 1996; Volume 96, pp. 226–231.
23. Kryszkiewicz, M.; Skonieczny, L. *Faster Clustering with DBSCAN. Advances in Soft Computing*; Springer: Berlin/Heidelberg, Germany, 2005; Volume 31, pp. 605–614.

engineering proceedings

MDPI

Proceeding Paper

A Preliminary Study on the Satisfaction Survey of Online Cultural Self-Guide with 360-Degree Panoramic Photography †

Ya-Ling Cheng [1,*] and Lai-Chung Lee [2]

1 College of Design, National Taipei University of Technology, Taipei 10608, Taiwan
2 Department of Multimedia and Game Development, Minghsin University of Science and Technology, Hsinchu 30401, Taiwan; lclee@must.edu.tw
* Correspondence: zeroya.cheng@gmail.com

† Presented at the 2024 IEEE 4th International Conference on Electronic Communications, Internet of Things and Big Data, Taipei, Taiwan, 19–21 April 2024.

Abstract: During the COVID-19 epidemic, countries enacted autonomous measures to suspend long-distance travel. As a result, people used online platforms to share perspectives and disseminate their knowledge and skills. Internet learning content thus emerged as a primary solution. This study was conducted to assess the reactions of users to virtual tours. Participants were introduced to the 360-degree panoramic photography system of cultural monuments of the Taipei City Government and participated in an online cultural tour. A closed-ended questionnaire was distributed for their response. After compiling data from 31 participants, we analyzed the link between users' demographic characteristics and their satisfaction levels with the online panoramic tour system. We discovered higher satisfaction rates of people with incomes exceeding that of the average participant. 83% of participants stated a willingness to explore scenic attractions virtually instead of physically traveling when unable to do so. The results of this study contribute to understanding the context of users' post-visit satisfaction. The information gathered can be used to improve cultural heritage websites in terms of design, navigation, and cultural education, enabling virtual access to cultural sites and enriching users' knowledge from home.

Keywords: 360-degree panoramic; cultural heritage; online cultural tour; user satisfaction; virtual exploration

Citation: Cheng, Y.-L.; Lee, L.-C. A Preliminary Study on the Satisfaction Survey of Online Cultural Self-Guide with 360-Degree Panoramic Photography. *Eng. Proc.* **2024**, *74*, 75. https://doi.org/10.3390/engproc2024074075

Academic Editors: Shu-Han Liao, Teen-Hang Meen and Cheng-Fu Yang

Published: 24 October 2024

1. Introduction

The pandemic of COVID-19 brought the self-sufficiency of individuals in each locale. With the suspension of transport and travel, alternative ways for learning about distant cities, sharing life experiences, and disseminating knowledge have been changed. The Internet offers the most viable methods for such changes. Nonetheless, a textual narrative accompanied by static images presents a one-dimensional understanding. Interactive elements transform webpage consumption into an empowering and comprehensive experience. Recent advancements in the research and development of visual tools offer opportunities for such enhanced interaction.

In this context, we conducted a satisfaction survey about an existing municipal tourism website for the design of related digital platforms. We measured user experiences of a 360-degree photographic tour system of cultural sites, launched by the Taipei City Government. We investigated the correlation between user characteristics and their satisfaction with the online panoramic tour. The result of this study guides the enhancement of design frameworks, navigational methodologies, and the dissemination approach of knowledge-based websites dedicated to cultural heritage. Such improvements also provide means to virtually tour cultural sites, stimulate dynamic reading, and enrich their knowledge.

2. Methods

2.1. Cultural Travel

Before the pandemic, according to the World Travel & Tourism Council, tourism was one of the large and growing sectors of the global economy despite some shocks and crises, contributing around 10.3% to global GDP [1]. Traditional tourism is characterized by visiting places, engaging with residents, savoring regional cuisines, experiencing diverse climates and customs, and exploring the natural terrains of the architectural heritage. These facets are integral to the tourism experience. In 2019, the United Nations Educational, Scientific and Cultural Organization (UNESCO) documented a surge in tourism primarily directed towards sites of natural and cultural heritage [2]. Cultural tourism has become a new trend in international tourism [3]. It has gained unprecedented prominence in the 21st century, as global demographic expansion has been beyond the Earth's carrying capacity. This scenario, along with fortified economic activities and a soaring education rate, has increased affluence and knowledge, accompanied by highly accessible transportation networks. This milieu fosters the desire of individuals to empirically validate their educational learnings through travel, which is a highly attractive proposition. However, with the increase in tourist arrivals, environmental issues such as the preservation and maintenance of related cultural industries and greenhouse gas emissions have arisen [4]. Consequently, the phenomenon of over-tourism has emerged and is proliferating at an alarming pace worldwide (Table 1).

Table 1. Types of Cultural Tourists. (McKercher and Du Cros, 2002) [5].

Travel	Type
Complete Cultural Tourism	Those who seek a deeper cultural experience use cultural tourism as their main motivation for visiting.
Cultural Tourism	Although the purpose and primary motivation of the visit is cultural tourism, they do not seek a deeper experience.
Cultural Discoverer	These tourists do not necessarily travel for cultural reasons but end up making profound cultural discoveries.
Cultural Leisure	Some cultural activities are sought in their travels, though not necessarily the main demand.
Cultural Accidents	The primary motivation for these tourists to travel was not cultural, but rather incidental and non-profound participation in cultural activities.

The strong growth of the tourism sector in recent years has led to the sustainability of this industry being widely addressed in the literature [6]. In the 1970s, experts identified over-tourism and three issues stemming from the excessive growth of tourism: (1) an overabundance of tourists, (2) significant disturbances such as noise pollution, and (3) extensive physical impacts, including the transformation of communities for tourist purposes and the degradation of natural environments [7]. This hyper-development of tourism endangers the lifestyles of residents in tourist destinations and disrupts environmental sustainability. For instance, strolling through the streets of Paris, one encounters fewer locals and more tourists dressed in casual attire. In the congested waterways of Venice, the chatter is not in Italian but in English and Chinese. Groundwater near Angkor Wat is lacking, signaling a crisis. Recent issues of over-tourism cause environmental destruction and pollution. The COVID-19 pandemic was a significant disaster and prompted countries to restrict transportation and movement, inadvertently allowing the Earth a chance to recuperate.

2.2. Online Tour

For over-tourism, governments have contemplated alternatives, including online self-guided cultural tours to simulate travel experiences (Table 1). Before the pandemic, television programs and Internet video content enabled virtual travel. During the pandemic, tourism was immediately impacted. In Japan, local travel guides started online tourism programs in various languages. Offering real-time interaction, these virtual tours allowed 'tourists' to experience locations and even receive souvenirs. On the inaugural day, the guide presented each attraction in a live broadcast, engaging 'tourists'. This approach gained immense popularity, with audiences from Europe and the United States participating irrespective of time zone differences [8]. It can be seen that if the restrictions of locomotion limited in-person interactions and traveling, consumers' behavior toward online and digital solutions increased even more amid the crisis [1]. For those who prefer to travel independently, technologies such as online 360-degree photography and interactive exhibits are particularly well-suited for self-guided tours, enabling 'tourists' to explore at their discretion.

2.3. 360-Degree Panoramic Photography

The concept of the panoramic view was proposed by Hendrik Willem Mesdag and his colleagues in 'Panorama Mesdag': a panoramic painting displayed on a circular wall with a diameter of approximately 40 m. The painting stretched 120 m in length and 14 m in height (Figure 1).

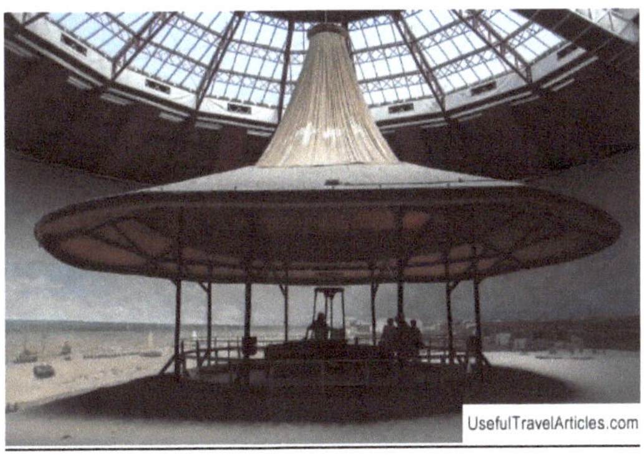

Figure 1. "Panorama Mesdag" panoramic painting created by Dutch painter Hendrik Willem Mesdag and others. "https://usefultravelarticles.com (accessed on 28 June 2021)".

With advancements in digital photography software and hardware, Apple introduced the QuickTime VR (QTVR) format in 1994 (Figure 2); it allows the creation and viewing of VR photography, photographically captured panoramas, and the viewing of objects photographed from multiple angles [9]. This innovation allows for the commercialization and widespread use of panoramic technology, which develops 360-degree panoramic views to encompass spherical panoramas. Panoramic photography is used widely on platforms such as Google Maps, offering photographic collages. Aerial cameras have enabled travel photography enthusiasts to capture 360-degree videos, integrating timeline elements to enhance the viewing experience. Currently, 360-degree photography is also applied in virtual reality (VR) and augmented reality (AR), broadening the scope and application of this technology (Figures 3–5).

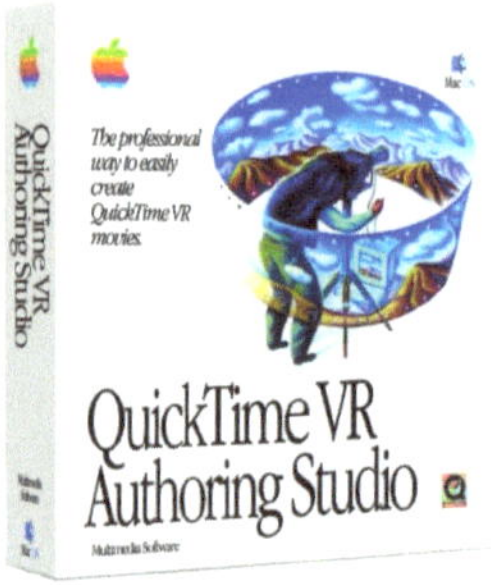

Figure 2. QTVR "www.amazon.de (accessed on 29 June 2021)".

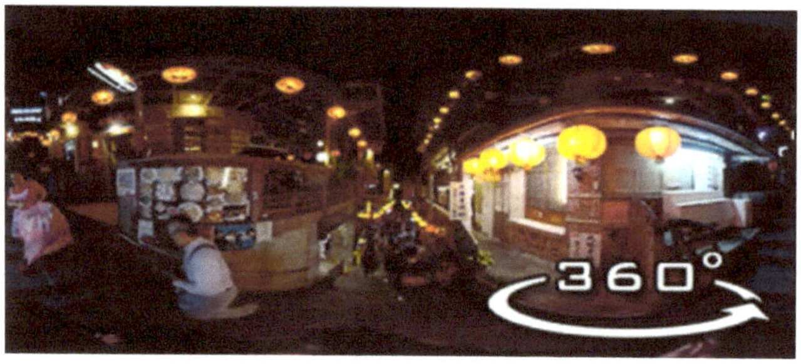

Figure 3. Advanced to spherical panoramic photography. "www.markwen.com (accessed on 24 June 2021)".

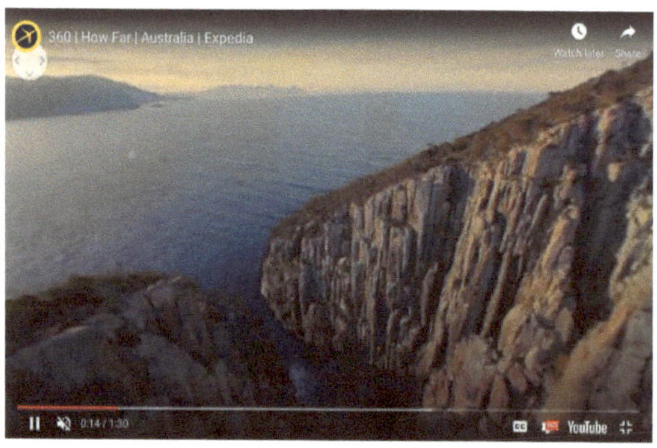

Figure 4. Online panoramic photography video. "www.phocuswire.com (accessed on 30 June 2021)".

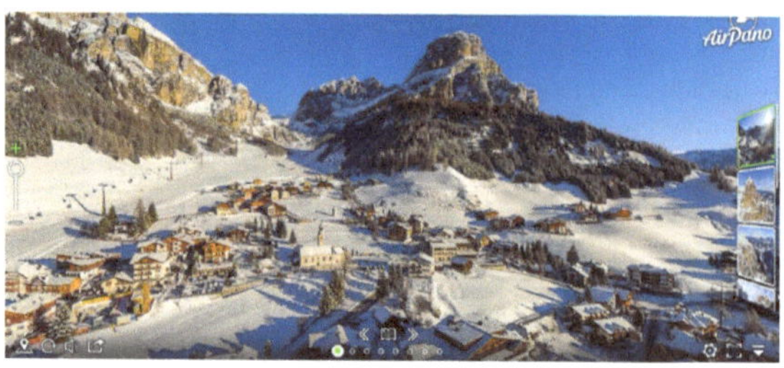

Figure 5. Multi-viewpoint stitching video. "www.airpano.com (accessed on 30 June 2021)".

3. Materials and Methods

3.1. Taipei Lin An Tai Ancient House

This historic mansion was constructed during the Qing Dynasty by Lin Zhineng, a native of Anxi, Fujian, China. Lin Zhineng amassed wealth through his business in Menga and subsequently constructed a mansion in the Da'an District of Taipei City. The construction was initiated during the Qianlong period and completed in 1785 AD. The side rooms flanking the mansion were finalized in 1823 and named 'An Tai Cuo' (安泰厝) (Figure 6). This mansion stands as one of the oldest extant residential dwellings in Taipei City. The original design of the Lin Antai historic house adopted Feng Shui, oriented northeast and southwest, embodying the concept of 'the snake surrounds the Beidou Cave in the south, with the snake head facing the seven stars' (Figure 7). It represents a unique and finely crafted ancient residence featuring two halls and five rooms. This cultural relic is at risk of demolition due to urban development projects. Fortunately, preservationists proposed a relocation plan, which led to the transposition of the entire structure to its current site for conservation. In recognition of the significance of the Lin An-Tai Ancient House's heritage in Taipei City, a 360-degree panoramic navigation system was constructed [10]. This virtual tour allows visitors to experience the site remotely and provides an avenue for users to feedback regarding their virtual visit and satisfaction.

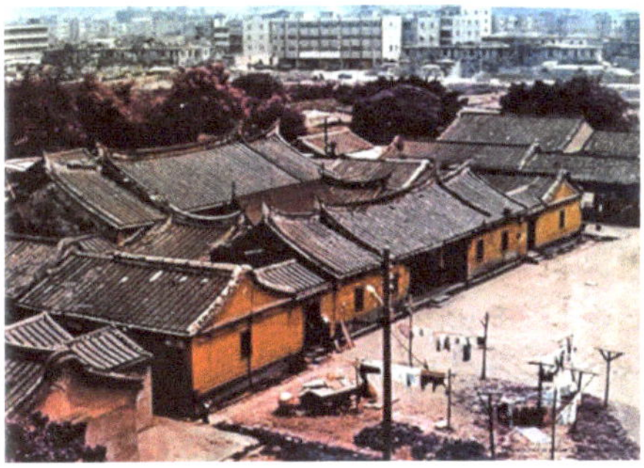

Figure 6. Photos of Lin Antai's ancient residence before reconstruction (source: Taipei Civil Affairs Bureau website).

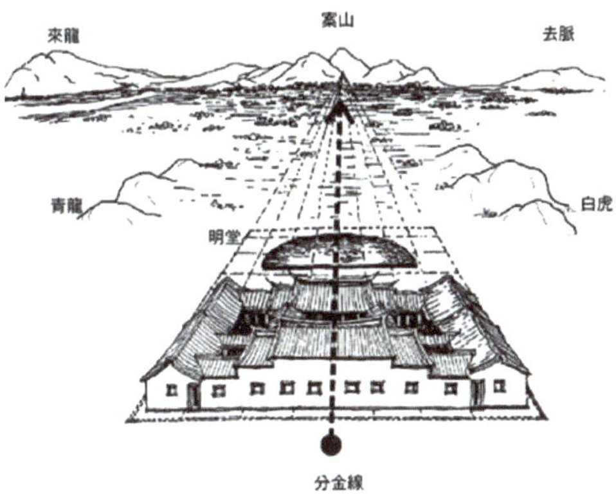

Figure 7. The Feng Shui Pattern of Antai Ancient House (source: Taipei Civil Affairs Bureau website). In the picture above: "案山" (An Shan) refers to the mountain or landform directly in front of a site in feng shui. 來龍 (Lai Long) refers to the flow of energy (or "chi") that comes from the distant mountains or terrain and converges onto the site in question. 去脈 (Qu Mai) refers to the flow or pathway that energy (chi) follows as it leaves a location. It represents the continuation or dissipation

of energy after it passes through the site. The "青龍" means the left side of a site or property when facing outward from the front of the location. The "白虎" represents the right side of a site or property when facing outward. This side is often kept lower than the "青龍" to maintain balance and avoid overbearing energy. The White Tiger is associated with yin energy and can represent protection and potential danger if unbalanced. "分金線" is a specific line used in feng shui to denote the precise alignment or division of space according to directions or energies. It plays a key role in determining the exact positioning of structures, entrances, or features on a property to ensure optimal energy flow and balance.

3.2. Research Methods

Using panoramic photography or video tours, visitors can explore natural attractions or cultural and historical monuments without the constraints of time or space. These tools do not require any wearable technology, allowing individuals to easily pursue their interests. Paired with explanatory narratives or audio commentaries of the scenic locations, visitors can understand the landscape's features or its historical background. We distributed a questionnaire to participants who used a 360-degree panoramic photography online navigation system. This system was devised by the Taipei Civil Affairs Bureau to provide public access to browse classic cultural assets. The participants received instructions before navigating the "Taipei Lin An Tai Ancient House 360-degree Surround View Photography Guide System" at least for five minutes. We assessed user preferences for four designated stopping points from the entrance to the interior of the site. These points included the sacred table in the hall, the gateway to the main hall, the front yard outside the entrance, and the west wing. Each point featured multiple points of interest (POIs) to prompt user exploration. The navigation system's appeal was assessed to users based on the breadth and depth of engagement from the ingress point. The 3D panoramic tour contents of the Lin Antai Ancient House were derived from the Taipei Civil Affairs Bureau website (Figures 8–12).

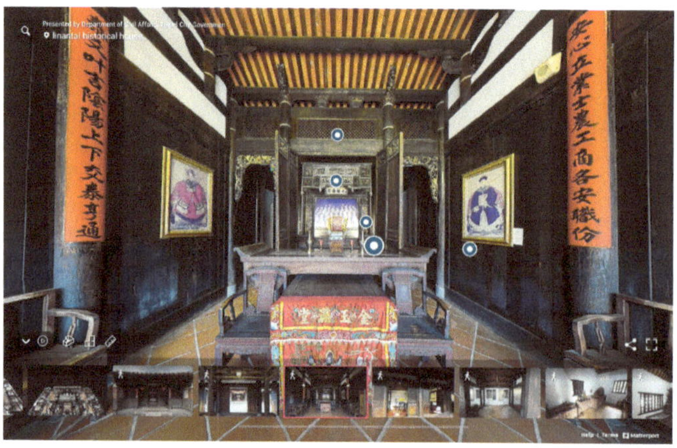

Figure 8. Interest point 01 god table (POI 01). Above the hall, a horizontal inscribed board is hanged, carved with "Outstanding descendants inherit the honors of forefathers". Besides, the characters of "An" and "Tai" are smartly used as beginnings in the couplet.

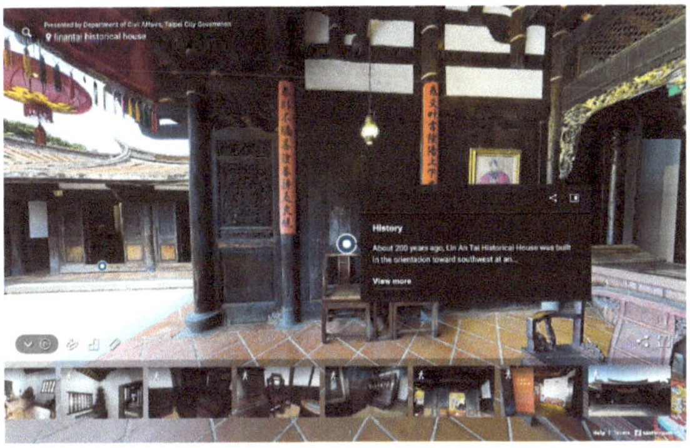

Figure 9. Openwork window at the point of interest 02 (POI 02). About 200 years ago, Lin An Tai Historical House was built in the orientation toward the southwest at an auspicious location in terms of good Feng Shui. It was a very refined 2-partitioned and 5-annex old house with a square.

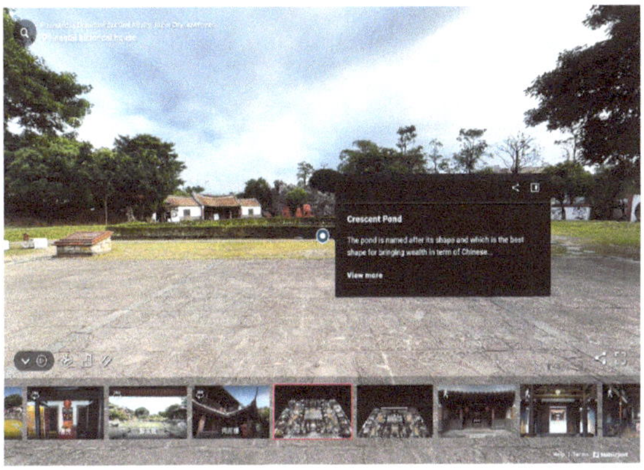

Figure 10. Point of Interest 03 Half Moon Pool (POI 03). The pool is named after its shape and which is the best shape for bringing wealth in term of Chinese Feng Shui study.

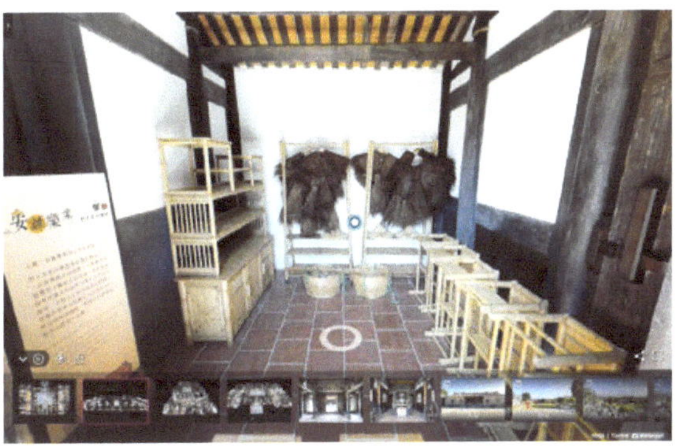

Figure 11. Point of Interest 04 (POI 04). In a side room, there are two coir raincoats and some bamboo furniture.

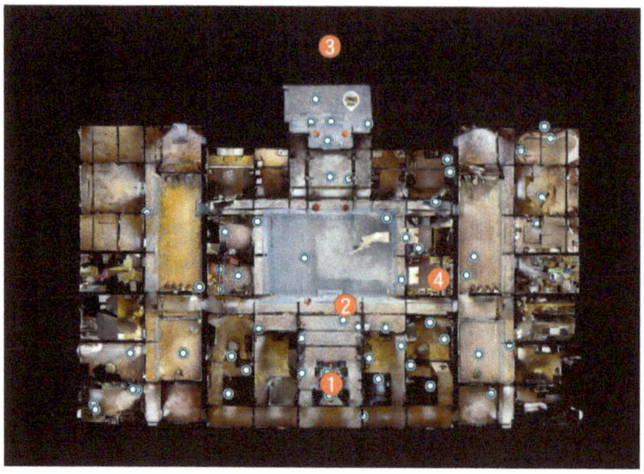

Figure 12. The entire map of the navigation system and the locations of 4 stopping points. Each stopping point has more than two points of interest. (The blue circles are viewing points of interest provided to viewers in the program).

Visitors provided the basic information and responded to the questionnaire after utilizing the navigation program. The questionnaires were collected online. To assess user satisfaction with the website's navigation system, a five-point Likert scale was employed, where 1 point indicated "very dissatisfied" and 5 points indicated "very satisfied". The content of the questionnaire is displayed in Table 2.

Table 2. Questionnaire questions "https://forms.gle/Q4fW87dvNL55ZVTQA (accessed on 20 August 2021)".

Questions	Answer Type
Is this your first time using online 360-degree panoramic photography to visit scenic spots?	YES/NO
Which objects did you discover during your tour? Divine Table/Half Moon Pond/ Coir raincoat/Openwork Window	Please check the items.
In addition to the objects and landscapes mentioned above, what else did you discover?	Short answer
While using 360-degree panoramic viewing online, do you want to see more everywhere?	YES/NO
I don't think this website system needs to be so complicated.	Likert Scale 1–5
I think this kind of tour is such as fresh and fascinating.	Likert Scale 1–5
I think this site is easy to use.	Likert Scale 1–5
I think the features of this tour site are well integrated.	Likert Scale 1–5
I feel like this site has a lot of inconsistencies.	Likert Scale 1–5
I feel I need help from someone experienced before I can use this website.	Likert Scale 1–5
I think most people can learn to use this site quickly.	Likert Scale 1–5
I feel confident using this system.	Likert Scale 1–5
There's a lot I need to learn to use this site.	Likert Scale 1–5
How would you rate your satisfaction after use?	Likert Scale 1–5
When you cannot travel, would you like to browse attractions in this way instead of traveling?	willing/unwilling
If you have any ideas after the online tour, please provide them. Thank you very much.	Short answer

3.3. Results

A total of 31 volunteers participated in the study, comprising 12 males and 19 females. One response was invalid. Two were high school students, and five held master's degrees or higher. The rest were college students or university graduates; four participants earned an annual salary exceeding TWD 1 million, 11 earned TWD 500,000 to TWD 990,000, and the rest earned less than TWD 500,000.

14 participants were using online 360-degree panoramic photography to visit scenic spots for the first time. The following were the key findings from the analysis:

(1) Of the 30 valid questionnaires, 63% of respondents were female and 37% were male. 80% had obtained at least a college degree, and 90% expressed interest in the system.
(2) A total of 47% of respondents were first-time users of the online 360-degree panoramic photography tour system.
(3) The satisfaction rates were 83% for females and 95% for males.
(4) Younger individuals with a college education showed higher satisfaction compared to those with a high school education or less.
(5) A total of 10% of respondents preferred not to explore attractions in this manner and reported lower satisfaction levels.
(6) The three least satisfied participants mentioned the red lantern in the scene, which others did not highlight.
(7) The participants with higher incomes indicated high satisfaction rates.
(8) A total of 80% were willing to use this method to browse scenic spots as an alternative to traveling when unable to do so.

4. Discussion

The results of this study indicated that male was satisfied more than females. This difference might stem from higher male engagement with websites and games. A total of 45% were first-time users, and the novelty of the experience generated interest for female participants and those with higher educational attainment. Participants with high incomes were more satisfied with new cultural experiences of "complete cultural tourism". Participants exhibiting lower satisfaction typically showed less interest in the activity's theme and demonstrated an unwillingness to spend extended periods within the navigation system. Interestingly, the participants who expressed lower satisfaction noticed the conspicuous red lantern within the scene. This "visual attention" needs to be considered in the future design of the system to enhance user engagement.

5. Conclusions

In the 1990s, 360-degree photography was popular among researchers and hobbyists. Presently, institutions including Google are developing street-level information in diverse regions. Leveraging its considerable resources, Google captures 360-degree panoramic photographs to construct vivid street views. Recently, dynamic navigation systems have been introduced for street view services, and panoramic tours of prominent museums have become cultural and art initiatives. The panoramic photography enables virtual experiences of different environments, ranging from wilderness areas to coastlines, through users' screens or AR and VR platforms. During the pandemic, personal mobility was restricted, which brought applications and websites of panoramic images for the public to virtually visit and enjoy natural landscapes and artistic displays and explore digital media. To enrich the virtual experience beyond mere stimulation or the impression, it is necessary to incorporate explanatory knowledge text and audio guides. By replicating natural sounds or providing expert commentary, the experience can be more engaging and holistic. This approach attracts prospective tourists and makes the design of navigation systems robust for immersive experiences, cultural asset comprehension, and education. The findings of this study can be used for the development of future online travel. Real-time voice navigation via AR and VR has the potential to craft exceptional experiences for users with the 360-degree navigation system. Such experiences help users understand cultural heritages. Future research is demanded to assess whether virtual tours inspire users to visit the actual sites for cultural engagement and economic growth. As the tourism industry is reviving after the pandemic, it is necessary to provide visitors with cultural explorations, educational content, and information on local cultural heritage.

Author Contributions: Conceptualization, Y.-L.C.; methodology, Y.-L.C. and L.-C.L.; data curation, Y.-L.C.; formal analysis, Y.-L.C., investigation, Y.-L.C.; writing—original draft, Y.-L.C.; writing—review and editing, L.-C.L. All authors have read and agreed to the published version of the manuscript.

Funding: This research received no external funding.

Institutional Review Board Statement: This study received no other committee approval.

Informed Consent Statement: Not applicable.

Data Availability Statement: The original data supporting the conclusions of this article were provided by the authors based on the questionnaire.

Conflicts of Interest: The authors declare that they have no conflicts of interest.

References

1. de Pinho, V.M.; Monteiro, J.; Binhote, J. Wanderlust without Wandering: Managing a Travel Blog during the COVID-19. *J. Contemp. Adm.* **2021**, *25*, e200243. [CrossRef]
2. UNESCO. International Conference "Innovative Policies for Heritage Safeguarding and Cultural Tourism Development". 2005. Available online: https://whc.unesco.org/en/events/258/ (accessed on 15 November 2019).
3. Chu, Y.-C.; Tung, C.-L. A forward-looking Prospective Analysis of the Cultural Tourism Development in Macao. *J. Dev. Prospect.* **2020**, *29*, 97–108.
4. Lu, S.-C. To integrate Miaoli's cultural landscape resources into environmental education and evaluating visitor satisfaction and environment awareness. *J. Environ. Art* **2019**, *20*, 59–74.
5. McKercher, B.; Du Cros, H. *Cultural Tourism: The Partnership between Tourism and Cultural Heritage Management*; Routledge: Abingdon, UK, 2002.
6. Huete-Alcocer, N.; López-Ruiz, V.R.; Grigorescu, A. Measurement of Satisfaction in Sustainable Tourism: A Cultural Heritage Site in Spain. *Sustainability* **2019**, *11*, 6774. [CrossRef]
7. Rosenow, J.E.; Pulsipher, G.L. *Tourism: The Good, the Bad, and the Ugly*; Century Three Press: Lincoln, NE, USA, 1979; ISBN 0939644088.
8. Global News. Available online: https://www.youtube.com/watch?v=z_bWYruZ0lI (accessed on 15 January 2021).
9. QuickTime VR. In Wikipedia, The Free Encyclopedia. Available online: https://zh.wikipedia.org/w/index.php?title=QuickTime_VR&oldid=76767325 (accessed on 15 January 2019).
10. Lin An Tai Historical House & Museum Website. Available online: https://mpembed.com/show/?m=umdSnRjzeML&mpu=718 (accessed on 15 November 2021).

engineering proceedings

Proceeding Paper

Magnetic Properties of Melanin Doped with Copper Oxide Nanoparticles †

Nawal Madkhali

Department of Physics, Imam Muhammed ibn Saud Islamic University (IMSIU), P.O. Box 90905, Riyadh 11623, Saudi Arabia; namadkhali@imamu.edu.sa

† Presented at the 2024 IEEE 4th International Conference on Electronic Communications, Internet of Things and Big Data, Taipei, Taiwan, 19–21 April 2024.

Abstract: In this study, the analysis of XRD patterns reveals that both natural melanin and copper oxide-doped melanin exhibit amorphous structures. The absence of new peaks for Cu_2O confirms that the copper oxide nanoparticles are effectively integrated into the melanin matrix. Utilizing Scherrer's equation, we calculated the crystallite size, which increased from 2.02 nm for natural melanin to 3.01 nm after doping, suggesting a significant influence of copper ions on melanin structure. Additionally, the VSM measurements demonstrate a shift from ferromagnetic behavior in the natural melanin to paramagnetism in the doped samples, highlighting the impact of copper oxide on the magnetic properties of melanin. These findings provide valuable insights into the biological and functional transformations of natural melanin, furthering our understanding of its role in various medical applications.

Keywords: natural melanin; nanocomposites; paramagnetism; copper oxide-doped melanin

Citation: Madkhali, N. Magnetic Properties of Melanin Doped with Copper Oxide Nanoparticles. *Eng. Proc.* **2024**, *74*, 76. https://doi.org/10.3390/engproc2024074076

Academic Editors: Shu-Han Liao, Teen-Hang Meen and Cheng-Fu Yang

Published: 8 November 2024

1. Introduction

Natural eumelanin is a hybrid bio-polymer found in various living organisms. It protects humans' skin. Melanin can be categorized into different types based on its molecular precursors. Eumelanin, or black melanin, consists primarily of oligomers originating from 5,6 di-hydroxy-indole and 5,6 dihydroxy-indole-2-carboxylic acid. It demonstrates remarkable antioxidant capabilities in lipid peroxidation inhibition and in standard chemical assays. In contrast, pheomelanin, known for its orange-red color, is formed from benzothiazine ring units [1–3]. Neuro-melanin, a dark type, is believed to be a combination of dihydroxy-indole and benzothiazine.

One of the primary biological functions of melanin is its capacity to chelate metals, which helps reduce oxidative stress in the human body. By binding to reactive metal ions, melanin exhibits high antioxidant activity [4,5]. The amine, carboxyl, and hydroxyl groups within melanin are crucial for its metal-binding properties. It is essentially a reservoir for metal ions that permits their exchange, re-release, and storage. Moreover, it effectively sequesters reactive metals, thereby mitigating their potential to induce oxidative stress.

Melanin demonstrates a high binding capacity for ions such as Ca and Zn ions [6]. Sepia melanin can release heavier metals, functioning as a sink [7,8]. The Fenton and Haber–Weiss reactions are two processes that catalyze transition metals to produce reactive oxygen species (ROS). Our previous research has shown that natural melanin can bind to transition metals such as zinc, iron, and copper, with their binding capacities determined [8,9]. These metals can interchangeably bind to the carboxyl groups in melanin. Notably, the binding capacity for certain transition metals (TMs) is often used as an indicator of the ratio amount of dihydroxy- carboxylic acid molecules in natural melanin. As individuals age [10], a decrease in binding capacity suggests a reduction in carboxyl groups or DHICA content, leading to diminished antioxidant efficiency.

2. Materials and Methods

Copper oxide nanoparticles were synthesized using the chemical co-precipitation technique. In a typical procedure, 5 g of $CuCl{\cdot}2H_2O$ and 10 g of $Cu_2Cl_3{\cdot}6H_2O$ were combined in distilled water under a nitrogen gas vacuum. The mixture was subjected to vigorous stirring and heated to 100 °C. Subsequently, 10 mL of NaOH was gradually introduced. The mixture was continuously stirred for 1 h. Afterward, the nanoparticles were repeatedly rinsed with distilled water and dried under vacuum for 24 h. Herbal eumelanin in this work was extracted from black seed (*Nigella sativa*). A total of 10 gm of seeds was solubilized in a solution of NaOH (pH 10) for 1 h then this was stirred with copper oxide for 3 h. The resulting nanoparticles were then washed twice with distilled water and dried in an oven for 48 h. For the XRD results for the nanoparticles, a Bruker D8 Discover diffractometer (Bruker, Karlsruhe, Germany) with Cu-Kα radiation of wavelength 1.54 Å was used. Magnetic measurements were performed by using a vibrating sample magnetometer (VSM, 7404 model-1.8T magnets, Lake Shore Cryotronics, Westerville, OH, USA).

3. Results and Conclusions

Figure 1 presents the XRD curves of both the melanin and copper oxide-doped (Cu_2O) melanin samples. The XRD pattern shows both samples have a broad peak, indicating an amorphous structure. The peak at ($2\theta = 22°$) indicates the formation of melanin. Furthermore, no new peaks for Cu_2O appear in the XRD result, confirming that the Cu_2O nanoparticles bonded well to the melanin molecules. The Scherrer equation is used to calculate the crystallite size ($D = \frac{k\lambda}{\beta cos\theta}$), where D is the crystallite size of the nanoparticles, (k = 0.9) is the constant for the spherical particles, λ is the wavelength of the XRD (~0.154 nm), and β is the FWHM of the Bragg angle. The average crystallite size of the melanin nanoparticles before doping with copper oxide is 2.02 nm and the average size increased significantly to 3.01 nm. The significant increase in the crystallite size of the melanin doped with copper oxide is related to the size of copper ions [8].

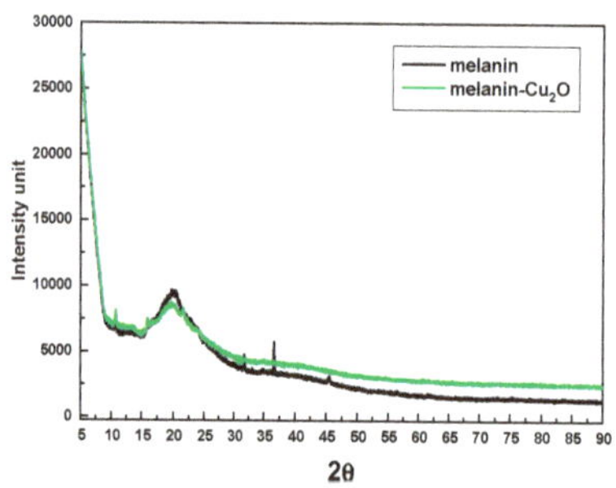

Figure 1. XRD pattern of natural melanin and natural melanin doped with Cu_2O.

Figure 2 shows a hysteresis loop at 300K°. The measured magnetization (M) per gram of all the samples was measured as a function of the magnetic field (H). The results show the ferromagnetic behavior of natural melanin becomes paramagnetic after doping with copper oxide. This change in magnetic behavior allows us to gain insight into certain biological and vital transformations of melanin.

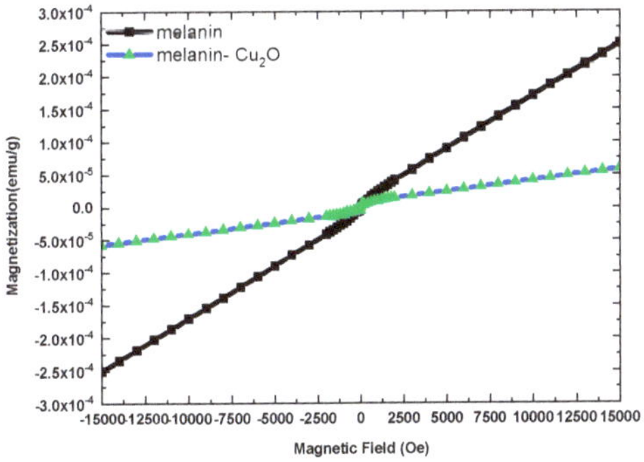

Figure 2. Magnetization hysteresis loops of natural melanin and natural melanin after it was doped with Cu_2O versus applied magnetic field at room temperature.

Funding: This research received no external funding.

Institutional Review Board Statement: Not applicable.

Informed Consent Statement: Not applicable.

Data Availability Statement: The data presented in this work are available on request from the corresponding author. Data are not publicly available due to privacy.

Conflicts of Interest: The author declares no conflicts of interest.

References

1. Ambrico, M.; Ambrico, P.F.; Ligonzo, T.; Cardone, A.; Cicco, S.R.; D'Ischia, M.; Farinola, G.M. From commercial tyrosine polymers to a tailored polydopamine platform concepts, issues and challenges en route to melanin-based bioelectronics. *J. Mater. Chem. C* **2015**, *3*, 6413–6423. [CrossRef]
2. Riley, P.A. Melanin. *Int. Biochem. Cell Biol.* **1997**, *29*, 1235–1239. [CrossRef] [PubMed]
3. Tran, M.L.; Powell, B.J.; Meredith, P. Chemical & structural disorder in eumelanins: A possible explanation for broadband absorbance. *Biophys. J.* **2006**, *90*, 743–752. [PubMed]
4. Bridelli, M.G.; Crippa, P.R. Theoretical analysis of the adsorption of metal ions to the surface of melanin particles. *Adsorption* **2008**, *14*, 101–109. [CrossRef]
5. Liu, Y.; Simon, J.D. Metal-ion interactions and the structural organization of Sepia eumelanin. *Pigment. Cell Res.* **2005**, *18*, 42–48. [CrossRef] [PubMed]
6. Okazaki, M.; Kuwata, K.; Miki, Y.; Shiga, S.; Shiga, T. Electron relaxation of synthetic melanin and melanin conaining human tissues as studied by electron spin echo and electron spin resonance. *Arch. Biochem. Biophys.* **1985**, *242*, 197–205. [CrossRef] [PubMed]
7. Liu, Y.; Hong, L.; Kempf, V.R.; Wakamatsu, K.; Ito, S.; Simon, J.D. Ion exchange & adsorption of Fe (III) by Sepia melanin. *Pigment. Cell Res.* **2004**, *17*, 262–269. [PubMed]
8. Madkhali, N.; Algessair, S. Exploring the optical properties of metal-modified melanin following ultra-violet irradiation: An experimental and theoretical study using density functional theory. *Heliyon* **2024**, *10*, e10088. [CrossRef]
9. Madkhali, N.; Alqahtani, H.R.; Al-Terary, S.; Laref, A.; Haseeb, A. The doping effect of Fe, Cu and Zn ions on the structural and electrochemical properties and the thermostability of natural melanin extracted from *Nigella sativa* L. *J. Mol. Liq.* **2019**, *285*, 436–443. [CrossRef]
10. Liu, H.; Yang, Y.; Liu, Y.; Pan, J.; Wang, J.; Man, F.; Zhang, W.; Liu, G. Melanin like nanomaterials for advanced biomedical applications: A versatile platform with extraordinary promise. *Adv. Sci* **2020**, *7*, 1903129. [CrossRef] [PubMed]

engineering proceedings

MDPI

Proceeding Paper

Effect of Exercise on Children with Autism Based on a Meta-Analysis †

Li-Xin Lin [1] and Kuei-Shu Hsu [2,*]

[1] School of Physical Education, Putian University, Putian 351100, China; ptxyllx@163.com
[2] Department of Recreation and Health Care Management, Chia Nan University of Pharmacy & Science, Tainan City 717, Taiwan
* Correspondence: kshsu888@mail.cnu.edu.tw; Tel.: +886-6-2904921

† Presented at the 2024 IEEE 4th International Conference on Electronic Communications, Internet of Things and Big Data, Taipei, Taiwan, 19–21 April 2024.

Abstract: How exercise influences the treatment of autistic children is explored in this paper to provide a reference for their treatment. The relevant data were collected from the results of research on campaigns and autism published in 2006–2018 using computer search methods. The data include 282 research objects in five groups. The Jadad scale scores were 0–2. The result of the meta-analysis conducted using Stata12.0 showed a significant improvement in the symptoms of autistic children. For moderate autism, the effect of exercise was consistent with high credibility, while for severe autism, the effect was not consistent with low credibility. It was found that the symptoms of moderately autistic children showed improvement with exercise, but not in severely autistic children, although the effect of exercise on severe autism is prospective. Thus, more research is required on the effect of exercise on severe autism.

Keywords: autistic children; controlled trial; meta-analysis

Citation: Lin, L.-X.; Hsu, K.-S. Effect of Exercise on Children with Autism Based on a Meta-Analysis. *Eng. Proc.* **2024**, *74*, 77. https://doi.org/10.3390/engproc2024074077

Academic Editors: Shu-Han Liao, Teen-Hang Meen and Cheng-Fu Yang

Published: 11 November 2024

1. Introduction

Autistic children are defined as having autism spectrum disorder (ASD), which causes difficult communication, language problems, limited interests, and repetitive behaviors. It is a serious mental and intellectual disability of children found all over the world [1]. The prevalence of childhood autism has been increasing for several decades. There has been much research on the development of diagnostic measures [2]. Untreated autism prognosis may lead to lifelong disability, and several patients exhibit disorders in behavior and even juvenile delinquency. Autism pressures the parents of patients in terms of expenses and feelings, and puts a heavy burden on schools [3].

Autism in children has been researched extensively from medical and psychological perspectives as well as from educational perspectives. Communication disorders, limited interests, and hobbies of autistic children especially affect the patient's lives. However, research has revealed that physical exercise improves the mood and personality of autistic children and relieves depression from stress and anxiety significantly [4]. Recent research by Taiwanese scholars has proved that exercise effectively mitigates childhood autism. These studies provide an important basis for verifying that physical exercise is effective in treating autistic children.

However, such research conclusions need further confirmation, as the scales adopted in the research on childhood autism are different. In addition, the research subjects are from different regions, and the intervention measures and methods are different. The degree of autistic symptoms of the children examined is also different. Considering such limitations, in this paper, research on the influence of exercise on autistic children with different symptoms is conducted using meta-analysis as a statistical analysis tool. The effect of exercise is quantitatively evaluated and explained to provide a reference for further exploration of how to improve the symptoms of childhood autism.

2. Data and Method

2.1. Data Retrieval

Data for this research was retrieved from the Database of Chinese Academic Journal (CNKI), Wanfang, and VIP. Relevant journals, theses, conference papers, non-randomized controlled trials, case studies, reports, reviews, data information, and periodic publications published from 2006 to 2018 were included in the retrieval list. The references in the documents were also used for data retrieval. Keywords such as exercise, physical exercise, autistic disorder, and autism were used for collecting data. The criteria for retrieval included control attributes, research objects (only children), and prescribed physical exercise. The "Childhood Autism Rating Scale" or "Autism Behavior Checklist" was adopted as the scale for measuring the level of childhood autism. The CARS scale was used with the criteria of 0–30 for non-autism, 30–36 for mild to moderate autism, and higher than 36 for severe autism. The ABC scale adopted in this research had the criteria of $\geq$31 for suspected autism and $\geq$62 for diagnosed autism.

2.2. Method

Two researchers independently read the documents to extract data that included authors, time of publication, implementation method of physical exercise, the difference in experimental and control groups, and the difference in the average scores and standard deviations of the scales before and after physical exercise. Differences in retrieving data were discussed or consulted with experts. To evaluate the quality of the retrieved data, the Jadad scale was used [5]. The scoring criteria included randomization and concealment, blind method, withdrawal, and missing visits. On a scale of 0–5, 0–2 points were classified as low quality, while 3–5 points were classified as high quality.

3. Results and Discussion

3.1. Retrieval Result

In total, 116 relevant documents were chosen from the database search. Among them, 63 were eliminated as they were duplicated, and 19 were not included as they were irrelevant. Out of the remaining 34 documents, 5 were finally selected following the selection criteria (Table 1). The final data contained 282 autistic children, among whom 164 were males, 78 were females, and 40 were unidentified. In Ref. [6], three experimental groups were defined with different interpersonal interactions. The experimental period in Refs. [6,7] was 4–8 weeks. The experimental period for one document was 3 months. The experimental period in two documents was 6 months. Reference [8] included mild autistic symptoms, Refs. [9,10] researched moderate autistic symptoms, and the remaining two documents explored severe symptoms of autism. All of the five articles had similar autism levels before the interventions with the same population.

Table 1. Data of selected documents in this study.

Date	Sample Size		Sample Size	Autistic Level before Intervention		Autistic Level after Intervention		Test Scale	Level
	Test	Control	Gender (Male/Female)	Test	Control	Test	Control		
2017	18	14	28/4	49.66 ± 28.506	47.71 ± 25.43	42.556 ± 26.27	57.214 ± 23.671	ABC	**Moderate**
2016	40	40	50/30	36.54 ± 6.58	35.98 ± 5.54	31.37 ± 4.24	34.84 ± 3.94	CARS	**Mild**
2017	30	30	35/25	37.96 ± 7.03	37.27 ± 10. 69	30.25 ± 7. 92	35. 91 ± 6. 23	CARS	**severe**
2018	35	35	51/19	39.33 ± 7.29	39.40 ± 7.34	29.71 ± 5.23	34.80 ± 6.19	CARS	**severe**
2018	30	10	—	60.34 ± 1.25	60.56 ± 1.12	54.98 ± 1.63	59.95 ± 1.33	ABC	**Moderate**

The five documents were published in Chinese and had a definitive scale of autistic symptoms, with comparability between the experimental and the control groups according to the baseline data. No study mentioned the implementation of a blinded experiment. Reference [7] only mentioned withdrawal and missing visits without a specific description. On the Jadad scale, the documents with 0–2 points were classified as low-quality documents with bias.

3.2. Meta-Analysis Results

We carried out a meta-analysis to investigate the influence of physical exercise on autistic children with moderate symptoms. They belonged to the experimental groups in three documents. The result of the heterogeneity test was statistically significant, indicating that there was obvious heterogeneity among the three groups. Therefore, the standardized mean difference (SMD) was calculated to understand the combined random effect. The combined effect size of SMD for autistic children with moderate symptoms showed a significant difference between the groups with and without physical exercise. The confidence level of SMD of 95% implied that the score of autistic children with physical exercise was significantly lower than those without physical exercise. This showed a significant improvement in symptoms. For autistic children with severe symptoms, physical exercise had a certain effect, but was not statistically proven. Although the scores were different between the groups with and without physical exercise, the difference was not high enough to be accepted as significant.

3.3. Meta-Regression Analysis

The test showed obvious heterogeneity among the group of autistic children with moderate symptoms with and without physical exercise. The results of the single-factor meta-regression analysis are presented in Table 2. The standard probability of heterogeneity increased from 0.05 to 0.1, which was high enough to select for the influencing factors. The probability of the heterogeneity for sample size, autism scale, intervention time, and intervention intensity was greater than 0.1. Such a result indicates that the four factors do not influence the heterogeneity of the selected documents. However, the document quality showed $p = 0.034 < 0.01$, and it was the only factor that affected the heterogeneity. The τ^2 of document quality also showed its influence on heterogeneity. The regression coefficients of the factors showed that document quality also had an obvious effect on heterogeneity, which was related to the effect of physical exercise on the moderate symptoms of autistic children.

Table 2. Results of heterogeneous single-factor meta regression analysis for the literature included in the research.

Heterogeneity Factor	Non-Covariate tau^2	Covariate tau^2	Constant	Coefficient	SE	t	p
Document quality	0.7604	0.259	−0.689	−0.673	0.298	−2.29	0.034
Sample size		0.89	−1.297	−0.0001	0.005	−0.03	0.76
Autism scale		0.8361	−2.19	0.547	0.417	1.31	0.188
Intervention time		0.913	−1.27	−0.001	0.021	−0.06	0.928
Intervention intensity		0.9512	−1.569	0.13	0.532	0.24	0.817

3.4. Publication Bias Analysis

It can be seen from Table 3: Moderate autism: $t = -1.46$, $p = 0.159 > 0.05$, and the 95% confidence interval is [−6.45, 1.21] including 0. It shows that the difference is not statistically significant, that is, there is no publication bias in the three literatures included in this study on exercise intervention for children with moderate autism symptoms. Meta analysis shows that the results are relatively stable and credible; severe autism: $t = -22.65$, $p = 0.026 < 0.05$, and the 95% confidence interval is [−6.18, −1.73] and does not contain 0.

Table 3. Evaluation of publication bias in the included the literature.

Degree of Autism	Correlation Coefficient	Standard Error	T Value	P > |t|	95% CI
Moderate autism	−2.59	1.68	−1.46	0.159	(−6.45, 1.21)
Severe autism	−3.87	0.16	−22.65	0.026	(−6.18, −1.73)

For autistic children with moderate symptoms, the bias in the three documents was not significant statistically. That is, the documents showed similar results for the effect of physical exercise on autistic children with moderate symptoms. This coincided with the meta-analysis result. For autistic children with severe symptoms, the bias in the documents was statistically significant, with a publication bias in two documents. This result, alongside the meta-analysis result, indicates that further research is needed on the effect of physical exercise on autistic children with severe symptoms.

4. Discussion

The pathogenesis of autism in children is not clarified yet. The disease may be related to environmental factors (genetics), social factors (social psychology), and/or health factors (immunology, brain, endocrine, and others). The results of the second survey of disabled children in Taiwan stated that 1.10% of children with mental disabilities were aged 0–6 years old, which is 111,000 patients. In total, 36.9% of them were autistic, which is 41,000 patients [11]. It has been suggested that systematic and active physical exercise stimulates body functions and therefore improves the physical condition of patients [12]. Sports programs improve the physical conditions of children with mild intellectual disability, showing that sports play an important role in enhancing the health of children with intellectual disability in terms of body shape, quality of life, and metabolic function [13]. These studies verified the effectiveness of sports for children with autism. As differences are found in various research results due to different competencies, conditions, methods, and subjects of research, more quantitative and comprehensive analyses and interpretations of the results are demanded. A meta-analysis was used in this research to evaluate the relevant research results quantitatively and comprehensively. Especially to explain the influence of physical exercise on autistic children with severe symptoms, more precise and objective research methods and frameworks are required to obtain quantitative results that can be an important basis for the treatment of autistic children.

The results of the meta-analysis of the five selected documents are as follows. The documents had a random selection of research subjects without explaining the method. Allocation concealment and blinded methods were not used, also, except for one document which explained the withdrawal of missing visits. As the quality of the documents was not high enough, the quality and the interpretation of their results may not be adequate for further implications. The results of the meta-regression analysis also show a lower quality due to heterogeneity. Therefore, more randomized and controlled object selection and grouping are required to investigate the effect of physical exercise on autistic children with various degrees of symptoms.

5. Conclusions

The results of the meta-analysis in this research show that physical exercise significantly improves the moderate symptoms of autistic children. The total SMD, confidence interval, and standard deviation changes prove that physical exercise has a significant effect on the mitigation of moderate symptoms in autistic children. A similar effect was confirmed for the severe symptoms in autistic children, but the statistical significance was not high enough to accept it as a firm proof. In total, four out of the five selected documents show that autistic symptoms still existed with physical exercise, but with their symptoms significantly improved. This implies that the treatment of autistic children requires physical exercise. However, it is still necessary to investigate if physical exercise allows for curing autism in children, and if the symptom of various degrees of autism in children worsens without the continuation of physical exercise.

Author Contributions: Conceptualization, L.-X.L.; formal analysis, K.-S.H.; data curation, L.-X.L.; writing—original draft preparation, K.-S.H.; writing—review and editing, K.-S.H. All authors have read and agreed to the published version of the manuscript.

Funding: This research received no external funding.

Institutional Review Board Statement: Not applicable.

Informed Consent Statement: Not applicable.

Data Availability Statement: The data that support the findings of this study are available from the corresponding author upon reasonable request.

Conflicts of Interest: The authors declare no conflict of interest.

References

1. Duan, G.; Yao, M.; Ma, Y.; Zhang, W. Perinatal and background risk factors for childhood autism in central China. *Psychiatry Res.* **2014**, *220*, 410–417. [CrossRef] [PubMed]
2. El-Ansary, A.K.; Ben Bacha, A.; Kotb, M. Etiology of autistic features: The persisting neurotoxic effects of propionic acid. *J. Neuroin Flammation* **2012**, *9*, 74. [CrossRef] [PubMed]
3. Jing, J. Early diagnosis and early intervention of autism in children. *Chin. J. Child Health Care* **2007**, *5*, 453–454. (In Chinese)
4. Wang, C.-S.; Huang, Y.-M.; Hsu, K.-S. The design and development of a mobile color mixing game. *Adv. Mech. Eng.* **2017**, *9*, 1–6.
5. Jadad, A.R.; Moore, R.A.; Carroll, D.; Jenkinson, C.; Reynolds, D.J.; Gavaghan, D.J.; McQuay, H.J. Assessing the quality of reports of randomized clinical trials: Is blinding necessary? *Control. Clin Trials* **1996**, *17*, 1–12. [CrossRef] [PubMed]
6. Hou, X.-H.; Feng, Y.-Q.; Pan, H.-L.; Wu, Y.-D.; Ma, Z.-M.; Zhu, Z.-P. Effects of Aquatic Therapy on Behaviors of Children with Autism: Based on Halliwick Technology. *J. Tianjin Univ. Sport* **2017**, *32*, 429–433. (In Chinese)
7. Ren, Q. Effect of Motion Sensing Game Rehabilitation Therapy on Impaired Social Interaction, Activities of Daily Living and Emotional Behaviors of Children with Autism. *China J. Health Psychol.* **2018**, *26*, 509–513.
8. Ang, F.; Xu, D. Intervention effect of Physical Exercise on Autistic Children—Taking Nanjing Ningxin Service Center as an Example. *Sichuan Sports Sci.* **2018**, *37*, 51–54.
9. Zhang, Z.J.; Yang, J.-Q. Effects of sports intervention on behavior and quality of life of children with autism. *Chin. J. Clin. Res.* **2017**, *30*, 1244–1246.
10. Yi, Y.; Yang, Y. Effect analysis of exercise intervention in autistic children. *China Mod. Med.* **2016**, *23*, 29–31.
11. Hao, C.-P.; Xi, W. A Case Study of the Impact of Sports Games on Moderate Mentally Retarded Children's Physique. *J. Beijing Union Univ. (Nat. Sci.)* **2014**, *28*, 84–88.
12. Miao, Y.-Y. Experimental Research on Sports Game Activities to Promote Children's Physique. Master's Thesis, Capital University of Physical Education and Sports, Beijing, China, 2011.
13. Zheng, W.; Hao, C.-P.; Zhang, B. Effects of exercise intervention on the physical fitness of slightly retarded children. *J. Phys. Educ.* **2014**, *21*, 124–127.

engineering proceedings

Proceeding Paper

Delicious Cyber Ghost: Using Pepper's Ghost in Computer-Aided Design to Enhance Cantonese Morning Tea Education †

Song Xu [1], Peng-Wei Hsiao [2], Chen Li [1,*] and Jin-Yu Zhang [1]

1 School of Design and Art, Beijing Institute of Technology, Zhuhai 519088, China; xusong@bitzh.edu.cn (S.X.); zhangjinyu2025@gmail.com (J.-Y.Z.)
2 Department of Visual Arts, Macao Polytechnic University, Macau 999078, China; pwhsiao@ipm.edu.mo
* Correspondence: lichen@bitzh.edu.cn

† Presented at the 2024 IEEE 4th International Conference on Electronic Communications, Internet of Things and Big Data, Taipei, Taiwan, 19–21 April 2024.

Abstract: Cantonese morning tea drinking is a cherished intangible cultural heritage in the Guangdong–Hong Kong–Macao Greater Bay Area in China and embodies Guangdong's culinary tradition. In the digital era, innovative design techniques and digital technology have been applied to preserve and promote this tradition. To enhance heritage education, we designed an augmented reality device for Cantonese morning tea using Pepper's Ghost technique. Employing field investigations, literature research, and experiments, we showcased Cantonese morning tea drinking. For further developments, affordable materials and professional photos are essential for constructing the model.

Keywords: Cantonese morning tea; Pepper's ghost; augmented reality; heritage education; design practice

Citation: Xu, S.; Hsiao, P.-W.; Li, C.; Zhang, J.-Y. Delicious Cyber Ghost: Using Pepper's Ghost in Computer-Aided Design to Enhance Cantonese Morning Tea Education. *Eng. Proc.* **2024**, *74*, 78. https://doi.org/10.3390/engproc2024074078

Academic Editors: Shu-Han Liao, Teen-Hang Meen and Cheng-Fu Yang

Published: 21 November 2024

1. Introduction

According to a Chinese saying, "Food is the people's priority". Food culture has long been seen as important in Chinese culture. During the last century, Guangdong, Hong Kong, and Macao of the Greater Bay Area (the GBA) in China have gradually embraced morning tea drinking into their daily lives. Cantonese morning tea drinking has become popular due to its sumptuous side dishes and relaxed market setting. Morning tea drinking is an important part of the culture of the Bay Area people despite the challenges of social advancement and urbanization. However, traditional tea businesses are facing difficulties in this modern era. Nevertheless, the majority of people in the GBA still appreciate the value of morning tea. As the modern and traditional versions of the morning tea experience differ in terms of dining options, cultural hubs, leisure activities, and other factors, there is an opportunity to embrace change and find ways to preserve the essence of morning tea while adapting to the changing times.

In today's fast-paced digital world, it is important to keep up with the changing habits of the younger generation. While it may be challenging to encourage young people to adopt the practice of having morning tea, it is crucial to make it more appealing to them. Similarly, traditional tea houses need to adapt to the changing landscape and embrace new technologies to stay relevant. By utilizing central kitchens, pre-prepared meals, and other innovative methods, tea houses can serve their customers efficiently and effectively. It is important to balance between tradition and innovation to ensure that tea culture is preserved. The popularity of new media tools such as TikTok has provided the younger generation with an abundance of information and news. It is remarkable how easily accessible information is, enabling people to stay up to date with the latest news and social trends from their homes.

Thus, using the cutting-edge technology Pepper's Ghost, we created an augmented reality (AR) Cantonese morning tea drinking experience to encourage pupils to share their stories. Additionally, the elements of Cantonese morning tea drinking were integrated into the video assets using a scripted story and young local actors, thereby promoting the local cultural heritage.

2. Literature Review

2.1. Study and Protection of Cantonese Morning Tea Drinking

The GBA is witnessing a surge in cultural research activities, thanks to the expanding coastal economy of China. While the study of morning tea drinking is not commonly known, relevant research findings have been published every year. Through a literature review, we compiled the latest research results regarding topics such as immigrant life, cultural identity, Cantonese culture, and cultural space. In a comparison study conducted over two decades ago, scholars found that children's linguistic backgrounds played a significant role in their interactions. Thus, teachers must encourage communication between children of similar linguistic backgrounds to promote interactions between children from varied language backgrounds. These findings help us to understand communities better and create more inclusive spaces [1]. Various research has been conducted on the hobbies and social networks of the population in the GBA, highlighting the role of Guangzhou-style morning tea drinking in helping immigrants feel more at home and integrated into Cantonese society, which leads to stronger social connections with locals and immigrants [2]. Additionally, several Hong Kong scholars have researched traditional Cantonese tea culture to expand understanding of the history and current state of tea facilities. Overall, these studies provide information on the lifestyles and cultural practices of the people in the Greater Bay Area.

Researchers have highlighted the cultural significance of traditional cuisine and its experiential value for consumers. They emphasized the influence of Cantonese morning tea drinking in shaping the dining experience and how it continues to inspire similar meals [3]. Additionally, the elements of the Cantonese morning tea drinking were integrated into artworks, showcasing the richness of traditional Cantonese culture. However, there are challenges faced by traditional Cantonese morning tea houses due to economic development, and there is an urgent need to preserve this cultural heritage and raise awareness about the importance of preserving and promoting traditional cultural practices [4]. Cantonese morning tea drinking is popular and has seen an increased presence in restaurants despite its decline in teahouses. The cultural significance of Cantonese morning tea drinking, particularly in the GBA, was researched to understand how urban cultural space has evolved in the region with morning tea culture playing a crucial role in shaping it. The authors examined the potential for expanding urban cultural space based on the growth dimension of cultural space. Their findings help preserve and promote the cultural heritage of Cantonese morning tea drinking [5].

2.2. Pepper's Ghost and Augmented Reality (AR)

Pepper's Ghost is an optical illusion. John explained its scientific principles in detail [6]. The illusion has been successfully integrated into a European museum by an Italian research team, who designed holographic cabinets for improving visitor experience [7]. Thomas explored the potential of Pepper's Ghost and AR to examine social systems through media forms. He observed the current revival of Pepper's Ghost as a promising way to create modern 'holograms' for the 21st century [8]. Researchers in Spain developed a highly economical multi-view display using the Pepper's Ghost technique. They encountered issues with the holographic display's thickness, which made it difficult for users to read text, and its inability to perform well in bright light conditions. However, comparing the monitor with commercial optical field monitors, a multi-view display was developed [9]. Pepper's Ghost was used to create virtual presentations of large or delicate antiques in art museums. A device with sensors enables users to interact with the images using holographic displays and related applications [10].

2.3. Three-Dimensional Modeling for Live Performance

Three-dimensional materials and various optical imaging technologies have been used to display cultural heritage content in recent years. Researchers combine live performances with cultural heritage by modeling cultural resources in three dimensions. Starting with manual modeling, semi-automatic computer-aided modeling is presently used with scanning drones to preserve and showcase cultural heritage [11]. The potential of 3D modeling in cultural heritage education was researched by identifying three significant challenges to ensure the efficacy of digital 3D modeling technology. These challenges include usage scenarios and user cognition for technical processes and user experience, and legislation and infrastructure. Overcoming these challenges contributes to the preservation of traditional culture [12]. Digital cultural treasures are accessible to visually impaired people by using interactive touch recognition techniques and traditional 3D scanning, modeling, and printing, which can be used to preserve and promote cultural heritage [13]. Live broadcasts and e-commerce are also used to preserve intangible cultural property. These innovative approaches to preserving cultural heritage are crucial in ensuring that future generations continue to learn and appreciate rich cultural heritage [14].

3. Study Design

3.1. Field Investigation

Although there are not many traditional Cantonese morning tea drinking businesses still in operation, the pandemic and quarantine regulations presented a unique opportunity for this research. Despite the challenges, we found six seafood restaurants serving Guangzhou-style morning tea in a three-kilometer radius (Table 1). They were easily accessible, so thorough research could be conducted. They were selected from 15 restaurants by carefully filtering out unsuitable options and focusing on relevant venues. Many restaurants had irregular operating hours, which made it difficult to carry out an effective study. We found that the three restaurants had storefronts facing the street, which was their success factor. We selected the morning tea offered at "Li Yuan Seafood Restaurant" and sampled five morning tea delights to ensure accuracy and fairness. Shrimp dumplings were selected for the experiment.

Table 1. List of teahouses within 3 km of the research team.

Restaurant	Distance (km)	Parking	Average Consumption Per Person	Other
Liyuan Seafood Restaurant	1.9	FREE	CNY78	
Tai SAN (St Wong Tau Street Shop)	2.3	N/A	CNY98.8/Set	
Jin Feng Sheng Restaurant	2.3	N/A	CNY69	
Gaozhou Lao Food City (Xiangzhou shop)	2.6	N/A	CNY58	
Yue Lanxuan Restaurant	3.0	CHARGE	N/A	Business hours were not fixed during the pandemic
Yijian Taste Room	3.1	FREE	CNY84	Business hours were not fixed during the pandemic

3.2. Story Design

The story's narrative structure started from the actors' perspective and moved on to the third person (Figure 1). With the help of Pepper's Ghost technique, we created an immersive dream-like experience for viewers. The story is set in the GBA, where a young man embarks on an exciting adventure by ship. The story introduces the iconic Cantonese morning tea, which unexpectedly comes to life to communicate with the protagonist. The virtual scenes in the story show the prominent landmarks of the GBA, including the famous Dancing Lion to support the characters. The story is exciting and engaging and captures the essence of the GBA. The story serves traditional Cantonese morning tea. The characters' dreams are displayed using a combination of real steamer props and computer-generated visuals. The protagonist, Brother Hao, and a virtual character named Shrimp Dumpling have a conflict, through which they introduce the principles of Cantonese morning tea drinking in a fun and engaging way. The story's climax is a creative representation of the protagonist's satiation with an endless supply of shrimp dumplings. The story is unique in showcasing the themes of traditional Cantonese morning tea culture. The story concludes when the protagonist is brought back to reality by the Dancing Lion. Pepper's Ghost illusion, resembling a live performance, adds value to the tale. This type of storytelling is unique in terms of the performances it stages, setting it apart from popular movie and television scripts. We present an example of how similar the montage editing technique is to film and television works in this article. The limitations of technology for stage performances encourage creativity and uniqueness in the form and content.

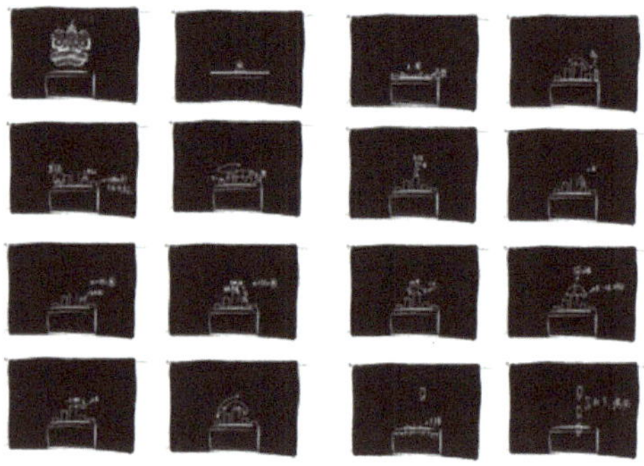

Figure 1. Storyboard.

3.3. *Pepper's Ghost Device*

We developed a device prototype for the innovative Pepper's Ghost illusion effect (Figure 2). We used lightweight corrugated paper and white, translucent acrylic panels as the main structure for the device. To ensure high-quality imaging, we experimented with two imaging sources: a portable laser projector and a 27-inch LCD screen. The LCD screen provided a superior imaging effect for the experiment. We selected lightweight corrugated paper for the prototype's main frame due to its affordability, ease of cutting, and wide availability. We created the prototype system to meet high standards. The projector's surface is made of standard acrylic sheets as a reflective film. Shrimp dumplings and traditional Cantonese morning tea were used to test the system.

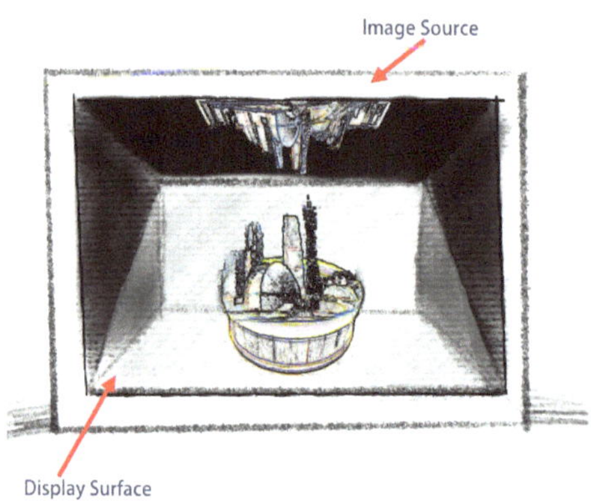

Figure 2. The Pepper's Ghost device's conceptual design.

4. Results

4.1. Virtual Scenes

Virtual scenes were essential in the story development process for "Brother Hao". These scenes were designed and rendered using digital tools to ensure that they appear in frame at the right moment (Figure 3). We used the line draft technique to create realistic and detailed virtual scenes to help the audience be immersed in the hero's dream world. Black with white lines presented a functional purpose by making use of the Pepper's Ghost technique. This technique allowed the audience to see only the white-image information. When the black background was removed, a more realistic and immersive experience was obtained. Constructing the virtual scene's material and animating it frame by frame took an enormous time. By introducing a video editing tool, the task was completed quickly and efficiently. We created the virtual character "Shrimp Dumpling" by freehand drawing in two dimensions for the resulting special effects. Colored avatars were more identifiable than standard visual elements to incorporate this.

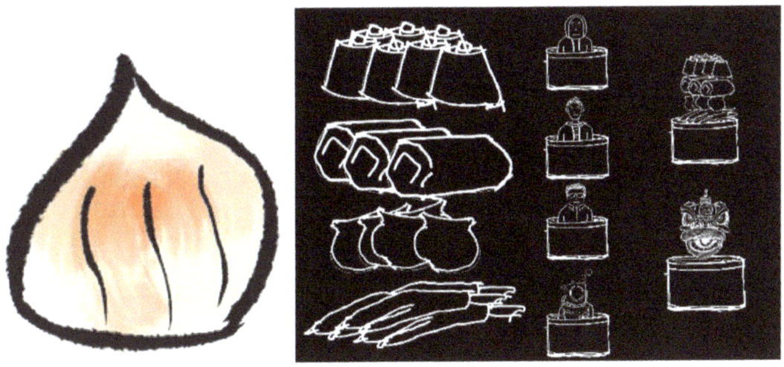

Figure 3. Virtual character "Shrimp Dumpling" and characters in Brother Hao's dream.

4.2. Real-Scene Content

In the recorded live concert, LED lights were used for a better film effect. Two lights illuminated the green screen, and another two lights focused on the main character, which resulted in a more uniform green background (Figure 4). The narrator's Cantonese and the protagonist's accent presented authenticity. Moreover, the protagonist treated the virtual character Shrimp Dumpling as if it were human for an engaging presence and live concert experience. There was no physical performance due to the character being virtual. The actor's experience and skills were critical for delivering a good performance. Marionettes were also used for the lion dance. To ensure the best outcome, we created a skilled puppeteer to direct the motion of the lion dance (Figure 5).

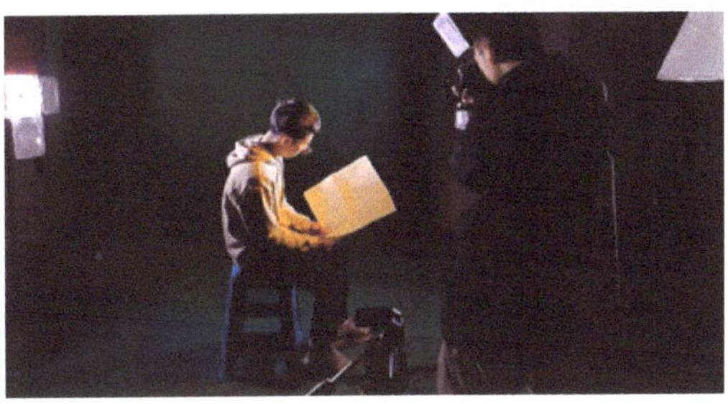

Figure 4. Filming the performance of the main character "Brother Hao".

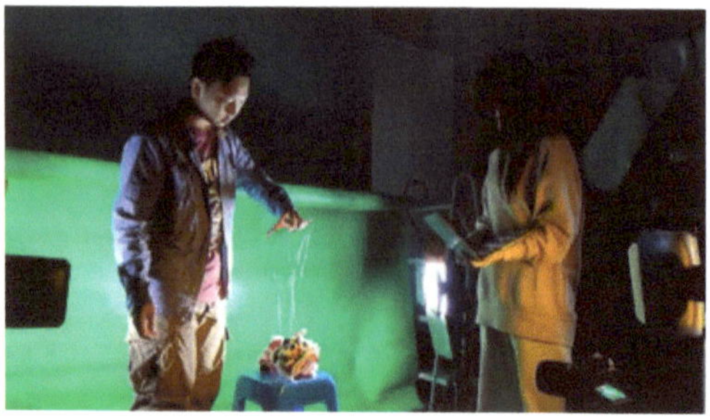

Figure 5. Filming the lion dance performance.

4.3. *Digital Effects and Post-Editing*

Once all the virtual video and live performance parts were recorded, the post-special effects were added and editing process commenced. For non-linear editing, Adobe Premiere 2018 was used, while Adobe Media Encoder 2018 was used for composite coding. We found that Adobe After Effects 2018 was the best post-production tool to bring all the elements together. The interactions between Brother Hao, the shrimp dumplings, and the Dancing Lion were challenging for special effects production. A real human needed to interact with the animation frame by frame. We animated the shrimp dumplings frame by frame in Adobe After Effects before importing the main character's image with a transparent channel and producing a new video track. We combined the real person and the performance video with special effects. We edited the lion dance video using a transparent channel and then imported the video of the actual protagonist. After incorporating the scripted story, we applied the appropriate effects to each shot to make it visually appealing. Finally, we exported the edited video in 720 P MP4 format to enhance the overall quality of the video and make it more engaging for the audience (Figures 6 and 7).

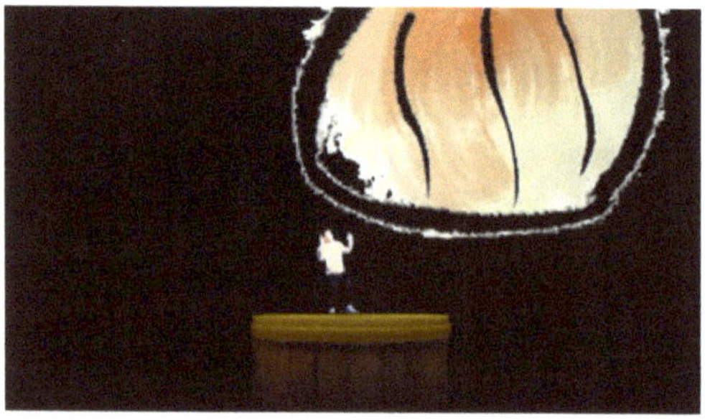

Figure 6. Scene compositing of real person and virtual character "Shrimp Dumpling".

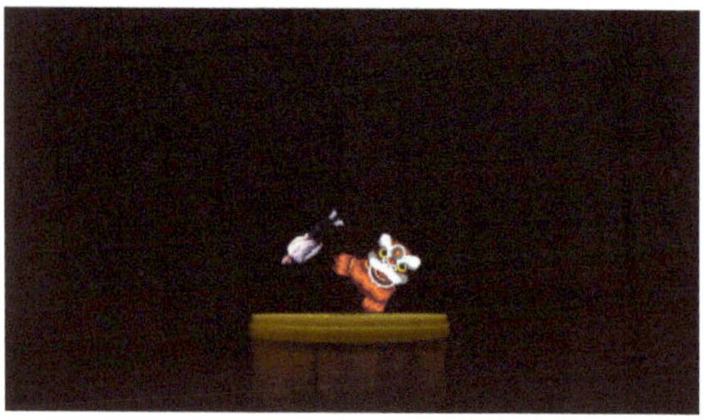

Figure 7. Scene compositing of real person and virtual characters "Dancing Lion".

4.4. Pepper's Ghost Device Assembling

We integrated accessibility and environmental protection via the use of Pepper's Ghost technique. Corrugated paper was chosen as the principal structure of the imaging device because this study's target population is lower-grade undergraduates and popular in colleges and universities. The basic structure sustained a 27″ LCD. Load bearings were used for the experimental apparatus. Acrylic sheets were used as the imaging medium and mounted at a 45-degree angle by grooving the left and right cardboard edges. In the construction of the entire gadget, the steamer props were positioned in the center of the bottom. It was important to place the steamer in front of the clear acrylic plate for the image effect (Figure 8).

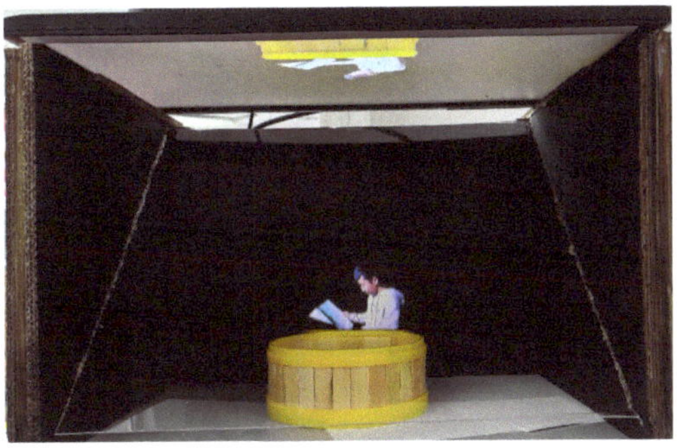

Figure 8. Effect of the Pepper's Ghost device.

5. Conclusions

To promote and meet the need for traditional Cantonese morning tea drinking, the establishment of culinary culture through its essence is important for the experience in dining and the cultural identity of locals. Cantonese morning tea drinking's essence is inextricably linked to its physical form and the distinctive cultural setting of the GBA. The culture of Cantonese morning tea drinking must be passed down and needs to be enhanced with expression forms as cultural heritage. Even though traditional Cantonese morning tea drinking is disappearing, its superior culinary standards and distinctive cultural practices of "one cup and two pieces" must be preserved. Even though Pepper's Ghost is an old technique with a history dating back more than a century, it still has a strong vitality even amongst new technologies like AR, virtual reality, and mixed reality. Even though human society has been at the threshold of the meta-universe, conventional 3D modeling technologies are used widely. The development of new media livestreaming platforms provides more e-commerce possibilities for intangible cultural heritage protection. In GBA, Pepper's Ghost was used as the imaging technology to set up a real-life performance experiment platform for local young people's cognition and emotional expression in this study.

In addition, there are limitations in the production of imaging devices. Live performances necessitate an upscaled studio and a larger venue compared to conventional 3D models. The Pepper's Ghost device requires a space ten times smaller than studios, and its projections can be cast with synthetic clips of digitally hand-painted materials and live performance materials. The artists' humanistic sentiments are added to the equivalent scale so that the virtual images can display cultural highlights on the real objects. This can be a way of ensuring traditional culture's ongoing survival. The developed "light field" imaging device with improved imaging performance and larger interaction potential can be used for a wide range of research in the future.

Author Contributions: Conceptualization, S.X., P.-W.H., C.L. and J.-Y.Z.; methodology, S.X. and C.L.; software, S.X.; validation, S.X. and C.L.; formal analysis, S.X.; investigation, S.X. and J.-Y.Z.; resources, S.X. and P.-W.H.; data curation, S.X.; writing—original draft preparation, S.X. and C.L.; writing—review and editing, S.X. and C.L.; visualization, S.X., C.L. and J.-Y.Z.; supervision, C.L.;

project administration, C.L. and P.-W.H.; funding acquisition, C.L. and P.-W.H. All authors have read and agreed to the published version of the manuscript.

Funding: This study was supported by the School of Design and Art, Beijing Institute of Technology, Zhuhai (ZX-2020-031) and the Department of Visual Arts, Macao Polytechnic University (RP/FAD-02/2022).

Institutional Review Board Statement: Not applicable.

Informed Consent Statement: Not applicable.

Data Availability Statement: Not available due to privacy restrictions.

Acknowledgments: We would like to extend our gratitude to the School of Design for their generosity in lending us the experiment venue and to Liang Yonghao and Zhou Meiyi who took time out of their busy schedules to participate in shooting the scenes and without whom this research would not have been completed successfully.

Conflicts of Interest: The authors declare no conflicts of interest.

References

1. Oi-Ling Leung, L.; Lewis, G.F. The Effect of Ethnolinguistic Differences on Proximity between Cantonese and Mandarin Speaking Children. *Early Child Dev. Care* **1999**, *159*, 135–144. [CrossRef]
2. Zhang, Y.; Long, M. The role of Yum Cha (Cantonese Morning Tea Drinking) in the integration process among interprovincial migration in China. *Leis. Stud.* **2015**, *34*, 59–66. [CrossRef]
3. Chen, Z. A pilot study of the co-creation experience in traditional Cantonese teahouses in Hong Kong. *J. Herit. Tour.* **2018**, *13*, 506–527. [CrossRef]
4. Liu, Y. Cantonese Cultural Center: Guangzhou China. Ph.D. Thesis, University of Georgia, Athens, GA, USA, 2019.
5. Xudong, G.; Fang, C.; Xiaowen, F.; Haiming, C. Growth and Function of Urban Cultural Space Seen from Guangfu Morning Tea Culture. *J. Landsc. Res.* **2021**, *13*, 112–116.
6. Greenslade Jr, T.B. Pepper's Ghost. *Phys. Teach.* **2011**, *49*, 338–339. [CrossRef]
7. Pietroni, E.; Ferdani, D.; Forlani, M.; Pagano, A.; Rufa, C. Bringing the illusion of reality inside museums—A methodological proposal for an advanced museology using holographic showcases. *Informatics* **2019**, *6*, 2. [CrossRef]
8. Conner, T. Pepper's Ghost and the AR of modernity. *J. Sci. Pop. Cult.* **2020**, *3*, 57–79. [CrossRef]
9. Ezcurdia, I.; Arregui, A.; Ardaiz, O.; Ortiz, A.; Marzo, A. Content adaptation and depth perception in an affordable multi-view display. *Appl. Sci.* **2020**, *10*, 7357. [CrossRef]
10. Andress, W. Virtual Presentation Methods for Physical Artifacts. Ph.D. Thesis, Worcester Polytechnic Institute, Worcester, MA, USA, 2022.
11. Barrile, V.; Bernardo, E.; Bilotta, G. An experimental HBIM processing: Innovative tool for 3D model reconstruction of morpho-typological phases for the cultural heritage. *Remote Sens.* **2022**, *14*, 1288. [CrossRef]
12. Muenster, S. Digital 3D Technologies for humanities research and education: An overview. *Appl. Sci.* **2022**, *12*, 2426. [CrossRef]
13. Montusiewicz, J.; Barszcz, M.; Korga, S. Preparation of 3D models of cultural heritage objects to be recognised by touch by the blind—Case studies. *Appl. Sci.* **2022**, *12*, 11910. [CrossRef]
14. Lu, Z.; Annett, M.; Fan, M.; Wigdor, D. "I feel it is my responsibility to stream" Streaming and Engaging with Intangible Cultural Heritage through Livestreaming. In Proceedings of the 2019 CHI Conference on Human Factors in Computing Systems, Glasgow Scotland, UK, 4–9 May 2019.

engineering proceedings

Proceeding Paper

Theoretical Model and Practical Pathway for Digital Transformation of Classroom Teaching in Health Education Using Big Data Technology †

Haoyu Wang

Beijing No. 27 High School, Beijing 100006, China; wanghaoyu09@163.com

† Presented at the 2024 IEEE 4th International Conference on Electronic Communications, Internet of Things and Big Data, Taipei, Taiwan, 19–21 April 2024.

Abstract: This study aims to reveal the characteristics of the digital transformation of classroom teaching in health education. The key links of the digital transformation process in classroom teaching were identified to determine an implementation pathway. Based on the results, theoretical and practical guidance for the implementation of digital transformation in health education was proposed.

Keywords: digital transformation; health education; classroom teaching; theoretical model; practical pathway

Citation: Wang, H. Theoretical Model and Practical Pathway for Digital Transformation of Classroom Teaching in Health Education Using Big Data Technology. *Eng. Proc.* **2024**, *74*, 79. https://doi.org/10.3390/engproc2024074079

Academic Editors: Shu-Han Liao, Teen-Hang Meen and Cheng-Fu Yang

Published: 28 November 2024

1. Introduction

Digital transformation and innovation are fundamental issues in educational reform and practice. In 2022, the Ministry of Education of China announced the implementation of the initiative for digitalization and smart education on the public service platform [1]. Digital transformation is a revolutionary and systematic approach to education innovation and reform [2], during which it is important to use data. This allows for the shared development of technology and education and effective talent cultivation [3]. The classroom is regarded as the front line of digital transformation in education. The utilization of data flow is a significant driving force for the structural transformation of classroom teaching as a necessary option to reduce the academic burden and improve the quality and efficiency of teaching [4]. Data flow is also important in the modernization and development of education [5]. Therefore, the digital transformation of classrooms based on data is emphasized.

Health is fundamental and necessary for humans [6]. Effective health education helps to improve the perspective on life, health, and safety. It also fosters the development of health, virtue, habits, and lifestyles, and the adoption and practice of healthy behaviors. These are a solid foundation for lifelong health [7]. The health education curriculum is crucial in implementing moral education and cultivating talents. It is important to foster talents for the possession of the necessary skills and qualities.

On this basis, the characteristics of digital transformation in classroom teaching in health education under the initiatives of digital transformation were studied in this research. A theoretical model was constructed to elucidate the key links of the digital transformation process and propose an implementation pathway for such transformation. Theoretical and practical guidance were also suggested for the implementation of digital transformation in the classroom.

2. Digital Transformation in Teaching of Health Education

The characteristics of digital transformation in classrooms are important for research and practice in education. Such transformation emphasizes the collaboration between teachers and students based on data accumulation, exchange, processing, and analyses using smart technologies that automate teaching processes on demand and intelligent learning [8]. Digital transformation in education is characterized by data collection, representation, and use.

2.1. Data Collection

For digital transformation in the classroom, classroom data need to be collected on a large scale. Data collection in health education is essential in addressing the problems and difficulties of using the Internet of Things (IoT), big data, and blockchain in teaching and ensuring a smooth and efficient connection between classrooms.

2.2. Use of Data for Objective Representation

The digital transformation in health education is based on the personalized processing and representation of data. Data are crucial in the teaching environment using smart technologies and are a foundation for adjusting teaching methods and adapting learning approaches.

2.3. Agile Adjustment of Collaborative Data

The digital transformation is based on the intelligent analysis and application. Therefore, the data are crucial to conducting teaching activities to meet the related needs and development of individual students. This approach significantly reduces irrelevant teaching activities and maximizes the efficiency of dynamic and creative classroom teaching.

3. Model for Digital Transformation

It is essential to facilitate digital transformation and data vitality and understand the concept of the transformation of health education to enhance the quality and efficiency of health education. Digital transformation and data vitality are also essential for the education of talents for competence and innovative capability in a digital society (Figure 1).

3.1. Health Education: Data Awareness

As an action plan and implementation guide for teaching activities in health education, classrooms play a strategic, guiding, and leading role. Successful digital transformation in health education demands classroom data and their analysis. The results are used to facilitate the data flow and use the attributes and factors of data. The digital transformation in health education demands fundamental theories and principles of education and teaching. Innovative thinking with digitalization and intelligence is the fundamental principle for the development of health education. The data allow for educational outcomes by enhancing the effectiveness of talent cultivation in the classroom. The data are also used to empower students and provide guidance on personalized growth, focusing on individual needs and adaptive development. This approach enhances the quality and efficiency of health education, stimulates the transformation of the classroom and student learning, and cultivates talents with advanced competence and key abilities for problem-solving and knowledge transfer.

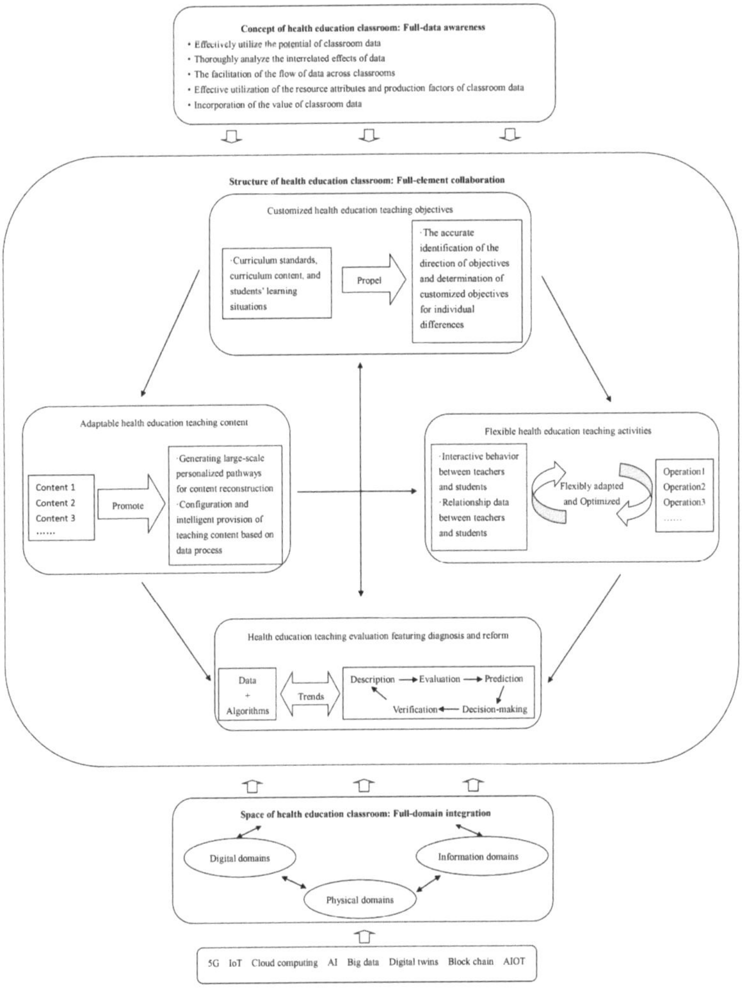

Figure 1. Theoretical model for digital transformation in health education.

3.2. Domain Integration of Classroom

The classroom encompasses material, spiritual, and social entities [9]. It consists of teacher–student communication, interaction, and collaboration. The incorporation and application of digital technologies allow for teaching in classrooms with integrated domains. Those also lead to the data-driven, platform-supported, resource-allocated, and intelligent adaptation of digital technologies. The incorporation of digital transformation into the classroom is based on the educational infrastructure. It needs the integration and interoperability of classroom data to remove the barriers between the physical, information, and digital domains and connect them in teaching. It is necessary to construct the digital twins of the classroom entity, teaching process, and learning using models for data analyses and prediction. The models are used to assist health education.

3.3. Structure of Classroom

The classroom in health education is important for the evolution of the teaching system. The classroom demands a scientific design to connect and interact between various elements including teachers, students, teaching objectives, teaching content, teaching activities, and teaching evaluation. The classroom structural reform in health education demands data and technologies such as AI and big data to improve teaching objectives, content, activities, and evaluation.

3.3.1. Teaching Objectives

The objectives of health education are important for the evaluation. Teachers establish teaching objectives following curriculum standards, content, and learning situations. The identification of objectives is challenging when considering individual differences. To improve the quality and efficiency of teaching, digital transformation with replication, connection, simulation, and feedback is demanded. It is also necessary to define knowledge points, classroom profiles, and personalized growth data of students. The relationship between teaching objectives and evaluation needs to be analyzed for customized teaching.

3.3.2. Teaching Content

The teaching content affects students' learning outcomes. Thus, the refinement, reconstruction, and adaptation of the content are needed for efficient teaching. Individual differences of students must be respected in the digital transformation of health education. Semantic networks and knowledge graphs are used to eliminate irrelevant content, while data are used as the basis for generating personalized pathways for content development to support the continued improvement in teaching content. In addition, technologies such as virtual reality, augmented reality, and extended reality are necessary for the continuous innovation of teaching content. The on-demand configuration of teaching content needs to be implemented based on the data according to students' learning needs and abilities to develop health education.

3.3.3. Teaching Activities

Based on the teacher–student bond and behavior, teaching activities are necessary according to teaching objectives to promote individual development. The diversification of teaching activities is a goal of traditional teaching to improve the quality and efficiency of teaching. The digital transformation of health education supports the integration of data, quantifies the relationship between teachers and students, and automates data collection, processing, analyses, application, and optimization. Then, teaching activities can be optimized through iteration for students' learning needs.

3.3.4. Teaching Evaluation

Evaluation is important in adjusting teaching activities and reviewing teaching objectives. Accurate teaching evaluation is necessary to improve the quality and efficiency of teaching. In the digital transformation of health education, the data must be used to process, integrate, process, optimize, diagnose, and reform teaching. Driven by the data, the transformation provides a new diagnostic and reform decision-making method to remove uncertainty in evaluation and transfer subjective evaluation to a data-driven decision. Then, the accurate verification of teaching is allowed to promote personalized and optimized configuration and student-centric education.

4. Key Links of Digital Transformation

For health education and its interdisciplinary practice, the systematic adjustment of teaching objectives, content, activities, and evaluation is important [10]. Based on the ideas and requirements of the Physical Education and Health Curriculum Standards for Compulsory Education (2022) [11], the classroom structure is constructed with the key links as shown in Figure 2.

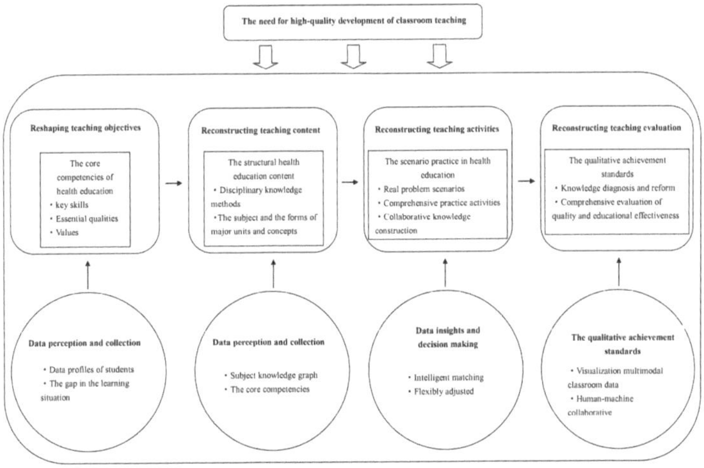

Figure 2. Key links for digital transformation of health education.

4.1. Reshaping Teaching Objectives

In health education, skills, qualities, and values are important for students' subject learning. It is important to develop the core competencies of students using data in the digital transformation and reshape teaching objectives based on the gap in the learning situation.

4.2. Reconstructing Teaching Content

The integrity and correlation of knowledge are crucial to develop students' core competencies. A subject knowledge graph can be used using data fusion and flow to integrate and reconstruct the existing teaching content.

4.3. Reconstructing Teaching Activities

It is important to conduct subject-specific and interdisciplinary practices based on real-world problems. In the digital transformation, smart technologies need to be used to create teaching scenarios and personalized learning resources through knowledge construction. Attention needs to be paid to students' deep learning trends to adjust teaching activities accordingly.

4.4. Reconstructing Teaching Evaluation

The standards of health education are described based on the performance of students and their core competencies. In the digital transformation, the standards of the curricula must be used to provide competency-based guidance. A method using machine learning can be developed based on multimodal data for the implementation of knowledge diagnoses and reform, and the evaluation of quality and educational effectiveness.

5. Implementation Pathway of Digital Transformation

There are implementation steps required to advance the digital transformation in health education. The digital transformation can be implemented from five aspects: the teaching concept, environment, design, process, and evaluation. These are used to develop health education (Figure 3). This approach is implemented by reforming the five aspects through the integration of digital and smart technologies.

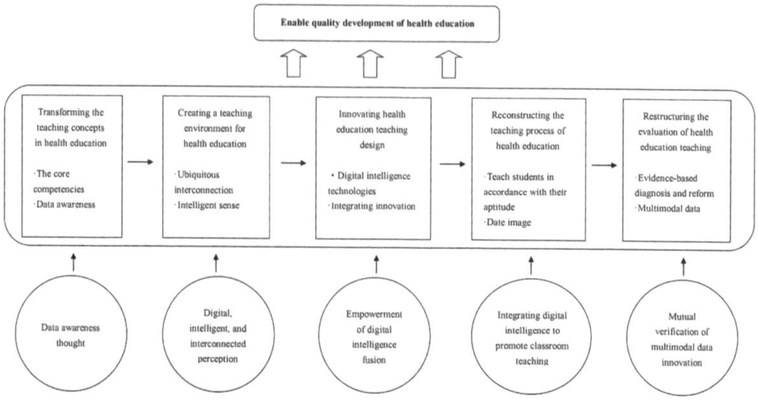

Figure 3. Pathway of digital transformation in health education classroom teaching.

5.1. *Data Awareness and Teaching Concepts*

It is important to increase data awareness and transform the teaching concept for the digital transformation of health education. Data are essential for digital transformation, and the resource attributes and production of classroom data are key to promoting the transformation of teaching concepts in health education. It is necessary to enhance quality and efficiency and reduce the academic burden. Students are independent individuals and personalized scenarios must be created for effective learning for training students' core competencies. It is important to understand data utility and its potential. The teaching process needs to be quantified and characterized, and technologies must be integrated with an innovative mindset to demonstrate the key links of the classroom teaching system. On this basis, teaching design and practice must be conducted based on human–technology collaboration to inspire students' motivation and enhance their engagement in learning. This can further increase the effectiveness of education and cultivate talents with digital awareness and innovative capabilities.

5.2. *Scenarios and Teaching Environment*

For the digital transformation of health education, it is important to create scenarios in teaching environments. The infrastructure is important in driving the digital transformation. The smart classroom can be constructed to connect smart devices and collect and use data generated from teaching to ensure multi-dimensional interconnection and intelligent perception. Learning scenarios and educational activities need to be constructed based on the problems and needs of health education. It is important to establish a digital classroom teaching environment online and offline using ubiquitous interconnectivity, human–machine collaboration, and reality–virtuality integration. This supports the development of teachers and students in the smart health education classroom.

5.3. *Digital Intelligence*

Digital intelligence helps to improve teaching design and support the digital transformation of health education for the improvement in quality and efficiency in the classroom. For innovative teaching design, it is necessary to establish the theoretical model by incorporating multimodal data and teachers' expertise. Then, accurate data on teachers, students, and classrooms can be created to design the model of health education.

5.4. *Digital and Smart Technologies*

To promote digital transformation in health education and reconstruct the teaching process, digital and smart technologies are used. The teaching process of health education consists of teaching activities, and the process demands an appropriate teaching environment. This entails the simulation, adjustment, and optimization of the existing teaching process, and the predetermination of the teaching process. On this basis, intelligent education is enabled to connect diverse teaching activities and manage data. The teaching process also enables personalized teaching through digital and intelligent integration, effectively improving the quality of health education.

5.5. Promoting Evidence-Based Diagnosis, Reform, and Evaluation

Evidence-based diagnoses, reform, and evaluation are important in the digital transformation as subjective recognition is changed to an objective one. It is also a new direction of development of the teaching evaluation in the digital transformation. Teachers must use smart technologies to collect and integrate academic, language, behavioral, psychological, and physiological data generated in teaching. Based on the data, dynamic interactive charts can be created to construct the digital profile of teachers and students and establish a feature–behavior–data mapping framework. This framework provides a credible, quantitative, and visual evaluation of health education and helps teachers and students effectively adjust their teaching strategies and activities.

6. Conclusions

The rapid development of smart technologies has led to digital transformation in education. Digital transformation with smart technologies is used to cultivate innovative talents. In this study, the characteristics of digital transformation in health education were explored to determine the initiatives of digital transformation and establish a theoretical model in education. The key links of the digital transformation in health education were determined for the implementation. Theoretical and practical guidance were proposed for the implementation of digital transformation in health education.

Author Contributions: Conceptualization, H.W.; methodology, H.W.; software, H.W.; validation, H.W.; formal analysis, H.W.; investigation, H.W.; resources, H.W.; writing—original draft preparation, H.W.; writing—review and editing, H.W.; visualization, H.W.; supervision, H.W.; project administration, H.W.; funding acquisition, H.W. All authors have read and agreed to the published version of the manuscript.

Funding: This research received no external funding.

Institutional Review Board Statement: Not applicable.

Informed Consent Statement: Not applicable.

Data Availability Statement: No new data were created or analyzed in this study. Data sharing is not applicable to this article.

Conflicts of Interest: The author declares no conflicts of interest.

References

1. Ministry of Education of the People's Republic of China. Highlights for the Work of the Ministry of Education of the People's Republic of China in 2022. Available online: http://www.moe.gov.cn/jyb_sjzl/moe_164/202202/t20220208_597666.html (accessed on 8 February 2022).
2. Zhu, Z.; Hu, J. The Logic of Practice and Opportunities for Digital Transformation in Education. *J. E-Educ. Res.* **2022**, *43*, 5–15.
3. General Office of the Central Committee of the CPC and the General Office of the State Council. Opinions on Further Reducing the Burdens of Homework and Off-Campus Training for Students during the Period of Compulsory Education. Available online: http://www.gov.cn/zhengce/2021-07/24/content_5627132.htm (accessed on 24 July 2021).
4. Huang, H.; Yang, J. Connotation and Implementation Pathway of Education Digital Transformation. *China Education News*, 6 April 2022; pp. 16–18.
5. Xie, Y.; Luo, W.; Zhang, R.; Liu, Y. Theoretical Exploration and Evolutionary Path of Digital Transformation of Classroom Teaching under the Background of "Double Reduction". *J. E-Educ. Res.* **2022**, *353*, 14–21.
6. Ministry of Education of the People's Republic of China. Notice on the Guidelines for Health and Safety Education in Primary and Secondary School Curriculum. Available online: http://www.moe.gov.cn/srcsite/A26/s8001/202111/t20211115_579815.html (accessed on 2 November 2021).

7. Ministry of Education of the People's Republic of China. National Guideline for Health Education in Primary and Secondary Schools. Available online: http://www.moe.gov.cn/srcsite/A17/moe_943/moe_946/200812/t20081201_80266.html (accessed on 1 December 2008).
8. Wang, H. Development and Future of Creativity Teaching-Intellectual Economy, Science and Technology, Neuroscience and Creativity. In Proceedings of the 3rd International Conference on Arts, Design and Contemporary Education (ICADCE 2017), Moscow, Russia, 29–30 May 2017; pp. 780–783. [CrossRef]
9. Xu, B. Reconsideration of the Implication and Value of Classroom Space from the Perspective of Sociology. *J. Educ. Res.* **2022**, *33*, 104–109.
10. Wang, H.; Liu, Y.; Han, Z.; Wu, J. Extension of media literacy from the perspective of artificial intelligence and implementation strategies of artificial intelligence courses in junior high schools. In Proceedings of the 2020 International Conference on Artificial Intelligence and Education (ICAIE2020), Tianjin, China, 26–28 June 2020; pp. 63–66. [CrossRef]
11. Ministry of Education of the People's Republic of China. *Physical Education and Health Curriculum Standards for Compulsory Education (2022)*; Beijing Normal University Publishing House: Beijing, China, 2022; p. 1.

engineering proceedings

Proceeding Paper

Analysis of the Package Tour Consumption Behaviors of Families in Taiwan, 2009–2019 †

Tzong-Shyuan Chen [1], Chi-Pei Ou Yang [2] and Jui-Yuan Chu [1,*]

1 Department of Leisure Services Management, Chaoyang University of Technology, Taichung 413310, Taiwan; jsmike@cyut.edu.tw
2 Department of Business Management, Chaoyang University of Technology, Taichung 413310, Taiwan; sam5008@hotmail.com
* Correspondence: jychu@cyut.edu.tw
† Presented at the 2024 IEEE 4th International Conference on Electronic Communications, Internet of Things and Big Data, Taipei, Taiwan, 19–21 April 2024.

Abstract: Destination platforms provide travel information and cheaper travel products, thus increasing the number of individual travelers. Therefore, travel agencies need to understand consumer behaviors toward family package tours and maintain and create new business opportunities. Using the cohort analysis method, we studied three variables in the time dimension: age, period, and cohort effects. A two-part model was combined to construct a model of family package tours in Taiwan, using data from the "Survey of Family Income and Expenditure in Taiwan" covering the period from 2009 to 2019. The results show that there were two peak periods when customers chose package tours: when the head of the household was between 46 and 50 years of age and between 66 and 70 years of age. A younger head of household had a higher willingness for such tours than an older one. The highest selection rate for these tours occurred in 2013, and then, it decreased gradually. Families with a head of household aged between 71 and 75 years had the highest expenditure on family package tours.

Keywords: cohort analysis; two-part model; package tour

Citation: Chen, T.-S.; Ou Yang, C.-P.; Chu, J.-Y. Analysis of the Package Tour Consumption Behaviors of Families in Taiwan, 2009–2019. *Eng. Proc.* **2024**, *74*, 80. https://doi.org/10.3390/engproc2024074080

Academic Editors: Shu-Han Liao, Teen-Hang Meen and Cheng-Fu Yang

Published: 28 November 2024

1. Introduction

The lives of human beings have been profoundly transformed by computer technology, which is evident in personal, social, economic, and medical aspects. The internet enables easy access to diverse information, thereby popularizing knowledge. The evolution of electronic commerce has revolutionized the shopping experience, allowing individuals to purchase goods and services online. This enhances convenience and broadens consumer choices and experiences, influencing people's travel behavior. With the rapid development of computer technology and mobile devices, travel information is available on online platforms, thus allowing users to access the latest travel information and book various travel products, such as package tours, accommodation, flight tickets, and amusement park tickets. The catalytic effect of the rapid growth of regional low-cost airlines has accelerated the trend of individuals planning overseas trips on their own.

According to data from the Tourism Bureau's survey on the travel habits of Taiwanese nationals, the proportion of outbound tourists participating in group tours decreased from 54.6% in 2011 to 44.1% in 2019. During the same period, the proportion of individuals planning overseas trips increased from 11.5 to 40.7%. The rapid advancement of technology is reshaping people's consumption habits and the way that they travel abroad.

Tourism plays a crucial role in the economies of countries. It stimulates economic growth and expands domestic markets, creates employment opportunities, catalyzes increased private investment, and enhances the participation in and quality of leisure life. According to statistics from the World Travel and Tourism Council in 2019, the global scale of tourism and sightseeing reached USD 8.90 trillion, contributing to 10.3% of the global gross domestic product (GDP). The global tourism industry employs 3.3 billion people, accounting for 10.0% of global employment. Considering its contributions to economic output and employment, it is evident that tourism is significant to economies.

In 2019, the outbreak of the COVID-19 pandemic significantly impacted the global tourism market. According to data from the World Tourism Organization, the number of global inbound tourist arrivals was 1.465 billion in 2019, but this dropped to 407 million in 2020, with a decrease of 72.2% compared to 2019. In 2022, the number of global tourist arrivals reached 963 million, representing 65.7% of that in 2019. As the pandemic subsided, borders reopened, and global tourism gradually returned to its former trend. Economic growth is now expected worldwide. Thus, it is important to seize opportunities in tourism-related businesses, create operational efficiencies, and understand the characteristics of people's travel consumption behaviors.

In Taiwan, tourism provides diverse activities for family leisure. From 2015 to 2019, more than half of annual leisure expenditures were allocated to package tours. In recent years, destination travel platforms have emerged, offering an abundance of travel information and a variety of affordable travel products and itineraries for consumer choice. This trend has increased the number of independent travelers, posing a significant challenge to traditional travel industry operators.

We identified three variables in the time dimensions of family package travel data using a cohort analysis. The effects of age, period, and cohort were analyzed through an observation of long-term changes in family package travel consumption. Package travel is not a necessity in daily life, and there was no data for several families, known as zero spending. If parameter estimation is conducted using ordinary least squares during these periods, then it may lead to biased and inconsistent results [1]. Thus, the double-hurdle model [2] and the Heckit model [3] were used to explore consumption behaviors, participation, and consumption decisions. A two-part model or two-stage decision model was used to address the issue of zero spending by analyzing the consumption behavior of tourists.

We combined the two-part model with the cohort analysis method to construct a model for the package tour consumption behavior of the Taiwanese population. We determined the factors influencing participation and expenditure decisions in family package travel, thus providing a reference for travel industry operators in formulating business strategies.

2. Literature Review

Previous research on tourism expenditures has been conducted in terms of macroeconomics and microeconomics. In macroeconomics, the impact of prices and income from tourist countries and destination countries on tourism expenditures were investigated. An analysis of tourist destination countries or regions, with a predominant emphasis on Europe as the primary subject, was used in the construction of an analysis model of a demand system [4], and the data were aggregated. In microeconomic studies, the optimal choice behavior of tourism demand, the influencing factors, and the construction of tourism price models were investigated [5]. The data used in these studies consisted of household or individual survey cross-sectional data, with traditional linear regression models being commonly employed [6].

2.1. Two-Part Model for Travel Expenditure

Weagley and Huh [7] used the double-hurdle (DH) model to explore the factors influencing the leisure consumption expenditures of households with older people who were either retired or nearing retirement in the United States. They compared the differences in the factors of decision-making on participation and consumption expenditure. The results revealed that, concerning the participation in decisions about active leisure activities, variables such as income, education level, and homeownership positively impacted the willingness of retired and near-retirement households to engage in leisure consumption. Variables such as the age of the household head, Black ethnicity, residence in the northwestern United States, and sources of income impacted the willingness of retired and near-retirement households to participate in active leisure activities. Regarding the expenditure decisions in active leisure, only income significantly impacted the willingness of retired and near-retirement households to spend money on active leisure activities.

Nicolau and Más [8] employed the Heckman model to analyze the factors influencing the participation and expenditure decisions of Spanish residents in tourism. Income, education level, and vacation preferences had a significantly positive impact on the willingness of individuals to participate in tourism. Family size negatively affected the willingness of Spanish families to participate in tourism. In terms of tourism expenditure, decisions, distance, accommodation location, family size, marital status, and income influenced the tourism expenditure of Spanish families. However, education level had no influence on the tourism expenditure of Spanish families.

Alegre, Mateo, and Pou [9] utilized data from the Spanish Household Survey from 2006 to 2010 and applied the Heckman model to investigate the factors influencing the participation in and expenditure on tourism for Spanish households. Income, the presence of children under 14 in the household, and education level positively affected the participation in and expenditure on family tourism. However, household size, renting a home, and unemployment of household members negatively affected participation in and expenditure on family tourism.

Bernini and Cracolici [10] used household expenditure data from Italy, spanning from 1997 to 2007, to explore the relationship between demographic characteristics, life cycle, and travel expenditure. Employing the double-hurdle model, they analyzed domestic and international travel participation decisions and consumption expenditure decisions and examined the significance of age and cohort effects. Demographics significantly impacted a household's travel behavior. For domestic or international travel, the willingness of Italian households to travel decreased gradually with age, while travel expenditures increased with age.

Lin, Qin, Li, and Wu [11] utilized data from the China Family Panel Studies (CFPSs) conducted in 2014, 2016, and 2018 and investigated the factors influencing the travel consumption behavior of Chinese households, employing the Heckman model. Household income, the number of family members aged over 65 years, ownership of a private car, education level, and general trust in others significantly influenced the participation in and expenditure on family tourism. Additionally, household size exhibited a significant negative impact on participation in and expenditure on family travel.

2.2. Cohort Travel Expenditure

Values, attitudes, and preferences shaped by generations are not easily changed with age and lifestyle [12]. Oppermann [13] used longitudinal data and explored the travel patterns of German residents. He analyzed differences in family life cycles and travel patterns between different generations. The family life cycle influences the travel patterns of German residents, affecting destination choices, travel expenditure, transportation, accommodation and group size, duration of stay, activities, and travel seasons. Pennington and Kerstetter [14] examined whether the travel preferences of two generations of elderly individuals in Canada changed over time using data from Statistics Canada and the Canadian Tourism Commission. Significant variations in travel preferences were found for older Canadian adults across different generations and periods.

Newbold et al. [15] investigated the travel behavior of the elderly population in Canada using data from the General Social Survey conducted in 1986, 1992, and 1998. Older Canadians traveled less frequently than younger generations. Chen and Shoemaker [16] analyzed time-series data to examine the psychological characteristics and travel behavior of elderly travelers from the Silent, Lucky Few, and Baby Boomer Generations in the United States, employing cohort theory, life course theory, and continuity theory. The results supported family life cycle theory and continuity theory in the U.S. senior travel market.

In explaining group differences in the travel market for seniors, age effects were more influential than cohort effects, suggesting limitations in using cohort theory to explain the elderly travel market.

Lin, Jiang, Li, and Qin [17] utilized five-year longitudinal data from the China Household Financial Survey to explore the impact of psychological factors, specifically risk aversion, on travel participation and expenditures. The results represented the integration of the hierarchical age–generation–period model and the Heckman model in analyzing the role of risk aversion in travel decision making. Risk aversion significantly influenced travel participation and expenditure. Individual willingness to travel and expenditure gradually decreased with the life cycle. Differences existed in the effects of period and cohort factors on travel participation and expenditure.

Travel is not a commodity that households regularly consume, making it crucial to choose appropriate models when exploring factors influencing family travel expenditure, especially in addressing zero expenditure. Additionally, it is necessary to understand the dynamic characteristics of family travel expenditure over time and introduce cohort analysis models to disentangle the effects of age, generation, and period for the prediction of changes in travel consumption patterns. In this study, the two-part, double-hurdle, dependent double-hurdle, and Heckman models were selected. The Voung test method was also employed to determine the appropriateness of the model for analyzing family package travel consumption behavior in Taiwan with factors influencing family package travel and its consumption patterns.

3. Methods

3.1. Data Collection

We utilized longitudinal data from 2009 to 2019, obtained from the "Taiwan Area Household Income and Expenditure Survey" of the Directorate General of Budget, Accounting, and Statistics, Executive Yuan [18], and investigated family package travel consumption behavior. The survey data included data on individuals and households in Taiwan. The total number of sampled households in this study was 126,312, with 46,596 households having zero expenditure on family package travel, accounting for 36.9% of all households.

3.2. Cohort Grouping

The term "cohort" originally referred to a military unit or soldiers, but now it denotes a group of people sharing common characteristics [19]. Cohort groups are classified based on shared experiences of historical events or by using birth years (birth cohort). In this study, birth years were used to distinguish cohorts. The range of years for cohort grouping can be arbitrarily determined [20], with intervals of five or ten years commonly used as the boundary points. We categorized cohorts based on the age of the head of household, with each cohort spanning five years across fourteen generations: 1926–1930, 1931–1935, 1936–1940, . . ., 1991–1995. Households with heads born before 1926 or after 1995 were excluded from the analysis.

3.3. Effects of Cohort, Age, and Period

As period (era) is equal to age plus birth year, it results in a perfect linear overlap with age, cohort, and period. Therefore, when estimating, it is necessary to introduce constraints to differentiate the effects of age, cohort, and period. Otherwise, the parameter estimation cannot be used to observe trends in consumption behavior. Thus, we employed the cohort–age–period linear decomposition model [21,22] to include age, cohort, and period variables. It was assumed that the long-term period effects were averaged to zero and were orthogonal to the linear trend.

3.4. Two-Part Model

3.4.1. Double Hurdle

The Tobit model is used to address the issue of zero expenditure in consumption [23]. It is used to analyze the observed data, assuming that zero expenditure represent the true consumption value of the goods. Zero expenditure is influenced by economic factors (corner solution), and the possibility that no consumption may result from a lack of willingness to participate can be overlooked. Crag [2] modified the Tobit model and suggested that the origin of zero observations was determined due to corner solutions and the fact that consumers had zero demand for the product, meaning that they chose not to consume. Cragg's double-hurdle (DH) model separates consumption into two components: the participation decision and the consumption decision. In the DH model, zero observations may occur either due to non-economic factors leading to non-participation in consumption in the first stage or due to economic factors resulting in zero expenditure in the second stage [24].

The primary distinction between the DH and Heckit models lies in the occurrence of zero observation. In the Heckit model, zero observation appears in the first stage of consumption choice, whereas in the DH model, it occurs in the first or second stage. Assuming independence between the error terms of the participation decision and consumption decision equations, the logarithmic likelihood function of the DH model is written as (1) [25,26]

$$lnL = \sum_0 ln[1 - \Phi(\alpha' z_i)\Phi(\frac{\beta' x_i}{\sigma})] + \sum_+ ln[\Phi(\alpha' z_i)\frac{1}{\sigma}\varphi(\frac{y_i - \beta' x_i}{\sigma})], \quad (1)$$

where z_i represents the variables affecting the participation decision, x_i represents the variables influencing consumption expenditure, and y_i is the observable consumption expenditure. In the DH model, the explanatory variables in the participation decision equation differ from those in the consumption decision equation, as shown in Equation (2) [27,28]:

$$\begin{pmatrix} \mu_i \\ v_i \end{pmatrix} \sim \left[\begin{pmatrix} 0 \\ 0 \end{pmatrix}, \begin{pmatrix} 1 & \rho\sigma \\ \rho\sigma & \sigma^2 \end{pmatrix}\right], \quad (2)$$

where ρ represents the correlation coefficient. The logarithmic likelihood function of the dependent double-hurdle model with the inclusion of the correlation coefficient is expressed as (3) [29]

$$lnL = \sum_0 ln[1 - \Phi(\alpha' z_i, \frac{\beta' x_i}{\sigma}, \rho)] + \sum_+ ln\left[\Phi\left(\frac{\alpha' z_i + \frac{\rho}{\sigma}\left(Y_i - \beta' x_i\right)}{\sqrt{1-\rho^2}}\right)\frac{1}{\sigma}\phi\left(\frac{y_i - \beta' x_i}{\sigma}\right)\right]. \quad (3)$$

3.4.2. Heckit Model

Heckman [3] proposed a sample selection model to address zero expenditure on unobservable goods, suggesting that zero expenditure results from consumer self-selection not to participate. If model parameter estimation is performed using only a subset of the sample, then the issue of sample selection bias may arise. The Heckit model assumes a correlation between the error terms (μ_i,v_i) of the decision equation and the consumption equation, with the degree of correlation denoted as ρ. The bivariate normal distribution of the errors in the two equations of the Heckit model is expressed in Equation (2). In addition to using a two-step estimation method, the Heckit model also employs maximum likelihood estimation for parameter estimation. The logarithmic likelihood function for the Heckit model is specified as follows [30,31]:

$$lnL = \sum_0 ln[1 - \Phi(\alpha' z_i)] + \sum_+ ln\left[\Phi\left(\frac{\alpha' Z_i + \frac{\rho}{\sigma}\left(y_i - \beta' x_i\right)}{\sqrt{1-\rho^2}}\right)\frac{1}{\sigma}\phi\left(\frac{y_i - \beta' x_i}{\sigma}\right)\right]. \quad (4)$$

4. Results and Discussion

4.1. Variables

The influencing variables on family package travel consumption behavior in Taiwan were categorized into four types, namely, economic factors, constraint factors, socio-demographic factors, and cohort factors, by summarizing the past literature on travel expenditure [6,8,10,32,33]. The economic factors included the household disposable income and the employment status of the homemaker. The constraint factors consisted of the presence of children under the age of 14, adults over the age of 65, and healthcare expenditure. The socio-demographic factors included the educational level, occupation, gender, and marital status of the head of the household. The cohort factors involved age groups such as 20–25 (AGE1), 26–30 (AGE2), . . ., 86–90 (AGE14), forming fourteen age categories and fourteen cohort groups. Variables such as household disposable income, package travel expenditure, and health expenditure were adjusted for inflation using the Consumer Price Index. Other variable explanations are detailed in Table 1. In the two-part model, there is currently no theoretical basis providing a reference for whether the explanatory variables must be the same in the two decision equations. Including the same explanatory variables in both decision equations may lead to an incorrect identification of model parameters [24]. Therefore, it is necessary to introduce exclusion constraints [24,26,29] to estimate accurate parameters in the model equations. In the decision-making process for family consumption in the market, the purchase decision is primarily influenced by non-economic factors. Hence, income variables were excluded from the purchase decision equation [24,26].

Table 1. Model for cohort analysis of family travel expenditure: explanation of variable names and descriptive statistics.

Variable	Description	Measurement		Statistics
LY	Household disposable income	Logarithmic household disposable income		9.09
WEMP	Women's employment per household	1: yes	0: no	39.31%
EDU1	Below middle school	Omitted variables		12.53%
EDU2	High school	1: yes	0: no	14.88%
EDU3	Junior college education	1: yes	0: no	32.22%
EDU4	College education	1: yes	0: no	33.50%
EDU5	Graduate education and above	1: yes	0: no	6.86%
OCU1	Not working	1: yes	0: no	10.40%
OCU2	Management level	1: yes	0: no	5.72%
OCU3	Professional	1: yes	0: no	33.34%
OCU4	Service	1: yes	0: no	15.40%
OCU5	Labor industry	1: yes	0: no	30.86%
OCU6	Agriculture	1: yes	0: no	3.61%
OCU7	Soldier	Omitted variables		0.67%
SEX	Gender	1: male	0: female	71.50%
MAR	Marital status	1: married	0: unmarried	79.97%
CH14	Number of children under 14	Number of children under 14		0.47 person
A65	Number of seniors aged over 65	Number of seniors aged over 65		0.42 person
HEL	Household healthcare expenditure	Expenditure on health and family care		5.07

4.2. Analysis Results

STATA statistical software (version 13) was used for the maximum likelihood estimation of the two-part models, namely, the DH, DDH, and Heckit models. The Voung test [34] was used to select the appropriate consumption behavior model for family package travel data. The test results are shown in Table 2, indicating that DDH was the most appropriate for analyzing family package travel consumption behavior in Taiwan.

Table 2. Test settings.

Model	Type of Test	Testing Value
Heckit vs. double hurdle	Vuong	3.31
Heckit vs. dependent double hurdle	Vuong	−30.89

4.2.1. Participation Decision

Table 3 presents the parameter estimation results for the dependent double-hurdle model. The participation of women in the workforce (WEMP) showed a significantly positive relationship with family participation in package travel, coinciding with the findings of Sun et al. [35]. Concerning the constraint factors, the number of individuals aged over 65 years in the household (A65), the number of individuals aged below 14 years (CH14), and health expenditure (HEL) exhibited a significant positive relationship with family willingness to participate in package travel. This indicates that, as the number of individuals aged 65 or over, the number of children aged below 14 years, and health expenditure in the household increased, the willingness of the family to participate in package travel also increased.

Table 3. Estimated coefficients of the cohort analysis model for family package travel expenditure.

Variable	Coefficient	Normalized Value	Variable	Coefficient	Normalized Value
			LY	1.1207	89.71 **
MAR	0.2493	17.19 **	MAR	−0.1475	−7.03 **
SEX	0.0155	1.75	SEX	−0.1120	−9.01 **
EDU2	0.1707	10.46 **	EDU2	0.3312	13.36 **
EDU3	0.2558	16.56 **	EDU3	0.5099	21.57 **
EDU4	0.3712	21.92 **	EDU4	0.7747	30.18 **
EDU5	0.4384	19.17 **	EDU5	1.0038	31.52 **
OCU1	−0.0648	−1.33	OCU1	0.5941	8.50 **
OCU2	0.6363	13.06 **	OCU2	1.0314	15.44 **
OCU3	0.4289	9.36 **	OCU3	0.6845	10.65 **
OCU4	0.2556	5.49 **	OCU4	0.4009	6.14 **
OCU5	0.2486	5.39 **	OCU5	0.3130	4.83 **
OCU6	0.2545	5.09 **	OCU6	0.2919	4.16 **
CH14	0.2851	39.91 **	CH14	−0.2315	−27.52 **
A65	0.0342	4.95 **	A65	−0.0957	−10.86 **
WEMP	0.1153	12.61 **	WEMP	0.0602	5.12 **
HEL	0.1166	24.07 **	HEL	−0.0041	−0.49
AGE2	0.0403	1.01	AGE2	0.3491	5.64 **
AGE 3	0.1208	2.81 *	AGE 3	0.5720	8.60 **
AGE 4	0.3796	8.37 **	AGE 4	0.7946	11.43 **
AGE 5	0.6975	14.66 **	AGE 5	1.0874	15.11 **
AGE 6	0.7626	15.40 **	AGE 6	1.2089	16.34 **
AGE 7	0.6970	13.61 **	AGE 7	1.4003	18.46 **
AGE 8	0.7085	13.31 **	AGE 8	1.6561	21.09 **
AGE 9	0.7953	14.11 **	AGE 9	1.8615	22.46 **
AGE 10	0.8656	13.66 **	AGE 10	2.1290	22.81 **
AGE 11	0.8399	11.63 **	AGE 11	2.1643	19.82 **
AGE 12	0.6885	8.57 **	AGE 12	2.0431	16.27 **
AGE 13	0.5272	5.76 **	AGE 13	1.7172	11.26 **

Table 3. *Cont.*

Variable	Coefficient	Normalized Value	Variable	Coefficient	Normalized Value
AGE 14	0.3733	3.31 *	AGE 14	1.6140	7.78 **
COH2	0.0381	0.65	COH2	0.0010	0.01
COH 3	0.1367	2.01 *	COH 3	0.0120	0.09
COH 4	0.2524	3.36 *	COH 4	0.1056	0.74
COH 5	0.2605	3.23	COH 5	0.1731	1.15
COH 6	0.3460	4.17v	COH 6	0.4049	2.64 *
COH 7	0.3528	4.18v	COH 7	0.5199	3.36 *
COH 8	0.4195	4.91v	COH 8	0.6481	4.16 **
COH 9	0.5105	5.90 **	COH 9	0.7578	4.83 **
COH 10	0.5633	6.43 **	COH 10	0.8586	5.45 **
COH 11	0.6106	6.88 **	COH 11	0.9705	6.12 **
COH 12	0.7408	8.22 **	COH 12	1.1932	7.44 **
COH 3	0.8594	9.25 **	COH 3	1.5218	9.27 **
COH 14	0.9796	9.72 **	COH 14	1.6986	9.74 **
YR3	0.0229	2.05 *	YR3	−0.0040	−0.27
YR4	0.0629	5.46 **	YR4	−0.0199	−1.3
YR 5	0.0793	6.69 **	YR 5	−0.0067	−0.43
YR 6	0.0327	2.79 *	YR 6	−0.0524	−3.38 *
YR 7	0.0456	3.90 **	YR 7	0.0159	1.03
YR 8	−0.0091	−0.79	YR 8	−0.0023	−0.15
YR 9	−0.0133	−1.18	YR 9	0.0268	1.83
YR 10	−0.0400	−3.71 *	YR 10	−0.0020	−0.14
YR 11	−0.0440	−4.29 **	YR 11	0.0014	0.1
Constant	−2.4431	−21.75 **	Constant	−8.8922	−42.83 **
ρ	0.6587	56.97 **			
Log likelihood		−208,619.43			

(**: $p < 0.01$, *: $p < 0.05$).

In terms of the socio-demographic factors, the education level of the head of the household (EDU) showed a positive relationship with the family's willingness to participate in package travel. The coefficients of the education level variables were not zero. As the education level of the head of the household increased, the willingness of the family to participate in package travel also increased, consistent with the findings of Nicolau and Más [8], Alegre et al. [9], Bernini and Cracolici [10], and Sun et al. [35].

Regarding the head of the household's occupation, the military profession (OCU7) was the baseline, and the coefficients for all five occupation variables, except for unemployment (OCU1), were not zero. By observing the estimated coefficients for the occupation variables, it was found that households with heads in managerial positions (OCU2) and professional occupations (OCU3) exhibited a higher willingness to participate in package travel. In contrast, households with unemployed heads (OCU1) demonstrated a lower willingness. Households with male heads (SEX) showed a significantly higher willingness to participate in package travel than households with female heads, although the estimated coefficient did not reach the significance level. Married households (MAR) exhibited a significantly higher willingness to participate in package travel than unmarried households, with the estimated coefficient being significantly different from zero.

In terms of the cohort factors, the Wald test results for the age, generation, and period coefficients revealed that age and cohort effects were significantly different from zero for participation and consumption decisions (Table 4). Regarding family participation in package travel decision making, as the age of the head of the household increased, the willingness to participate in package travel increased (Figure 1a).

Table 4. Wald test results of age, cohort, and period.

Equation	Age Effect	Cohort Effect	Period Effect
Participation	chi2 = 830.1 *p*-value = 0.000	chi2 = 231.5 *p*-value = 0.000	chi2 = 178.2 *p*-value = 0.000
Consumption	chi2 = 904.7 *p*-value = 0.000	chi2 = 457.6 *p*-value = 0.000	chi2 = 32.6 *p*-value = 0.000

Source of data: this study.

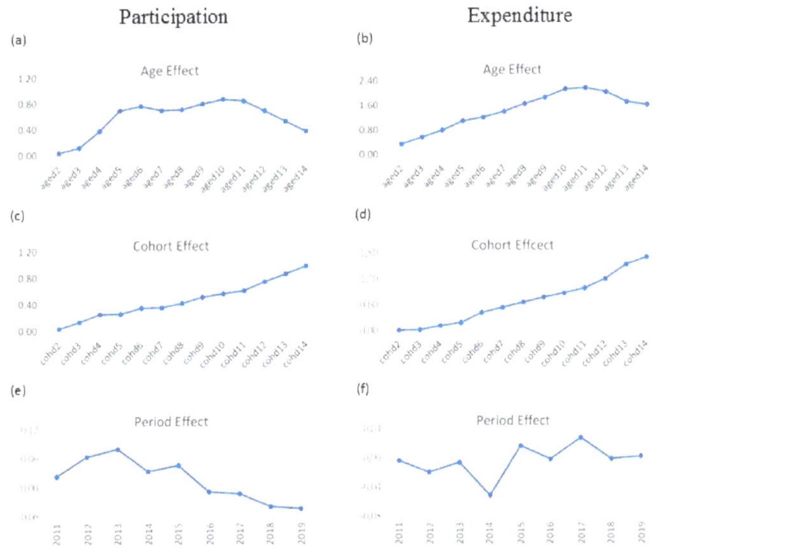

Figure 1. Effects of age, cohort, and period on household package travel consumption and expenditure decisions (**a**–**f**).

The first peak in travel willingness was observed around the age of 46–60 (AGE 6), followed by a decline and a gradual rise. Another peak in willingness to participate in family package travel was observed between the ages of 66 and 70 (AGE 10), with a subsequent decline in willingness for heads of households over 70 years old (Figure 1c). The cohort variable coefficients exhibited a monotonic increase, indicating that, as the generation became younger, the willingness of families to participate in package travel increased. In terms of the period variables, a peak in willingness to participate in family package travel was observed in 2013, followed by a gradual decline in subsequent years (Figure 1e).

4.2.2. Consumption Decision

Regarding family package travel expenditure decisions, the economic factor of disposable family income showed a significant positive relationship with package travel expenditure. As income increased, the amount that families allocated to package travel expenses also increased. This result aligns with the findings of previous studies [7,9,32–34,36–40]. The participation of females in the workforce (WEMP) in the household also significantly impacted package travel expenditure [34]. As a limiting factor, household health expenditure (HEL) showed a negative relationship with package travel expenditure, although the coefficient was not significant. The number of adults aged 65 or over (A65) showed a negative relationship with package travel expenditure, indicating that the higher the number of seniors aged 65 or over in the family, the less the family spent on package travel [35]. The number of individuals aged below 14 years (CH14) in the household had a significant negative relationship with package travel expenditure, suggesting that the higher the number of individuals aged below 14 years in the family, the less the family spent on package travel.

Regarding socio-demographic observations, there was a significant positive relationship between the educational level of the household head and package travel expenditure. As the educational level of the household head increased, the amount spent on package travel also increased. This finding aligns with the results of previous studies [7,9,10,32,33,35,38,40]. In terms of the household head's occupation, the coefficients of variables were not zero. Households with a management-level head (OCU2) and professional head (OCU3) tended to spend more on package travel. Conversely, households with a head employed in the military (OCU7) or engaged in agriculture (OCU6) spent less on package travel. Single households (MAR) exhibited significantly higher package travel expenditure than married households. Additionally, households with a female head (SEX) had significantly higher package travel expenditure than those with a male head.

In terms of cohort factors, with an increase in the household head's age, the expenditure on household package travel participation also increased (Figure 1b). The peak of household package travel expenditure was observed between the ages of 71 and 75 years (AGE11), and, over the age of 75 years, the expenditure gradually decreased. The coefficients of the cohort variables increased, indicating that the younger the age of the generation, the higher the household package travel expenditure (Figure 1d). In terms of period variables, household package travel expenditure fluctuated in response to changes in the economic environment (Figure 1f).

5. Conclusions

The COVID-19 pandemic in 2019 significantly impacted the global tourism industry. As the pandemic subsided and borders reopened, countries embraced the vast business opportunities with the recovery of tourism. The rapid development of computer technology has transformed people's lifestyles and consumption patterns. Destination travel platforms provide the latest and abundant travel information and affordable travel products, increasing the number of independent travelers. With this change, package tours are gradually losing their appeal and competitiveness. For traditional travel agencies, it is necessary to adopt these changes and maintain and create business opportunities. Therefore, it is essential to understand the characteristics of family package travel consumption behavior. We used longitudinal data from the Directorate-General of Budget, Accounting, and Statistics of the Executive Yuan, focusing on the "Family Income and Expenditure Survey Report." Employing the two-part model with the dependent double-hurdle and cohort–age–time linear decomposition models [21,22], we analyzed the consumption behavior of Taiwanese families regarding package travel. The results revealed two peaks in the willingness to participate among household heads aged 46–50 and 66–70 years, with the highest willingness observed in families with heads aged between 66 and 70 years. Younger household heads exhibited a higher willingness to participate in package travel than older household heads. The peak of willingness to participate in family package travel occurred in 2013, and, since then, it has declined. A higher propensity to participate in package travel was found for household heads who were male or married with higher education levels, who had managerial or professional occupations, who had family members aged 65 years or over and below 14 years, and who had higher health expenditure and working housewives. The respondents aged 71 to 75 years old spent the most on family package travel. Younger families had higher package travel expenditure than older generations, and family package travel expenditure fluctuated due to changes in the economic environment. Higher income, working housewives, female and single household heads, higher education levels of household heads, managerial or professional occupations, and fewer family members aged over 65 and below 14 years were demographic characteristics associated with higher package travel expenditure.

Family participation in packaged travel in Taiwan was mostly for outbound tourism. Younger families who were less familiar with travel abroad expressed a higher willingness to participate in package tours abroad and, consequently, exhibited higher travel expenditure. Travel industry operators need to consider the characteristics of the younger generation in planning travel itineraries and marketing to sustain the development of the package travel market. The willingness of families to participate in package travel peaked after a household head retired.

The results of this study serve as a basis for travel agencies in formulating market segmentation strategies. The willingness of families to participate in package travel has gradually declined since 2013, indicating an increase in independent travel. Regarding package travel expenditure, little change was observed in travel spending. Strategies for travel agencies are necessary to mitigate the impact of independent travel, explore the high-end package travel market, and address the challenges of slowing expenditure growth and a shrinking market share for the sustainable development of the tourism industry.

Author Contributions: Conceptualization, methodology, formal analysis, and writing—original draft, T.-S.C.; data curation, C.-P.O.Y.; formal analysis and writing—review and editing, J.-Y.C. All authors have read and agreed to the published version of the manuscript.

Funding: This research received no external funding.

Institutional Review Board Statement: Not applicable.

Informed Consent Statement: Not applicable.

Data Availability Statement: Analyses were conducted based on the information contained in the datasets on the Survey of Travel by R.O.C. (Taiwan) Citizens for the years 2009–2019. The information can be found in the reference list.

Conflicts of Interest: The authors declare no conflicts of interest.

References

1. Judge, G.G.; Hill, R.C.; Griffiths, W.E.; Lutkepohl, H.; Lee, T.C. *Introduction to the Theory and Practice of Econometrics*; John Wiley and Sons: Hoboken, NJ, USA, 1988.
2. Cragg, J.G. Some Statistical Models for Limited Dependent Variables with Application to the Demand for Durable Goods. *Econometrica* **1971**, *39*, 829–844. [CrossRef]
3. Heckman, J.J. Sample Select Bias as a Specification Error. *Econometrica* **1979**, *47*, 153–161. [CrossRef]
4. Li, G.; Song, H.; Witt, S.F. Recent developments in econometric modeling and forecasting. *J. Travel Res.* **2005**, *44*, 82–99. [CrossRef]
5. Wang, Y.; Davidson, M.C.G. A review of microanalyses of tourist expenditure. *Curr. Issues Tour.* **2010**, *13*, 507–524. [CrossRef]
6. Brida, J.G.; Scuderi, R. Determinants of tourist expenditure: A review of microeconometric models. *Tour. Manag. Perspect.* **2013**, *6*, 28–40. [CrossRef]
7. Weagley, R.O.; Huh, E. Leisure Expenditures of Retired and Near-Retired Households. *J. Leis. Res.* **2004**, *36*, 101–127. [CrossRef]
8. Nicolau, J.L.; Más, F.J. Heckit modelling of tourist expenditure: Evidence from Spain. *Int. J. Serv. Ind. Manag.* **2005**, *16*, 271–293. [CrossRef]
9. Alegre, J.; Mateo, S.; Pou, L. Tourism Participation and Expenditure by Spanish Household: The Effects of the Economic Crisis Unemployment. *Tour. Manag.* **2013**, *39*, 37–49. [CrossRef]
10. Bernini, C.; Cracolici, M.F. Demographic Change, Tourism Expenditure and Life Cycle Behavior. *Tour. Manag.* **2015**, *47*, 191–205. [CrossRef]
11. Lin, V.S.; Qin, Y.; Li, G.; Wu, J. Determinants of Chinese households' tourism consumption: Evidence from China family panel studies. *Int. J. Tour. Res.* **2021**, *23*, 542–554. [CrossRef]
12. Schewe, C.D.; Meredith, G. Segmenting global markets by generational cohorts: Determining Motivations by age. *J. Mark. Manag.* **1994**, *4*, 51–63. [CrossRef]
13. Oppermann, M. Travel Life Cycle. *Ann. Tour. Res.* **1995**, *22*, 535–552. [CrossRef]
14. Penning-Gray, L.; Kerstetter, D.L. Examining travel preferences of older Canadian adults over time. *J. Hosp. Leis. Mark.* **2001**, *8*, 131–145.
15. Newbold, K.B.; Scott, D.M.; Spinney JE, L.; Kanaroglou, P. Travel behavior within Canada's older population: A cohort analysis. *J. Transp. Geogr.* **2005**, *13*, 340–351. [CrossRef]
16. Chen, S.C.; Shoemaker, S. Age and Cohort Effects: The American Senior Tourism Market. *Ann. Tour. Res.* **2014**, *48*, 58–75. [CrossRef]

17. Lin, V.S.; Jiang, F.; Li, G.; Qin, Y. Impacts of risk aversion on tourism consumption: A hierarchical age-period-cohort analysis. *Ann. Tour. Res.* **2023**, *101*, 103607. [CrossRef]
18. *AG020001-20018*; Tourism Bureau, Ministry of Transportation and Communications (2009–2019). Survey of Travel by R.O.C. Citizens, 2005–2018. Executive Information System Tourism Administration, MOTC. Available online: https://srda.sinica.edu.tw/search/metadata/detail/AG020001 (accessed on 26 November 2024).
19. Glenn, N.D. *Cohort Analysis*, 2nd ed.; SAGE: Thousand Oaks, CA, USA, 2005.
20. Attanasio, O.P.; Blow, L.; Hamilton, R.; Leicester, A. Booms and Busts: Consumption, House Prices and Expectations. *Economica* **2009**, *76*, 20–50. [CrossRef]
21. Deaton, A.; Paxson, C.H. Saving growth aging in Taiwan. In *Studies in the Economics of Aging*; David, A.W., Ed.; Chicago University Press: Chicago, IL, USA, 1994.
22. Deaton, A. *The Analysis of Household Surveys: A Microeconometric Approach to Development Policy*; Johns Hopkins University: Baltimore, MD, USA, 1997.
23. Tobin, J. Estimation of Relationships for Limited Dependent Variables. *Econometrica* **1958**, *26*, 24–36. [CrossRef]
24. Newman, C.; Henchion, M.; Matthew, A. Infrequency of Purchase and Double-Hurdle Models of Irish Households' Meat Expenditure. *Eur. Rev. Agric. Econ.* **2001**, *28*, 393–412. [CrossRef]
25. Moffatt, P.G. *Hurdle Models of Loan Default*; East Anglia University: Norwich, UK, 2003.
26. Aristei, D.; Pieroni, L. A Double-Hurdle Approach to Modeling Tobacco Consumption in Italy. *Appl. Econ.* **2008**, *40*, 2463–2476. [CrossRef]
27. Jones, A.M.; Yen, S.T. A Box-Cox Double-Hurdle Model. *Manch. Sch.* **2000**, *68*, 203–221. [CrossRef]
28. Martínez-Espineira, R. A Box-Cox Double-Hurdle Model of Wildlife Valuation: The Citizen's Perspective. *Ecol. Econ.* **2006**, *58*, 192–208. [CrossRef]
29. Jones, A.M. A Note on Computation of The Double-Hurdle with Dependence with an Application to Tobacco Expenditure. *Bull. Econ. Res.* **1992**, *44*, 67–74. [CrossRef]
30. Aristei, D.; Perali, F.; Pieroni, L. Cohort, Age and Time Effect in Alcohol Consumption by Italian Households: A Double-Hurdle Approach. *Empir. Econ.* **2008**, *35*, 29–61. [CrossRef]
31. Wodjao, T.B. *A Double-Hurdle Model of Computer and Internet Use in America Households*; Western Michigan University: Kalamazoo, MI, USA, 2007.
32. Dardis, R.; Derrick, F.; Lehfeld, A.; Wolfe, K.E. Cross-section Studies of Recreation Expenditures in The United States. *J. Leis. Res.* **1981**, *13*, 181–194. [CrossRef]
33. Dardis, R.; Soberon-Ferrer, H.; Patro, D. Analysis of Leisure Expenditures in The United States. *J. Leis. Res.* **1994**, *26*, 309–321. [CrossRef]
34. Vuong, Q.H. Likelihood Ratio Tests for Model Selection and Non-Nested Hypotheses. *Econometrica* **1989**, *57*, 307–333. [CrossRef]
35. Sun, P.-C.; Lee, H.-S.; Chen, T.-S. Analysis of Relationship between Household Life Cycle and Tourism Expenditure in Taiwan: An Application of Infrequency of Purchase Model. *Tour. Econ.* **2015**, *21*, 1015–1033. [CrossRef]
36. Thompson, C.S.; Tinsley, A.W. Income Expenditure Elasticities for Recreation: Their Estimation and Relation to Demand for Recreation. *J. Leis. Res.* **1978**, *4*, 265–270. [CrossRef]
37. Davies, B.; Mangan, J. Family Expenditure on Hotels and Holidays. *Ann. Tour. Res.* **1992**, *19*, 691–699. [CrossRef]
38. Cai, L.A.; Hong, G.S.; Morrison, A.M. Household Expenditure Patterns for Tourism Products and Service. *J. Travel Tour. Marking* **1992**, *4*, 15–40.
39. Fish, M.; Waggle, D. Current Income Versus Total Expenditure Measures in Regression Models of Vacation and Pleasure Travel. *J. Travel Res.* **1996**, *35*, 70–74. [CrossRef]
40. Cai, L.A. Relationship of Household Characteristics and Lodging Expenditure on Leisure Trips. *J. Hosp. Leis. Marking* **1999**, *6*, 5–18. [CrossRef]

MDPI AG
Grosspeteranlage 5
4052 Basel
Switzerland
Tel.: +41 61 683 77 34

Engineering Proceedings Editorial Office
E-mail: engproc@mdpi.com
www.mdpi.com/journal/engproc

www.ingramcontent.com/pod-product-compliance
Lightning Source LLC
Chambersburg PA
CBHW041433210926
51850CB00013B/3420
9783725831050